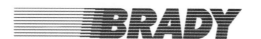

FIRST RESPONDER

A Skills Approach

FIFTH EDITION

Keith J. Karren, Ph.D.

Chair, Department of Health Sciences
Brigham Young University
Provo, Utah

Brent Q. Hafen, Ph.D.

Professor, Department of Health Sciences
Brigham Young University
Provo, Utah

Daniel Limmer, EMT-P

Paramedic, Colonie EMS Department, Colonie, New York
Training Officer, Colonie Police Department, Colonie, New York
Instructor, Hudson Valley Community College, Institute of Prehospital Emergency Medicine, Troy, New York

Medical Editor
Edward T. Dickinson, M.D., FACEP

BRADY

PRENTICE HALL   UPPER SADDLE RIVER, NEW JERSEY 07458

Library of Congress Cataloging-in-Publication Data

Karren, Keith J.
    First responder : a skills approach / Keith J. Karren, Brent Q.
Hafen, Daniel Limmer ; medical director, Edward T. Dickinson — 5th
ed.
        p.   cm.
    Includes index.
    ISBN 0-8359-5106-5
    1. Medical emergencies.   2. Emergency medical technicians.
I. Hafen, Brent Q.   II. Limmer, Daniel.   III. Title.
RC86.7.K365   1998
616.02'5—dc21   97-24631
                                                                     CIP

PUBLISHER: Susan Katz
MARKETING MANAGER: Judy Streger
MANAGING DEVELOPMENT EDITOR: Lois Berlowitz
DEVELOPMENT EDITOR: Josephine Cepeda
DIRECTOR OF PRODUCTION/MANUFACTURING: Bruce Johnson
MANAGING PRODUCTION EDITOR: Patrick Walsh
PRODUCTION LIAISON: Julie Boddorf
PRODUCTION EDITOR: Karen Fortgang, *bookworks*
CREATIVE DIRECTOR: Marianne Frasco
INTERIOR DESIGN: Wanda Kossak
COVER DESIGN: Bruce Kenselaar
MANAGING PHOTOGRAPHY EDITOR: Michal Heron
ASSISTANT PHOTOGRAPHY EDITORS: Baylen Leonard, Nancy Soares
PHOTOGRAPHERS: Stephen Agricola, Michael Gallitelli, Michal
    Heron, Richard Logan, Rick Nye
COVER PHOTOGRAPHY:
Photo Left: Howard M. Paul, Emergency! Stock
Photo Center: Michael Gallitelli
Photo Right: Michal Heron
PREPRESS/MANUFACTURING BUYER: Ilene Sanford

Notice: The authors and the publisher of this book have taken care to make certain that the equipment and schedules of treatment are correct and compatible with the standards generally accepted at the time of publication. Nevertheless, as new information becomes available, changes in treatment and in the use of equipment and procedures become necessary. The reader is advised to carefully consult the instruction and information material included in each piece of equipment or device before administration. First Responders are warned that the use of any techniques must be authorized by their medical director, where appropriate, in accord with local laws and regulations. The publisher disclaims any liability, loss, injury, or damage incurred as a consequence, directly or indirectly, of the use and application of any of the contents of this book.

© 1998 by Prentice-Hall, Inc.
A Simon & Schuster Company
Upper Saddle River, New Jersey 07458

All rights reserved. No part of this book may be reproduced, in any form or by any means, without permission in writing from the publisher.

Printed in the United States of America

10 9 8 7 6 5 4 3 2 1

ISBN 0-8359-5106-5

Prentice-Hall International (UK) Limited, *London*
Prentice-Hall of Australia Pty. Limited, *Sydney*
Prentice-Hall Canada Inc., *Toronto*
Prentice-Hall Hispanoamericana, S.A., *Mexico*
Prentice-Hall of India Private Limited, *New Delhi*
Prentice-Hall of Japan, *Tokyo*
Simon & Schuster Asia Pte. Ltd., *Singapore*
Editora Prentice-Hall do Brasil, Ltda., *Rio de Janeiro*

*Many who have had long, rewarding experiences in EMS can look back
with gratitude to the support and encouragement offered by friends
and colleagues, especially during the early years. I was fortunate
to have received guidance from a number of people. There are four
to whom I extend special thanks:*

Mal Rosen for a "foot in the door" of EMS
Francis X. "Chip" Beaudet for being a terrific mentor
Raymond Hughes III for helping me regain confidence at a time when it was fading
Jon Politis for wisdom shared over the years.

Thank you.

And, of course, to Beverly, Sarah Katherine, and Barney.

DL

CONTENTS

First Responder: A Skills Approach has been extensively revised to meet your needs as a student, as well as to conform to the U.S. Department of Transportation's 1995 "First Responder: National Standard Curriculum."

The role of a First Responder is a special one. While the emergency medical services system is comprised of a talented team of many individuals at different certification levels, you are the one who will arrive on the scene of an emergency first. This is a special responsibility for which you will receive special training. In addition to the training in emergency medical care, you also will receive training that will help you in the first few minutes at the scene, including how to stay safe.

FEATURES OF THE FIFTH EDITION

To help you in your role as a First Responder, the Fifth Edition of *First Responder: A Skills Approach* includes several valuable new features:

- Case Study—Each chapter contains one. These detailed scenarios describe scene safety, patient assessment, and patient care from the perspective of an on-scene First Responder. Each case study walks you through all the relevant steps of your patient assessment plan.
- First Responder Focus—This feature boils down the chapter to the ideas and insights that will be most important to you in the field.
- "Special Rescue Situations"—A new chapter provides an overview of the most up-to-date emergency care and rescue methods for rope rescue, helicopter operations, confined space rescue, and other situations where special teams may be required. Important topics such as identification of hazards to the First Responder and when to call specialized teams are highlighted.

First Responder: A Skills Approach continues

to maintain the clarity and depth of coverage that has been our trademark over the previous editions. It also offers the same easy-to-read, *step-by-step* format that students continue to applaud.

U.S. DOT'S 1995 "FIRST RESPONDER: NATIONAL STANDARD CURRICULUM"

You can rest assured that this course meets the U.S. Department of Transportation's 1995 "First Responder: National Standard Curriculum." Look at the lists of objectives that introduce each chapter. The DOT objectives that are met by chapter content are listed verbatim.

In addition, the Department of Transportation acknowledges that many instructors will add enrichment materials to their lessons. That is, materials not covered in the national curriculum may be covered in your class. This is due to state or regional mandates or to special situations in your area. There are many places where we have chosen to add these extra, or "enrichment," materials to this textbook. They include:

- *A full chapter on automated external defibrillation (AED)*—This life-saving skill is being taught to many First Responders. The ability of First Responders and EMTs to deliver an electrical current to the chest of a patient whose heart has stopped beating is the most significant advance in the emergency medical services in many years.
- *Expanded coverage of common medical emergencies*—Cardiac and respiratory complaints are two of the most frequent reasons you will be called as a First Responder. Though they are not covered in the DOT curriculum, you will find them in this text. Additionally, you will find coverage of diabetic emergencies, alcohol and drug emergencies, stroke, poisoning, seizure, and abdominal pain.
- *Expanded coverage of patient assessment*—If you

require information on how to take a patient's vital signs, including obtaining a patient's blood pressure, you will find it covered in the "Patient Assessment" chapter.

- *Oxygen administration*—This topic is covered in the "Airway" module.
- *Expanded coverage of communications and documentation*
- *Splinting and spinal immobilization*—These topics are presented in the "Illness and Injury" module.
- *Water emergencies*—Updated to meet current standards, a whole chapter is devoted to this topic, which also includes a new section on swift-water emergencies.
- *Other enrichment materials,* such as bites and stings; shock including anaphlactic shock; psychological emergencies and crisis intervention (including rape); farm and industrial emergencies; complications of pregnancy and childbirth; safety for ambulance driving and safety in traffic on foot.
- *Chapter review questions*—Organized by chapter section, these questions also offer references to pages where answers may be found or supported.
- *New vocabulary is bold-faced the first time used and taught*—New terms also are defined in text as often as appropriate. In addition, two new easy-to-use glossaries—a glossary of abbreviations and a glossary of terms—have been added.

We believe that you will be pleased with *First Responder: A Skills Approach*. We always welcome your comments, which may be mailed to:

Judy Streger, Marketing Manager
BRADY PUBLISHING
One Lake Street
Upper Saddle River, NJ 07458

The authors may be contacted via email at Danlimmer@aol.com

ACKNOWLEDGMENTS

This textbook results from the efforts and cooperation of many people. As authors we create a vision for our textbook, determine an organization, establish a writing style, and of course present the information. In the complex process of text development we look to many others for assistance.

Medical Editor
We would like to express special appreciation to our medical editor, Edward Dickinson, MD, FACEP, who provided essential review and advice to ensure accuracy throughout the text. He was always available for questions. His energy, dedication, and knowledge of medicine and field procedures were indispensable. Dr. Dickinson is a board certified emergency physician who began his career in EMS in 1979 as an EMT-firefighter. He is currently an assistant professor in the Department of Emergency Medicine of the University of Pennsylvania School of Medicine and Medical Director of the Town of Colonie (NY) Department of EMS. Dr. Dickinson remains active in EMS as a researcher and teacher and regularly rides in the field, maintaining his paramedic certification. He is a recipient of *Firehouse Magazine's* National Award for Heroism and Community Service.

Contributors
To those who contributed chapters to the text, thank you. Brenda Beasley, Rich Beebe, Jon Politis, Brent Ricks, and Andy Stern prepared material reflecting up-to-date standards. We are pleased to have each on our team of contributors.

Brenda Beasley
 EMS Program Director,
 Calhoun State Community College,
 Decatur, AL

Rich Beebe
 Instructor, Institute of Prehospital
  Emergency Medicine,
 Hudson Valley Community College
 Troy, NY

Jon Politis
 Director, Emergency Medical
  Services,
 Colonie, NY

Brent Ricks
 Instructor,
 Institute of Prehospital Emergency
  Medicine,
 Hudson Valley Community College,
 Troy, NY

Andy Stern
 Senior Paramedic,
 Colonie EMS Department,
 Colonie, NY

Brady
At Brady, a wonderful team exists to make book development and production possible. Susan Katz, our publisher, has been very supportive. The team she has assembled is a true credit to her leadership and vision. Lois Berlowitz as managing editor handles the details. And there were many of them. Without Lois there would be no schedules, no organization, no common thread. While this is a formidable task in itself, Lois elevates her work to an art form. Her organization is enhanced by her dedication and the positive attitude she brings to every project. Thank you, Lois.

Jo Cepeda, as editor and project director for this book, worked tirelessly to assure the clear presentation and readability of the material. Jo edited the previous edition of this text, too. Her editorial talents are many. In particular, Jo's conscientious orientation to detail and positive suggestions throughout the development process proved invaluable. Jo has been indispensable to preparation of this edition. We thank Jo for all of this and more.

Michal Heron is our managing photo editor. Michal's talent as a photographer is matched by her strength as a photo manager. Michal shot photographs, researched others, and managed photographers in various parts of the country, all of which has led to the high quality of photos you will find in this textbook. Stephen Agricola, Michael Gallitelli, Richard Logan, and Rick Nye contributed photographs to this book as well.

Production of *First Responder: A Skills Approach* was guided skillfully by Julie Boddorf and Karen Fortgang. Laurie Burton proofread the material with diligence. Pat Walsh led the production team expertly.

We continue with thanks to the following people. Carol Sobel, editorial assistant, corresponds with our reviewers and handles the paperwork that is part of the process. Judy Streger markets our book with great exertise. Judy Stamm and the sales reps sell our texts and, as importantly are a wonderful vehicle by which we receive feedback from our readers. We listen carefully to the sales group and incorporate the suggestions they receive from students and instructors.

Reviewers
The following reviewers provided helpful perspective and suggestions. Our thanks to all.

Donna Alogna
 Seymour Ambulance
 Teacher, Harding High School
 Bridgeport, CT

Jerry Brungardt, BS, NREMT-P
 Norfolk, NE

James A. Christopher NREMT-P
 EMS Coordinator
 St. Francis Hospital Health Centers
 Beach Grove, IN

John A. Lewin
 EMS Instructor/ Illinois State Police
 Director, Cullom Fire Protection
  District EMS

Robert L. Marnatti
 EMMCO East, Inc.
 Kersey, PA

Steve McGraw
 The George Washington University
 EMS Program
 Washington, DC

Gerald W. Otto
 EMS Coordinator
 Ridgewater College
 Willmar, MN

Sheldon Richardson
 Vice-Chancellor
 Southern Arkansas University Tech
 Camden, AR

Gina Riggs, EMT-P
 EMS Coordinator
 Kiamichi Vo-Tech
 Stigler, OK

Sherman K. Sowby, Ph.D., CHES
 Professor of Health Sciences
 California State University, Fresno

H. Jeffrey Turner, MSM, NREMT-P,
  CMA
 Department Chairperson
 Ivy Tech State College
 Muncie, IN

Mike Whooley
 SFDPHN Paramedic Division
 San Francisco, CA

R. Thony Windham
 PEE DEE Regional EMS
 Education Coordinator/ Deputy
  Director
 Florence, SC

Richard E. Wolfe
   Lieutenant Commander
   Reserve Education and Training– Naval
   School of Health Sciences
   Bethesda, MD

Photo Acknowledgments

Photo Sources Our thanks to the following individuals for providing photos for this edition:

Charles Stewart, M.D.: 18-1a,b; 20-11; 22-3 a,b,c,d; 27-19a, b
Howard Paul, Emergency Stock! CO32, 32-1, 32-2, 32-3

Companies We wish to thank the following companies for their cooperation in providing photos for the Fifth Edition of this book: Motorola, Inc.; Ferno; National Registry of EMTs

Organizations We wish to thank the following organizations for their assistance in creating the photo program for the Fifth Edition:

All Children's Hospital, Pediatric Emergency Center
   St. Petersburg, FL
Hillsborough County EMS
   Bob Goldhammer, Assistant Operations Chief
   Tampa, FL
Hillsborough County Fire & Rescue
   Chief Bill Nesmith
   Bill Kaplan, Training Chief
   Chris Reynolds, Personnel Officer
   Tampa, FL
Hillsborough County Sheriff's Office
   Sheriff Cal Henderson
   Tampa, FL
Hudson Valley Community College
   Troy, NY
AMR West Florida,
   Conrad T. Kearns, MBA, Paramedic
   Director of Government Affairs
   Largo, FL

Sarasota County Fire Department
   Chief Brian Gorsky
   Sarasota, FL
Florida Highway Patrol
   Capt. F.D. Pedrick
   Lt. Harry Mofield
   Tampa, FL
Town of Colonie Department of EMS
   Colonie, NY
Town of Colonie Police Department
   Colonie, NY
Town of Guilderland EMS
   Guilderland, NY
Town of Guilderland Police Department
   Guilderland, NY
Western Turnpike Rescue Squad
   Albany, NY

Technical Advisors Thanks to the following EMS professionals for providing valuable technical support during the photo shoots for this edition:

Richard W.O. Beebe, BS, RN, EMT-P, Instructor, Hudson
   Valley Community College
Ted Rogers, AMR West Florida
Merill Seabury, AMR West Florida
Herman Cortez, AMR West Florida
Carol Hawthorne, AMR West Florida
Tom Maiolo, AMR West Florida
Bob Goldhammer, Assistant Operations Chief, Hillsborough
   County EMS
Bob Marschall, EMS Training Officer, Hillsborough
   County EMS
Michael Van Hoek EMS Training Officer, Hillsborough
   County Fire & Rescue
Lt. Paul Dezzi, Sarasota County Fire Department
Hubert "Mac" McNeely, Moulage Specialist, Tampa, FL

CORRELATION
U.S. DOT *"First Responder National Standard Curriculum"* with *First Responder: A Skills Approach*

INTRODUCTION TO THE EMS SYSTEM

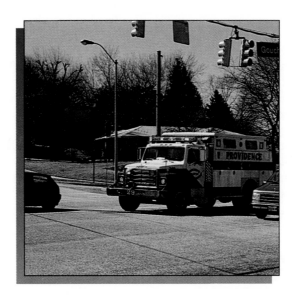

INTRODUCTION

You are about to join a vitally important profession. Every year thousands of people in this country die or are permanently injured because they did not receive emergency care in time. As a First Responder, you can make a difference.

This course will help you gain the knowledge, skills, and attitudes you need. To begin, your instructor will describe what you can expect in the course. He or she will inform you of required immunizations and physical exams, and outline your state and local certification requirements. Your instructor also will explain state and local policies concerning the Americans with Disabilities Act (ADA) and the implications of harassment in the classroom environment.

Cognitive, affective, and psychomotor objectives are from the U.S. DOT's 1995 "First Responder: National Standard Curriculum." Enrichment objectives, if any, identify material that is supplemental to the DOT curriculum.

Cognitive

1-1.1 Define the components of Emergency Medical Services (EMS) systems. (pp. 2–3)

1-1.2 Differentiate the roles and responsibilities of the First Responder from other out-of-hospital care providers. (pp. 5–7)

1-1.3 Define medical oversight and discuss the First Responder's role in the process. (pp. 8–9)

1-1.4 Discuss the types of medical oversight that may affect the medical care of a First Responder. (pp. 8–9)

1-1.5 State the specific statutes and regulations in your state regarding the EMS system. (p. 9)

Affective

1-1.6 Accept and uphold the responsibilities of a First Responder in accordance with the standards of an EMS professional. (pp. 7–8)

1-1.7 Explain the rationale for maintaining a professional appearance when on duty or when responding to calls. (p. 8)

1-1.8 Describe why it is inappropriate to judge a patient based on a cultural, gender, age, or socioeconomic model, and to vary the standard of care rendered as a result of that judgment. (p. 8)

Psychomotor

No objectives are identified.

Enrichment

* Describe the various methods by which the public can access EMS. (pp. 4–5)

SECTION 1: EMERGENCY MEDICAL SERVICES (EMS)

An ill or injured patient may need immediate medical care to prevent permanent disability or death. Too often those who arrive first at the scene of the emergency are not trained to give proper care. As a result, patients who might have been saved die.

The Maryland Institute for Emergency Medical Services describes the time immediately after an accident as the "Golden Hour." This is when lives that hang in the balance can be saved by proper emergency care.

In general, the **emergency medical services (EMS) system** is a network of resources linked together for one purpose. That purpose is to provide emergency care and transport to victims of sudden illness or injury (Figure 1–1). For example, when an emergency occurs, a citizen at the scene recognizes it and calls for help. If the citizen has dialed 9-1-1 or another emergency number, he or she will receive patient care instructions from an EMS dispatcher. When First Responders arrive, they will assess the situation and take over care. When necessary, they inform dispatch of the need for additional EMS resources. Usually, EMS rescuers with higher levels of training are called to the scene. They continue care and transport the patient to the hospital. There patient care is transferred to emergency medical department personnel and, finally, to the in-hospital care system.

CLASSIC COMPONENTS OF EMS

Each state in the U.S. has control of its own EMS system. However, standards are set by the National Highway Traffic Safety Administration, U.S. Department of Transportation (DOT). Those standards include ten classic components of any EMS system:

* *Regulation and policy.* Each state must have laws, regulations, policies, and procedures that govern its EMS system. It also is required to provide leadership to local jurisdictions.

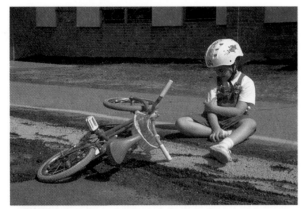

Figure 1-1a Patient.

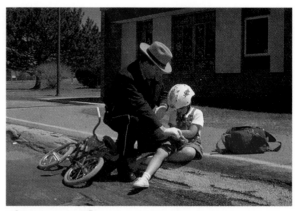

Figure 1-1b First Responder.

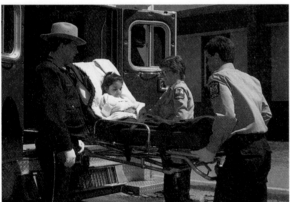

Figure 1-1c EMT-Basics or other EMS responders.

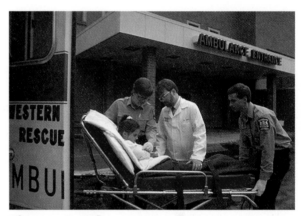

Figure 1-1d Hospital emergency department staff.

- *Resources management.* Each state must have central control of EMS resources so all patients have equal access to acceptable emergency care.
- *Human resources and training.* All personnel who staff ambulances and transport patients must be trained to at least the EMT-Basic level.
- *Transportation.* Patients must be safely and reliably transported by ground or air ambulance.
- *Facilities.* Every seriously ill or injured patient must be delivered in a timely manner to an appropriate medical facility.
- *Communications.* A system for public access to the EMS system must be in place. Communication among dispatcher, ambulance crew, and hospital also must be possible.

- *Public information and education.* EMS personnel should participate in programs designed to educate the public. The programs are to focus on the prevention of injuries and how to properly access the EMS system.
- *Medical oversight.* Each EMS system must have a physician as a medical director.
- *Trauma systems.* Each state must develop a system of specialized care for trauma patients, including one or more trauma centers and rehabilitation programs. It must also develop systems for assigning and transporting patients to those facilities.
- *Evaluation.* Each state must have a quality improvement system in place for continuing evaluation and upgrading of its EMS system.

CASE STUDY

DISPATCH

We were dispatched to a woman with chest pain at 426 Clifford Street. I had not been on many calls, but my partner has been on hundreds. I felt very nervous, especially with the lights and siren on.

SCENE SIZE-UP

When we approached the scene, my partner turned off the lights and siren. We grabbed protective gloves, and when we saw it was safe, left our rig. We both kept alert for signs of danger as we got closer to the house.

INITIAL ASSESSMENT

Inside the house, we saw our patient sitting on a chair. Our general impression was that she was pale and sweaty. I also remember thinking that she looked really sick. Almost immediately we began to assess her ABCs—airway, breathing, and circulation.

My partner gave me a look, which let me know that he believed the patient could be in serious condition. I radioed the dispatcher to update the incoming unit and requested the EMT-Paramedics. My partner administered oxygen to the patient while keeping her and her husband calm.

> You will encounter a wide range of calls as a First Responder. Some may be medical calls such as this one. Others may involve trauma (injury). You will learn how these First Responders handled their patient's emergency at the end of this chapter.

ACCESS TO EMS

There are two general systems by which the public can access EMS: *9-1-1* and *non-9-1-1*. Often called the "universal number," 9-1-1 is used in many areas to access police, fire, rescue, and ambulance. Generally, calls are received at a public safety answering point. There a dispatcher decides which service is to be activated and alerts that service (Figure 1–2).

There are two main benefits of a universal number. First, the public safety answering point generally is staffed by trained technicians. They may offer medical advice over the phone while the patient waits for rescuers to arrive. This is referred to as "emergency medical dispatching." The second benefit of a universal number is that it minimizes delay. Callers do not have to look up a number and it is easy enough to remember by even the youngest caller.

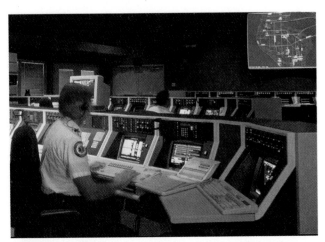

Figure 1-2 The emergency medical dispatcher (EMD) is an important member of the EMS team.

With enhanced 9-1-1, or E-9-1-1, the EMS dispatcher is able to see the street address and phone number of the caller on a computer screen. This is valuable when a patient becomes unconscious before giving an address.

In areas not served by 9-1-1, callers either call a dispatch center or the specific service they need (police, fire, etc.). Probably the most serious drawback of a non-9-1-1 system is the delay in reaching the appropriate services.

LEVELS OF TRAINING

There are four levels of **emergency medical services** training: **First Responder, EMT-Basic, EMT-Intermediate,** and **EMT-Paramedic.** (EMT is short for emergency medical technician.) Note that responsibilities for each level may vary from state to state. However, the minimum certification guidelines are published by the U.S. Department of Transportation (DOT).

- *First Responder* (Figure 1–4). The First Responder is the first person on the scene with emergency medical training. He or she may be a police officer or firefighter, a truck driver or school teacher, an industrial health officer, or a community volunteer. Training includes:
  - Airway care and suctioning
  - Patient assessment
  - Cardiopulmonary resuscitation (CPR)

  - Bleeding control
  - Stabilization of injuries to the spine and extremities
  - Care for medical and trauma emergencies
  - Use of a limited amount of equipment
  - Assisting other EMS providers
  - Other skills and procedures as permitted by local or state regulations
- *EMT-Basic* (Figure 1–5). The EMT-B can do all that the First Responder does. He or she also can perform complex immobilization procedures, restrain patients, and staff and drive ambulances.
- *EMT-Intermediate* (Figure 1–6). The EMT-I can do all that the two previous levels do. He or she also can perform a limited number of advanced techniques and administer a few medications. In some states, the EMT-I may also be trained as a cardiac technician.
- *EMT-Paramedic* (Figure 1–7). The paramedic has the most advanced EMS training. He or she can do all that the three previous levels do, plus administer more medications and perform more advanced techniques such as cardiac monitoring.

The National Registry of Emergency Medical Technicians was formed in 1970. It offers examinations for certification of First Responders and EMTs. If your state does not recognize or require national registration, it may still be help-

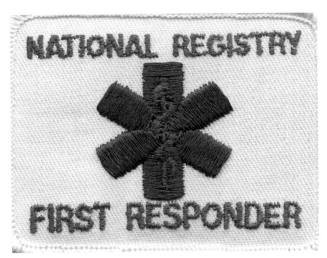

Figure 1-3 The National Registry First Responder patch.

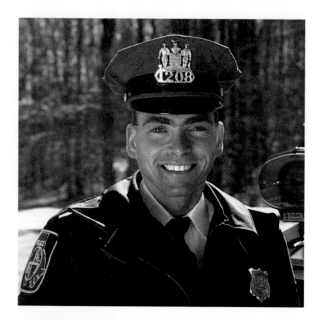
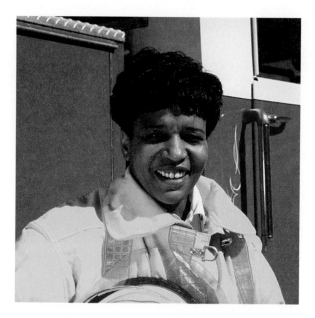
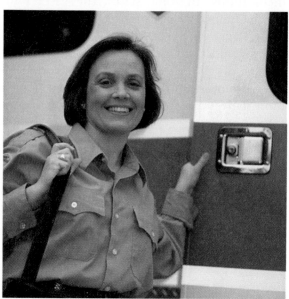
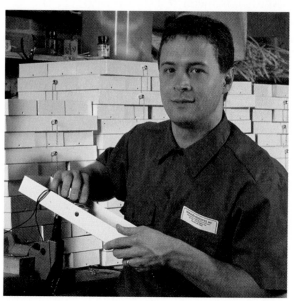

Figure 1-4 First Responders may be police officers, firefighters, educators, truck drivers, industrial workers, or community volunteers.

ful if you move to another state. It also is considered desirable by private employers. Ask your instructor about getting national certification or contact:

National Registry of Emergency Medical
  Technicians
6610 Busch Boulevard
Columbus, OH 43229
614-888-4484

IN-HOSPITAL CARE SYSTEM

First Responders and EMTs provide *prehospital care,* or emergency medical treatment, before transport to a medical facility. In some areas, the term *out-of-hospital care* is preferred. It reflects a trend toward providing care on the scene with or without transport to a hospital. (Your instructor will provide information on how these terms apply to your EMS system.)

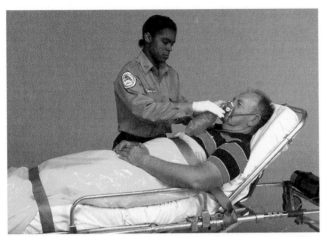

Figure 1-5   An EMT-Basic.

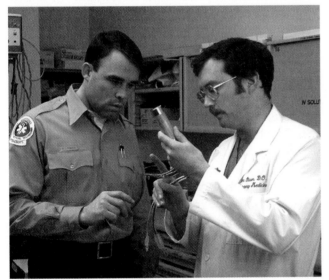

Figure 1-6   An EMT-Intermediate.

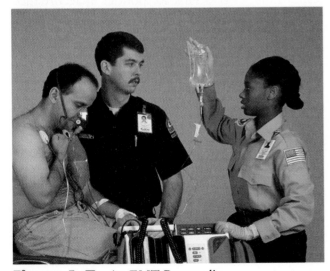

Figure 1-7   An EMT-Paramedic.

Specialized facilities to which some patients may be taken include:

- *Trauma center*—for injury treatment that may exceed what a general hospital can do.
- *Burn center*—for treatment of burns, often including long-term care and rehabilitation.
- *Pediatric center*—for treatment of infants and children.
- *Perinatal center*—for high-risk pregnant patients.
- *Poison center*—for information and advice on how to treat poisoning victims.

The most familiar destination of EMS patients is the local hospital emergency department. There a staff of physicians, nurses, and other allied health professionals stabilize the patient and prepare him or her for further care elsewhere in the hospital.

SECTION 2: THE FIRST RESPONDER

As a First Responder, you may be called to emergencies where you are the only trained rescuer on the scene. At other times, specialized rescue teams and fire personnel, as well as law enforcement, may all be involved.

YOUR ROLE

As a First Responder, your primary concern is your patient. Generally, your role includes the following:

- *Protect your safety and the safety of your crew, the patient, and bystanders.* This is your first and most important priority. Remember that you cannot help the patient if you are injured. You also do not want to endanger other rescuers by forcing them to rescue you. Once scene safety is assured, the patient's needs become your primary concern.
- *Gain access to the patient.* In some emergencies, you may need to move one patient in order to gain access to a more critically injured one.
- *Assess the patient to identify life-threatening problems.* Always perform an initial assessment

to help you identify life threats. Such problems may include a blocked airway, heart attack, or severe bleeding.

- *Alert additional EMS resources.* In cases where a patient needs medical care or transport to a medical facility, you must remain with the patient until other EMS personnel take over patient care.
- *Provide care based on assessment findings.* While you are waiting for EMS resources to arrive, you must provide patient care based on the needs you identified during patient assessment.
- *Assist other EMS personnel.* When requested, assist other EMS personnel with patient care as needed.
- *Participate in record keeping and data collection as required.* You may be required by state law or your local EMS system to document your calls, especially if a patient refuses care.
- *Act as liaison with other public safety workers.* These may include local, state, or federal law enforcement, fire department personnel, and other EMS providers.

YOUR RESPONSIBILITIES

The responsibilities of a First Responder vary from state to state. However, they always include assuring scene safety and maintaining a professional attitude, appearance, and up-to-date skills. Specifically, you should:

- *Guard your personal health and safety.* Drive safely at all times. Use a seat belt whenever you drive or ride. Remove yourself from hazards such as gas leaks, fires, chemical spills, and so on, and follow the directions of specialized rescuers at those scenes. Never enter a crime scene or an angry crowd until it has been controlled by the police. Locate or create a safe area in which you can care for patients. Stay away from high-traffic areas. Redirect traffic as needed. Always wear the proper personal protective equipment (PPE) including, when appropriate, a hard hat and leather gloves. (See Chapter 2 for more details.)
- *Maintain a caring attitude.* Often you will arrive at an emergency scene to find the patient, family, and bystanders in a state of panic or chaos. These are normal reactions. Reassure and

comfort them. Identify yourself, assure them that you will begin to stabilize the patient, and let them know that more help is on the way.

- *Maintain your own composure.* Many calls will be routine, and patient care will be simple. However, some calls will involve life-threatening or emotionally charged problems. In those cases, it is critical that you stay calm so you can get an accurate picture of the scene and properly establish your priorities.
- *Keep a neat, clean, professional appearance.* Excellent personal grooming and a crisp, clean appearance help instill confidence in patients. Being clean also helps to protect your patients from contamination from dirty hands or soiled clothing. Respond to every call in complete uniform or other appropriate dress. Portray the positive image you want to project. Remember that you are on a medical team. Your appearance can send the message that you are competent and trustworthy.
- *Maintain up-to-date knowledge and skills.* New research often shows us better ways of doing things. So take every opportunity to continue your education, including taking refresher courses offered through your local EMS system.
- *Maintain current knowledge of local, state, and national issues affecting the EMS system.* Attend conferences and read professional journals dedicated to EMS issues.

You will be expected to accept and uphold the responsibilities of a First Responder in accordance with the standards of an EMS professional. Note that as a First Responder you will come in contact with people of different genders, ages, cultures, and socioeconomic backgrounds. It is your responsibility to meet the standard of care for all your patients.

SECTION 3: MEDICAL OVERSIGHT

MEDICAL DIRECTOR

A formal relationship exists between a community's EMS providers and the physician who is responsible for out-of-hospital emergency medical care. This physician is often referred to as the system **medical director**. He or she is legally responsible for the clinical and patient-care aspects of an EMS system.

Every EMS system *must* have a medical director. He or she must provide guidance to all emergency care and rescue personnel. The medical director is also responsible for reviewing and improving the quality of care in an EMS system.

MEDICAL CONTROL

Two basic types of medical oversight are **direct medical control** and **indirect medical control**. Direct medical control occurs when the medical director or another physician directs an EMS rescuer at the scene of an emergency. This may be done via telephone, radio, or in person. This usually occurs when an EMS rescuer asks for help with a patient. Note that direct medical control is also called "on-line," "base station," "immediate," or "concurrent."

Indirect medical control may also be called "off-line," "retrospective," or "prospective." It includes such things as system design and quality management. Through indirect medical control, protocols spell out the accepted practice for First Responders in your area. They tell you things like whether or not you can give oxygen to a patient or how to respond to a family who refuses your help. They also tell you how to document each call, participate in reviews, gather feedback, and maintain your skills.

THE FIRST RESPONDER

In general, First Responders are the designated agents of the medical director. If this is true in your area, the care you render by law may be considered an extension of the medical director's authority. Your instructor will tell you what the law is in your area.

FIRST RESPONDER FOCUS

As a First Responder, you play a vital role in the emergency medical care of patients experiencing an illness or injury. Perhaps the most important reason your role is so crucial is that you are responsible for the first few minutes with the patient. The EMS system depends on your action during this time to set the foundation for the remainder of the call.

It is during this time that correcting a breathing problem or stopping bleeding will actually save a life. You also will help patients who are not in critical condition when you prevent further injury, perform the proper assessments, gather a medical history, and prepare for the arrival of the EMTs or paramedics. ■

CASE STUDY FOLLOW-UP

At the beginning of this chapter, you read that First Responders were caring for a patient with chest pain. To see how chapter material applies to this emergency, read the following. It describes how the call was completed.

PATIENT HISTORY

The woman told us she was 67 and her name was Paula McMaster. She said she had a heavy feeling in her chest for about two hours. It radiated to her left shoulder. The pain came on while she was watching TV. The patient told us that she had high blood pressure for many years. She had two heart attacks over the past five years. She took a blood pressure medication and a pill for diabetes. She denied any allergies. Her last meal was about two hours ago, when she had a sandwich and coffee.

PHYSICAL EXAMINATION

The patient denied any injury such as a fall or car crash earlier. Because of this we did not perform a hands-on, head-to-toe exam. We did check her chest, shoulders, and arms for pain. We took her vital signs and found that her pulse was 96, weak and irregular. Her respirations were 20 and labored. Blood pressure was 100/56. Listening to her chest we heard adequate air entering on both sides.

We applied oxygen and made sure the paramedics were on the way.

ONGOING ASSESSMENT

We remained concerned because the patient was pale and sweaty with some difficulty breathing. We verified that the patient was still alert and breathing adequately. Oxygen continued to flow through a nonrebreather mask. We made sure the patient was as comfortable as she could be and tried to reassure her and her husband. We finished another set of vitals just as the ambulance pulled up.

PATIENT HAND-OFF

Since my partner had responsibility for patient care during this call, he gave the EMTs the hand-off report:

> "We have a 67-year-old female patient, Mrs. McMaster. She began having heaviness in the chest and left shoulder about two hours ago while watching TV. She is pale and sweaty with some labored breathing. Her vital signs are 100/56, pulse is 96 weak and irregular, respirations are 20 and labored. She has a history of heart attack, high blood pressure, and diabetes. We tried to make her comfortable and gave her oxygen by nonrebreather mask."

After we made sure the EMTs didn't need us any longer, we radioed dispatch to say we were available for our next call and headed back to headquarters.

> It takes all of the resources of an EMS system working together to help a patient survive an illness or injury. As a First Responder, you are a valuable part of that system.

REVIEW QUESTIONS

Page references where answers may be found or supported are provided at the end of each question.

Section 1

1. What is the purpose of the EMS system? (p. 2)
2. What is the typical sequence of events that occurs from the time an accident occurs and EMS is activated? (p. 2)
3. What are five of the 10 classic components of an EMS system? (pp. 2–3)
4. What are two basic ways to access the EMS system? (pp. 4–5)
5. How many levels of training are offered in the EMS system? Briefly describe each one. (p. 5)

6. What are three types of medical facilities to which an EMS patient may be taken? (p. 6)

Section 2

7. What roles do First Responders play at the scene of an emergency? (pp. 5–6)
8. What are the First Responder's responsibilities? (pp. 8–9)

Section 3

9. What are the two types of medical oversight? Describe each one. (p. 9)

THE WELL-BEING OF THE FIRST RESPONDER

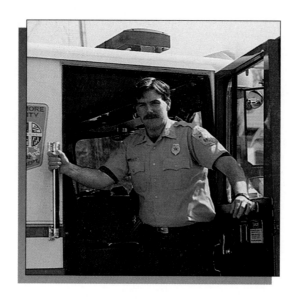

INTRODUCTION

As a rescuer, your safety always comes first. It comes before the patient and before any bystander at the scene. The reason is simple. If you are injured, you lose the ability to help those who need you. Instead of providing emergency care, you end up needing it.

Many elements make up rescuer safety. Most basic training programs teach how to react safely to a variety of environmental threats, such as fire and flood. But the most common threat to a rescuer is likely to be as simple as oncoming traffic.

This chapter outlines the basic steps you should take to maintain your well-being. It includes how to anticipate and handle the emotional aspects of emergencies and how to protect yourself against infection. It also introduces you to scene safety.

Cognitive, affective, and psychomotor objectives are from the U.S. DOT's 1995 "First Responder: National Standard Curriculum." Enrichment objectives, if any, identify material that is supplemental to the DOT curriculum.

Cognitive

1-2.1 List possible emotional reactions that the First Responder may experience when faced with trauma, illness, death, and dying. (pp. 13–14, 16–17)

1-2.2 Discuss the possible reactions that a family member may exhibit when confronted with death and dying. (pp. 14–15)

1-2.3 State the steps in the First Responder's approach to the family confronted with death and dying. (pp. 15–16)

1-2.4 State the possible reactions that the family of the First Responder may exhibit. (pp. 17–18)

1-2.5 Recognize the signs and symptoms of critical incident stress. (pp. 13–14, 16–17)

1-2.6 State possible steps that the First Responder may take to help reduce/alleviate stress. (pp. 17–19)

1-2.7 Explain the need to determine scene safety. (pp. 24–27)

1-2.8 Discuss the importance of body substance isolation (BSI). (pp. 19–21)

1-2.9 Describe the steps the First Responder should take for personal protection from airborne and bloodborne pathogens. (pp. 21–24)

1-2.10 List the personal protective equipment necessary for each of the following situations: (pp. 22–27)
- Hazardous materials
- Rescue operations
- Violent scenes
- Crime scenes
- Electricity
- Water and ice
- Exposure to bloodborne pathogens
- Exposure to airborne pathogens

Affective

1-2.11 Explain the importance of serving as an advocate for the use of appropriate protective equipment. (p. 23)

1-2.12 Explain the importance of understanding the response to death and dying and communicating effectively with the patient's family. (pp. 15–16)

1-2.13 Demonstrate a caring attitude towards any patient with illness or injury who requests emergency medical services. (pp. 14–16)

1-2.14 Show compassion when caring for the physical and mental needs of patients. (pp. 14–16)

1-2.15 Participate willingly in the care of all patients. (p. 21)

1-2.16 Communicate with empathy to patients being cared for, as well as with family members, and friends of the patient. (pp. 14–16)

Psychomotor

1-2.17 Given a scenario with potential infectious exposure, the First Responder will use appropriate personal protective equipment. At the completion of the scenario, the First Responder will properly remove and discard the protective garments. (pp. 21–23)

1-2.18 Given the above scenario, the First Responder will complete disinfection/cleaning and all reporting documentation. (pp. 21–22, 24)

SECTION 1: EMOTIONAL ASPECTS OF EMERGENCY MEDICAL CARE

Stress is any change in the body's internal balance. It occurs when outside demands are greater than the body's resources. High-stress situations include mass casualties, injury to an infant or child, death of a patient, an amputation, violence, abuse, and injury or death of a coworker.

A rescuer's emotional responses to high stress may include weakness, nausea, vomiting, or fainting. You can help avoid these reactions by using the following techniques:

- Remind yourself that the patient desperately needs you and your skills. You must be in control to give the best care.

CASE STUDY

DISPATCH

My partner and I are community volunteers associated with the fire department. We were on the 3-to-12 shift, and it was just about time to quit when dispatch called. There was a person bleeding at 1433 Magnolia.

We got in our unit. It was my partner's turn to drive. I got out the town map and located the residence. On the way, I mentally went over the procedures for body substance isolation and bleeding control.

SCENE SIZE-UP

We arrived at the patient's house in about four minutes. We approached carefully. Without any more information than "a person bleeding," we had to be ready for anything. When we got to the door, we waited a second and listened.

Men were yelling, and I heard glass breaking. Loud thumps and scuffling made it obvious that people were fighting in there.

> Caution will help you to recognize potential dangers at an emergency scene. But is violence the only kind of danger you may face? What precautions would you take in the situation described above? Consider your answer as you read Chapter 2.

• Close your eyes and take several long, deep breaths. Focus on counting each breath. When you feel more in control, return to giving emergency care.

• Change your thought patterns. Very quietly hum or mentally sing a peaceful song.

• Eat properly to maintain your blood sugar. Low blood sugar can add to a fainting problem.

DEATH AND DYING

Death and dying are inherent parts of emergency medical care. When your patient is dying, you must care for his or her emotional needs as well as the injury or illness. If the patient dies suddenly, help the family or bystanders deal with their grief.

The Grieving Process

There are five general stages that dying patients—and those close to them—experience. The five stages are called the **grieving process.** Each person progresses through the stages at his or her own rate and in his or her own way.

Patients with nonfatal emergencies also may go through a grieving process. For example, a patient who loses both legs in a factory accident will grieve the loss of his limbs.

As a First Responder, you will not witness all five stages during emergency care. For example, a critically injured patient who is aware that death is imminent may just begin the process. A terminally ill patient who is more prepared may be at the final "acceptance" stage. The key is to accept all emotions as real and necessary. Respond accordingly.

The stages of the grieving process occur as follows:

- *Denial ("Not me!").* At first the patient may refuse to accept the idea that death is near. This refusal creates a buffer between the shock of approaching death and the need to deal with the illness or injury. Families of dying patients often are at the denial stage.
- *Anger ("Why me?").* Watch out. You may be the target of this anger. But remember that it is a normal part of the grieving process. Do not take it personally. Be tolerant. Try to understand, and use your best listening and communication skills.
- *Bargaining ("Okay, but first let me . . .").* In the patient's mind a bargain, or agreement of sorts, will postpone death. For example, a patient may mentally determine that if he is allowed to live, he will patch up a long-standing break with his parents.
- *Depression ("Okay, but I haven't . . .").* As reality settles in, the patient may become silent, distant, withdrawn, and sad. He usually is thinking about those he leaves behind and all the things left undone.
- *Acceptance ("Okay, I am not afraid.").* Finally, the patient may appear to accept the fact that he is dying, though he is not happy about it. At this stage, the family usually needs more support than the patient does.

Dealing with the Dying Patient

It is one of your jobs to help a patient and his or her family through the grieving process. Keep in mind that they may progress through the stages of grief at different rates. Whatever stage they are in, their needs include dignity, respect, sharing, communication, privacy, and control. To help reduce their emotional burden, consider the following:

- *Do everything possible to maintain the patient's dignity.* Avoid negative statements about the patient's condition. Even an unresponsive patient may hear what you say and feel the fear in your words. Talk to the patient as if he is fully alert. Explain the care you are providing.

- *Show the greatest possible respect for the patient.* Do this especially when death is imminent. Families will be extra sensitive at this time. Even attitudes and unspoken messages are perceived. So explain what you are doing. Assure family members that you are making every possible effort to help the patient. It is important for them to know with certainty that you never simply "gave up."
- *Communicate.* Help the patient become oriented to the surroundings. If necessary, explain several times what happened and where. Explain who you are and what you and others are planning. Assure the patient that you are doing everything possible and that you will see that he gets to a hospital as quickly as possible. Without interrupting care, communicate the same message to the family. Explain any procedure you need to carry out. Answer their questions. Do not guess. Report only what you know to be true.
- *Allow family members to express rage, anger, and despair.* They should be able to scream, cry, or vent grief but in a way that is not dangerous to you or others. Be tolerant. If they vent their anger at you, do not get angry or hostile.
- *Listen with empathy.* Many dying people want messages delivered to survivors. Take notes. Assure the patient that you will do whatever you can to honor his requests. Then follow through on your promise. If possible, stay with the family to listen to their concerns and answer their questions.
- *Do not give false assurances, but allow for some hope.* Be honest but tactful. If the patient asks if he is dying, do not confirm it. Patients who do the most poorly are often the ones who feel hopeless. Instead, say something like "We are doing everything we can. We need you to help us by not giving up." If the patient insists that death is imminent, say "That might be possible, but we can still try the best we can, can't we?"
- *Use a gentle tone of voice.* Be kind to both the patient and the family. Explain the scope of the injury, your medical care, and when necessary, the suspected cause of death to the best of your ability. Do so as gently and kindly as you can in terms they will understand.

- *Let the patient know that everything that can be done will be done.* Emphasize that you are not going to give up. Say that you are doing everything possible and you will see that the patient gets to a hospital as quickly as possible for further care.
- *Use a reassuring touch,* if appropriate. In addition, if family members want to touch or hold the body after death, and local protocol allows it, arrange for it. Do what you can to improve the appearance of the body. If the body is mutilated, warn the family first. Tell them you covered the badly injured parts.

  Note that at a possible crime scene, *never* clean the patient or remove any blood from the patient or the scene.
- *Do what you can to comfort the family.* Arrange for them to briefly see or talk to the patient. However, do not interrupt your emergency care or delay transport. If the patient is deceased and the family asks you to pray with them, do so. Stay with the family until the medical examiner or coroner arrives.

STRESS MANAGEMENT

Many First Responders expose themselves to a great deal of stress in order to meet the needs of their patients. They feel completely responsible for everything that happens at the scene, even things clearly out of their control. Some become so involved that their self-image is actually based on job performance.

Chronic stress at work plus an emotionally charged environment can lead to a state of exhaustion and irritability. Beware. That state can markedly decrease your effectiveness. Even some of the very best EMS workers have had to leave the system because of it.

Recognize Warning Signs

One of the best ways to manage chronic stress and prevent burnout is to be aware of the warning signs. The earlier they are spotted, the easier they are to remedy. The warning signs include (Figure 2–1):

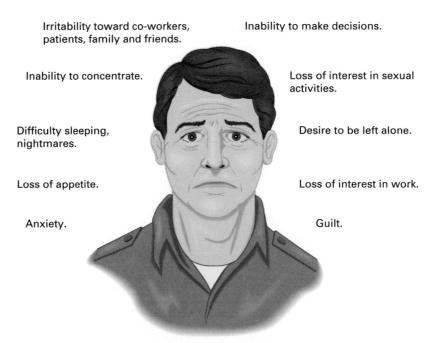

Irritability toward co-workers, patients, family and friends.

Inability to concentrate.

Difficulty sleeping, nightmares.

Loss of appetite.

Anxiety.

Inability to make decisions.

Loss of interest in sexual activities.

Desire to be left alone.

Loss of interest in work.

Guilt.

Figure 2-1 The warning signs of stress.

- Irritability with coworkers, family, and friends
- Inability to concentrate
- Difficulty sleeping, nightmares
- Anxiety
- Inability to make decisions
- Guilt
- Loss of appetite
- Loss of sexual desire
- Isolation
- Loss of interest in work

In addition, the following general signs and symptoms have been identified with stress:

- *Cognitive*—confusion, inability to make judgments or decisions, loss of motivation, memory problems, loss of objectivity
- *Psychological*—depression, excessive anger, negativism, hostility, defensiveness, mood swings, feelings of worthlessness
- *Physical*—constant exhaustion, headaches, stomach problems, dizziness, pounding heart
- *Behavioral*—overeating, increased use of drugs or alcohol, grinding teeth, hyperactivity, lack of energy
- *Social*—frequent arguments, decreased ability to relate to patients

Make Lifestyle Changes

Certain lifestyle changes can be helpful in dealing with chronic stress. One change you can make is in your diet. Certain foods increase the body's response to stress. So cut down on sugar, caffeine, and alcohol. Avoid fatty foods, and eat more low-fat carbohydrates. While at work, eat often but in small amounts.

Avoid alcohol and other kinds of self-medication. Reaching for a drink or pills will not help you cope with stress. In fact, they increase stress. And remember, problems will still be there when you wake from your stupor. They may even be worse, because you did not act on them right away.

Exercise more often, too (Figure 2–2). Exercise has all kinds of benefits, including physical release for pent-up emotions.

Finally, learn to relax. Meditation and visual imagery are helpful techniques. You also may

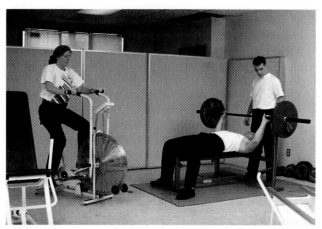

Figure 2-2 As a First Responder, you must safeguard your own health.

want to try to cut loose a little bit. Watch a funny movie, read a good book, or go dancing or to a concert.

Keep Balance in Your Life

One way to balance work, recreation, family, and health is to assess your priorities. Take a few minutes to list all your activities on paper. Write "1" beside your first priority. Write "2" beside your second, and so on. Then perform those activities—all of them—in the order you assigned.

Be sure to share your worries with someone else. Talk to someone you trust and respect. It can help relieve stress and help you discover alternatives. A good confidante listens well and asks questions that help you explore your ideas honestly.

Still another way to help keep balance in your life is to accept the fact that you will sometimes make mistakes. Admit to yourself that no person is right all the time. Understand that a mistake does not reduce your value. You do not have to be perfect to do a good job.

Remember that the support of your family and friends is essential to helping you manage stress. Keep in mind, though, that they suffer from stress related to your job, too. Their stress factors include the following:

- *Lack of understanding.* Families typically have little if any knowledge about prehospital emergency care.

- *Fear of separation or of being ignored.* Long hours can take their toll and increase your family's distress over your absences. You may hear, "Your job is more important to you than your family!"
- *Worry about on-call situations.* Stress at home may increase because your family may focus on the danger you face when you respond to emergency calls.
- *Frustrated desire to share.* It may be too difficult for you to talk about what happened on certain calls. Even though your family and friends understand that, they may still feel frustrated in their desire to help and support you.

If at all possible, you can help to keep balance in your life by changing your work environment. Request work shifts that allow for more time to relax with family and friends. Ask for a rotation of duty to an assignment that is less stressful. Take periodic breaks to exercise and to support and encourage coworkers.

Seek Professional Help

Mental health professionals, social workers, and clergy can help you realize that your reactions are normal. They can also mobilize your best coping strategies and suggest more effective ways to deal with stress.

CRITICAL INCIDENT STRESS DEBRIEFING (CISD)

A **critical incident** is any event that causes unusually strong emotions that interfere with your ability to function either during the incident or later. This type of stress requires aggressive and immediate management, including:

- Pre-incident stress education
- On-scene peer support
- One-on-one support
- Disaster support services
- Follow-up services
- Spouse and family support
- Community outreach programs
- Other general health and welfare programs, such as wellness programs

In addition, a system has been developed to help rescuers cope with critical incident stress. It is called **critical incident stress debriefing (CISD).** CISD combines a team of peer counselors with mental health professionals (Figure 2–3). It is successful because it helps rescuers vent their feelings quickly. Its nonthreatening environment also encourages rescuers to feel free to air their concerns and reactions.

CISD includes anyone involved in an incident—police, firefighters, EMS personnel, dispatchers, doctors, and so on. In some cases, it may also include their families. After mass casualties (such as earthquakes or explosions), a number of CISD meetings may be needed.

There are two basic CISD techniques: **defusing** and **debriefing.**

Defusing

Much shorter and less formal than a debriefing, a defusing is usually held within hours of the critical incident. It is attended only by those most directly involved and lasts only 30 to 45 minutes. A defusing gives rescuers a chance to vent their feelings and get information they may need before the larger group meets. It may either eliminate the need for a formal debriefing, or it may enhance a later debriefing.

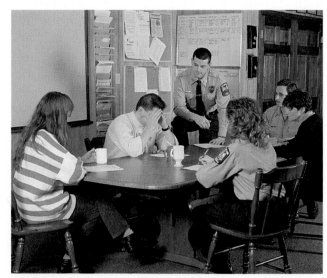

Figure 2-3 The critical incident stress debriefing (CISD) helps rescuers deal with particularly stressful incidents.

Debriefing

Ideally, a debriefing is held within 24 to 72 hours of a critical incident. It is not an investigation or an interrogation. Everything that is said at a debriefing is confidential. Rescuers are urged to explore any physical, mental, or emotional symptoms they are having. CISD counselors and mental health professionals then evaluate the information and offer suggestions on how to cope with the stress resulting from the incident.

Accessing CISD

Generally, your agency or organization will organize a CISD. Attend if you have been involved in:

- Serious injury or death of a rescuer in the line of duty
- Multiple-casualty incident
- Suicide of an emergency worker
- An event that attracts media attention
- Injury or death of someone you know
- Any disaster

Also access CISD after any event that has unusual impact on you. That may include an incident in which injury or death of a civilian was caused by a rescuer (an ambulance colliding with a car, for example). A death of a patient, child abuse or neglect, an event that threatens your life, or one that has distressing sights, sounds, or smells—all may be cause for accessing CISD.

Ask your instructor about the CISD programs available through your EMS system.

SECTION 2: PREVENTING DISEASE TRANSMISSION

As a First Responder, you will come in contact with patients who are sick. If you are worried about "catching" their diseases, you are justified. However, don't despair. The following section will explain how diseases are transmitted and describe the ones of most concern to EMS personnel. It also will outline proven ways for you to protect yourself.

HOW DISEASES ARE TRANSMITTED

Diseases are caused by **pathogens,** microorganisms such as bacteria and viruses. An **infectious disease** is one that spreads from one person to another (Figure 2–4). It can spread *directly* through blood-to-blood contact (bloodborne), contact with open wounds or exposed tissues, and contact with the mucous membranes of the eyes and mouth. An infectious disease also can spread

HOW INFECTIOUS DISEASES CAN SPREAD

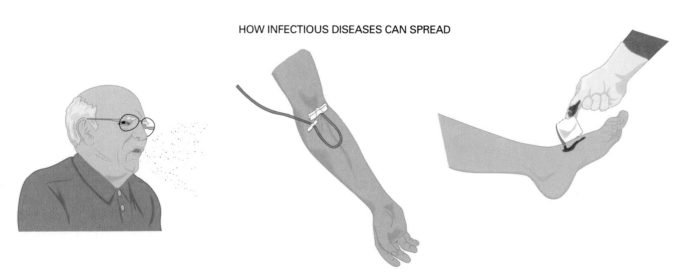

a. Droplet infection.   b. Blood-to-blood contact.   c. Open wounds/exposed tissue.

Figure 2-4   How infectious diseases can spread.

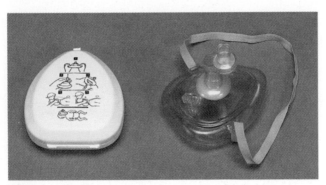

Figure 2-5 A pocket face mask with one-way valve and carrying case.

indirectly by way of a contaminated object, such as a needle or by way of infected droplets breathed into the respiratory tract (airborne).

Some pathogens are transmitted easily, such as the viruses that cause the common cold. Others need specific routes of contact. The tuberculosis bacteria, for example, is transmitted by droplets from a cough or sneeze of an infected patient. Poor nutrition, poor hygiene, crowded or unsanitary living conditions, and stress all make infection from any disease easier.

In order to protect yourself, you must *always* make use of the appropriate personal protective equipment. That includes using a barrier device such as a pocket face mask *every time* you ventilate a patient (Figure 2–5). Make sure the device has a one-way valve that prevents fluid from backing up.

DISEASES OF CONCERN

As a First Responder, you can be exposed to infectious diseases whenever you treat a patient. Three diseases of most concern are described below.

Hepatitis B

Hepatitis B (HBV) is a virus that directly affects the liver. It can be fatal. A serious disease that can last for months, HBV is contracted through blood and body fluids. A major source of the virus is the "chronic carrier." This person can carry the virus for years. He or she usually has no

signs or symptoms and is often unaware of being ill. When signs and symptoms do appear, they may include:

- Fatigue
- Nausea
- Loss of appetite
- Abdominal pain
- Headache
- Fever
- Yellowish color of the skin and whites of eyes

If you suspect you have been exposed to HBV, report the incident to your supervisor. Immediately contact a physician or your local public health agency for care. Care may include injections of HBIG (hepatitis B immunoglobulin). You also may receive a vaccination if you have not already had one.

Note that the most effective way to deal with HBV is prevention. Employers and most agencies offer HBIG free of charge. Medical authorities strongly recommend this vaccine.

Tuberculosis

Tuberculosis (TB) almost vanished once. But it is back. In fact, researchers are worried because new drug-resistant strains are developing. The pathogen that causes TB is found in the lungs and other tissues of the infected patient. You can be infected from droplets in a patient's cough or from infected sputum. The main signs and symptoms of TB include:

- Fever
- Cough
- Night sweats
- Weight loss

The U.S. Occupational Safety and Health Administration (OSHA) has adopted standards for rescuers' protection against TB. They include the use of special masks. One type of mask is called the **N-95 respirator** (Figure 2–6). The other type is called the high efficiency particulate air respirator, or the **HEPA respirator.** Wear one whenever you suspect TB. Perform ventilation only with OSHA-approved equipment.

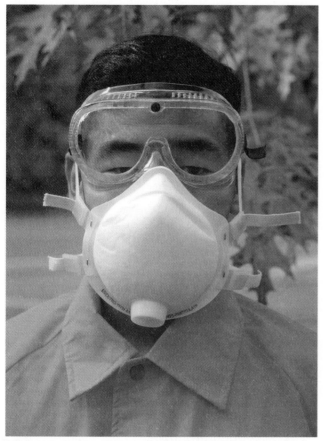

Figure 2-6 The N-95 respirator should be worn when you suspect a patient of TB infection.

Acquired Immune Deficiency Syndrome (AIDS)

Fortunately, AIDS is not spread through casual contact. It cannot be spread by touching the skin, coughing, sneezing, sharing eating utensils, or other indirect ways. *Transmission requires intimate contact with the body fluids of infected persons.* Infection may occur with:

- Sexual contact involving the exchange of semen, saliva, blood, urine, or feces.
- Infected needles.
- Infected blood or blood products.
- Mother to child during pregnancy, birth, or breast-feeding.

Simply stated, the human immunodeficiency virus (HIV) knocks out the body's ability to fight infection. HIV leads to AIDS. AIDS victims get infections caused by viruses, bacteria, parasites, and fungi. These are serious illnesses that do not occur (or occur only mildly) among people with healthy immune systems. They involve many organs of the body, causing a countless array of signs and symptoms.

Not everyone infected by HIV has developed AIDS. However, people who carry HIV are still able to spread the infection to others. So, because any patient could be infected with HIV or other diseases, follow all the precautions described below at all times and with all patients.

BODY SUBSTANCE ISOLATION

For many years, OSHA guidelines required EMS personnel to take steps to protect themselves against diseases transmitted by way of blood. They were called "universal precautions." In the late 1980s, the Centers for Disease Control (CDC) published guidelines that set a new standard. That standard says *assume all blood and body fluids are infectious.* It requires EMS personnel to practice a strict form of infection control with *all* patients. It is called **body substance isolation (BSI)**.

With BSI precautions, it is possible to take care of all patients safely, even those with infectious diseases. BSI precautions include handwashing; proper cleaning, disinfection, or sterilization of equipment; and use of personal protective equipment (PPE).

Handwashing

Handwashing is the single most important thing you can do to prevent the spread of infection. According to the U.S. Public Health Service, most contaminants can be removed from the skin with 10 to 15 seconds of vigorous lathering and scrubbing with plain soap.

Always wash your hands after caring for a patient, *even if you were wearing gloves.* For maximum protection, begin by removing all jewelry from your hands and arms. Then lather up and rub together all surfaces of your hands. Pay attention to creases, crevices, and the areas between your fingers. Use a brush to scrub under and around your fingernails (Figure 2–7). (Note that it is a good idea

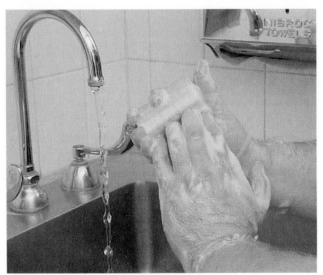

Figure 2-7 The first line of protection against infectious disease is handwashing.

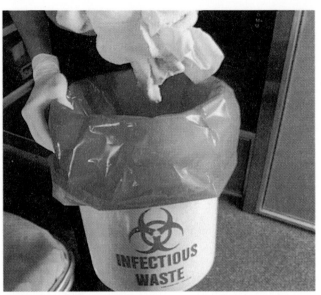

Figure 2-8 Be sure to discard contaminated items properly.

for you to keep your nails short and unpolished.) If your hands are visibly soiled, spend more time washing them. Wash your wrists and forearms, too. Rinse thoroughly under a stream of water and dry well. Use a disposable towel if possible.

If you do not have access to soap and running water, you can use a foam or liquid washing agent. As soon as you can, wash your hands again using the procedure described above.

Cleaning Equipment

Cleaning, disinfecting, and sterilizing are related terms. **Cleaning** is simply the process of washing a soiled object with soap and water. **Disinfecting** is cleaning plus using a chemical like alcohol or bleach to kill many of the microorganisms on an object. **Sterilizing** is a process in which a chemical or other substance (like superheated steam) kills all of the microorganisms on an object.

Generally, disinfecting is used on items that come in contact with the intact skin of a patient. Items that come in contact with open wounds or mucous membranes should be sterilized.

Whenever possible, use disposable equipment. *Never reuse disposable items.* Instead, place them in a plastic bag that is clearly labeled "infectious waste" (Figure 2–8). Then seal the bag. Disposable items used with patients who have HBV or HIV should be double-bagged.

After each use, clean non-disposable equipment. Wash off all blood, mucus, tissue, and other residue. Be sure to wear a good pair of utility gloves while doing so. Then disinfect or sterilize it as per local protocols.

Wash items that do not normally touch the patient. Rinse them with clear water and dry thoroughly. Clean walls or window coverings in an ambulance or rescue vehicle when they get soiled. Then use a hospital-grade disinfectant or a solution of household bleach and water to clean up any blood or body fluids.

If your clothes get soiled with body fluids, remove, bag, and label them. Wash them in hot soapy water for at least 25 minutes. Take a hot shower yourself and rinse thoroughly.

Personal Protective Equipment (PPE)

Always use **personal protective equipment (PPE)** as a barrier against infection. Such items will keep you from coming into contact with a patient's blood and body fluids. They include eye protection, gloves, gowns, and masks (Figure 2–9).

* *Eye protection.* Use eye shields to protect you from blood and body fluids splashing into your eyes. Several types are available. Clear plastic shields cover the eyes or the whole face. Safety

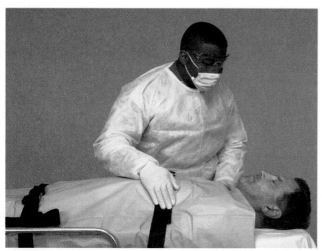

Figure 2-9 Personal protective equipment (PPE) includes safety glasses or goggles, face mask or shield, gown or apron, gloves, cap, and shoe coverings.

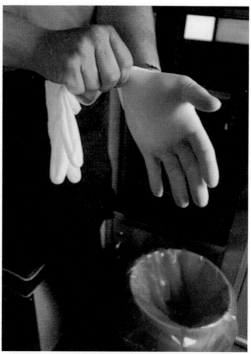

Figure 2-10 Wear protective gloves whenever you care for a patient.

glasses have side shields. If you wear prescription glasses, attach removable side shields. Form-fitting goggles are also available but are not required.

- *Gloves* (Figure 2–10). Wear high-quality vinyl or latex gloves whenever you care for a patient. Never reuse them. Put on a new pair for each patient to avoid exposing one patient to another's infection. Soiled gloves must be changed as soon as it is practical to do so. If a glove accidentally tears, remove it as soon as you can do so safely. Then wash your hands and replace the torn glove with a new one.

- *Gowns.* Wear a gown when there might be significant splashing of blood or body fluids. Generally, you will need a gown during childbirth or major injury. Whenever possible, use a disposable one. It also is recommended that you change your clothes if the gown gets soiled.

- *Masks.* Wear a disposable surgical-type face mask to protect against possible splatter of blood or body fluids. An N-95 or HEPA respirator is recommended for use with suspected tuberculosis patients.

Use personal protective equipment yourself and be sure to remind other EMS personnel at the scene to wear it, too. Make gloves and other PPE available to others who arrive to help.

Immunizations

Before you start active duty, have a physician make sure you are adequately protected against common infectious diseases. The following immunizations are recommended for active-duty First Responders:

- Tetanus prophylaxis (every 10 years).
- Hepatitis B vaccine.
- Influenza vaccine (every year).
- Polio.
- Rubella (German measles).
- Measles.
- Mumps.

Because some immunizations offer only partial protection, have your physician verify your immune status against rubella, measles, and mumps. Remember *always* practice BSI precautions—even after being vaccinated.

Have a tuberculin skin (tine) test at least once every year you are on duty. It will tell you if you have been exposed to TB. Your agency's medical director or your physician can advise you.

Reporting Exposures

In general, report any suspected exposure to blood or body fluids. Report the incident as soon as possible to your supervisor and to medical control. Report especially if the patient is HIV-positive, has hepatitis B, or is in a high-risk category for infection. Include in your report the date and time of the exposure, the type of body fluid involved, the amount, and details of the incident. State laws vary, so be sure to follow all local protocols.

SECTION 3: SCENE SAFETY

Be very sure to protect yourself at scenes involving hazardous materials, car crashes, or violence (Figure 2–11). It is imperative that you do not fall victim to the same problems that affect your patients.

As you approach a scene, turn off your lights and siren to avoid broadcasting your arrival, if it is safe to do so. Take a good look at the neighborhood. If possible, do not park directly in front of the call address. This is so you can size up the scene unnoticed and save a place for an ambulance to park.

Then decide whether or not it is safe to approach the patient. If any of the following exists on scene, you may need to call for help:

- Motor vehicle or airplane crashes.
- Presence of toxic substances or low levels of oxygen.
- Crime scenes.
- Presence of a weapon of any kind.
- Possible drug or alcohol use.
- Arguing, threats, violent behavior, broken glass, overturned furniture.
- Unstable surfaces, such as water and ice.

While each emergency scene is unique, a general rule applies to all. *If the scene is unsafe, make it*

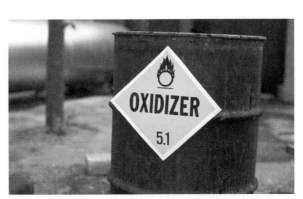

a Hazardous materials

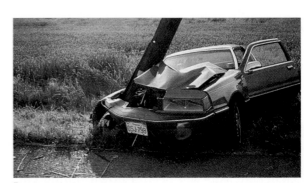

b Motor-vehicle crash

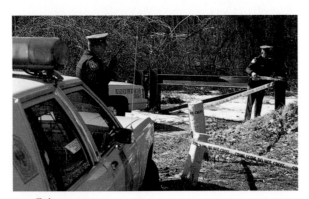

c Crime scene

Figure 2-11 Always be alert to potential hazards as you approach an emergency scene.

safe before you enter. Otherwise, wait for help to arrive. Specialized personnel will have the training, equipment, and protective gear needed to enter an unstable scene safely.

Once a scene is secure, take measures to protect the patient from hazards. That includes fire, structural instability, gasoline leaks, chemical spills, oncoming traffic, and extremes in temperature. Bystanders should also be protected from illness or injury.

HAZARDOUS MATERIALS

Do not enter a hazardous materials scene. Call a specialized team of rescuers to secure the scene first. Provide emergency care only after the scene is safe and patient contamination is limited. In general, rescuers should wear protective clothing, such as a self-contained breathing apparatus (Figure 2–12) and a "hazmat" suit (Figure 2–13). Check with your instructor about the availability of training for hazmat situations. Also learn how to access your local hazmat team. (Hazardous materials are discussed in more detail in Chapter 28.)

MOTOR VEHICLE CRASHES

Some car crashes lead to situations that threaten the life of both patients and rescuers. For example:

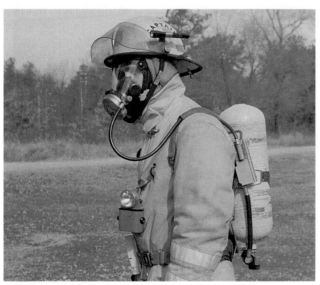

Figure 2-12 Self-contained breathing apparatus (SCBA).

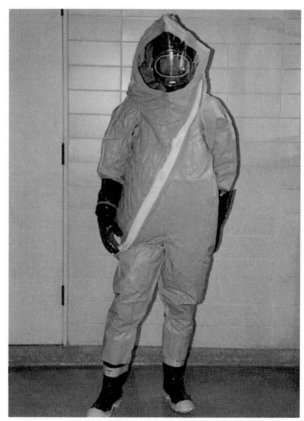

Figure 2-13 Typical hazardous materials protective suit.

- Downed power lines or other potential sources of electrocution.
- Fire or the potential for fire such as leaking gasoline.
- Explosion or the potential for explosion.
- Hazardous materials.
- Oncoming traffic.

When there is life-threatening danger on scene, call for specially trained personnel before you enter. Also call for special teams when a complex or extensive rescue is needed. Once a scene is safe, make sure you are wearing the proper personal protective equipment before you enter. That may include turnout gear, puncture-proof gloves, helmet, and eye protection (Figure 2–14). Follow local protocols.

Many traffic accidents occur in the dark or in bad weather. So be sure to wear reflective clothing. Depending on the scene, you might also consider waterproof boots and slip-resistant

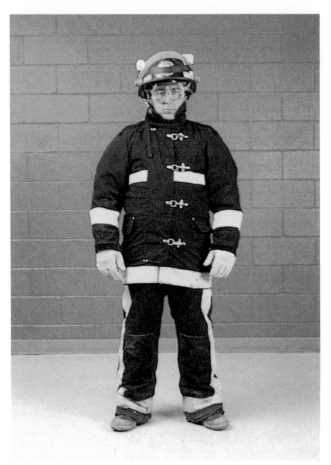

Figure 2-14 Turnout gear, plus helmet, eye wear, puncture-proof gloves, and boots.

gloves in wet weather. Wear gloves, a warm hat, and long underwear in cold weather. An impact-resistant helmet with reflective tape and a chin strap is also useful for risk of falling debris.

VIOLENCE

You may face violence without warning, from a patient, bystander, or perpetrator of a crime. If you suspect potential violence, *call law enforcement before you enter the scene.* Never enter the scene to give patient care until it has been adequately controlled by the police.

Always call for law enforcement in cases of domestic disputes, street or gang fights, bar fights, or potential suicide. Call them for any type of crime scene and for scenes that involve angry family or bystanders.

No matter where you work, consider using **body armor** (Figure 2–15). It is made of Kevlar™ or other synthetic materials that resist penetration by bullets. The amount of protection it offers depends on the tightness of the weave and the number of layers. While it will protect you, body armor will not make you invincible. You are still vulnerable in the areas not covered, and you can still be killed by the blunt force of a bullet, even if it does not penetrate the armor. Never take chances you would normally avoid just because you are wearing armor.

If you need to treat patients at a crime scene, you must preserve the chain of evidence needed for investigation and prosecution. A general rule is to avoid disturbing the scene unless absolutely necessary for medical care. Basic guidelines include:

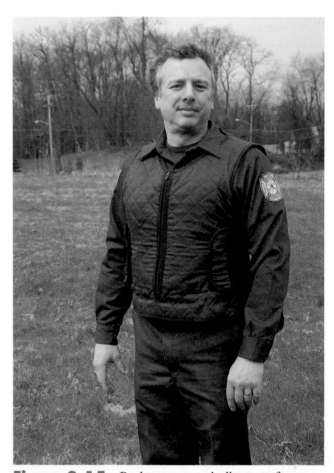

Figure 2-15 Body armor, or bullet-proof vest.

- Never wipe away blood. It can be used as evidence.
- Touch only what you need to touch to provide patient care.
- Move only what you need to move to protect the patient and to provide proper care.
- Do not use the telephone unless the police give you permission to do so.
- Observe and document anything unusual at the scene.

- If possible, do not cut through holes in the patient's clothing that could have been caused by bullets or other penetrating weapons.
- Do not cut through any knot in a rope or tie. Knots are used as evidence. Cut the rope or tie somewhere away from the knot.
- If the crime is rape, do not wash the patient or allow the patient to wash. Do not allow the patient to change clothing, use the bathroom, or take anything by mouth. Any of these actions could damage valuable evidence.

FIRST RESPONDER FOCUS

Television has led us to believe that it is okay to rush into calls without regard for your own well-being. This is not true. This is not real life. The fact is that if you become ill or injured, you will not be able to perform what you set out to do—help patients.

One of the most important factors to be considered in the first 10 minutes of a call is your own personal safety. Practice body substance isolation (BSI) precautions on every call. And always remain alert for violence, hazardous materials, and other unsafe conditions.

It is easy to understand that all you want to do so early in your career is focus on information about illness and injury. However, do not underestimate the importance of the information in this chapter. Just to make sure you realize how important it is, there will be reminders in every chapter in this book. ■

CASE STUDY FOLLOW-UP

At the beginning of this chapter, you read that First Responders were at a violent and potentially dangerous scene. To see how chapter skills apply to this emergency, read the following. It describes how the call was completed.

SCENE SIZE-UP *(Continued)*
My partner and I looked at each other. We returned to our vehicle and immediately called the police. I'm glad we did, or we would have been right in the middle of a fight.

We moved our vehicle out of sight, and waited. When the police arrived, we reported what we knew and they went in. After a few minutes, they radioed to tell us the scene was secure. But we still approached very cautiously.

The officers told us that two brothers had been in a fist fight. One of the brothers said his hands went through a window. Both of the brothers appeared to be intoxicated.

INITIAL ASSESSMENT
After we put on eye protection and gloves, we introduced ourselves to Mike, the brother who needed medical help. He seemed calm. Mike had moderate bleeding from his right forearm. His airway and breathing were good. He denied any other injuries or falls.

PHYSICAL EXAMINATION
Even though Mike denied other injuries, we decided to do a physical exam anyway. Sometimes people get into fights and get so excited, they

CASE STUDY FOLLOW-UP *(Continued)*

don't know they're hurt. Since there were two of us, my partner controlled the bleeding while I checked Mike's head, neck, chest, abdomen, and extremities.

While we were waiting for an ambulance, Mike's brother became loud and abusive to the police. We had the patient walk outside with us to get away from the potential danger. There we checked his pulse and respirations.

PATIENT HISTORY
Mike admitted to drinking six or eight cans of beer before the fight started. He told us that he had asthma, but wasn't feeling any respiratory distress or problems. He took an inhaler for his asthma, but didn't have it with him. He continued to deny any injuries other than the cut to his forearm.

ONGOING ASSESSMENT
We checked Mike's airway and breathing. They were okay. Mike didn't have any changes in mental status. The bleeding was controlled and the bandages were secure. We didn't get to recheck the vitals before the ambulance arrived.

PATIENT HAND-OFF
We advised the EMTs:

"The patient's name is Mike. He's a 22-year-old male who had sustained a laceration to his right forearm from going through a window. The wound has been dressed and bandaged. The bleeding was moderate and was easily controlled. Mike has been drinking but has been alert and oriented throughout the call. His airway and breathing are good. He denies any other injuries. He has a history of asthma and uses an inhaler. The physical exam was negative for injuries anywhere other than his arm. His pulse is 88, strong, and regular. His respirations are 18 and adequate. We were about to recheck his vitals as you pulled up."

Your safety and well-being are your top priorities. Without them, you cannot be an effective First Responder. Throughout this textbook, you will find reminders about taking BSI and other safety precautions. Make note of them.

REVIEW QUESTIONS

Page references where answers may be found or supported are provided at the end of each question.

Section 1

1. What are four techniques you can use to help you avoid responses like nausea or fainting in an emergency situation? (pp. 13–14)
2. What are the five stages of the grieving process? (p. 15)
3. What can you do to help a dying patient, in addition to providing medical care? (pp. 15–16)
4. What are five signs of chronic stress and burnout? (pp. 16–17)
5. What are some of the negative feelings a First Responder's family may have about the job? (pp. 17–18)

6. What are three examples of situations that may cause critical incident stress? (p. 19)
7. What is a critical incident stress debriefing (CISD)? (p. 18)

Section 2

8. How does an infectious disease spread from person to person? (pp. 19–20)
9. What equipment is needed to take BSI precautions? (pp. 22–23)

Section 3

10. What rule applies to all unsafe emergency scenes? (pp. 24–25)

CHAPTER 3

LEGAL AND ETHICAL ISSUES

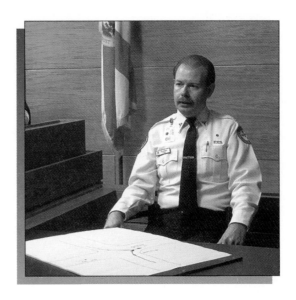

INTRODUCTION

Legal and ethical issues are a vital element of a First Responder's life, both on and off duty. You may already have some questions. For example, should you stop to treat an accident victim when you are off duty? Should patient information be released to an attorney over the phone? May a child be treated without a parent's consent?

This chapter will help you answer your questions. It will describe your scope of practice and what it means to have a duty to act. It will define patient consent and explain advance directives. It also will give you an overview of various other legal issues that will affect you in the field.

OBJECTIVES

SECTION 1: SCOPE OF CARE

Emergency care has changed a lot since its early days. One improvement has been in the quality of EMS training. People have come to expect a competent First Responder, one who understands and accepts his or her responsibilities to patients and to the public.

LEGAL DUTIES

Each state defines a First Responder's **scope of care** (actions that are legally allowed). All First Responders are to provide for the well-being of their patients as outlined in the scope of care. For example, providing CPR when needed is within your scope of care. However, stitching up a deep wound is not and, for you, it is illegal.

State law is enhanced by your local medical director. In fact, your legal right to act as a First Responder depends on medical oversight. State law is further enhanced by the "First Responder: National Standard Curriculum," established by the U.S. Department of Transportation.

When providing medical care, you should:

* Follow standing orders and protocols as approved by medical direction.
* Consult medical direction via phone or radio any time there is a question about the scope of care.
* Communicate clearly and completely with medical direction.
* Follow orders the medical director gives.

CASE STUDY

DISPATCH
Our first response unit was dispatched to a child who fell. I remember thinking how calls involving kids get to me. I hoped we could help this child.

SCENE SIZE-UP
We arrived to find the patient sitting up and crying. It appeared that he had fallen from his bike when it hit a tree. The bike's front tire was flat, the front end was bent in, and there were several yards of obvious skid marks. The patient had been wearing a helmet.
*   A police officer was kneeling, and talking to the boy quietly. The officer motioned us to approach. He said, "A dog jumped onto the path. Mark here did his best to avoid hitting it. But then that darn tree got in the way."*
*   We introduced ourselves to the patient. He said he was nine years old. While my partner began an initial assessment, I spoke to the police officer to see if contact had been made with the boy's parents.*

> Why are they looking for the child's parents? Can't they just treat the child's injuries? These questions revolve around the issue of consent—one of many legal and ethical issues you will face as a First Responder. As you read Chapter 3, consider how you might answer them.

ETHICAL RESPONSIBILITIES

A code of ethics is a list of the rules for ideal conduct. Basically, if you place the welfare of a patient above all else during emergency care, you rarely will do anything unethical.

Your ethical responsibilities are:

- Make the physical and emotional needs of the patient a priority. Serve those needs with respect for human dignity and with no regard to nationality, race, gender, creed, or status.
- Practice your skills to the point of mastery.

Show respect for the competence of other medical workers.
- Continue your education and take refresher courses. Stay on top of changes in EMS. Help define and uphold professional standards.
- Critically review your performance. Seek ways to improve response time, patient outcome, and communication.
- Report with honesty. Hold in confidence all information obtained in the course of your work, unless required by law to share it.
- Work in harmony with other First Responders, EMTs, and other members of the health care team.

SECTION 2: PATIENT CONSENT AND REFUSAL

PATIENT COMPETENCE

A **competent** adult is one who is lucid and able to make an informed decision about medical care. He understands your questions. He also understands the implications of decisions made about medical care. A patient must be competent in order to refuse treatment. Therefore, you must determine competence in every adult you want to treat.

Generally, consider an adult incompetent if he or she . . .

- Is under the influence of alcohol or drugs.
- Has an altered mental status.
- Has a serious illness or injury that could affect judgment.
- Is mentally ill or mentally retarded.

PATIENT CONSENT

By law, you must get a patient's **consent,** or permission, before you can provide emergency care. In order for that consent to be valid, the patient must be competent and the consent must be informed. It is your responsibility, therefore, to fully explain the care you plan to give, as well as the related risks.

There are two general types of consent: **expressed consent** and **implied consent.**

Expressed Consent

Expressed consent may consist of oral consent, a nod, or an affirming gesture from a competent adult. To get it you must explain your plan for emergency care *in terms that the patient can understand.* Be sure to include the risks, too. In other words, the patient needs a clear idea of all the factors that would affect a reasonable person's decision to either accept or refuse treatment.

You must get a responsive, competent adult's expressed consent before you render treatment. To do so, first tell the patient who you are. Identify your level of training, and then carefully explain your plan for emergency care. Make sure you identify both the benefits and the risks. To make sure the patient understands, question him or her briefly.

Implied Consent

In an emergency when an unresponsive patient is at risk of death, disability, or deterioration of condition, the law assumes that he or she would agree to care. This is called *implied consent.* It applies when you assume that a patient who cannot consent to life-saving care, would if he or she were able to.

Implied consent also applies to a patient who refuses care but who then becomes unresponsive and to a patient who is not competent to refuse care.

Children and Mentally Incompetent Adults

Depending on state law, a **minor** usually is any person under the age of 18 or 21. A parent or legal guardian must give consent before you can treat a minor. The same is true for a mentally incompetent adult. However, if a life-threatening condition exists and the parent or guardian is not available, provide emergency care under the principle of implied consent.

An emancipated minor is one who is married, pregnant, a parent, a member of the armed forces, or financially independent and living away from home with permission of the courts. You do not need the consent of a parent or legal guardian to treat this patient. You only need the patient's consent.

ADVANCE DIRECTIVES

There may be a time when you are called to treat a terminally ill patient. He may ask you to let him die if his heart or lungs stop working. Legally, if the patient is competent, he or she has the right to make this request.

An **advance directive** is written in advance of an emergency. It must be signed by both the patient and a physician. Legal in many states, it is commonly called a "living will" or a **Do Not Resuscitate (DNR) order** (Figure 3–1). It documents the wish of the chronically or terminally ill patient not to be resuscitated. It also allows the First Responder to withhold resuscitation legally.

PREHOSPITAL DO NOT RESUSCITATE ORDERS

ATTENDING PHYSICIAN

In completing this prehospital DNR form, please check part A if no intervention by prehospital personnel is indicated. Please check Part A and options from Part B if specific interventions by prehospital personnel are indicated. To give a valid prehospital DNR order, this form must be completed by the patient's attending physician and must be provided to prehospital personnel.

A) _____ **Do Not Resuscitate (DNR):**
No Cardiopulmonary Resuscitation or Advanced Cardiac Life Support be performed by prehospital personnel

B) _____ **Modified Support:**
Prehospital personnel administer the following checked options:
_____ Oxygen administration
_____ Full airway support: intubation, airways, bag/valve/mask
_____ Venipuncture: IV crystalloids and/or blood draw
_____ External cardiac pacing
_____ Cardiopulmonary resuscitation
_____ Cardiac defibrillator
_____ Pneumatic anti-shock garment
_____ Ventilator
_____ ACLS meds
_____ Other interventions/medications (physician specify)
_____

Prehospital personnel are informed that (print patient name)_____
should receive no resuscitation (DNR) or should receive Modified Support as indicated. This directive is medically appropriate and is further documented by a physician's order and a progress note on the patient's permanent medical record. Informed consent from the capacitated patient or the incapacitated patient's legitimate surrogate is documented on the patient's permanent medical record. The DNR order is in full force and effect as of the date indicated below.

_____   _____

_____
Attending Physician's Signature

_____   _____
Print Attending Physician's Name   Print Patient's Name and Location
                                             (Home Address or Health Care Facility)

_____
Attending Physician's Telephone

_____   _____
Date   Expiration Date (6 Mos from Signature)

Figure 3-1 Example of an EMS "Do Not Resuscitate" order.

When you are given an advance directive, you must determine to the best of your ability if it is valid. Usually it is accompanied by a doctor's written instructions. Check to see that they are written clearly and concisely. They also should be typed or written legibly on professional letterhead. Phrases like "no heroics" or "no extraordinary treatment" are *not* clear enough to be legal.

In many areas, a standard form is used for a DNR order. In some states, the law also requires that patients wear some sort of DNR insignia on their bodies where emergency personnel will be sure to find it.

By its very nature, a DNR order is best suited to a hospital or nursing home. There all personnel know the patient and his or her physician. If the DNR order is needed, it can be found and verified quickly. However, in the field there may be problems. In many areas, for example, a second physician must verify the patient's condition. This can be difficult in an emergency situation, even if the DNR order is on hand. Another problem is the time it takes to verify a DNR order. Precious, life-saving moments can be lost.

There are varying degrees of DNR orders. For example, one may explain that a patient allows all medical care except long-term life support. Another might say that the patient specifically does not allow the use of a respirator.

If you are ever in doubt about the validity of an advance directive, you must begin full resuscitation immediately. However, always consult your medical director or the hospital emergency department physician before you decide to follow or put aside a DNR order.

Be sure to review all state law and local protocols on this issue.

PATIENT REFUSAL

A competent adult has the right to refuse treatment for himself or his child. Under the law, he must first be informed of the treatment, fully understand it, and completely comprehend the risks involved in refusing it. He may refuse verbally, by pulling away, shaking his head, gesturing, or pushing you away.

A competent adult has the right to withdraw from treatment after it has started. This is true for a patient who initially gave consent but then changes his mind. It is also true for the patient who at first was unresponsive, but then wakes and asks you to stop.

A patient's legal refusal of treatment or transport must follow the rules of expressed consent. That is, the patient must be mentally competent and of legal age. The patient also must be informed of all the risks *in terms he or she can fully understand*. When in doubt, always err in favor of providing care.

Make every reasonable effort to persuade the patient or guardian to give consent for care. If he still refuses, insist that additional EMS personnel evaluate the patient.

Complete and accurate records are key to protecting yourself from liability. So before you leave the scene:

- *Try again to persuade the patient to accept treatment or transport.* Tell him clearly why it is essential. Be especially clear when you explain what could happen if he refuses care. Write down what you tell him. Then have the patient read it aloud to see if he understands.
- *Be sure the patient is able to make a rational, informed decision.* Note that a patient who is seriously ill or injured may only appear to be competent. Such a patient may be emotionally, intellectually, or physically impaired and may not be able to absorb all the information you give.
- *Consult medical direction as required by local protocol.*
- *Have the patient sign a refusal or "release from liability" form* (Figures 3–2 and 3–3). It must be signed by the patient and a witness. If the patient refuses to sign, indicate that on the form and have a witness sign it. Many areas use official documents for patients to sign. Check local protocols.
- *Before you leave, encourage the patient to seek help if certain symptoms develop.* Be specific. Avoid using terms the patient may not understand. For example, you might tell a patient to go to the hospital emergency department "if you get a burning pain in your stomach" or "if you start having shortness of breath." Then document the fact that you did.
- Advise the patient to call EMS again immediately if he changes his mind.

SECTION 3: OTHER LEGAL ASPECTS OF EMERGENCY CARE

▼

ASSAULT AND BATTERY

There is no single definition of assault and battery. Traditionally, threatening physical harm is *assault*. Actual unlawful physical contact is *battery*. In the context of emergency medical care,

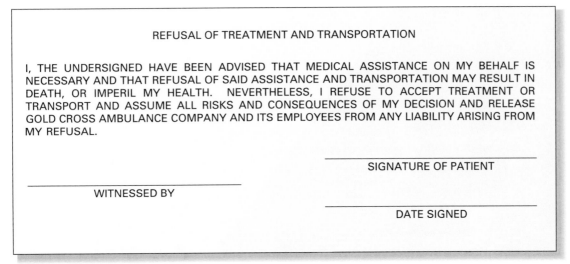

Figure 3-2   Example of a patient refusal statement.

you can be charged with assault and battery if you touch a patient's body or clothing without first getting consent.

ABANDONMENT AND NEGLIGENCE

Simply stated, **abandonment** means you stopped providing care for a patient without making sure that the same or better care would be provided. Under the law, once you start giving emergency care to a patient, you must continue until another health care professional with at least as much expertise as you takes over or until the police order you to leave the scene.

Negligence is defined as carelessness, inattention, disregard, inadvertence, or oversight that was accidental but avoidable. You may be charged with negligence if your care deviates from the accepted standard of care and results in further injury to the patient.

To establish negligence, the court must decide that all four of the following are true:

- *The First Responder had a duty to act.* The concept known as **duty to act** refers to your contractual or legal obligation to provide care. That is, while you are on duty, you must care for a patient who needs it and consents to it.
- *There was a breach of duty.* A breach of duty exists when a First Responder either fails to act or fails to act appropriately. That is, the First

Responder violated the standard of care reasonably expected of a First Responder with similar background and training.
- *The patient was injured physically or psychologically.*
- *The First Responder caused the injury.* It must be proven that the First Responder's breach of duty is what caused or contributed to the patient's injury.

Note that your duty to act also means that you must render care to a patient to the best of your ability. You must follow accepted guidelines for care and act as any other prudent person would in the same situation.

In some cases a duty to act refers to an implied contractual or legal obligation. For example, a patient may call for EMS. The dispatcher confirms that help will be sent. All EMS members that respond—including First Responders—then have a legal obligation to provide treatment to the patient.

In most states, you do not have a duty to act when you are off duty or driving an emergency vehicle outside your company's service area. (Check your state laws.) However, you may feel a certain moral or ethical obligation to help. In such cases, take extra steps to protect yourself against legal risk. Carefully document all aspects of the call and treatment you give, including a patient's refusal of care.

In general, your best defense against negligence is to have a professional attitude, to provide a

---

EMS PATIENT REFUSAL CHECKLIST

PATIENT NAME: _____ AGE: _____

LOCATION OF CALL: _____ DATE: _____

AGENCY INCIDENT #: _____ AGENCY CODE: _____

NAME OF PERSON FILLING OUT FORM: _____

I.   ASSESSMENT OF PATIENT (Circle appropriate response for each item)

    1.   Oriented to: Person?   Yes   No

                               Place?   Yes   No

                               Time?   Yes   No

                               Situation?   Yes   No

    2.   Altered level of consciousness?   Yes   No

    3.   Head injury?   Yes   No

    4.   Alcohol or drug ingestion by exam or history?   Yes   No

II. PATIENT INFORMED (Circle appropriate response for each item)

    Yes   No   Medical treatment/evaluation needed

    Yes   No   Ambulance transport needed

    Yes   No   Further harm could result without medical treatment/
                    evaluation

    Yes   No   Transport by means other than ambulance could be
                    hazardous in light of patient's illness/injury

    Yes   No   Patient provided with Refusal Information Sheet

    Yes   No   Patient accepted Refusal Information Sheet

III. DISPOSITION

    _____   Refused all EMS services

    _____   Refused field treatment, but accepted transport

    _____   Refused transport, but accepted field treatment

    _____   Refused transport to recommended facility

    _____   Patient transported by private vehicle to _____

    _____   Released in care or custody of self

    _____   Released in care or custody of relative or friend

              Name: _____   Relationship: _____

    _____   Released in custody of law enforcement agency

              Agency: _____   Officer: _____

    _____   Released in custody of other agency

              Agency: _____   Officer: _____

IV. COMMENTS: _____

    _____

    _____

Figure 3-3   Sample patient refusal checklist from Spokane County EMS, Washington State.

consistently high standard of care, and to correctly and completely document the care you provide.

CONFIDENTIALITY

A patient's history, condition, and emergency care are confidential. To release this information, you must have a written form signed by the patient or legal guardian. Never release any patient information on request unless you are authorized to do so in writing.

By law, you are allowed to release information without a patient's or guardian's permission only if:

- Another health-care provider needs it in order to continue medical care.
- You are requested by the police to provide it as part of a crime investigation. State laws, for example, require the reporting of rape, abuse, gunshot wounds, and certain other crimes.
- You are required by legal subpoena to provide it in court (Figure 3–4).

GOOD SAMARITAN LAWS

Many states have "Good Samaritan" laws. The first of these laws was enacted in 1959 in California. It was designed to protect doctors who render emergency care from civil suits. Most states now have laws of their own, some of which cover EMS personnel. Be sure to learn your local laws.

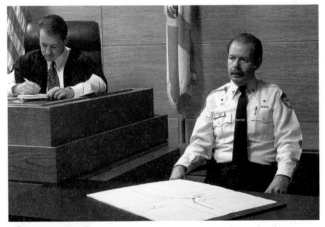

Figure 3-4 First Responders may be asked to testify in court.

Generally, these laws protect a First Responder from liability for acts performed in good faith unless those acts are grossly negligent. Under these laws, the person suing must prove that emergency care was markedly below the **standard of care.** Standard of care is defined as the care that would be expected to be provided to the same patient under the same conditions by another First Responder who had received the same training. (This is referred to as the "reasonable man" test.)

If you are sued and the case goes to court, a *tort* proceeding will be held. This is a civil court action, not a criminal one. It determines whether or not the natural rights of an individual have been violated. In a tort proceeding, it must be proven that you are guilty of gross negligence.

A Good Samaritan law does not prevent you from being sued. But it may give you some protection against losing the lawsuit if you have performed according to the standard of care for a First Responder. So while on and off duty, your best defense against lawsuits is prevention. Always render care to the best of your ability. Do no more or less than your scope of care allows. If you keep your patient's best interests in mind, you will seldom—if ever—go wrong.

PRESERVATION OF EVIDENCE

Whenever a First Responder is called to a potential crime scene, dispatch should also notify the police. In general, a potential crime scene is any scene that may require police support. That includes a potential or actual suicide, homicide, drug overdose, domestic dispute, abuse, hit-and-run, riot, robbery, or any scene involving gunfire or a weapon.

Your first concern should always be your own safety. *If you suspect that a crime is in progress or a criminal is active at the scene, do not try to provide care to any patient.* Wait until the police arrive and tell you that the scene is safe. Once the scene is safe, your priority is patient care.

When on scene, do not disturb any item that may be evidence. Basic guidelines include:

- Observe and document anything unusual at the scene.
- Touch only what you need to touch.

- Move only what you need to move to protect the patient and provide emergency care.
- Do not use the telephone unless the police give you permission to do so. They may wish to find out who the last caller was.
- Move the patient only if he or she is in danger or must be moved in order for you to provide emergency care.
- If possible, do not cut through holes in the patient's clothing. They may have been caused by bullets or stabbing.
- Do not cut through any knot in a rope or tie. Knots are often used as evidence.
- If the crime is rape, do not wash the patient or allow the patient to wash. Ask him or her not to change clothing, use the bathroom, or take anything by mouth. Doing any of these things could destroy evidence.

SPECIAL DOCUMENTATION

In general, physicians must report suspected child, elderly, and spouse abuse. Some states require others—such as teachers and First Responders—to report them as well. Related state laws often grant immunity from liability for libel, slander, or defamation of character as long as the report is made in good faith.

EMS personnel may be required to report an injury that may be the result of a crime. That includes gunshot wounds, knife wounds, and poisonings. Your state may also want you to report any injury that you suspect was caused by sexual assault.

In some areas EMS workers must report all suspected infectious disease exposure. That includes TB, hepatitis B, and AIDS. Other situations to report may include use of restraints on a patient, attempted suicides, and dog bites. Learn your local and state requirements.

SPECIAL SITUATIONS

Medical Identification Tags

Some patients may wear or carry a medical identification tag (Figure 3–5). Such tags may be found on bracelets, necklaces, or cards carried in

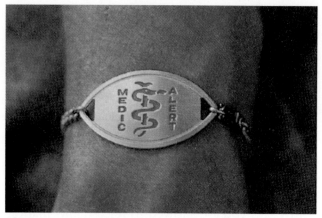

Figure 3–5 A medical identification tag.

a wallet. They identify a specific medical condition such as an allergy, epilepsy, or diabetes. Look for them whenever you examine a patient. Many list a phone number you can call for detailed information.

Donor and Organ Harvesting

In general, organs can be donated only if there is a signed document giving permission to harvest them. A signed donor card is a legal document. So is the sticker on the reverse side of some driver licenses.

A potential organ donor should be treated the same as any other patient. Remember, the person is a patient first, an organ donor last. So, in addition to providing the appropriate emergency medical care, you can:

- *Identify the patient as a potential donor.* Patients who are about to die or who have died within hours may be organ donors. In each case, the hospital staff and the patient's family must make the ultimate decision.
- *Communicate with medical direction.* You can begin the process by alerting the EMTs who take over patient care. They will in turn alert the hospital emergency staff.
- *Provide life-saving emergency care,* such as CPR. It will help to maintain vital organs. This is best accomplished by treating every patient equally well.

FIRST RESPONDER FOCUS

Legal issues are a large part of the first few minutes of a call. For example, it is during this time that you must obtain consent from your patient. You also may be faced with legal documents such as "DNR" orders.

Consider this scenario: You walk into a house and find a patient lying on a couch. The relative who meets you says, "I think he's dead. He's had cancer, and we got this paper from his doctor so he can die in peace." Picture the situation. You have a patient who needs CPR, and a relative who presents you with some type of form. Every second you spend trying to figure out what it is and what to do about it is time you could be using to help the patient.

This does not have to happen to you. Learn well the regulations that affect your duties as a First Responder, before you find yourself in a situation like this. ■

CASE STUDY FOLLOW-UP

At the beginning of this chapter, you read about a nine-year-old patient who had fallen from his bike. To see how chapter information applies to this emergency, read the following. It describes how the call was completed.

INITIAL ASSESSMENT

My partner confirmed that the patient's ABCs—airway, breathing, and circulation—were adequate. There was no obvious external bleeding. Our initial impression was that of a nine-year-old boy who had hit a tree with his bike. He complained of pain to his arm.

Just then, Mark's mother arrived on scene. She gave consent for his care, and my partner continued his assessment.

PHYSICAL EXAMINATION

The mother's presence calmed the boy. We checked Mark carefully. We examined his head, neck, chest, abdomen, and extremities. The only sign of injury was to Mark's arm. He wasn't thrown from the bike, so we did not suspect spinal injuries. His pulse was 88, strong and regular, and his respirations were 18 and adequate. My partner manually stabilized the arm to prevent further injury. I spoke to Mark's mother about his medical history.

PATIENT HISTORY

I was told that Mark was basically healthy. He had a heart murmur since birth, but no related problems or complications. He takes no medications. He had a full lunch consisting of spaghetti and meatballs. He has no allergies.

ONGOING ASSESSMENT

Mark continued to be responsive. He responded to his mother well, which is an important sign in a child. He was wondering if he was going to have a cast on his arm for his friends to sign. His ABCs were still fine. His pulse, respirations, and skin color and temperature were unchanged.

PATIENT HAND-OFF

We introduced Mark and his mom to the EMTs who would be taking him to the hospital. We told the EMTs that Mark hit a tree with his bicycle and fell. We went on with our report:

"He complains of pain to his right arm which we are now stabilizing. He was wearing a helmet. He does not complain of neck or back problems. Mark never lost consciousness and has no other complaints. His pulse is 88, respirations 18. He had spaghetti and meatballs for lunch. He has a heart murmur but no problems with it. No meds, no allergies."

CASE STUDY FOLLOW-UP *(Continued)*

The EMTs thanked us and took over care. My partner was asked to stay, since Mark felt comfortable with him. I manually stabilized Mark's arm while the EMT-B applied a splint. Mark's mom thanked us as she got into the ambulance with her son.

Mark did indeed need a cast for his broken arm, but he was expected to heal completely. While this might not have been a critical emergency, just by stabilizing Mark's arm, we prevented further injury or problems that would have been with him his whole life.

> Consent is one of many legal and ethical issues you will face as a First Responder. Learn the laws related to you and your EMS system.

REVIEW QUESTIONS

Page references where answers may be found or supported are provided at the end of each question.

Section 1

1. What is a First Responder's scope of care? (p. 30)

Section 2

2. What are two types of consent? Define each one. (p. 32)
3. What is a DNR order? What should a First Responder do if presented with one? (pp. 32–34)
4. How should you handle a patient's refusal of treatment? (p. 34)

Section 3

5. What must happen in order for a First Responder to be liable for abandonment or negligence? (p. 35)
6. What does it mean for a First Responder to have a duty to act? (p. 35)
7. Under what conditions may a First Responder release confidential patient information? (p. 37)
8. What are some ways a First Responder can help to preserve evidence at a crime scene? (pp. 37–38)
9. What are the situations a First Responder may be required to report? (p. 38)

CHAPTER 4

THE HUMAN BODY

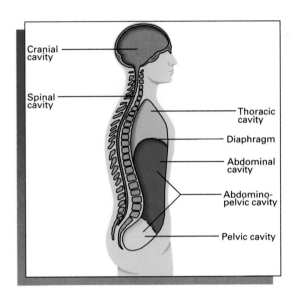

Cranial cavity

Spinal cavity

Thoracic cavity

Diaphragm

Abdominal cavity

Abdomino-pelvic cavity

Pelvic cavity

INTRODUCTION

As a First Responder, you must be able to recognize illness and injury and know how to care for each. You also must be able to tell other medical personnel about a patient's problem quickly and accurately. In order to do all this, you need a solid foundation of basic knowledge. In this chapter, you will study **anatomy** (the structure of the body) and **physiology** (how the body works). You also will be introduced to common anatomical terms.

Cognitive, affective, and psychomotor objectives are from the U.S. DOT's 1995 "First Responder: National Standard Curriculum." Enrichment objectives, if any, identify material that is supplemental to the DOT curriculum.

Cognitive

1-4.1 Describe the anatomy and function of the respiratory system. (pp. 46–47, 49)
1-4.2 Describe the anatomy and function of the circulatory system. (pp. 49, 51)
1-4.3 Describe the anatomy and function of the musculoskeletal system. (pp. 45–46)
1-4.4 Describe the components and function of the nervous system. (p. 51)

Affective

No objectives are identified.

Psychomotor

No objectives are identified.

Enrichment

* Use anatomical terms correctly, including terms of position, direction, and location. (pp. 42–44)
* Describe the main body cavities. (p. 44)
* Describe skin and its components. (pp. 51–56)
* Describe the digestive system and its components. (p. 56)
* Describe the urinary system and its components. (pp. 56–57)
* Describe the endocrine system and its components. (p. 57)
* Describe the reproductive system and its components. (p. 57)

SECTION 1: ANATOMICAL TERMS

It is important to describe a patient's position, direction, and location to other EMS personnel. Using correct terms will help you communicate the extent of a patient's injury quickly and accurately.

Terms of position include the following (Figure 4–1):

- **Anatomical position.** In this position, a patient's body stands erect with arms down at the sides, palms facing you. "Right" and "left" refer to the patient's right and left.
- **Supine position.** The patient is lying face up on his or her back.
- **Prone position.** The patient is lying face down on his or her stomach.
- **Lateral recumbent position.** In this position, the patient is lying on the left or right side. This is also known as the *recovery position*.

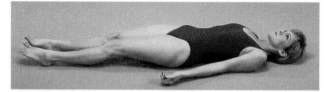

Figure 4–1a Supine position.

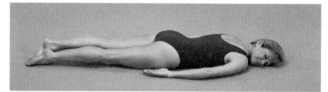

Figure 4–1b Prone position.

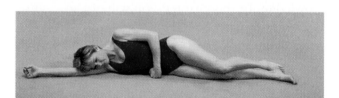

Figure 4–1c Right lateral recumbent position.

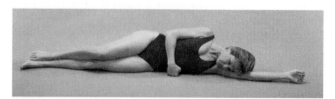

Figure 4–1d Left lateral recumbent position.

CASE STUDY

DISPATCH

My first response unit was called to the mall for a "person injured." A woman had missed a step on an escalator, fell, and hurt her left leg.

SCENE SIZE-UP

We scanned the small crowd as we approached, making sure there were no problems. The patient was clear of the escalator. I made a mental note to check with the patient about the mechanism of injury. Did she fall just a step or two or down the whole flight?

INITIAL ASSESSMENT

The woman was responsive and alert. She denied passing out or injuring her head or spine. She had no breathing problems and no obvious bleeding. She told us that her left shin bone hurt near her ankle.

PHYSICAL EXAMINATION

We conducted a head-to-toe exam, and found no injuries other than the left lower leg. It was deformed and swollen, but there was no bleeding. We stabilized the leg manually to prevent further damage. We checked her pulse and found it to be 88, strong and regular. Her respirations were 16, regular and deep; blood pressure 110/82. We checked to make sure there was a pulse, movement, and sensation below the injury.

> Knowing basic anatomy and physiology of the human body is key to this course. It is the foundation on which you will build all your skills. Consider the patient in this Case Study as you read Chapter 4. How would you communicate her condition to the responding EMTs?

Terms of direction and location are as follows:

- **Superior** means toward, or closer to, the head. **Inferior** means toward, or closer to, the feet.
- **Anterior** is toward the front. **Posterior** is toward the back.
- **Medial** means toward the midline, or center of the body. **Lateral** refers to the left or right of the midline.
- **Proximal** means close, or near the point of reference. **Distal** is distant, or far away from the point of reference. The point of reference is usually the torso. For example, a wound of the forearm is proximal to the wrist because it is closer to the torso than the wrist. That same wound is distal to the elbow because it is farther away from the torso than the elbow.
- **Superficial** is near the surface. **Deep** is remote, or far from the surface.

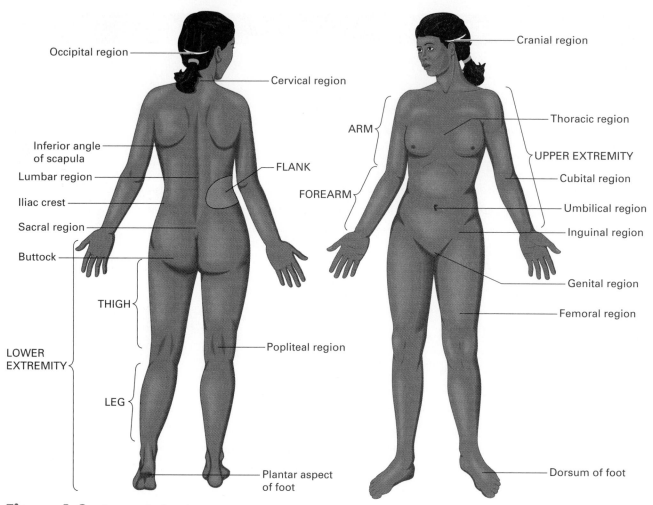

Figure 4-2 Anatomical regions.

- **Internal** means inside. **External** means outside.

Anatomical regions and topography are the internal and external landmarks of the body (Figures 4–2 and 4–3). During assessment of a patient, refer to these landmarks. They will help make the description of a patient's condition clear to others, particularly when you use a radio.

The organs of the body are located in certain body cavities (Figure 4–4). The main body cavities include:

- **Thoracic cavity.** Also called the chest cavity, the lungs and heart are found here. The **diaphragm,** a muscle that moves up and down during respiration, separates this cavity from the abdomen.

- **Abdominal cavity.** It contains organs of digestion and excretion, including the liver, gallbladder, spleen, pancreas, kidneys, stomach, and intestines.
- **Pelvic cavity.** It is bounded by the lower part of the spine, the hip bones, and the **pubis.** It protects the lower abdomen, including the bladder, rectum, and internal female organs.

Note that you can think of the abdomen as if it were divided into four parts or quadrants. Health-care workers often refer to it that way. The quadrants are formed by imaginary lines. One line is drawn horizontally through the navel. The other line is drawn vertically through the midline of the body. (See Figure 4–5, p. 47.)

TOPOGRAPHIC
ANATOMY

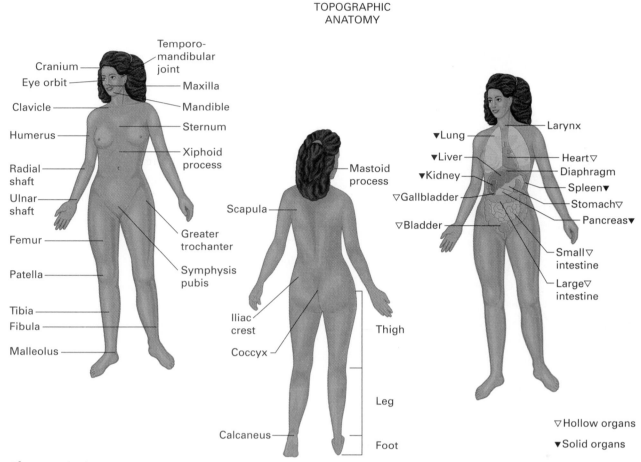

Figure 4-3 Topographic anatomy.

SECTION 2: BODY SYSTEMS

THE MUSCULOSKELETAL SYSTEM

The musculoskeletal system is made up of the skeleton and muscles. Each helps to give the body shape and protects internal organs. The muscles also provide for movement.

The Skeleton

The human body is shaped by its bony framework (Figure 4–6, p. 48). Bone is composed of living cells and nonliving matter. The nonliving matter contains calcium compounds that help make bone hard and rigid. Without bones, the body would collapse.

The adult skeleton has 206 bones. It must be strong to support and protect, jointed to permit motion, and flexible to withstand stress. It is held together mainly by **ligaments, tendons,** and layers of muscle. (Ligaments connect bone to bone. Tendons connect muscle to bone.) Bone ends fit into each other at joints. The three kinds of joints are: immovable like the skull, slightly movable like the spine, and freely movable like the elbow or knee. (See Figure 4–7, p. 49.)

The major areas of the skeleton include the following:

• The **skull** has a number of broad, flat bones that form a hollow shell. The top (including the forehead), back, and sides of the shell make up the **cranium.** It houses and protects the brain. There are several small bones of the face. They give shape to the face and permit the jaw to move. The major features of the face are the nose, ears, eyes, cheeks, mouth, and jowls.

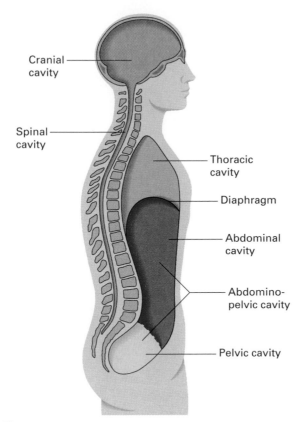

Cranial cavity

Spinal cavity

Thoracic cavity

Diaphragm

Abdominal cavity

Abdomino-pelvic cavity

Pelvic cavity

Figure 4-4 Main body cavities.

- The **spinal column** houses and protects the **spinal cord.** The spinal column is the central supportive bony structure of the body. It consists of 33 bones known as **vertebrae.** The spine is divided into five sections: the **cervical spine** (the neck, formed by 7 vertebrae) the **thoracic spine** (the upper back, formed by 12 vertebrae), the **lumbar spine** (the lower back, formed by 5 vertebrae), the **sacrum** (the lower part of the spine, formed by 5 fused vertebrae), and the **coccyx** (the tail bone, formed by 4 fused vertebrae).
- The **thorax,** or rib cage, protects the heart and lungs—vital organs of the body. They are enclosed by 12 pairs of ribs that are attached at the back to the spine. The top 10 are also attached in front to the **sternum,** or breastbone. The lowest portion of the sternum is called the **xiphoid process.**
- The **pelvis,** or hip bones, consists of the **ilium, pubis,** and **ischium.** Iliac crests form the

"wings" of the pelvis. The pubis is the anterior portion of the pelvis. The ischium is in the posterior portion.
- The **shoulder girdle** consists of the **clavicle** (the collarbone) and the **scapulae** (shoulder blades).
- The upper **extremities** extend from the shoulders to the fingertips. The arm (shoulder to elbow) has one bone known as the **humerus.** The bones in the forearm are the **radius** and **ulna.** The lower extremities extend from the hips to the toes. The bone in the thigh, or upper leg, is known as the **femur.** The bones in the lower leg are the **tibia** and **fibula.** The knee cap is called the **patella.**

The Muscles

Movement of the body depends on the work performed by the muscles. Muscles have the ability to contract (become shorter and thicker) when stimulated by a nerve impulse. Each muscle is made up of long threadlike cells called fibers, which are closely packed or bundled. Overlapping bundles are bound by connective tissue. (See Figure 4–8, p. 50.)

There are three basic kinds of muscles (Figure 4–9, p. 51):

- **Skeletal muscle,** or **voluntary muscle** makes possible all deliberate acts such as walking and chewing. It helps shape the body and form its walls. In the trunk this type of muscle is broad, flat, and expanded. In the extremities, it is long and rounded.
- **Smooth muscle,** or **involuntary muscle,** is made of longer fibers. It is found in the walls of tubelike organs, ducts, and blood vessels. It also forms much of the intestinal wall. A person has little or no control over this type of muscle.
- **Cardiac muscle** makes up the walls of the heart. It is able to stimulate itself into contraction, even when disconnected from the brain.

THE RESPIRATORY SYSTEM

The body may get enough nutrition from food to last for several weeks. It can store water to last for several days. But it can only store oxygen for a

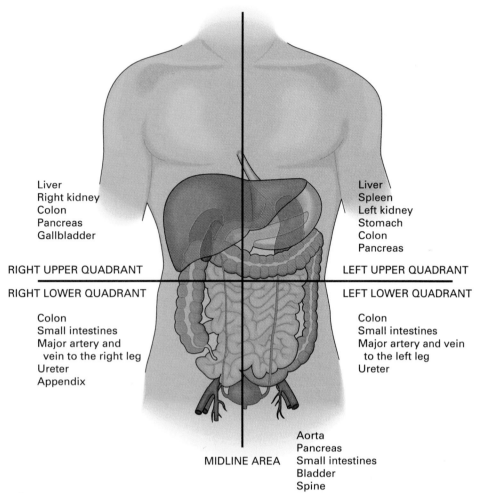

Liver
Right kidney
Colon
Pancreas
Gallbladder

Liver
Spleen
Left kidney
Stomach
Colon
Pancreas

RIGHT UPPER QUADRANT

LEFT UPPER QUADRANT

RIGHT LOWER QUADRANT

LEFT LOWER QUADRANT

Colon
Small intestines
Major artery and
  vein to the right leg
Ureter
Appendix

Colon
Small intestines
Major artery and vein
  to the left leg
Ureter

MIDLINE AREA

Aorta
Pancreas
Small intestines
Bladder
Spine

Figure 4–5 The abdominal area in quadrants.

few minutes. The body depends on a constant supply of oxygen. The respiratory system delivers oxygen to the body, as well as removes carbon dioxide from the body.

The passage of air into and out of the lungs is called **respiration.** Breathing in is called **inspiration** or inhaling. Breathing out is called **expiration** or exhaling.

During inspiration, the muscles of the thorax contract, moving the ribs outward and up. The diaphragm contracts and lowers. These movements expand the chest cavity and cause air to flow into the lungs. During exhalation the opposite happens. The muscles of the chest relax and

cause the ribs to move inward. The diaphragm relaxes and moves up.

The respiratory system consists of the organs that let us breathe (Figure 4–10, p. 52). When air enters the body, it does so through the mouth and nose. The area posterior to the mouth and nose is called the **pharynx,** which is divided into the **oropharynx** and **nasopharynx.** Air then travels down through the **larynx** (voice box) and into the **trachea** (windpipe). The trachea is the air passageway to the lungs. It is made of cartilage rings and is visible in the anterior portion of the neck. The **epiglottis** is a leaf-shaped structure that prevents foreign objects from entering the trachea

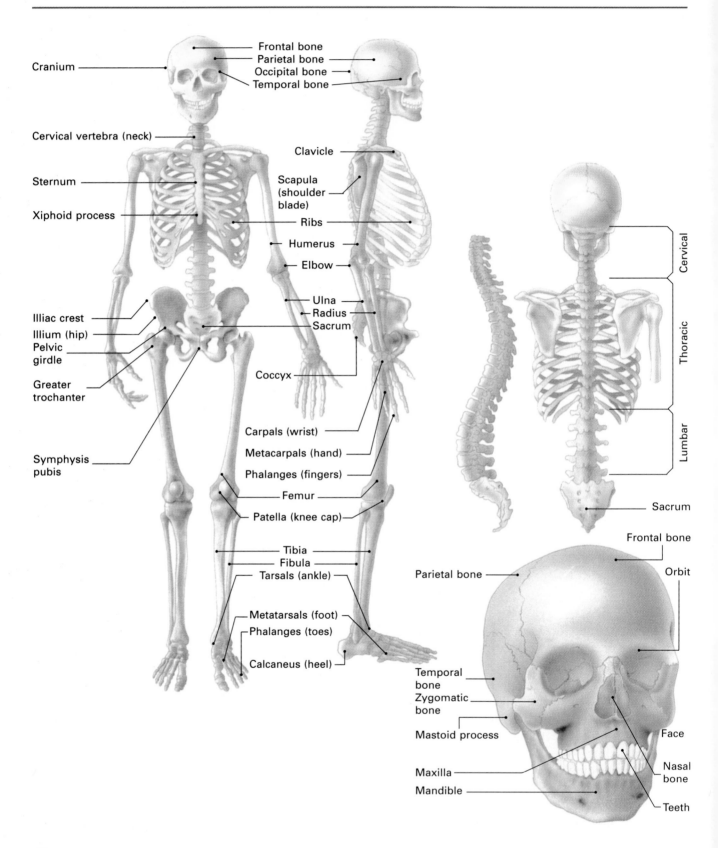

Figure 4-6 The skeletal system.

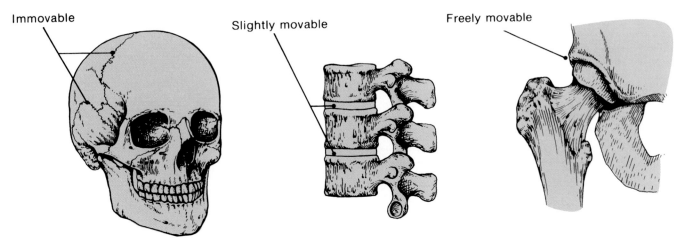

Immovable   Slightly movable   Freely movable

Figure 4–7 Three types of joints.

during swallowing. The trachea splits into two **bronchi.** These air passages gradually become smaller and smaller until they reach the **alveoli,** where carbon dioxide and oxygen are exchanged with blood.

It is important to remember that the respiratory structures of infants and children differ from those of adults. While the structures all have the same names, they may be smaller or less developed in infants and children. These differences are very important:

- All structures, including the mouth and nose, are smaller in children. They are more easily obstructed by even small objects, blood, or swelling. Pay extra attention to an infant or child to be sure the airway stays open.
- The tongue of an infant or child takes up proportionally more space in the pharynx than the tongue of an adult. As a result, it can block the airway more easily.
- The trachea of an infant or child is narrower, softer, and more flexible. So, tipping the head too far back or allowing the head to fall forward can close the trachea. Whenever needed, place a folded towel or similar item under the shoulders to keep the airway aligned and open.
- The primary cause of cardiac arrest in infants and children is an uncorrected respiratory problem. Because the chest wall is softer, infants and children tend to rely more heavily

on the diaphragm for breathing. So watch for excessive movement of the diaphragm. It can alert you to respiratory distress in an infant or child.

THE CIRCULATORY SYSTEM

The circulatory system delivers oxygen and nutrients to the body's tissues and removes waste products. It consists of the heart, blood vessels, and blood. (See Figure 4–11, p. 53.)

The heart is a muscular organ that is responsible for pumping blood through the body. The adult heart contracts between 60 and 80 times per minute when at rest and faster when under stress. Problems with the heart account for many of the emergencies you will encounter as a First Responder.

The heart is divided into four chambers. The upper chambers are called **atria.** The lower chambers are called **ventricles.** The heart has a left and right side, each of which has an atrium and a ventricle. The right side of the heart receives blood from the body and pumps it to the lungs. The left side of the heart receives oxygenated blood from the lungs and pumps it to the body.

When the heart pumps blood from the left ventricle, blood enters the arteries. This pumping action causes a wave of pressure that can be

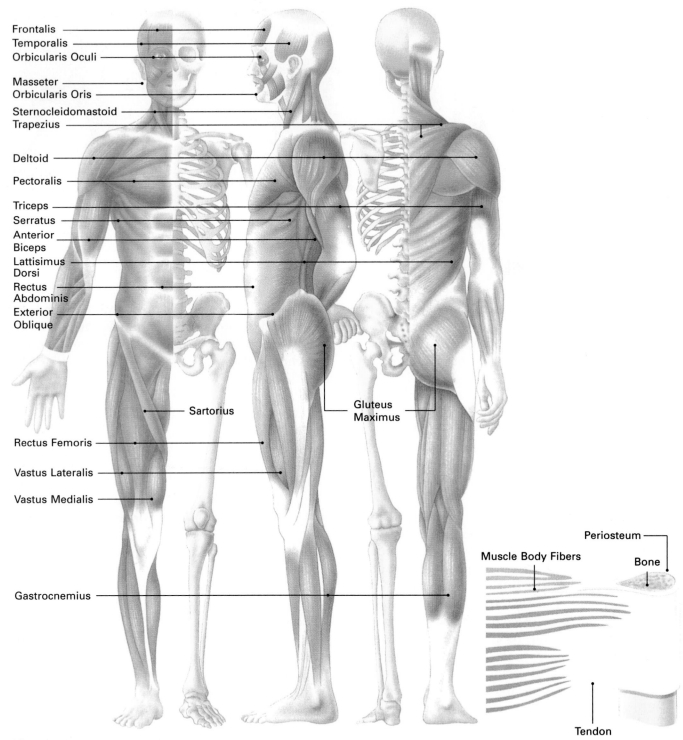

Frontalis
Temporalis
Orbicularis Oculi

Masseter
Orbicularis Oris
Sternocleidomastoid
Trapezius

Deltoid

Pectoralis

Triceps
Serratus
Anterior
Biceps
Lattisimus
Dorsi
Rectus
Abdominis
Exterior
Oblique

Sartorius

Rectus Femoris

Vastus Lateralis

Vastus Medialis

Gastrocnemius

Gluteus
Maximus

Periosteum

Muscle Body Fibers

Bone

Tendon

Figure 4-8 The muscular system.

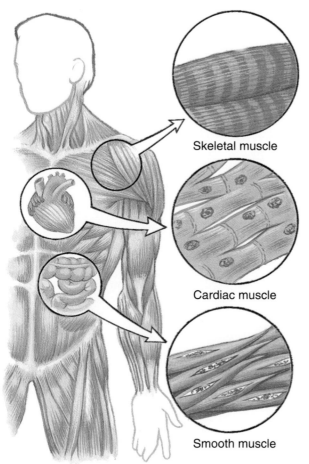

Figure 4-9 Three types of muscles.

felt as a pulse. There are many points where a pulse can be felt in the body. The most common are:

- The **carotid pulse point,** felt on either side of the neck.
- The **brachial pulse point,** felt on the inside of the arm between the elbow and the shoulder.
- The **radial pulse point,** felt on the thumb side of the wrist.
- The **femoral pulse point,** felt in the area of the groin in the crease between the abdomen and thigh.

The **blood vessels** are a closed system of tubes through which blood flows. **Arteries** and **arterioles** take blood away from the heart. The **capillaries** are distributors. They are the smallest vessels through which the exchange of fluid, oxygen, and

carbon dioxide takes place between blood and tissue cells. The **venules** and **veins** are collectors. They carry blood back to the heart from the rest of the body.

THE NERVOUS SYSTEM

The nervous system is composed of the brain, the spinal cord, and nerves (Figure 4–12, pp. 54-55). It has two major functions—communication and control. It lets a person be aware of and react to the environment. It coordinates the body's responses to stimuli and keeps body systems working together.

The nervous system has two main parts—the **central nervous system** and the **peripheral nervous system.** The central nervous system consists of the brain and spinal cord. The peripheral nervous system consists of the nerves. They carry information back and forth from the body to the spinal cord and brain.

The nervous system may also be broken down by function, or voluntary and involuntary components. Voluntary components are under our control. They are responsible for activities such as movement. Involuntary components are handled by the **autonomic nervous system.** This system is a network of nerve tissue that regulates functions we normally pay no attention to, such as how quickly or slowly the heart beats.

THE SKIN

The skin separates the human body from the outside world. It protects the deep tissues from injury, drying out, and invasion by bacteria and other foreign bodies. The skin helps to regulate body temperature. It aids in getting rid of water and various salts, as well as helps to prevent dehydration. It acts as the receptor organ for touch, pain, heat, and cold. (See Figure 4–13, p. 56.)

The **epidermis** is the outermost layer of skin. It contains cells that give the skin its color. The **dermis,** or second layer, contains a vast network of blood vessels. The deepest layers of the skin contain hair follicles, sweat and oil glands, and

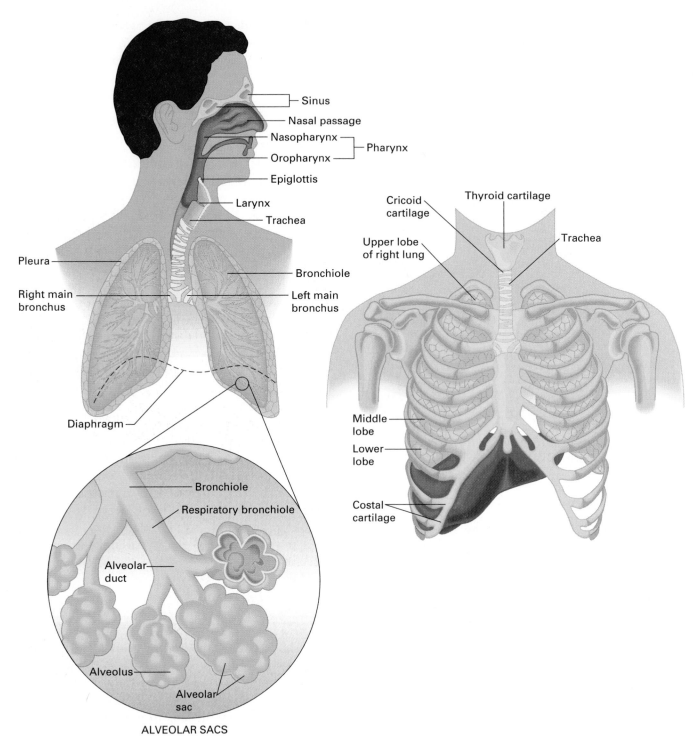

ALVEOLAR SACS

Figure 4-10 The respiratory system.

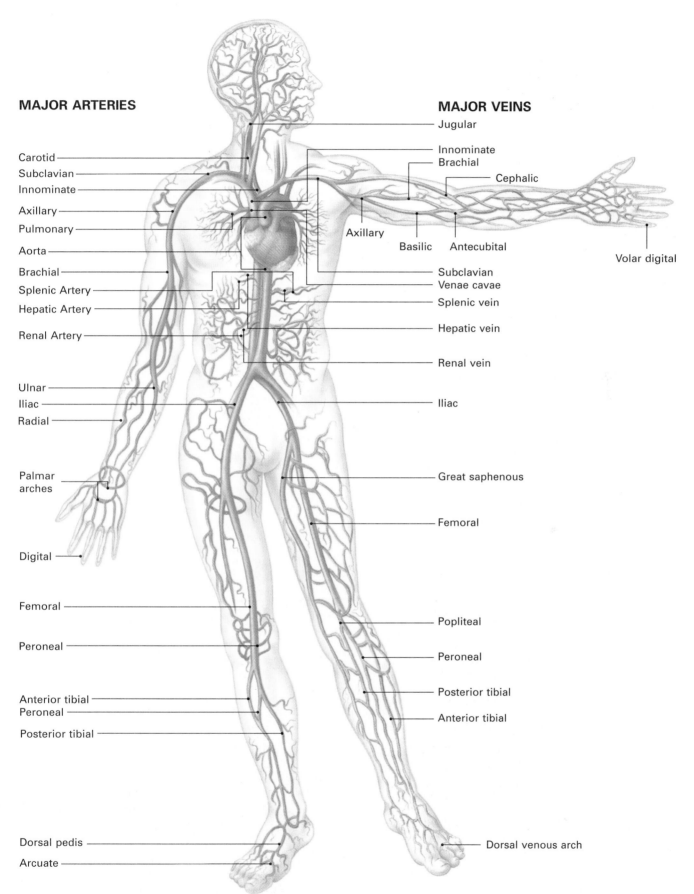

MAJOR ARTERIES

Carotid
Subclavian
Innominate
Axillary
Pulmonary
Aorta
Brachial
Splenic Artery
Hepatic Artery
Renal Artery
Ulnar
Iliac
Radial
Palmar arches
Digital
Femoral
Peroneal
Anterior tibial
Peroneal
Posterior tibial
Dorsal pedis
Arcuate

MAJOR VEINS

Jugular
Innominate
Brachial
Cephalic
Axillary
Basilic
Antecubital
Volar digital
Subclavian
Venae cavae
Splenic vein
Hepatic vein
Renal vein
Iliac
Great saphenous
Femoral
Popliteal
Peroneal
Posterior tibial
Anterior tibial
Dorsal venous arch

Figure 4-11 The circulatory system.

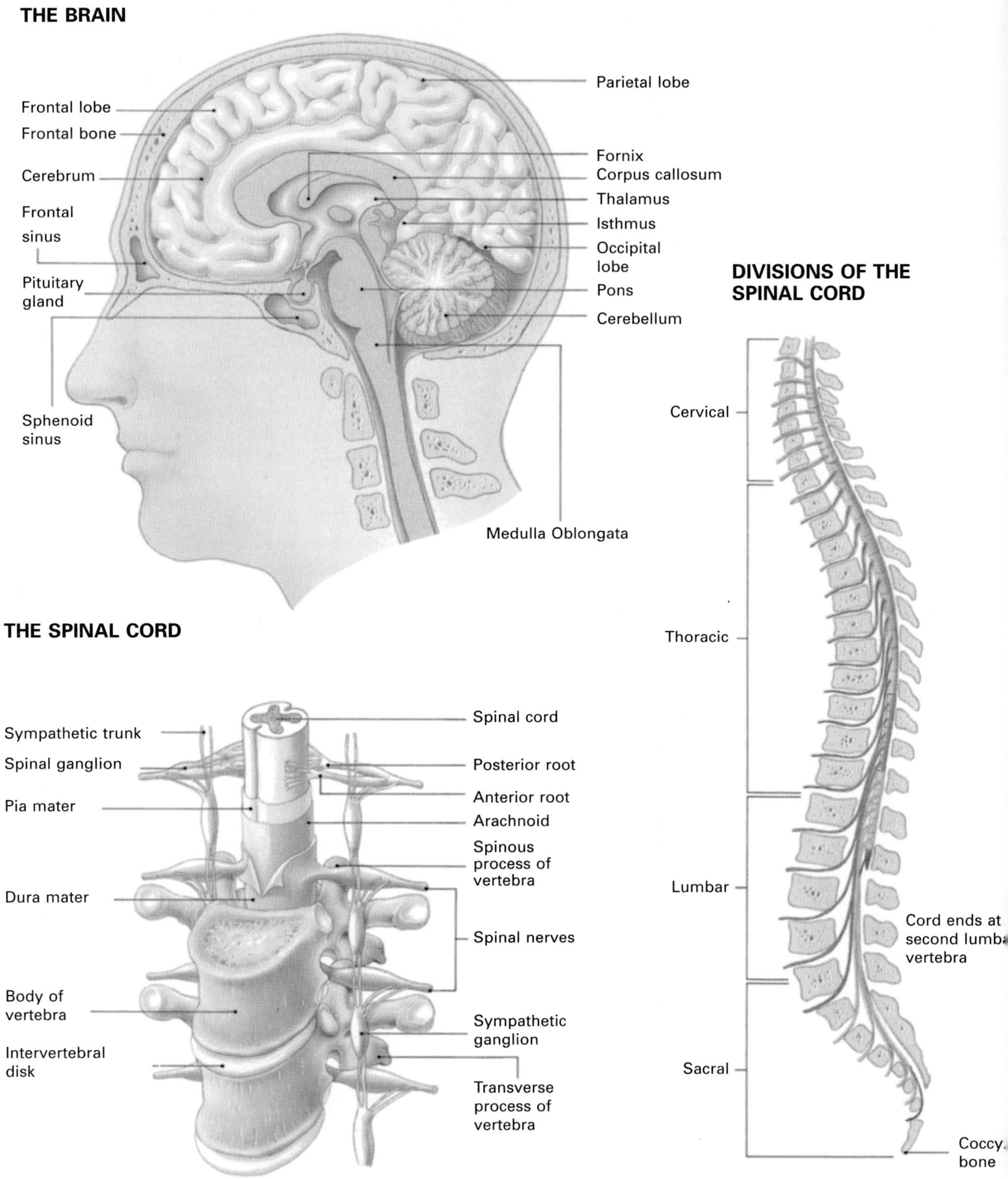

THE BRAIN

Frontal lobe

Frontal bone

Cerebrum

Frontal sinus

Pituitary gland

Sphenoid sinus

Parietal lobe

Fornix

Corpus callosum

Thalamus

Isthmus

Occipital lobe

Pons

Cerebellum

Medulla Oblongata

DIVISIONS OF THE SPINAL CORD

Cervical

Thoracic

Lumbar

Sacral

Cord ends at second lumbar vertebra

Coccyx bone

THE SPINAL CORD

Sympathetic trunk

Spinal ganglion

Pia mater

Dura mater

Body of vertebra

Intervertebral disk

Spinal cord

Posterior root

Anterior root

Arachnoid

Spinous process of vertebra

Spinal nerves

Sympathetic ganglion

Transverse process of vertebra

Figure 4-12 The nervous system.

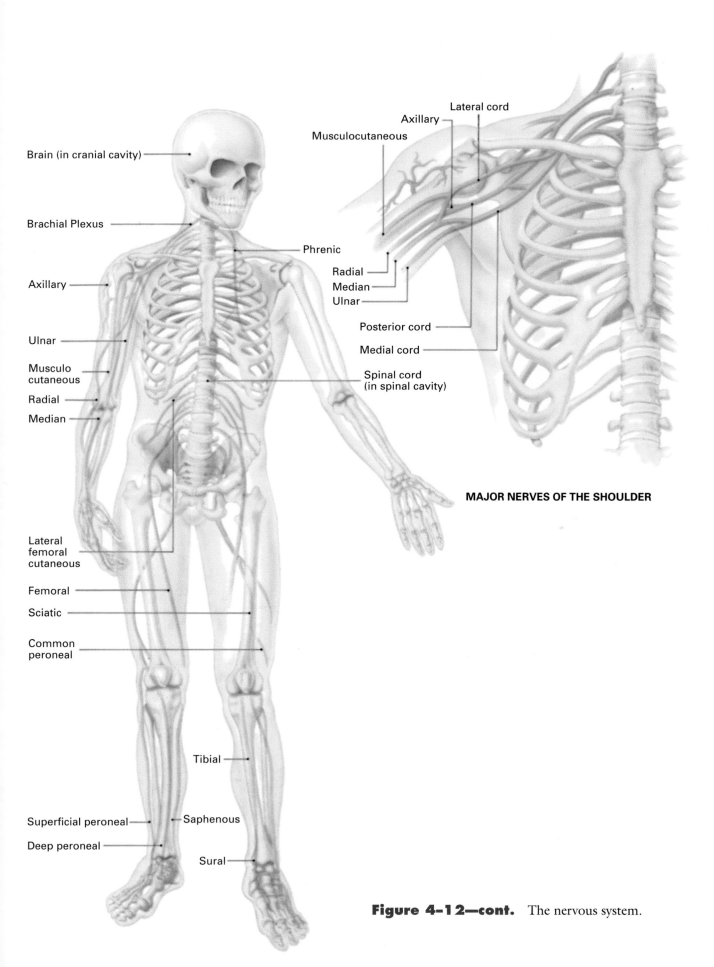

Brain (in cranial cavity)

Brachial Plexus

Axillary

Ulnar

Musculo cutaneous

Radial

Median

Lateral femoral cutaneous

Femoral

Sciatic

Common peroneal

Tibial

Superficial peroneal

Deep peroneal

Saphenous

Sural

Phrenic

Spinal cord (in spinal cavity)

Musculocutaneous

Axillary

Lateral cord

Radial

Median

Ulnar

Posterior cord

Medial cord

MAJOR NERVES OF THE SHOULDER

Figure 4-12—cont. The nervous system.

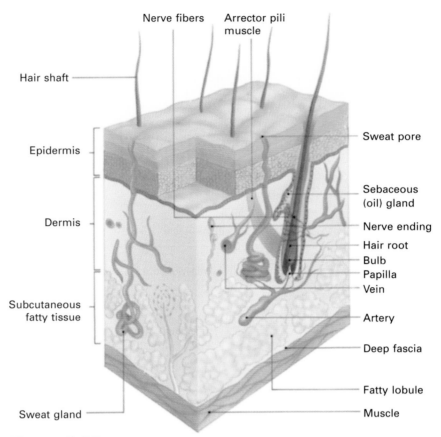

Nerve fibers

Arrector pili muscle

Hair shaft

Epidermis

Dermis

Subcutaneous fatty tissue

Sweat gland

Sweat pore

Sebaceous (oil) gland

Nerve ending

Hair root

Bulb

Papilla

Vein

Artery

Deep fascia

Fatty lobule

Muscle

Figure 4-13 Structure of normal skin.

sensory nerves. Just below the skin is a layer of fatty tissue, which varies in thickness. For example, it is extremely thin in the eyelids, but thick over the buttocks.

THE DIGESTIVE SYSTEM

The digestive system is composed of the **alimentary tract** (food passageway) and accessory organs (Figure 4–14). Its main functions are to ingest food and get rid of waste. Digestion consists of two processes—mechanical and chemical.

The mechanical process includes chewing, swallowing, the rhythmic movement of matter through the tract, and defecation (the elimination of waste). The chemical process consists of break-

ing food into simple components that can be absorbed and used by the body.

Except for the mouth and **esophagus,** the organs of this system are in the abdomen. They include the stomach, pancreas, liver, gallbladder, small intestine, and large intestine.

THE URINARY SYSTEM

The urinary system filters and excretes waste from the body. It consists of two kidneys and two ureters, one urinary bladder, and one urethra (Figure 4–15). The ureters take urine from the kidneys to the next part of the system, the bladder. The bladder stores urine until it is passed through the urethra and excreted from the body.

THE DIGESTIVE SYSTEM

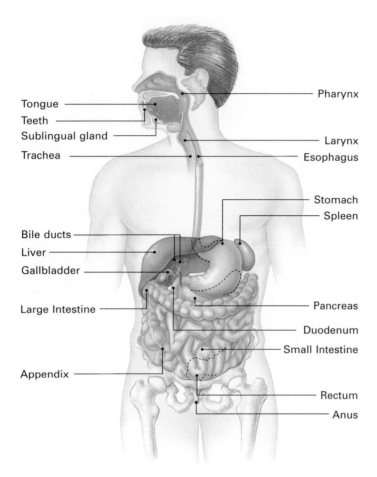

Tongue
Teeth
Sublingual gland
Trachea

Pharynx

Larynx
Esophagus

Stomach
Spleen

Bile ducts
Liver
Gallbladder

Large Intestine

Pancreas

Duodenum

Small Intestine

Appendix

Rectum
Anus

Figure 4-14 The digestive system.

The urinary system helps the body maintain the delicate balance of water and chemicals needed for survival. During the process of urine formation, wastes are removed and useful products are returned to the blood.

THE ENDOCRINE SYSTEM

The endocrine glands regulate the body by secreting hormones directly into the bloodstream. They affect physical strength, mental ability, stature, reproduction, hair growth, voice pitch, and behavior. How people think, act, and feel depends largely on these tiny secretions. Each gland produces one or more hormones. The glands include the thyroid, parathyroids, adrenals, ovaries, testes, islets of Langerhans, and the pituitary.

THE REPRODUCTIVE SYSTEM

The reproductive system of the male includes two testes, a duct system, accessory glands, and the penis. The reproductive system of the female consists of two ovaries, two fallopian tubes, the uterus, vagina, and external genitals. (See Figure 4–16.)

ORGANS OF THE URINARY SYSTEM

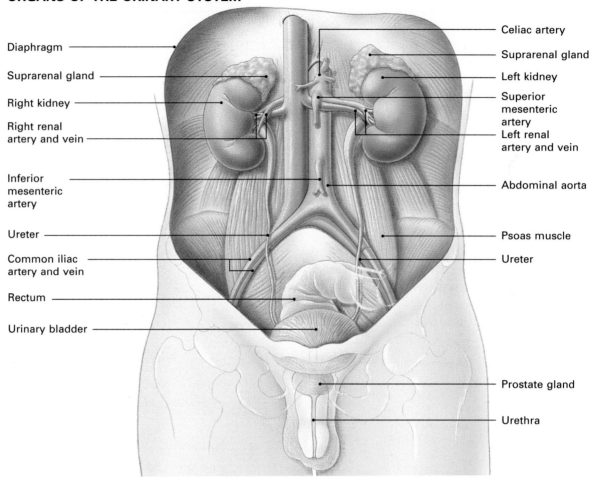

Diaphragm

Suprarenal gland

Right kidney

Right renal
artery and vein

Inferior
mesenteric
artery

Ureter

Common iliac
artery and vein

Rectum

Urinary bladder

Celiac artery

Suprarenal gland

Left kidney

Superior
mesenteric
artery

Left renal
artery and vein

Abdominal aorta

Psoas muscle

Ureter

Prostate gland

Urethra

Figure 4-15 The urinary system.

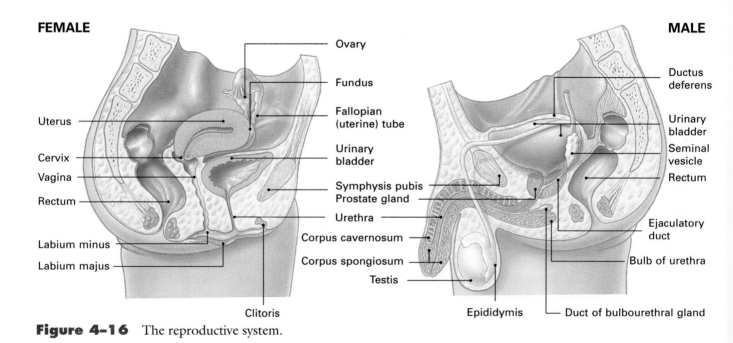

FEMALE

MALE

Ovary

Fundus

Fallopian
(uterine) tube

Urinary
bladder

Symphysis pubis

Prostate gland

Urethra

Corpus cavernosum

Corpus spongiosum

Testis

Uterus

Cervix

Vagina

Rectum

Labium minus

Labium majus

Clitoris

Ductus
deferens

Urinary
bladder

Seminal
vesicle

Rectum

Ejaculatory
duct

Bulb of urethra

Epididymis

Duct of bulbourethral gland

Figure 4-16 The reproductive system.

FIRST RESPONDER FOCUS

Consider these important tasks: opening an airway, examining a patient for the ability to move a part of his or her body, updating incoming EMS personnel via radio. Each task requires a knowledge of the human body.

To open an airway or examine a patient for breathing, you must know how the body breathes and how to recognize when it is not doing so adequately. To examine for injuries to the spine or certain bones, you may wish to check for the patient's ability to wiggle his or her fingers and toes. Your knowledge of the human body will let you know why that is important. When reporting a patient's condition, you must be able to describe it accurately to the incoming EMTs. Again, it is your knowledge of the body that will allow this to happen. ■

CASE STUDY FOLLOW-UP

At the beginning of this chapter, you read that First Responders were providing emergency care to a patient who "hurt her left leg." To see how chapter information applies to this emergency, read the following. It describes how the call was completed.

PATIENT HISTORY

I asked the patient to describe what happened. She said she mis-stepped as she was getting off the escalator. She didn't fall the entire length. She said that she felt a twisting and then a sudden pain in her lower left leg. She denied allergies. She told us that she doesn't take any medications or have any medical problems. She ate a burger for lunch at the food court in the mall.

ONGOING ASSESSMENT

We rechecked the pulse, movement, and sensation below the injury. They were all present and the same as the first time we checked. We repeated her vital signs. Pulse was 84, strong, and regular. Respirations were 16, regular, and deep. Blood pressure was 114/78. We made sure she was comfortable and continued to monitor her carefully.

PATIENT HAND-OFF

When the EMTs arrived, my partner gave them the hand-off report:

"This is Ellen Levine, who is 43 years old. She was getting off the elevator and mis-stepped. She felt a twisting in her left lower leg. She never lost consciousness and denies any other injury from the fall. She has pain, swelling, and deformity in the distal third of her tib/fib. There is adequate pulse, motor function, and sensation distal to the injury. The remainder of the physical exam was negative. We've held manual stabilization on the injured leg. Ellen's vital signs are pulse 84 strong and regular, respirations 16 and adequate, blood pressure 114/78."

While the EMTs immobilized the patient's leg in a splint, we helped keep onlookers from invading the patient's privacy. It wasn't long before the EMTs and the patient were ready to head for the ambulance. We walked with them to make sure the way was clear. Then, at the ambulance, we helped to get the stretcher loaded.

It was an exciting night. We were glad that everyone turned out to be okay.

> It is of the utmost importance that you have a basic knowledge of the human body. It is just as important for you to be able to use that knowledge to communicate a patient's condition to other health-care professionals. Learn the language. Speak it and write it every chance you get. You will need it throughout this course and in the field.

REVIEW QUESTIONS

Page references where answers may be found or supported are provided at the end of each question.

Section 1

1. How does a patient appear when he or she is in the anatomical position? The lateral recumbent position? Supine? Prone? (p. 42)
2. What are definitions of the terms *anterior, medial, distal, superficial,* and *external*? (pp. 43–44)

Section 2

3. What is the anatomy and function of the musculoskeletal system? Give a brief description. (pp. 45–46)
4. What is the anatomy and function of the respiratory system? Give a brief description. (pp. 46–47, 49)
5. What is the anatomy and function of the circulatory system? Give a brief description. (pp. 49, 51)

CHAPTER 5

LIFTING AND MOVING PATIENTS

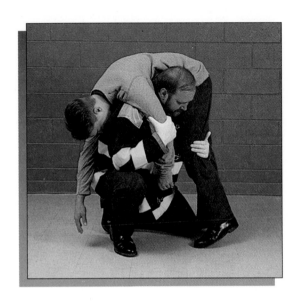

INTRODUCTION

After receiving emergency care, a patient may need to be handled or transported. If this is done improperly, the patient may be injured further. It is your responsibility to see that the patient is not subjected to unnecessary pain or discomfort.

Each EMS system defines if and when First Responders may move patients. Generally, you may only move patients who are in immediate danger. You may position patients to prevent further injury. You also may assist other EMS workers in moving patients. Learn and follow your local protocols.

SECTION 1: BODY MECHANICS

BASIC PRINCIPLES

As an EMS worker, you may be asked to lift and carry patients and heavy equipment. If you do it incorrectly, you could cause yourself injury, strain, and life-long pain. With planning, good health, and skill, you can do your job with minimum risk to yourself.

Apply the principles of proper lifting and moving every day. Practice enough for them to become automatic. Make them a habit that increases your safety and performance, even in the most stressful emergency situations.

Body mechanics refers to the safest and most efficient methods of using your body to gain a mechanical advantage. It includes:

- *Use your legs to lift, not your back.* To move a heavy object, use the muscles of your legs, hips, and buttocks, plus the contracted muscles of your abdomen. These muscles let you safely generate a lot of power. Never use the muscles in your back to help you move or lift a heavy object.
- *Keep the weight of the object as close to your body as possible.* Reach a short distance to lift a heavy object (Figure 5–1). Back injury is much more likely to occur when you reach a long distance to lift an object.
- *"Stack."* That is, visualize your shoulders stacked on top of your hips, and your hips on top of your feet. Then move as a unit. If your shoulders, hips, and feet are not aligned, you could create twisting forces that can harm your lower back.
- *Reduce the height or distance you need to move the object.* Get closer to the object, or reposition it before you try to lift. Lift in stages if you need to.

CASE STUDY

DISPATCH

My partner and I were returning from a call in our first response vehicle when we saw the scene of a car crash. It really took us by surprise. At least when you are dispatched, you have time to prepare for what you might see.

SCENE SIZE-UP

We parked a safe distance away from the scene. As we were about to exit our vehicle, we saw smoke billow out from under the hood of the car. The fire must have been fueled by grease. We called the dispatcher to notify the fire department.

We had turnout gear on, so we carefully approached the car. A woman was in the driver's seat. She seemed dazed. The smoke was filling the car. The windshield was turning black. Then we saw flames. Before long we were sure the passenger compartment would be on fire.

Lifting and moving patients is an important responsibility. Many lifts and moves are routine while others require quick thinking and skill. Consider this patient as you read Chapter 5. Is it within the First Responders' scope of care to move her? If so, how can they do it without causing further injury?

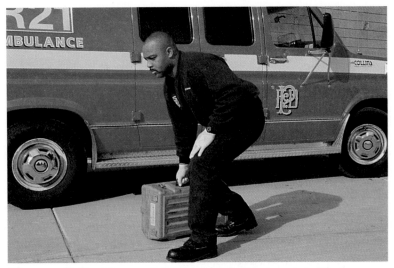

Figure 5-1   Keep weight close to the body as it is lifted.

POWER LIFT

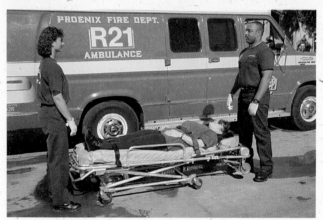

Figure 5-2a Get in position.

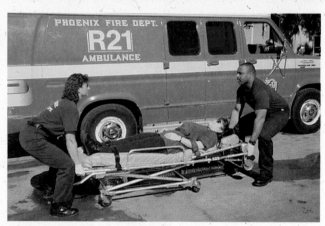

Figure 5-2b Lift in unison, keeping your back locked and feet flat.

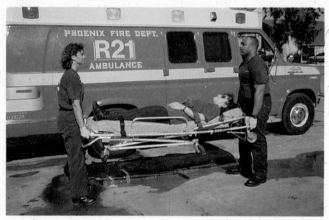

Figure 5-2c Stand, making sure your back remains locked.

Apply the principles of body mechanics to lifting, carrying, moving, reaching, pushing, and pulling. Key to preventing injury during all those tasks is correct alignment of the spine. Keep a normal inward curve in the lower back. Keep wrists and knees in normal alignment, too. Whenever possible, use equipment to do the lifting for you.

In an emergency, teamwork is essential. Just as a football coach positions players according to ability, rescuers should too. It can help capitalize on their abilities to ensure the best outcome in any emergency.

All members on a team should be trained in the proper techniques. Problems can occur when teams members are greatly mismatched. The stronger partner can be injured if the weaker one fails to lift. The weaker one can be injured if he tries to do too much. Ideally, partners in lifting and moving should have adequate and equal strength and height. So know your physical ability and limitations. Respect them. Consider the weight of the patient and recognize the need for help.

Team members also need to communicate during a task, clearly and frequently. Use commands that are easy for team members to understand. Verbally coordinate each lift from beginning to end.

THE POWER LIFT

The power lift is a technique that offers you the best defense against injury. It also protects the patient on a stretcher with a safe and stable move. It is especially useful for rescuers who have weak knees or thighs. Remember that in performing the power lift, keep your back locked and avoid bending at the waist (Figure 5–2). Follow these steps:

1. Place your feet a comfortable distance apart. For the average-size person, this is usually about shoulder width. Taller rescuers might prefer a little wider stance.
2. Turn your feet slightly outward. Most people find that this helps them feel more comfortable and more stable.
3. Bend your knees to bring your center of gravity closer to the object. As you bend your knees, you should feel as though you are sitting down, not falling forward.
4. Tighten the muscles of your back and abdomen to splint the vulnerable lower back. Your back should remain as straight as you can comfortably manage, with your head facing forward in a neutral position.
5. Keep your feet flat with your weight evenly distributed and just forward of the heels.
6. Place your hands a comfortable distance from each other to provide balance to the object as it is lifted. This is usually at least 10 inches apart.
7. Always use a power grip to get maximum force from your hands. That is, your palms and fingers should come in complete contact with the object and all fingers should be bent at the same angle. (See Figure 5–3.)
8. As lifting begins, your back should remain locked as the force is driven through the heels and arches of your feet. Your upper body should come up before the hips do.
9. Reverse these steps to lower the object.

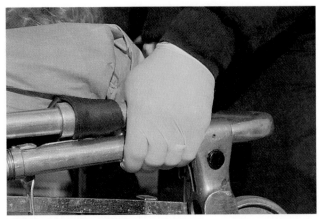

Figure 5-3 The power grip.

POSTURE AND FITNESS

Posture is a much overlooked part of body mechanics. When people spend a great deal of time sitting or standing, poor posture can easily tire back and stomach muscles. This can only make back injury more likely.

One extreme of poor posture is the swayback (Figure 5–4). In it the stomach is too far forward and the buttocks too far back, causing extreme stress on the lower back. Another extreme is the slouch. In it the shoulders are rolled forward, putting increased pressure on every region of the spine.

Be aware of your posture. While standing, your ears, shoulders, and hips should be in vertical alignment. Your knees should be slightly bent, and your pelvis slightly tucked forward (Figure 5–5).

When sitting, your weight should be evenly distributed on both *ischia* (the lower portion of your pelvic bones). (See Figure 5–6.) Your ears, shoulders, and hips should be in vertical alignment. Your feet should be flat on the floor or crossed at the ankles. If possible, your lower back should be in contact with the support of the chair.

Finally, proper body mechanics will not protect you if you are not physically fit. A proactive, well balanced physical fitness program should include flexibility training, cardiovascular conditioning, strength training, and nutrition.

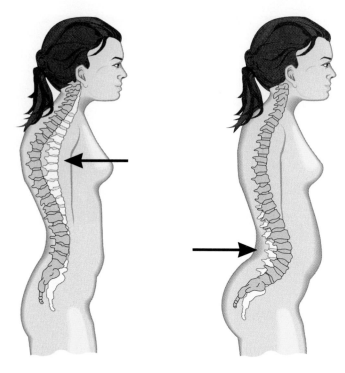

Excessive kyphosis
(slouch)

Excessive lordosis
(swayback)

Figure 5-4 Slouch and swayback are extremes of poor posture.

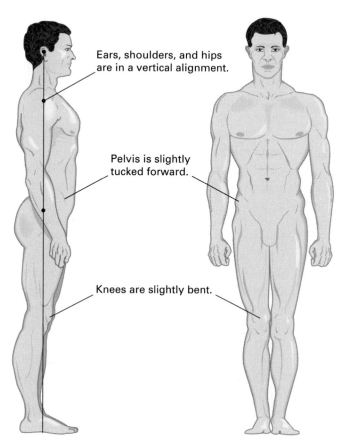

Ears, shoulders, and hips are in a vertical alignment.

Pelvis is slightly tucked forward.

Knees are slightly bent.

Figure 5-5 Proper standing position.

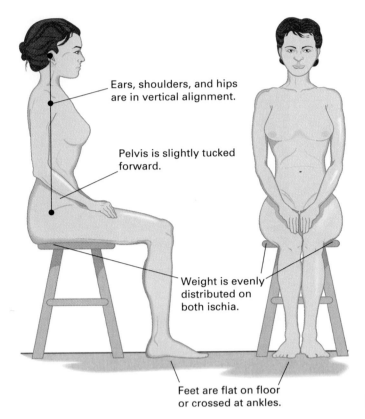

Ears, shoulders, and hips are in vertical alignment.

Pelvis is slightly tucked forward.

Weight is evenly distributed on both ischia.

Feet are flat on floor or crossed at ankles.

Figure 5-6 Proper sitting position.

SECTION 2: PRINCIPLES OF MOVING PATIENTS

EMERGENCY MOVES

The top priority in emergency care is to maintain a patient's airway, breathing, and circulation. However, if the scene is unstable or poses an immediate threat, you may have to move the patient first. Follow local protocols.

In general, when there is no threat to life, provide emergency medical care and wait for the EMTs to move the patient. Make an **emergency move** only when there is an immediate danger to the patient. Examples of situations in which you may make an emergency move are:

- *Fire or threat of fire.* Fire should always be considered a grave threat, not only to patients but also to rescuers.
- *Explosion or the threat of explosion.*
- *Inability to protect the patient from other hazards at the scene.* Examples of hazards include an unstable building, a rolled over car, spilled gasoline and other hazardous materials, an unruly or hostile crowd, and extreme weather conditions.
- *Inability to gain access to other patients who need life-saving care.* For example, this may occur at the scene of a car crash involving two or more patients.
- *When life-saving care cannot be given because of the patient's location or position.* For example, a patient in cardiac arrest must be supine on a flat, hard surface in order for you to perform CPR properly. If that patient is sitting on a chair, an emergency move must be made in order for you to provide life-saving care.

The greatest danger in an emergency move is the possibility of making a spine injury worse. So to provide as much protection to the spine as possible, pull the patient in the direction of the long axis of the body.

It is impossible to move a patient from a vehicle quickly and, at the same time, protect the spine. So move a patient from a vehicle immediately only if one of the five conditions described above exist.

If the patient is on the floor or the ground, use one of the following emergency moves. But be sure never to pull the patient's head away from the neck and shoulders. If there is time, you may wish to bind the patient's wrists together with a cravat or gauze. This will make the patient easier to move, and it will help protect the hands and arms from injury.

Shirt Drag

To perform a shirt drag, do the following (Figure 5–7). First, fasten the patient's hands or wrists loosely with a cravat or gauze to protect them during the move. Then grasp the shoulders of the patient's shirt (not a tee shirt). Pull the shirt under the patient's head to form a support. Then, using the shirt as a "handle," pull the patient toward you. Be careful not to strangle the patient. The pulling should engage the patient's armpits, not the neck.

Blanket Drag

To perform a blanket drag, do the following (Figure 5–8). First, spread a blanket alongside the patient. Gather half of it into lengthwise pleats. Roll the patient away from you onto his side, and tuck the pleated part of the blanket as far under him as you can. Then roll the patient back onto the center of the blanket, preferably on his back. Wrap the blanket securely around the patient. Grabbing the part of the blanket that is under the patient's head, drag the patient toward you.

If you do not have a blanket, you can use a coat in the same way.

Shoulder or Forearm Drag

To perform a shoulder drag, do the following (Figure 5–9). First, stand at the patient's head. Then slip your hands under the patient's armpits from the back. If you must drag the patient a long distance and need a better grip, the perform a forearm drag. That is, position yourself as you would in a shoulder drag. After you slip your

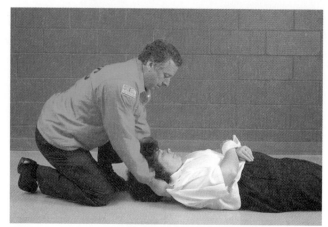

Figure 5-7   Shirt drag.

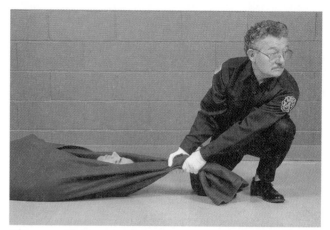

Figure 5-8   Blanket drag.

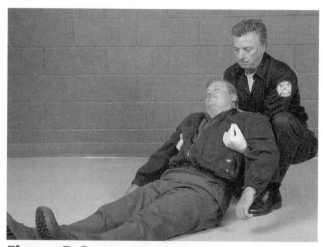

Figure 5-9   Shoulder drag.

hands under the patient's armpits, grasp the patient's forearms and drag the patient toward you. Use your own forearms as a support to keep the patient's head, neck, and spine in alignment.

Other Emergency Moves

Other emergency moves include the piggyback carry, one-rescuer crutch, one-rescuer cradle carry, firefighter's drag, and others. (See Figures 5–10 and 5–11.)

NON-EMERGENCY MOVES

Non-emergency moves, or non-urgent moves, are generally performed with other rescuers. They require no equipment and may take less time than moves such as a blanket drag. However, do not use them with possible spine-injured patients, since they offer no spinal protection.

Non-emergency, or non-urgent, moves include the direct ground lift and extremity lift.

Direct Ground Lift

The direct ground lift requires two or three rescuers. It is valuable when the patient cannot sit in a chair and when a stretcher cannot be brought close to the patient. It is difficult if the patient weighs more than 180 pounds, is on the ground or some other low surface, or is uncooperative.

Position the stretcher as close to the patient as possible. Undo the stretcher straps, lower the railings, and clear any equipment off the mattress. Tell the patient what you are going to do. Then warn him that he must remain still in order to protect your balance. Place the patient's arms on his chest if possible.

To perform a direct ground lift, follow these steps (Figure 5–12, p. 72):

1. Line up on one side of the patient. If at all possible, line up on the least injured side.
2. Kneel on one knee, preferably the same knee for all rescuers.
3. Have the first rescuer cradle the patient's head by placing one arm under the neck and shoulder. He must place his other arm under the patient's lower back.

4. Have the second rescuer place one arm under the patient's knees, and the other arm above the buttocks.
5. If a third rescuer is available, have him place both arms under the patient's waist. The other two rescuers should slide their arms up to the middle of the back and down to the buttocks as appropriate.
6. On signal, all rescuers should lift the patient to their knees as a unit. Then, with a gentle rocking motion, roll the patient as a unit toward your chests until he or she is cradled in the bends of your elbows. Tuck the patient's head in toward your chests.
7. On signal, the rescuers should stand and carry the patient to the stretcher.
8. To lower the patient onto the stretcher, reverse the steps.

Extremity Lift

Do not use the extremity lift if the patient has injuries to his arms or legs. Use this lift to move an unresponsive patient from a chair to the floor. Two rescuers are needed to perform the lift (Figure 5–13, p. 73):

1. Take a position at the patient's head. The other rescuer should kneel at the patient's side by the knees.
2. Place one hand under each of the patient's shoulders, reaching through to grab the patient's wrists.
3. The second rescuer should slip his hands under the patient's knees.
4. On signal, both of you then can move the patient to the desired location.

POSITIONING THE PATIENT

How you position a patient depends on the patient's condition. General guidelines include:

- An unresponsive patient who is not injured should be placed in the recovery position. This is done by rolling the patient onto his or her side, preferably the left side.
- Unless there is a life-threatening emergency, a patient who has been injured should not be

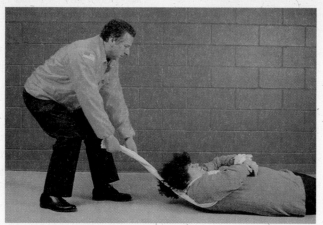

Figure 5-10a Sheet drag.

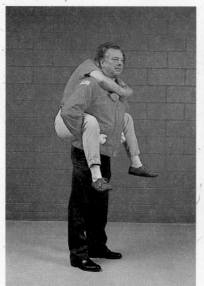

Figure 5-10b Piggyback carry.

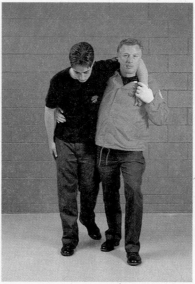

Figure 5-10c One-rescuer crutch.

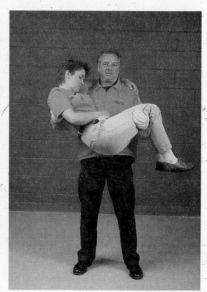

Figure 5-10d Cradle carry.

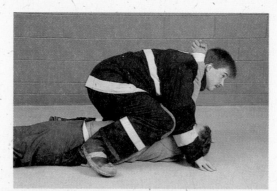

Figure 5-10e Firefighter's drag.

FIREFIGHTER'S CARRY

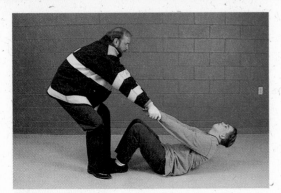

Figure 5-11a Grasp the patient's wrists.

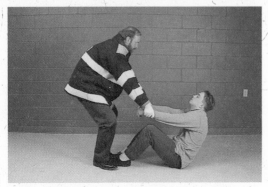

Figure 5-11b Stand on the patient's toes and pull.

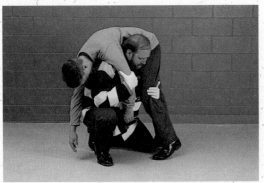

Figure 5-11c Pull the patient over a shoulder.

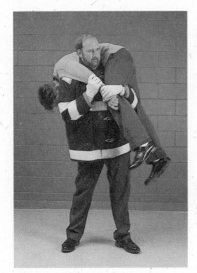

Figure 5-11d Pass an arm between the legs and grasp the arm nearest you.

moved. The EMTs will evaluate, stabilize, and move the patient as necessary.

- A patient who shows signs of shock may be placed in the shock position. If it will not aggravate injuries to the legs or spine, this is done by elevating the supine patient's legs 8-12 inches.
- A patient who has pain or breathing problems may get in any position that makes him more

comfortable, unless his injuries prevent it. Generally, a patient who has breathing difficulties will want to sit up. A patient with abdominal pain will want to lie on his side with knees drawn up.

- A responsive patient who is nauseated or vomiting should be allowed to remain in a position of comfort. However, you should always be positioned so you can manage the patient's airway if needed.

DIRECT GROUND LIFT

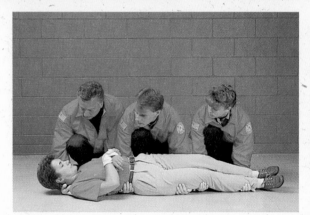

Figure 5-12a Kneel on one knee on the least injured side.

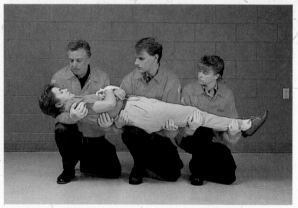

Figure 5-12b In unison, lift the patient to knee level.

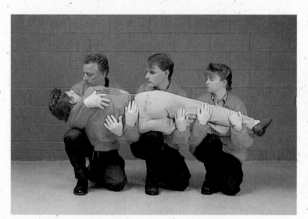

Figure 5-12c Slowly turn the patient toward you.

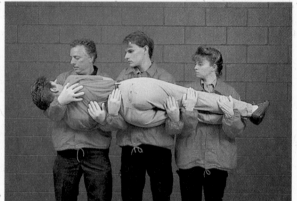

Figure 5-12d In unison, rise to a standing position.

SECTION 3: EQUIPMENT

Become completely familiar with the equipment used to move patients in your EMS system. To decide which to use, base your decision on the patient's condition, the environment in which he is found, and the resources available. Generally, the best way to move a patient is the easiest way that will not cause injury or pain.

Let your equipment do the work whenever possible. Drag or slide the patient (not lift), whenever you can. If you must lift a patient, do it with a device designed for that purpose. As a rule, carry a patient only as far as absolutely necessary. Make sure you have adequate help. If you do not, get it. Never risk injuring yourself.

Typical equipment used in EMS includes: various types of stretchers, the stair chair, and backboards.

EXTREMITY LIFT

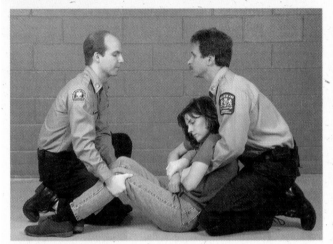

Figure 5-13a Get in position at the head and feet of the patient.

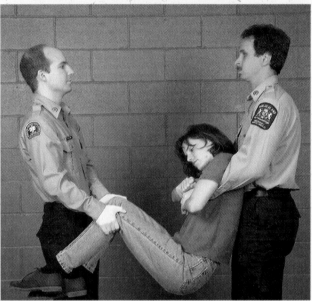

Figure 5-13b Move up to a crouch and then to a standing position.

STRETCHERS

A standard stretcher, or cot, has wheeled legs. It also has a collapsible undercarriage that makes it possible to load it into an ambulance. (See Figure 5–14.)

A portable stretcher is lightweight, folds compactly, and is easy to clean. It does not have an undercarriage and wheels. It is comfortable to rest on, especially if the head is padded. It is valuable when there is not enough space for a standard stretcher or when there are multiple patients. There are a variety of styles. The most common has an aluminum frame with canvas fabric. (See Figures 5–15 and 5–16.)

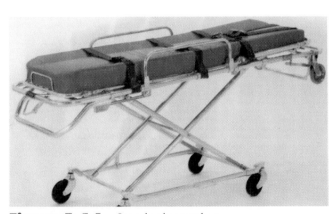

Figure 5-14 Standard stretcher.

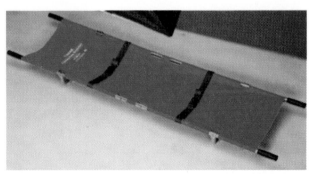

Figure 5-15 Pole stretcher.

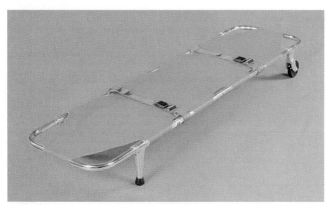

Figure 5–16 Portable ambulance stretcher.

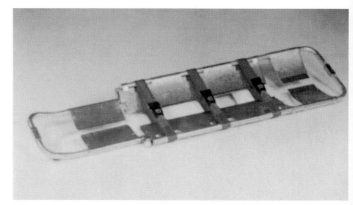

Figure 5–17 Scoop or orthopedic stretcher.

A scoop, or orthopedic, stretcher splits in two or four sections (Figure 5–17). Each section can be fitted around a patient who is lying on a relatively flat surface. It is used in confined areas where larger stretchers will not fit. Once secure in a scoop stretcher, a patient can be lifted and moved to a standard one. To operate a scoop stretcher, split it apart lengthwise. Carefully slide it under the patient from both sides. Then lock the brackets at each end, and lift the patient.

A stretcher also can be improvised with a blanket, canvas, brattice cloth, or a strong sheet and two 7- to 8-foot poles. To improvise a stretcher with two poles and a blanket, follow these steps (Figure 5–18):

1. Place one pole about one foot from the center of the unfolded blanket.
2. Fold the short side of the blanket over a pole.
3. Place the second pole on top of the two folds of blanket. It should be about two feet from the first pole and parallel to it.
4. Fold the remaining side of the blanket over the second pole. When the patient is placed on the blanket, the weight of the body secures the poles.

Cloth bags or sacks may be used as stretchers. Make holes in the bottoms of bags or sacks so that the poles pass through them. Enough bags should be used to provide the required length.

IMPROVISED STRETCHER

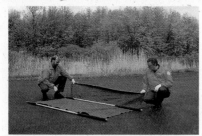

Figure 5–18a Fold the short side of the blanket over the first pole.

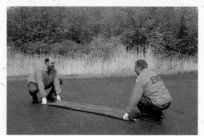

Figure 5–18b Fold the remaining side over the second pole.

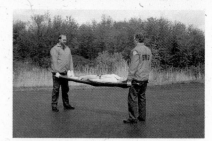

Figure 5–18c The weight of the patient should secure the poles.

USING A STAIR CHAIR

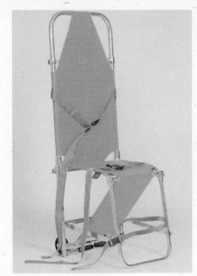

Figure 5-19a Stair chair.

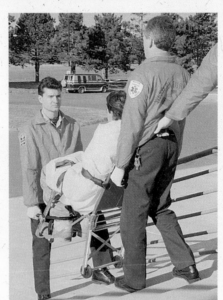

Figure 5-19b Moving a patient up steps with a third rescuer as spotter.

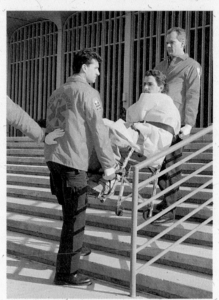

Figure 5-19c Moving a patient down steps with a third rescuer as spotter.

A stretcher can also be made from three or four coats or jackets. First turn the sleeves inside out. Then fasten the jacket with the sleeves inside the coat. Place a pole through each sleeve.

STAIR CHAIR

Moving patients up or down stairs dramatically increases the potential for rescuers to be injured. The safest way to do it is with a stair chair. A stair chair is a lightweight folding device. It has straps to confine the patient, wheeled legs, a grab bar below the patient's feet, and handles that extend behind the patient's shoulders.

When you use a stair chair (Figure 5–19), make sure as many people as necessary are helping. A "spotter" is needed to help maneuver the stair chair down stairs. He should continually tell how many stairs are left and what conditions are ahead. A spotter also can place his hand on the back of the rescuer who is moving backward to help steady him.

Rescuers carrying a patient in a stair chair should keep their backs in a locked position. They should flex at the hips instead of at the waist, bend at the knees, and keep arms (and the weight of the chair) as close to their bodies as possible. Once off the stairs, the patient can be transferred to a more conventional stretcher.

Stair chairs work well for patients in respiratory distress who must be moved up or down stairs. The sitting position does not worsen the patient's breathing problems.

BACKBOARDS

There are both long and short backboards (Figure 5–20). A long backboard may be 6 to 7 feet long, which means it can stabilize the patient's entire body. It is used for patients with suspected spine injury who are lying down.

BACKBOARDS

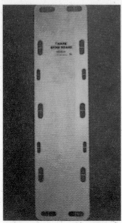

Figure 5-20a
Traditional wooden
long backboard.

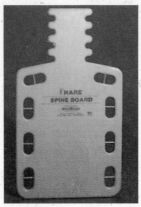

Figure 5-20b
Short backboard.

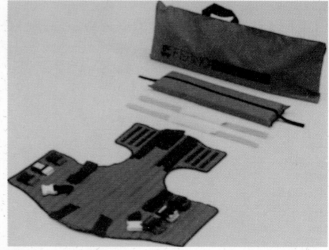

Figure 5-20c Vest-type immobilization device.

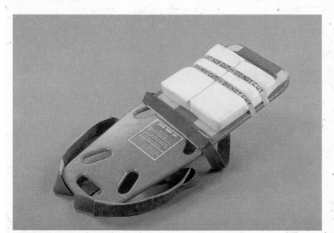

Figure 5-20d Short backboard.

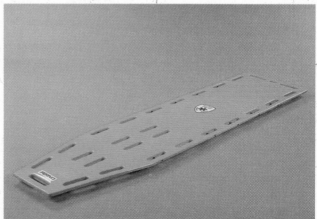

Figure 5-20e Long backboard.

A short backboard is 3 to 4 feet long and can stabilize the patient down to the hips. It is used to stabilize a patient with suspected spine injuries who is in a sitting position.

Both the long and short backboards feature handholds and straps. Most are made of synthetic material that will not absorb blood and is easy to clean. Regardless of whether you use a long or short backboard, always maintain manual support of the patient's head and neck in the normal anatomical position. Maintain that support until the patient is *fully* secured to the backboard.

FIRST RESPONDER FOCUS

▼

You will find most patients are in safe locations. Others have problems that would be worsened by movement. So in most cases, you will not move a patient until the EMTs arrive on scene.

However, when moving a patient means the difference between life and death, your ability to do so safely and properly is key. For example, a patient in a burning vehicle must be moved. If you have a sound knowledge of lifting and moving skills, you could move that patient without causing further injury to the spine or other parts of his or her body.

Study and practice the skills presented in this chapter. You will use them more than you think. ■

CASE STUDY FOLLOW-UP

At the beginning of this chapter, you read that the First Responders were at the scene of a collision. They were faced with a patient with unknown injuries and in serious danger from smoke and fire. To see how chapter skills apply to this emergency, read the following. It describes how the call was completed.

SCENE SIZE-UP *(Continued)*
We glanced at each other. We both knew the patient was in mortal danger and had to be moved immediately. While we were concerned about her possible injuries, we knew it would do no good to leave her in the smoke-filled, flaming car.

I grabbed her under her shoulders and began the move. I cradled her head in my arms to help minimize problems with her spine. My partner grabbed her legs. We moved her a safe distance from the car, and set her down carefully.

INITIAL ASSESSMENT
My partner stabilized her head as I assessed her responsiveness. She moaned when I spoke loudly. My partner kept an eye on her airway. She was breathing adequately and had no foreign material in her mouth, but that could change quickly. She had no signs of external bleeding.

Our general impression was that this woman was about 50 years old and in potentially serious condition. She may have had injuries from the crash and from the smoke. We had oxygen available, so we applied a nonrebreather immediately.

We updated the incoming units of our suspicions so they could be prepared when they arrived on scene.

PHYSICAL EXAMINATION
Based on the mechanisms of injury, any type of injury was possible. The patient was not alert and could not tell us what hurt. Palpation of her head and neck were negative for signs of injury. I palpated her chest and she groaned, indicating that she felt pain from an injury there. I listened to her chest and found unequal breathing sounds, diminished on the right where she had the pain. She had some abrasions on her lower legs and no other injuries that I could find. As I finished the exam, my partner told me that respirations were becoming inadequate. My partner began to assist them. I checked the patient's pulse, which was 112, regular and weak. Her respirations were 28 and shallow.

PATIENT HISTORY
We didn't notice any medical information devices on the patient. She couldn't tell us anything about her condition and no family members were present.

ONGOING ASSESSMENT
We continued to assist her ventilations. They remained shallow and rapid. Her pulse increased slightly to 120 and remained weak. We concentrated on ventilating the patient until the EMTs arrived.

CASE STUDY FOLLOW-UP *(Continued)*

PATIENT HAND-OFF
We told the EMTs about the situation we found on arrival. They agreed that the patient had to be moved fast. We told them:

"This is a female, about 50 years of age, involved in a motor vehicle crash. She responds only by moaning. We are currently assisting ventilations because of inadequate breathing. We are stabilizing the spine because of the mechanism of injury. We noted pain in her chest while we palpated. Breath sounds on the right are diminished compared to the left. Her pulse increased from 112 to 120 and is weak. Her respirations are shallow and 28. We have no information on history. We'll give you a hand with the backboarding so you can get off the scene quickly."

It turns out the patient experienced a collapsed lung in the crash. The smoke from the fire really didn't help. The EMTs told us they corrected the lung problem right in the emergency department and the patient improved dramatically. She was expected to recover fully. Our actions at the scene were an important part of her doing so well.

> When to move a patient is determined by the patient's condition and the environment in which he or she is found. How to move a patient is determined by considering his or her condition, location, and resources. Remember, in general, a First Responder does not move a patient unless an emergency move must be made or the EMTs ask for assistance. When you do move a patient, be sure to follow the rules of good body mechanics.

REVIEW QUESTIONS

Page references where answers may be found or supported are provided at the end of each question.

Section 1

1. Why should you follow the principles of body mechanics? (p. 62)

Section 2

2. What are five situations in which you should perform an emergency move of a patient? (p. 67)
3. Who should move a patient when there is no immediate threat to the patient's life? (p. 69)
4. How would you perform a shirt drag? (p. 68)

5. How would you perform a blanket drag? (p. 68)
6. How would you perform a direct ground lift? (p. 69)
7. How would you perform an extremity lift? (p. 69)
8. What is the preferred position for a patient who is unresponsive? A patient who had difficulty breathing? A patient who is nauseated or vomiting? (pp. 69, 71)

Section 3

9. How is a stair chair used? (p. 75)
10. How is a scoop stretcher used? (p. 74)

CHAPTER 6

THE AIRWAY AND VENTILATION

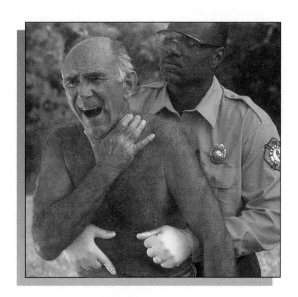

INTRODUCTION

The most important part of your job as a First Responder involves a patient's airway. No matter what a patient's problem may be, you must determine whether or not the airway is open and clear first. That can spell the difference between life and death—for a business executive who chokes on a piece of steak, a child who falls into a swimming pool, or an unresponsive patient whose tongue is blocking her airway.

OBJECTIVES

Cognitive, affective, and psychomotor objectives are from the U.S. DOT's 1995 "First Responder: National Standard Curriculum." Enrichment objectives, if any, identify material that is supplemental to the DOT curriculum.

Cognitive

2-1.1 Name and label the major structures of the respiratory system on a diagram. (p. 82)

2-1.2 List the signs of inadequate breathing. (pp. 94–95)

2-1.3 Describe the steps in the head-tilt chin-lift. (pp. 85–86)

2-1.4 Relate mechanism of injury to opening the airway. (pp. 85–87)

2-1.5 Describe the steps in the jaw thrust. (pp. 86–87)

2-1.6 State the importance of having a suction unit ready for immediate use when providing emergency medical care. (pp. 92–94)

2-1.7 Describe the techniques of suctioning. (pp. 92–94)

2-1.8 Describe how to ventilate a patient with a resuscitation mask or barrier device. (pp. 95–102)

2-1.9 Describe how ventilating an infant or child is different from an adult. (pp. 100–101)

2-1.10 List the steps in providing mouth-to-mouth and mouth-to-stoma ventilation. (pp. 99–100)

2-1.11 Describe how to measure and insert an oropharyngeal (oral) airway. (p. 88)

2-1.12 Describe how to measure and insert a nasopharyngeal (nasal) airway. (pp. 89–90)

2-1.13 Describe how to clear a foreign body airway obstruction in a responsive adult. (pp. 110–112)

2-1.14 Describe how to clear a foreign body airway obstruction in a responsive child with complete obstruction or partial airway obstruction and poor air exchange. (p. 116)

2-1.15 Describe how to clear a foreign body airway obstruction in a responsive infant with complete obstruction or partial airway obstruction and poor air exchange. (pp. 114–115)

2-1.16 Describe how to clear a foreign-body airway obstruction in an unresponsive adult. (pp. 112, 114)

2-1.17 Describe how to clear a foreign body airway obstruction in an unresponsive child. (pp. 116–117)

2-1.18 Describe how to clear a foreign body airway obstruction in an unresponsive infant. (pp. 115–116)

Affective

2-1.19 Explain why basic life support ventilation and airway protective skills take priority over most other basic life support skills. (pp. 81, 94, 117)

2-1.20 Demonstrate a caring attitude towards patients with airway problems who request emergency medical services. (p. 84)

2-1.21 Place the interests of the patient with airway problems as the foremost consideration when making any and all patient care decisions. (p. 117)

2-1.22 Communicate with empathy to patients with airway problems, as well as with family members and friends of the patient. (p. 84)

Psychomotor

2-1.23 Demonstrate the steps in the head-tilt chin-lift. (pp. 85–86)

2-1.24 Demonstrate the steps in the jaw thrust. (pp. 86–87)

2-1.25 Demonstrate the techniques of suctioning. (pp. 92–94)

2-1.26 Demonstrate the steps in mouth-to-mouth ventilation with body substance isolation (barrier shields). (pp. 98–99)

2-1.27 Demonstrate how to use a resuscitation mask to ventilate a patient. (pp. 101–102)

2-1.28 Demonstrate how to ventilate a patient with a stoma. (pp. 99–100)

2-1.29 Demonstrate how to measure and insert an oropharyngeal (oral) airway. (p. 88)

2-1.30 Demonstrate how to measure and insert a nasopharyngeal (nasal) airway. (pp. 89–90)

2-1.31 Demonstrate how to ventilate infant and child patients. (pp. 100–101)

2-1.32 Demonstrate how to clear a foreign body airway obstruction in a responsive adult. (pp. 110–112)

2-1.33 Demonstrate how to clear a foreign body airway obstruction in a responsive child. (p. 116)

2-1.34 Demonstrate how to clear a foreign body airway obstruction in a responsive infant. (pp. 114–115)

2-1.35 Demonstrate how to clear a foreign body airway obstruction in an unresponsive adult. (pp. 112, 114)

2-1.36 Demonstrate how to clear a foreign body airway obstruction in an unresponsive child. (pp. 116–117)

2-1.37 Demonstrate how to clear a foreign body airway obstruction in an unresponsive infant. (pp. 115–116)

OBJECTIVES

Enrichment

* Describe how to perform bag-valve-mask ventilation. (pp. 101–102)
* Describe the oxygen cylinders, oxygen delivery equipment, and oxygen administration guidelines. (pp. 103–108)
* Describe the special considerations related to administering oxygen to patients with chronic obstructive pulmonary diseases (COPD). (p. 109)

SECTION 1: THE RESPIRATORY SYSTEM

The body can store food for weeks and water for days, but it can only store enough oxygen for a few minutes. When oxygen is cut off, brain cells begin to die in about 5 minutes. The respiratory system supplies the body with the oxygen it needs. It also removes carbon dioxide.

ANATOMY OF THE RESPIRATORY SYSTEM

The major components of the respiratory system are the nose and mouth, pharynx (throat), epiglottis, trachea (windpipe), larynx (voice box), and the bronchi, lungs, and diaphragm. (See the upper airway in Figure 6–1. You also may wish to review the diagrams in Chapter 4.)

Nose and Mouth

Air normally enters the body through the nose and mouth. There it is warmed, moistened, and filtered as it flows over the damp, sticky mucous membranes.

Pharynx

From the back of the nose and mouth, the air enters the pharynx (throat), the passageway for both food and air. Air from the mouth enters through the oral portion of the pharynx, or the oropharynx. Air from the nose enters through the nasal portion of the pharynx, or the nasopharynx. At its lower end, the pharynx divides in two. One division is the esophagus, which leads to the stomach. The other is the trachea (windpipe), which leads to the lungs.

Epiglottis

The trachea is protected by a small leaf-shaped flap called the epiglottis. Normally, this flap covers the entrance of the larynx during swallowing so food and liquid cannot enter. However, with injury or illness, that reflex may not work properly. As a result, a patient could **aspirate** (inhale) liquid, blood, or vomit into the trachea and lungs, causing suffocation.

Trachea and Larynx

The trachea (windpipe) carries air from the nose and mouth to the lungs. Immediately above it is the larynx (voice box) or "Adam's apple." The larynx can be easily felt with your fingertips at the front of the throat.

Bronchi and Lungs

The lower end of the trachea divides into two tubes called bronchi. The bronchi lead to the lungs. Each bronchus divides into the smaller bronchioles, somewhat like the branches of a tree. At the ends of the bronchioles are thousands of tiny air sacs called alveoli. Each alveolus is enclosed in a network of capillaries and is responsible for the exchange of oxygen and carbon dioxide.

The principal organs of respiration are the lungs. The lungs are two large lobed organs that house thousands of tiny alveoli.

Diaphragm

The diaphragm is a powerful dome-shaped muscle essential to breathing. It separates the thoracic cavity from the abdominal cavity. If it cannot contract

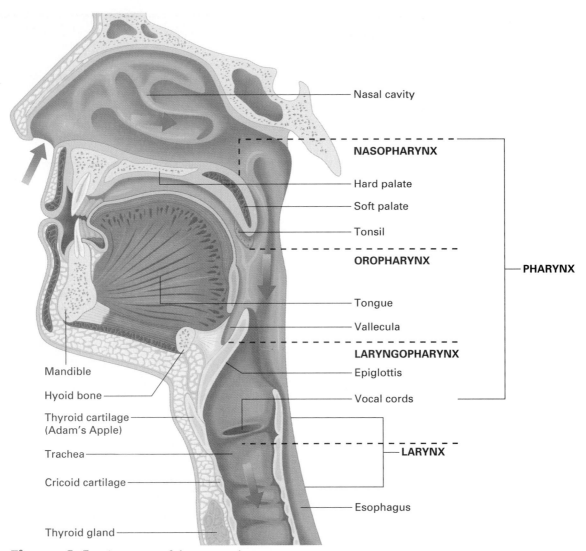

Figure 6-1 Anatomy of the upper airway.

effectively because of illness or injury, a patient will breathe inadequately and develop significant respiratory distress.

HOW RESPIRATION WORKS

During inhalation, the diaphragm and the muscles between the ribs contract. This increases the size of the thoracic cavity, making it possible for the lungs to expand. The diaphragm moves down slightly, flaring the lower portion of the rib cage, which then moves upward and outward. This decreases pressure in the chest and causes air to flow into the lungs. (See Figure 6–2.)

In the lungs gases pass through the thin walls of the alveoli and capillaries. Oxygen enters the alveoli during inhalation and passes through the capillary walls into the bloodstream. Carbon dioxide and other waste gases pass from the blood through the capillary walls into the alveoli so they can be exhaled.

During exhalation the diaphragm and the muscles between the ribs relax. This decreases the size of the thoracic cavity. The diaphragm moves up, the ribs move down and in, and air flows out of the lungs.

CASE STUDY

DISPATCH
Our first response unit was dispatched to an "unresponsive person."

SCENE SIZE-UP
We moved to the house carefully as we always do. A man came to the door. He looked very concerned. He explained that his wife slumped over in her chair minutes ago. "She looks bad," he told us. "She's not breathing right. Please help her."

As we approached the patient, we asked her husband if she had sustained any falls or injuries. He assured us that she had not.

INITIAL ASSESSMENT
We already had our gloves and eye wear on when we reached the patient's side. She was unresponsive with snoring respirations.

> The patient in this scenario requires immediate attention. No matter what the underlying reason for her condition, she will not survive without adequate respirations. Perhaps the most important part of her care will be the care she receives for her airway. Consider this patient as you read Chapter 6. What do you think the First Responders should do for her?

With some respiratory diseases, a patient has a hard time moving air out of the lungs. He or she has to use muscles not only to draw air in but also to force air out. As a result, both inhalation and exhalation require energy. Such patients tend to get exhausted quickly and will deteriorate rapidly.

Adequate breathing occurs at a normal rate (Table 6–1). For adults, that is 12 to 20 breaths per minute. For children, it is 15 to 30 breaths per minute. For infants, it is 25 to 50 breaths per minute. Adequate breathing is regular in rhythm and free of unusual sounds, such as wheezing or whistling. The chest should expand adequately and equally with each breath. The depth of the breaths should be adequate, too.

Breathing should be virtually effortless. It should be accomplished without the use of accessory, or additional, muscles in the neck, shoulders, and abdomen.

TABLE 6-1
NORMAL BREATHING RATES

Infant	25-50 breaths per minute
Child	15-30 breaths per minute
Adult	12-20 breaths per minute

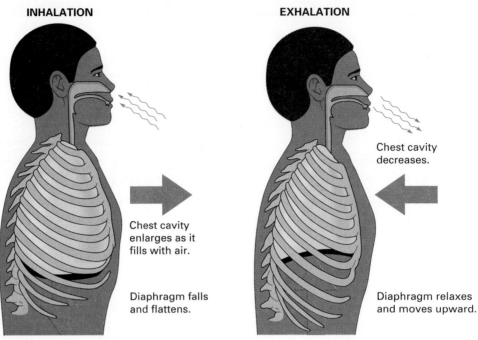

HOW RESPIRATION WORKS

INHALATION

Chest cavity enlarges as it fills with air.

Diaphragm falls and flattens.

Air pressure inside the chest cavity is less than outside, so air rushes into lungs to balance the pressure.

EXHALATION

Chest cavity decreases.

Diaphragm relaxes and moves upward.

Air pressure inside the chest cavity is greater than outside, so air is pushed out of the lungs.

Figure 6-2   How respiration works.

INFANTS AND CHILDREN

When treating infants and children, remember the anatomical differences in their respiratory systems. They include the following (Figure 6–3).

- All structures, including the mouth and nose, are smaller than those of adults. They are more easily obstructed even by small objects, blood, or swelling. Take extra care to keep the airway of infants and children open.
- The tongue of an infant or child takes up proportionally more space in the pharynx than the tongue of an adult. It can therefore block the airway more easily.
- The trachea of an infant or child is narrower than an adult's. It also is softer and more flexible. So tipping the head too far back or allow-

ing it to fall forward can close the trachea. Because the head of an infant or young child is quite large relative to the body, a folded towel or similar item under the shoulders may be needed to keep the airway aligned and open.

- Because the chest wall is softer, infants and children tend to rely on the diaphragm for breathing. So watch for excessive movement there. It can alert you to respiratory distress in an infant or child. Remember, the primary cause of cardiac arrest in infants and children is an uncorrected respiratory problem.

Just a reminder: whether your patient is an infant, child, or adult, remember that family members also need you. Be calm and caring as well as professional. Place the patient's interests first, but in this respect, consider the family too.

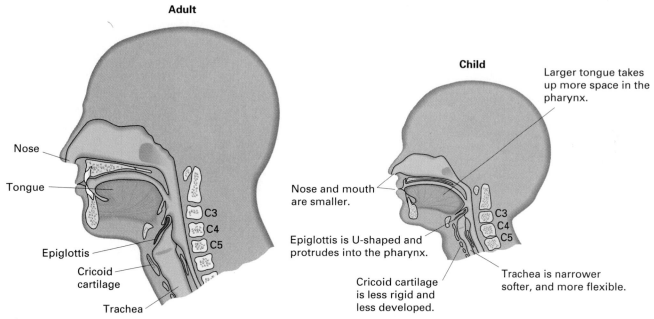

Figure 6-3 Comparison of airways of adult and infant or child.

Labels in figure:

Adult

Nose

Tongue

Epiglottis

Cricoid cartilage

Trachea

C3
C4
C5

Child

Larger tongue takes up more space in the pharynx.

Nose and mouth are smaller.

Epiglottis is U-shaped and protrudes into the pharynx.

Cricoid cartilage is less rigid and less developed.

Trachea is narrower softer, and more flexible.

C3
C4
C5

SECTION 2: PATIENT ASSESSMENT GUIDELINES

OPENING THE AIRWAY

The tongue is the most common cause of airway obstruction in an unresponsive patient. A patient who loses consciousness will lose muscle tone. When that happens, the base of the tongue can fall back and **occlude** (block) the airway. The patient's effort to breathe then creates negative pressure, which pulls the tongue, epiglottis, or both into the throat.

In some cases, patients require **ventilation** (assisting breathing by forcing air into the patient's lungs). Before a patient who is breathing inadequately can receive it, he must have an open airway.

There are two maneuvers commonly used to open an airway: the **head-tilt/chin-lift maneuver** and the **jaw-thrust maneuver.** Both techniques move the tongue from the back of the throat and allow air to pass into the lungs. (The tongue is attached to the lower jaw. So moving the lower jaw forward will relieve the obstruction.)

Head-tilt/Chin-lift Maneuver

The head-tilt/chin-lift maneuver is the method of choice for opening the airway of an uninjured patient. The American Heart Association (AHA) recommends it for opening the airway of patients who do not have injuries to the head, neck, or spine. Use it first for unresponsive patients who are not injured.

To perform the maneuver (Figure 6–4):

1. Place your hand on the patient's forehead. Use the hand that is closest to the patient's head.
2. Apply firm, backward pressure with the palm of your hand to tilt the head back.
3. Place the fingertips of your other hand under the bony part of the patient's lower jaw. (If the patient is an infant or child, place only your index finger under the jaw.)
4. Lift the chin forward. At the same time, support the jaw and tilt the head back as far as possible. The patient's teeth should be nearly together. (If the patient is an infant or child, tilt the head back only slightly, as if the child is "sniffing." Remember not to overextend the head.)

ADULT

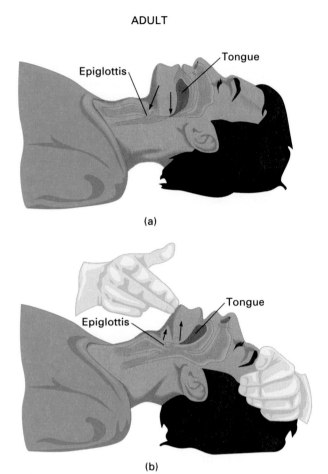

(a)

(b)

Figure 6-4a   Head-tilt/chin-lift maneuver for an adult.

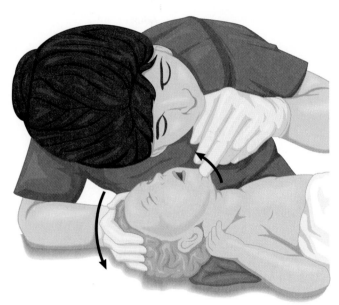

Figure 6-4b   Head-tilt/chin-lift maneuver for an infant.

5. Continue to press the other hand on the patient's forehead to keep the head tilted back.

There are several important precautions to remember when performing the head-tilt/chin-lift:

- Never let your fingers press deeply into the soft tissues under the chin. You could block the patient's airway.
- If necessary, use your thumb to press in the patient's lower lip, keeping the patient's mouth slightly open. Never use your thumb to lift the patient's chin.
- Do not let the patient's mouth close.
- If the patient has dentures (false teeth), try to hold them in place. It will help prevent the patient's lips from interfering with breathing. If you are unable to manage the dentures, remove them.

Jaw-Thrust Maneuver

A jaw-thrust maneuver may be used instead of the head-tilt/chin-lift. Note, however, that it is tiring and technically difficult. It is the safest approach to opening the airway in a patient with suspected spine injury. With it, the patient's head and neck are brought into a neutral position. This means the head is not turned to the side, tilted forward, or tilted back.

Use the jaw-thrust maneuver on unresponsive patients who are injured or who have suspected spine injury. To perform it (Figure 6–5):

1. Kneel above the patient's head. Place your elbows on the surface where the patient is lying. Place one hand on each side of the head.
2. Grasp the angles of the patient's lower jaw on both sides. (If the patient is an infant or child, place two or three fingers of each hand at the angle of the jaw.)
3. Use a lifting motion to move the jaw forward with both hands. This pulls the tongue away from the back of the throat.
4. Keep the patient's mouth slightly open. If necessary, pull back the lower lip with the thumb of your gloved hand.

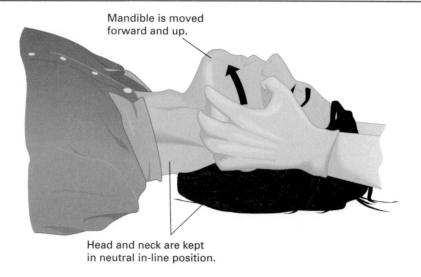

Mandible is moved forward and up.

Head and neck are kept in neutral in-line position.

Figure 6-5 Jaw-thrust maneuver.

If the jaw-thrust maneuver does not open the patient's airway, try again. Reposition the jaw and determine whether or not the airway is open. If repositioning does not work, insert an airway adjunct (described later in this chapter).

INSPECTING THE AIRWAY

Assess the airway of each and every one of your patients. A clear and open airway, or **patent airway,** is absolutely necessary for adequate breathing.

You can determine that a patient's airway is patent if he is alert, responsive, and talking to you in a normal voice. If you see that his mental status is altered, however, you have to look more closely. A patient who is drowsy, disoriented, confused or unresponsive may have blood, vomit, or excess saliva in the airway.

To inspect the airway of an unresponsive patient, first open the patient's mouth with a gloved hand. If necessary, use a **cross-finger technique.** That is, kneel above the patient. Then cross the thumb and forefinger of one hand. Place the thumb on the patient's lower incisors and the forefinger on the upper incisors. Then use a scissors-like or finger-snapping motion to open the patient's mouth. When the mouth is open, look inside for fluids and solids, including broken teeth or dentures that may be blocking the airway. Finally, listen for unusual sounds.

Sounds that may indicate an airway obstruction include:

- Snoring—may indicate the upper airway is blocked by the tongue or by relaxed tissues in the throat.
- **Crowing**—like the cawing of a crow, may mean the muscles around the larynx are in spasm.
- Gurgling—blood, vomit, mucus, or another liquid may be in the airway.
- **Stridor**—a harsh, high-pitched sound during inhalation, may indicate the larynx is swollen and blocking the upper airway.

AIRWAY ADJUNCTS

Once the airway is open, it may be necessary to insert an **airway adjunct** (an artificial airway). There are two kinds—the **oropharyngeal airway** and the **nasopharyngeal airway.** Both extend down to, but do not pass through, the larynx. They often are used when patients are being artificially ventilated.

When using airway adjuncts, remember the following:

- The airway adjunct must be clean and clear of any obstructions.
- The proper size must be used to be effective and to prevent complications.

- A patient with an airway adjunct can still aspirate (inhale) secretions, blood, vomit, or other foreign substances into the lungs.
- The patient's mental status and gag reflex will tell you if an airway adjunct is appropriate. That is, in general, if the patient is unresponsive with no gag reflex, use the oropharyngeal airway. If the patient is responsive or has a gag reflex, use the nasopharyngeal airway.
- You must continually and carefully monitor the patient's mental status. If he becomes completely responsive or gags, you must remove the airway adjunct.

Oropharyngeal Airway

The oropharyngeal, or oral, airway is a semicircular device made of hard plastic or rubber (Figure 6–6). It is designed to hold the tongue away from the back of the throat at the level of the pharynx. It also allows secretions to drain in a patient without a gag reflex.

There are two common types. One is tubular, and the other has a channeled side. Both types are disposable and come in a variety of adult, child, and infant sizes.

The oral airway can be used to help maintain and open the airway of an unresponsive patient who has no gag reflex. Do not use this device on a patient who is responsive or has a gag reflex. If you do, it may cause vomiting or spasm of the vocal cords, which will further compromise the airway.

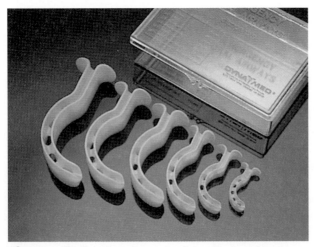

Figure 6-6 Oropharyngeal (oral) airways.

To insert an oropharyngeal airway, follow these steps (Figure 6–7).

1. *Select the proper size.* It should extend from the corner of the lip to the angle of the jaw or to the tip of the earlobe. Note that if the device is too long, it can push the epiglottis over the opening of the trachea, closing off the airway completely.
2. *Open the patient's mouth.* If necessary, use the cross-finger technique.
3. *Insert the adjunct upside down.* Be sure the tip is pointing toward the roof of the patient's mouth.
4. *Advance the adjunct gently.* Stop when you encounter resistance. This will happen when the device comes in contact with the soft back of the roof of the mouth.
5. *Turn the airway 180°.* Do so while continuing to advance it until the flat flange at the top rests on the patient's front teeth. The airway follows the natural curve of the tongue and the oropharynx.

If the patient gags at any time during insertion, *remove the oropharyngeal airway.* It may then be necessary to use a nasopharyngeal (nasal) airway or no airway adjunct at all. If the patient tries to dislodge the device, remove it by gently pulling it out and down. Do not rotate the device during removal. Be prepared for vomiting.

If the patient is an infant or child, a preferred alternative is to use a tongue depressor (blade) to help insert the device. Proceed as follows (Figure 6–8):

1. Select the proper size.
2. Open the patient's mouth.
3. Insert the tongue depressor. Stop when its tip is at the base of the tongue. Press the tongue depressor, and therefore the tongue, down towards the floor of the mouth and away from the opening of the throat.
4. Insert the airway in its normal upright position. Stop when the flange is seated on the patient's teeth. (Do not insert it upside down as you would in an adult. If you do, it could cause bleeding in the airway.)

INSERTING AN OROPHARYNGEAL AIRWAY

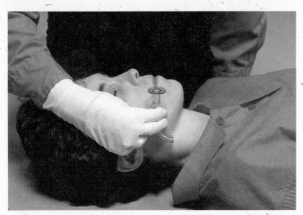

Figure 6-7a Measure to assure correct size.

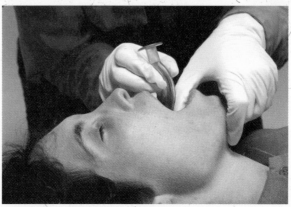

Figure 6-7b Insert with top pointing up toward the roof of the mouth.

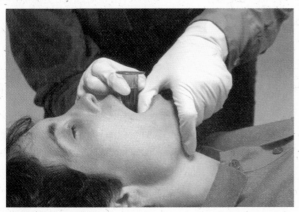

Figure 6-7c Gently rotate it until it reaches proper position.

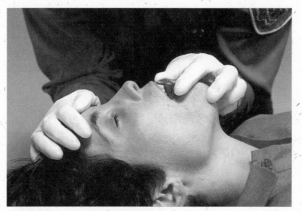

Figure 6-7d Continue until the flange rests on the patient's teeth.

Nasopharyngeal Airway

The nasopharyngeal, or nasal, airway is a curved hollow tube of soft plastic (Figure 6–9). It has a flange or flare at the top and a bevel at the bottom. It comes in a variety of sizes.

Nasal airways are less likely to cause vomiting than oral airways. This is because the soft tube moves and gives when the patient swallows. Use it to keep the tongue from blocking the airway in patients who are not fully responsive or who have a gag reflex. Use it also when the patient cannot take the oral airway or if the teeth are clenched tightly and will not open.

Even though a nasal airway is lubricated before insertion, it can be painful and may cause the lining of the nose to bleed into the airway.

To insert, follow these steps (Figure 6–10):

1. *Select the proper size.* It should extend from the tip of the patient's nose to the tip of the earlobe. Also, the diameter should fit inside the nostril without **blanching** (losing color from)

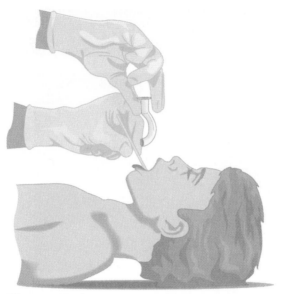

Figure 6-8 Inserting an oropharyngeal airway in an infant or child.

the skin of the nose. If it is too long, it could send air into the stomach instead of the lungs, causing massive **gastric distention** (inflation of the stomach) and inadequate ventilation.

2. *Lubricate the device.* Use a sterile, water-soluble lubricant. This makes the airway easier to insert. It also reduces the chances of injuring the nasal lining. Do not use petroleum jelly, which can damage the lining of the nose and throat.

3. *Insert the airway posteriorly.* The bevel should point toward the **septum** when it is inserted into the right nostril. (The septum is the wall

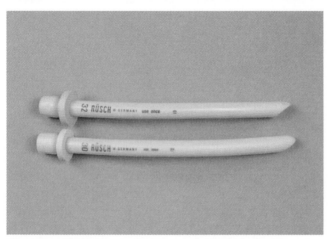

Figure 6-9 Nasopharyngeal (nasal) airways.

dividing the two nostrils.) Insert the device close to the midline, along the floor of the nostril, and straight back into the nasopharynx. When the airway is properly inserted, the flange should lie against the flare of the nostril.

4. If the airway cannot be inserted in one nostril, try the other nostril. Do not force a nasal airway into place. If you meet resistance, gently rotate it from side to side. If you still feel resistance, remove the airway.

After insertion, check to see that air is flowing through the airway as the patient breathes. If the patient is breathing spontaneously but no air movement is felt through the tube, remove it immediately and try inserting it in the other nostril.

Note that it is still necessary to maintain a head-tilt/chin-lift or jaw-thrust once the device is inserted.

CLEARING THE AIRWAY

There are three ways a First Responder can clear an airway of secretions—by the **recovery position, finger sweeps,** or **suctioning.** These techniques are not performed sequentially. The technique you choose depends on the patient's condition.

Recovery Position

If the patient is breathing adequately and has a pulse, the American Heart Association (AHA) recommends that you place him in the recovery position. It is the first step in maintaining an open airway.

This position uses gravity to keep the airway clear. It allows fluids to drain from the mouth instead of into the airway. The patient's airway is likely to remain open and airway obstructions are less likely to occur. Note that even though the patient is in a recovery position, you should continue to monitor him until the EMTs arrive and assume care.

Do not move the patient into the recovery position if you suspect trauma or spinal injury. It

INSERTING A NASOPHARYNGEAL AIRWAY

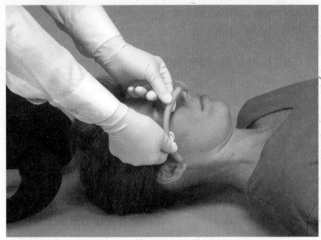

Figure 6-10a Measure the nasopharyngeal airway.

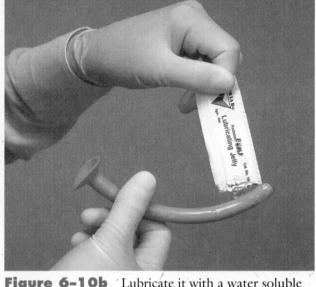

Figure 6-10b Lubricate it with a water soluble lubricant.

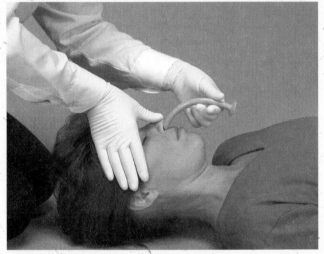

Figure 6-10c Insert the adjunct.

should be used for an unresponsive, uninjured patient who is breathing adequately. He or she should stay in that position until the ambulance arrives. (If the patient is not breathing or breathing inadequately, he or she must be supine so you can provide artificial ventilation.)

To move a patient into the recovery position, perform the following (Figure 6–11):

1. Lift the patient's left arm above his head. Then cross the patient's right leg over the left leg.
2. Support the patient's face as you grasp his right shoulder.
3. Roll the patient toward you onto his side (the left side, preferably). Then place his right hand under the side of his face. If possible,

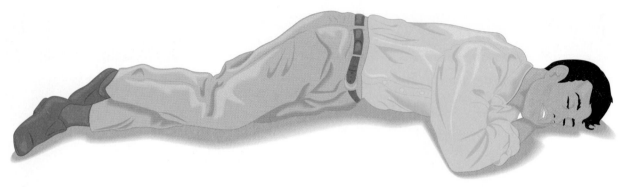

Figure 6-11 The recovery position.

move the patient's head, shoulders, and torso simultaneously as a unit without twisting. The head should be in as close to a midline position as possible.

4. Flex the patient's top leg at the knee.

Finger Sweeps

A finger sweep is performed only on unresponsive patients. In a finger sweep, you use your finger to remove solid objects from the airway. Always wear latex gloves when performing a finger sweep. Foreign material or vomit in the mouth should be removed quickly. Never probe deeply with your fingers in an infant's or child's mouth. (This is called a "blind" finger sweep.) If you do not see an object in the infant's or child's mouth, do not perform a finger sweep.

To perform a finger sweep on an uninjured unresponsive patient (Figure 6–12):

1. Roll the patient onto his left side. This position allows material to drain out of the mouth. It also helps to keep the tongue away from the back of the throat.
2. Open the patient's mouth and look inside. If you see liquids or semi-liquids, cover your gloved index and middle fingers with a cloth.
3. Wipe out the patient's mouth. Insert your index finger. Pass it along the inside of the cheek and into the throat at the base of the tongue. (Use your little finger for an infant or child.) Hook your finger to dislodge and remove any foreign object. Take extreme care that you do not force an object deeper into the patient's throat.

Suctioning

Suction devices use negative pressure to keep the airway clear. They remove blood, vomit, secretions, and other liquids from the mouth and airway. If you hear a gurgling sound during assessment or artificial ventilation, immediately suction the airway.

Most suction units cannot remove solid objects like teeth, particles of food, and other foreign bodies. Some cannot remove very thick vomit. In such situations, you may need to use an alternative piece of suction equipment or a finger sweep.

FINGER SWEEP

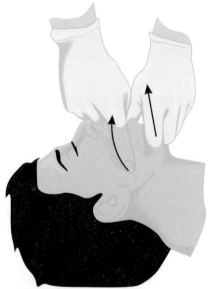

Figure 6-12 A finger sweep.

Suctioning Equipment. Portable suction units (Figure 6–13) can be manually or electrically powered. Some are oxygen- or air-powered. All produce a vacuum that can suction substances from the throat. Each should be inspected before a shift or on a regular basis.

Manual units do not require an energy source other than the person operating it. As a result, they lack some of the typical problems associated with electric- or oxygen-powered devices. They also can more effectively suction heavy substances, such as thick vomit.

Electric units must have fully charged batteries to function effectively. A low battery charge reduces the vacuum and the length of time the unit can be used. Some units allow for constant charging, so batteries remain full.

Any type of suction unit must have:

* Wide-bore, thick-walled, non-kinking tubing that fits a standard suction catheter.
* Several sterile disposable suction catheters. A "tonsil tip" (rigid plastic) is used to suction unresponsive patients. A soft and flexible one is generally used to suction the nose.
* An unbreakable collection bottle or container and a supply of water for rinsing and clearing tubes and catheters.
* Enough vacuum pressure and flow to suction substances from the throat effectively.

Principles of Suctioning. The procedure for suctioning varies, depending on the type of unit and catheter used. However, the following general principles apply (Figure 6–14):

1. Be sure to take body substance isolation precautions. Suctioning involves removal of body fluids. The potential for coughing and splatters is high. So wear protective eye wear, a mask, and gloves. If you suspect tuberculosis (TB), wear an N-95 or HEPA respirator the entire time you are in contact with the patient.
2. Use the correct type of catheter for your patient. Use a "tonsil tip" or "tonsil sucker" catheter to suction the mouth and throat of an unresponsive patient, or an infant or child. Use a flexible, or "French," catheter to suction the nose.

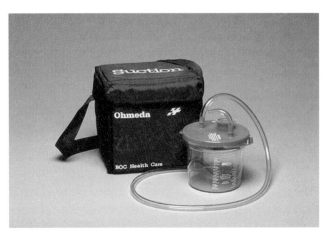

Figure 6-13 A portable suction unit.

3. Insert the catheter, without suction, only to the base of tongue. Place the convex (bulging) side of the catheter against the roof of the patient's mouth.
4. Apply suction by moving the catheter from side to side. Stop after 15 seconds in an adult, 10 seconds in a child, and 5 seconds in an infant.

Do not exceed the maximum times noted above. Air and oxygen are removed during suctioning, which can cause a quick drop in blood

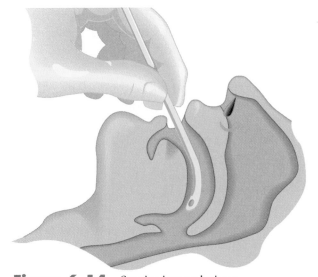

Figure 6-14 Suctioning technique.

oxygen levels and changes in heart rate. In an adult, watch for rapid, slow, or irregular heart rates. In an infant, watch for a decreased heart rate. If a decrease is noted, stop suctioning and reapply oxygen or ventilate for at least 30 seconds prior to suctioning again.

ASSESSING BREATHING

After you establish an open airway, determine if the patient's breathing is adequate. The brain, heart, and liver are most sensitive to inadequate oxygen. Brain cells start to die within minutes without an oxygen supply.

Determining the Presence of Breathing

Breathing should be effortless. Watch to determine whether or not the chest rises and falls as the patient breathes. Also check to see if the patient is using accessory muscles to breathe. Look for excessive use of the neck muscles or pulling inward of the muscles between the patient's ribs.

Observe a responsive patient for the ability to speak. This ability means the air is moving past the vocal cords. If the patient can only make sounds or can speak just a few words, breathing may be inadequate. Patients who can speak full sentences without showing signs of distress or obstruction are breathing adequately.

In an unresponsive patient, use the cross-finger technique, if needed. Then open the airway with the head-tilt/chin-lift or jaw-thrust maneuver. Place your ear close to the patient's mouth and nose for 3 to 5 seconds, and:

- *Look* for the rise and fall of the patient's chest.
- *Listen* for air coming out of the patient's mouth and nose.
- *Feel* for air coming out of the patient's nose and mouth.

If the airway is obstructed, the patient's chest may still rise and fall. However, air will not be moving in and out of the patient's nose or mouth.

Note that "agonal" respirations (reflex gasping with no regular pattern or depth) may occur with cardiac arrest. They may also be a late sign of impending respiratory arrest. These reflex gasps should not be confused with breathing.

Signs of Inadequate Breathing

It is very important for you to recognize the signs of inadequate breathing. Some are subtle and require careful evaluation. If you are not sure that a patient needs breathing assistance, it is better to err on the side of safety and provide ventilations.

Inadequate breathing is characterized by the following signs (Figure 6–15). Note, however, that not all of the signs will be present at the same time. Any one of them may be reason enough to ventilate a patient without delay.

- *Too fast or too slow breathing rate.* Rates of less than 8 respirations per minute in an adult, less than 10 in a child, and less than 20 in an infant are ominous signs of inadequate breathing.
- *Inadequate chest wall motion.* Adequate breathing is normally accompanied by the rise and fall

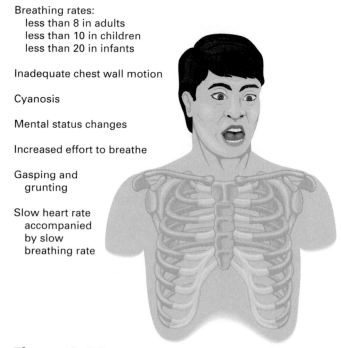

Breathing rates:
  less than 8 in adults
  less than 10 in children
  less than 20 in infants

Inadequate chest wall motion

Cyanosis

Mental status changes

Increased effort to breathe

Gasping and grunting

Slow heart rate accompanied by slow breathing rate

Figure 6-15   Signs of inadequate breathing.

of the chest. If the chest wall is not rising and falling as it should, or if the sides of the chest rise and fall unequally, breathing is inadequate.

- *Cyanosis.* This is a bluish discoloration of the skin and mucous membranes. It is a sign that body tissues are not receiving enough oxygen.
- *Mental status changes.* Remember that the mental status of a patient typically correlates with the status of his airway and breathing. A patient who becomes drowsy, disoriented, confused, or unresponsive may not be breathing adequately.
- *Increased effort to breathe.* Normal breathing is effortless. When you see a pronounced use of abdominal muscles to breathe, the patient is pushing on the diaphragm to force air out of the lungs. An infant also may develop a "see-saw" motion in which the abdomen and chest move in opposite directions. You may note retractions (pulling inward) between the ribs, above the collarbone, around the muscles of the neck, and below the rib cage as the patient inhales. Flaring of the nostrils during inhalation is another sign more commonly seen in infants and children.
- *Gasping and grunting.* These sounds mean the patient is having a difficult time moving air through the respiratory tract. Be alert for other abnormal sounds, such as snoring, crowing, gurgling, or stridor.
- *Slow heart rate accompanied by slow breathing rate.*

SECTION 3: GUIDELINES FOR EMERGENCY CARE

ARTIFICIAL VENTILATION

If a patient is breathing inadequately or is not breathing at all, that patient needs your immediate assistance. **Artificial ventilation** is a way of breathing for these patients.

The air we inhale contains about 21% oxygen. Only 5% is used by the body. The remaining 16% is exhaled. Since the air you breathe into a patient contains more than enough oxygen to keep him alive, artificial ventilation is sufficient to support life until high-concentration oxygen is available.

When performing artificial ventilation, monitor the patient continuously to make sure your breaths are adequate. Indications of adequate ventilations include:

- Rate of respiration is adequate—once every 3 seconds for infants and children, once every 5 seconds for adults.
- The force of air is consistent. It also is sufficient to cause the chest to rise during each ventilation.
- The patient's heart rate decreases or returns to normal. However, underlying medical conditions may prevent this from happening even when ventilations are adequate.
- The patient's color improves.

Inadequate ventilation may occur because of problems with the patient's airway or because of improper use of a ventilation device. Indications of inadequate ventilations include:

- The chest does not rise and fall with each ventilation.
- The ventilation rate is too fast or too slow.
- The heart rate does not decrease or return to normal.

The risk of coming in contact with a patient's secretions, blood, or vomit while ventilating are high. Therefore, you must take BSI precautions. At a minimum, use gloves, eye wear, and a pocket face mask or other barrier device with a one-way filter. If large amounts of blood or secretions are present, use a face mask.

There are many techniques for artificial ventilation. A First Responder must be competent in three, listed here in order of preference: **mouth-to-mask**, **mouth-to-barrier device**, and **mouth-to-mouth**.

Mouth-to-Mask Ventilation

The most effective First Responder technique for ventilation is mouth-to-mask. A pocket face mask with a one-way valve is used to form a seal around the patient's nose and mouth (Figure 6–16). You

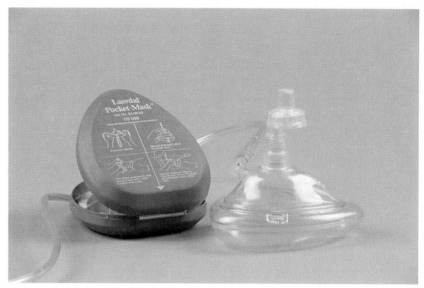

Figure 6-16   A pocket face mask with one-way valve and oxygen port.

blow into a port at the top of the mask to deliver the ventilation. The one-way valve diverts the patient's exhaled breath.

Mouth-to-mask is the preferred technique because it eliminates direct contact with the patient's nose, mouth, and body fluids. It prevents exposure to the patient's exhaled air. It also allows you to deliver ventilations of adequate force. The mask you use should have the following characteristics.

- It should be transparent, so you can see vomit, blood, or other substances in the patient's mouth.
- It must fit snugly enough on the patient's face to form a good seal.
- It should be available in an average adult size and in additional sizes for infants and children.
- It must have a one-way valve, or it must be able to connect to a one-way valve at the ventilation port.
- If you have oxygen available, the mask must have an oxygen inlet port.

Mouth-to-mask ventilation is very effective because both your hands are used to create a seal around the mask. To perform the technique, position yourself at the top of the patient's head.

Attach oxygen to the mask, if available. Then follow these steps (Figures 6–17 and 6–18).

1. *Position the mask on the patient.* The narrower top portion of the mask should be seated on the bridge of the nose. The broader portion should fit in the cleft of the chin. The position of the mask is critical. If it is wrong, it will leak and prevent you from delivering adequate ventilations.

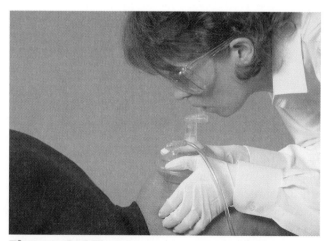

Figure 6-17   You must maintain a jaw-thrust during artificial ventilation of a patient with suspected spinal injury.

ARTIFICIAL VENTILATION

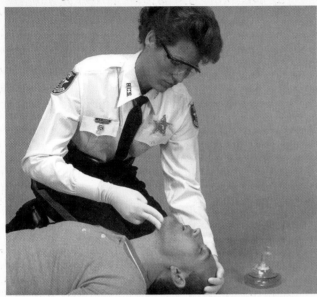

Figure 6-18a Open the airway with a head-tilt/chin lift maneuver.

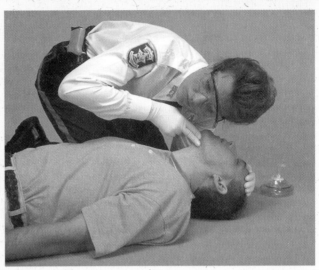

Figure 6-18b Look, listen, and feel to establish breathlessness.

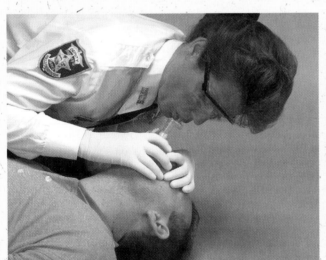

Figure 6-18c Deliver two slow intial breaths.

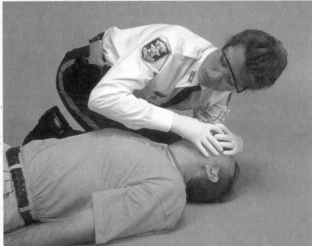

Figure 6-18d If successful, you will see the chest fall and feel the exhaled air on your cheek after each breath. If successful, continue ventilations at the proper rate.

2. *Seal the mask.* Place both thumbs on the top portion. Place the heels and palms of both hands along the sides. Compress the mask firmly around the edges to form a good seal.

3. *Open the patient's airway.* Place your index fingers on the part of the mask that covers the chin. Using your middle and ring fingers of both hands, grasp along the mandible (the bony part of the jaw). Pull upward to perform the maneuver. Use a jaw-thrust maneuver if trauma is suspected.

4. *Deliver two slow initial breaths.* Place your mouth around the one-way valve and blow into the ventilation port. Each breath should be slow (delivered over 1.5 to 2 seconds for an adult and 1 to 1.5 seconds for an infant or child). It also should be steady and of sufficient volume to make the chest rise (usually 800 to 1200 ml in an average adult). Make sure that you do not deliver too much air too fast, or you will force air into the patient's stomach.

5. *Determine if ventilations are adequate.* Watch the chest rise and fall. Listen and feel for air escaping when the patient exhales.

6. *Continue ventilations at the proper rate* (Table 6–2). For adults, deliver 10–12 breaths per minute with each lasting 1.5 to 2 seconds. For infants and children, deliver 20 breaths per minute with each lasting 1 to 1.5

seconds. For a newborn, deliver 40 breaths per minute with each breath lasting 1 to 1.5 seconds.

7. *If you cannot ventilate the patient or if the chest does not rise adequately,* position the patient's head and try again. (Improper head position is the most common cause of difficulty with ventilation.) If the second try also fails, assume the airway is blocked by a foreign object. Then follow the guidelines (later in this chapter) for removing it.

Mouth-to-Barrier Device Ventilation

A barrier device, such as a face shield, can be used during ventilation (Figure 6–19). It provides some of the same protection to the First Responder as a pocket face mask. A thin and flexible plastic face shield also can be folded and carried easily. Some are available in key-ring and belt-storage containers.

Barrier devices are thin enough to provide very low resistance to the ventilations you deliver to the patient. And they can provide some protection against contamination from body fluids. However, many do not have a one-way valve that diverts the patient's exhaled air.

To provide ventilations using a barrier device, kneel at the patient's head. Then follow these steps.

1. *Position the device on the patient.*
2. *Open the patient's airway.* Use a head-tilt/chin-lift or a jaw-thrust maneuver.
3. *Deliver two slow initial breaths.* Place your mouth over the barrier device and blow into

TABLE 6-2

ARTIFICIAL VENTILATION RATES

Newborn	40 breaths per minute at 1.0 to 1.5 seconds each
Infant	20 breaths per minute at 1.0 to 1.5 seconds each
Child	20 breaths per minute at 1.0 to 1.5 seconds each
Adult	10–12 breaths per minute at 1.5 to 2.0 seconds each

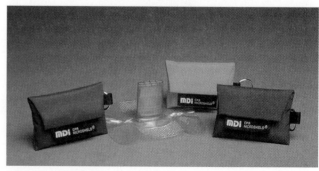

Figure 6-19 Example of a barrier device.

it. Each breath should be slow (delivered over 1.5 to 2 seconds for an adult and 1 to 1.5 seconds for an infant or child). It also should be steady and of sufficient volume to make the chest rise. Make sure that you do not deliver too much air too fast, or you will force air into the patient's stomach.

4. *Determine if ventilations are adequate.* Watch the chest rise and fall. Listen and feel for air escaping when the patient exhales.

5. *Continue ventilations at the proper rate.* For adults, deliver 10-12 breaths per minute, each lasting 1.5 to 2 seconds. For infants and children, deliver 20 breaths per minute, each lasting 1 to 1.5 seconds. For a newborn, deliver 40 breaths per minute, each breath lasting 1 to 1.5 seconds.

6. *If you cannot ventilate the patient or if the chest does not rise adequately,* position the patient's head and try again. If the second try also fails, assume the airway is blocked by a foreign object. Then follow the guidelines (later in this chapter) for removing a foreign body airway obstruction.

Mouth-to-Mouth Ventilation

The risk of contracting infectious diseases makes mouth-to-mouth ventilation too dangerous for regular use by First Responders. As described earlier, barrier devices and face masks with one-way valves are available. You should always use them as a BSI precaution. However, your decision is a personal one. Mouth-to-mask and mouth-to-barrier device techniques should not replace training in mouth-to-mouth ventilation.

Mouth-to-mouth ventilation is a quick, effective method of delivering oxygen to a nonbreathing patient. It involves ventilating the patient with your exhaled breath while making mouth-to-mouth contact. Use the mouth-to-mouth technique only in emergency situations in which no protective devices are available. For example, you may find that you need to perform mouth-to-mouth on a family member at home where a barrier device is not available.

In mouth-to-mouth, you form a seal with your mouth around the patient's mouth. The obvious risk to you is exposure to body fluids and thus to infectious disease.

To perform the technique, kneel at the patient's head. Then follow these steps.

1. *Open the patient's airway.* Use a head-tilt/chin-lift or a jaw-thrust maneuver.

2. *Form an airtight seal.* Gently squeeze the patient's nostrils closed with the thumb and index finger of the hand that is holding the patient's head tilt. Take a deep breath and form an airtight seal with your lips around the patient's mouth. If you are ventilating an infant or small child, cover both the nose and mouth with your lips.

3. *Deliver two slow initial breaths* (over 1.5 to 2 seconds for an adult and 1 to 1.5 seconds for an infant or child). Each should be steady and of sufficient volume to make the chest rise. Make sure that you do not deliver too much air too fast, or you will force air into the patient's stomach.

4. *Determine if ventilations are adequate.* Watch the chest rise and fall. Listen and feel for air escaping when the patient exhales.

5. *Continue ventilations at the proper rate.* For adults, deliver 10-12 breaths per minute, each lasting 1.5 to 2 seconds. For infants and children, deliver 20 breaths per minute, each lasting 1 to 1.5 seconds. For a newborn, deliver 40 breaths per minute, each breath lasting 1 to 1.5 seconds.

6. *If you cannot ventilate the patient or if the chest does not rise adequately,* position the patient's head and try again. If the second try also fails, assume the airway is blocked by a foreign object. Then follow the guidelines (later in this chapter) for removing a foreign body airway obstruction.

Mouth-to-Stoma Ventilation

A patient who has had all or part of the larynx surgically removed has had a laryngectomy (Figure 6–20). This patient will have a **stoma,** a permanent opening that connects the trachea directly to the front of the neck. These patients breathe only through the stoma.

To perform artificial ventilation on a patient with a stoma, remove all coverings such as scarves or ties from the stoma area. Then follow these steps (Figure 6–21):

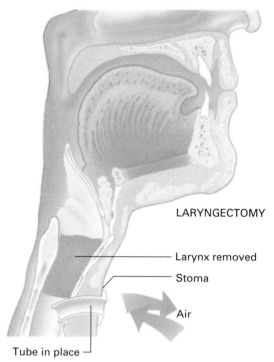

LARYNGECTOMY

Larynx removed

Stoma

Air

Tube in place

Figure 6-20   The neck breather's airway has been changed by surgery.

1. *Clear the stoma of any foreign matter.* Use a gauze pad or handkerchief. Do not use tissue, which can shred and cling.
2. *Form an airtight seal around the stoma.* Whenever possible, use a barrier device such as a pocket face mask or shield.

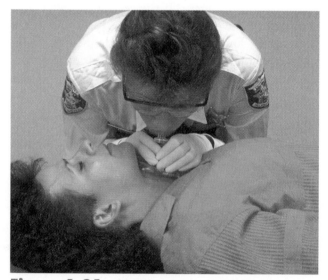

Figure 6-21   Mask-to-stoma ventilation.

3. *Blow slowly through the stoma* for 1.5 to 2 seconds. Use just enough force to make the patient's chest rise.
4. *Determine if ventilations are adequate.* Allow time for exhalation. Watch for the patient's chest to fall. Feel to make sure air is escaping back through the stoma as the patient exhales.
5. *Continue ventilations at the proper rate.* For adults, deliver 10-12 breaths per minute with each lasting 1.5 to 2 seconds. For infants and children, deliver 20 breaths per minute with each lasting 1 to 1.5 seconds. For a newborn, deliver 40 breaths per minute with each breath lasting 1 to 1.5 seconds.

If the chest does not rise, the patient may be a "partial neck breather." This patient has had only part of the larynx removed. He or she can breathe through both the stoma and the mouth and nose. Seal the patient's nose and mouth with one hand. Pinch off the nose between your third and fourth fingers. Seal the lips with the palm of the same gloved hand. Hook your thumb under the patient's chin, and press up and back. Continue ventilations through the stoma.

Infants and Children

Many of the steps involved in managing the airway of an infant or child are the same as those for an adult. However, remember there are important differences.

You must position the head carefully when preparing for artificial ventilation. Keep an infant's head in a neutral ("sniffing") position. You can extend the head slightly beyond neutral if the patient is older than one year. But do not extend the infant's or child's head too far. The airway is more flexible than an adult's and can be easily overextended, which can in itself block the airway.

Consider an oral airway for an infant or child. The primary cause of blocked airway in these patients is the tongue. Try positioning the head and pulling the jaw forward to move the tongue away from the back of the throat. If that is unsuccessful, use an oropharyngeal airway to keep the tongue away from the throat and the airway open.

Depending on the age and size of an infant, you may be able to form a seal with your mouth over the infant's mouth and nose. If an adult pocket face mask must be used, position the mask upside down (Figure 6–22).

Guard against gastric distention (inflation of the stomach). It is common in infants and children who are being ventilated. During artificial ventilation, air may get into the esophagus and stomach if ventilations are too forceful. Gastric distention may significantly impair your attempts at ventilation, because it forces the diaphragm up, limiting the amount of air that can enter the lungs. Monitor the infant or child carefully to make sure the chest is rising and falling with ventilations. Listen and feel for exhaled air. Watch carefully to make sure the abdomen does not start to extend.

The American Heart Association (AHA) recommends against pressing on the abdomen to relieve gastric distention. To help avoid gastric distention keep the following points in mind:

- Breathe slowly and with just enough force to make the chest rise. If you notice that the abdomen is starting to distend, reduce the force of your ventilations.
- Keep the infant's or child's head in a neutral position.
- Allow the infant or child to exhale between ventilations.
- Monitor against vomiting. If it looks like the infant or child is about to vomit, stop ventilat-

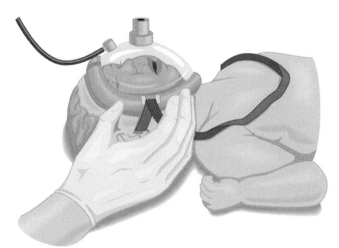

Figure 6-22 On an infant, the pocket face mask is reversed.

ing immediately and roll him onto his side. This position allows the vomit to flow from the mouth rather than into the lungs. If the infant or child vomits, suction or quickly wipe the mouth out with gauze pads. Wipe off the face, and return to ventilation.

Patients with Dental Appliances

If the patient has dentures that are secure in the mouth, leave them in place. It is much easier to create an airtight seal with them there. If the dentures are extremely loose, remove them so they do not block the airway. Partial dentures—plates and bridges—may become dislodged, too. If they are loose, remove them.

Reassess the mouth frequently in patients who have dental appliances to make sure they have not come loose.

Bag-Valve-Mask Ventilation

The bag-valve-mask (BVM) is a hand-operated device (Figure 6–23). It consists of a self-inflating bag, one-way valve, face mask, and oxygen reservoir. The BVM device has a volume of about 1600 milliliters. When used with oxygen, it can deliver almost 100% oxygen to the patient.

Note that two rescuers are highly recommended to operate a BVM. It is too difficult and tiring for one rescuer to work alone. If you are alone, we recommend that you use a pocket face mask, which is easier for one rescuer to create a seal.

The BVM is available in infant, child, and adult sizes. Whatever the size, it should have the following features:

- Self-refilling bag that is disposable or easily cleaned and sterilized.
- Non-jam valve that allows a maximum oxygen inlet flow of 15 liters per minute or greater.
- No pop-off valve. If there is one, it can be disabled. Failure to do so may result in inadequate ventilations.
- Standardized 15/22 mm fittings.
- Oxygen inlet and reservoir that allows for a high concentration of oxygen.
- True nonrebreather valve.
- Ability to perform in all environments and temperature extremes.

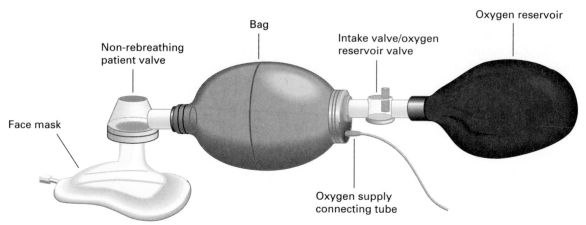

Figure 6-23 Bag-valve-mask unit.

To provide artificial ventilation by way of a BVM, follow these steps:

1. *Open the patient's airway.* Note that an oral or nasal airway may be necessary in conjunction with the BVM. Note, if you suspect injury to the head or spine, stabilize the patient's head between your knees or have an assistant manually stabilize it.
2. *Select the correct size mask*—adult, child, or infant size.
3. *Position the mask.* Place your thumbs over the top half of the mask. Index and middle fingers should be over the bottom half. Then put the narrow end (apex) of the mask over the bridge of the patient's nose. Lower the mask over the mouth and upper chin. If the mask has a large round cuff around a ventilation port, center the port over the patient's mouth. Use your ring and little fingers to bring the jaw up to the mask. Use the jaw-thrust, if you suspect head or spine injury. Be sure to avoid tilting the head or neck.
4. *Connect the mask to the bag*, if it has not already been done.
5. *Operate the bag* (Figure 6–24). Your partner should squeeze the bag with two hands until the patient's chest rises. For adults, deliver 10-12 breaths per minute with each lasting 1.5 to 2 seconds. For infants and children, deliver 20 breaths per minute with each lasting 1 to 1.5 seconds.

If you are alone, form a "C" around the ventilation port with your thumb and index fingers. Use your middle, ring, and little fingers under the jaw to maintain a chin lift and complete the seal. Squeeze the bag with your other hand while observing the chest rise and fall.

If the chest does not rise and fall with your ventilations, reposition the patient's head or jaw. Check again for an airway obstruction. If air is escaping from under the mask, reposition your fingers and check the position of the mask. If the patient's chest still does not rise, use an alternative method such as mask-to-mouth ventilation.

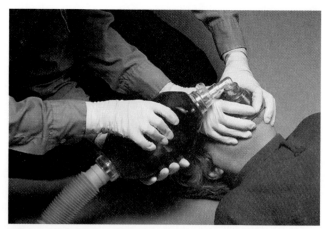

Figure 6-24 Two rescuers operating a bag-valve-mask unit.

Assisting Inadequate Breathing

If your patient is breathing but breathing inadequately, you must assist. Provide ventilations while the patient is inhaling or trying to breathe on his or her own.

Since inadequate breathing is often slower than usual, you will need to provide additional ventilations in between the patient's own attempts to breathe. If breathing is rapid and very shallow, and therefore inadequate, provide assisted ventilations when the patient begins a respiration. You will find that providing a ventilation while the patient is exhaling can create resistance or an unusual noise.

Simply continue to time your assisted ventilations as best you can with the patient's own respiratory effort. To recognize inadequate breathing and then to assist the patient with ventilations are among the best things you can do for your patient. Your intervention may prevent him or her from lapsing into complete respiratory and cardiac arrest.

OXYGEN THERAPY

Oxygen equipment can be an excellent tool for a well-trained First Responder. It allows you to deliver oxygen to patients who desperately need it. However, if you are not allowed to administer oxygen in your EMS system, do not wait for it to arrive before providing emergency care.

Indications

Conditions that may require oxygen therapy include injury, heart or breathing problems, shock, and any other condition that prevents the efficient flow of oxygen throughout the body. Signs and symptoms that indicate the need for oxygen are:

- Poor skin color (blue, gray, or pale).
- Unresponsiveness.
- Cool, clammy skin.
- Difficulty breathing.
- Blood loss.
- Chest pain.
- Trauma (injury).

Note that when you provide artificial ventilation, you can give a higher concentration of oxygen to the patient by connecting supplemental oxygen to your pocket face mask.

Oxygen Cylinders

All oxygen cylinders are manufactured according to strict governmental (U.S. Department of Transportation) regulations. According to those regulations, cylinders must be checked for safety at least once in 5 years. New cylinders should be checked every 10 years. (See Figure 6–25 for a portable oxygen cylinder.)

A number of different types of oxygen cylinders are available. They vary in size and volume. Even though the volume of oxygen may vary, all of the cylinders when full are at the same pressure, about 2000 psi. Cylinder sizes are identified by letter. The following are sizes used in emergency medical care:

- D cylinder — 350 liters.
- E cylinder — 625 liters.
- M cylinder — 3000 liters.
- G cylinder — 5300 liters.
- H cylinder — 6900 liters.

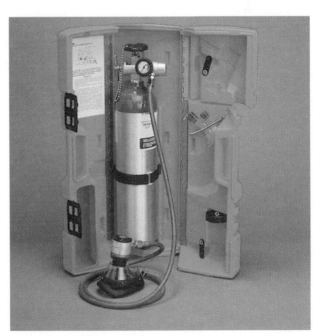

Figure 6-25 A basic portable oxygen cylinder.

Gas flow from an oxygen cylinder is controlled by regulators. They reduce pressure in the cylinder to a safe range of about 50 psi and control the flow to 15-25 liters per minute. Regulators are attached to the cylinder by a yoke. Each yoke fits only the cylinders made for one type of gas. In addition, all gas cylinders are color coded according to contents. Oxygen cylinders in the U.S. are generally steel green or aluminum gray.

Two types of regulators may be attached to oxygen cylinders. They are *high-pressure regulators* and *therapy regulators*.

The high-pressure regulator can provide 50 psi to power a demand-valve type resuscitator (flow-restricted oxygen-powered ventilation device) or a suction device. It has a threaded outlet and one gauge, which registers cylinder contents. It cannot be used interchangeably with the therapy regulator. It has no mechanism to adjust flow rate, and it is designed specifically for use with other equipment. To use a high-pressure regulator, attach the equipment supply line to the threaded outlet and open the cylinder valve fully. Then back off one-half turn for safety.

The therapy regulator can administer up to 15-25 liters of oxygen per minute. It has two gauges. One shows cylinder contents and the other allows you to provide a metered flow of oxygen to the patient. The cylinder is full when the pressure is 2000 psi or greater. This pressure drops in direct proportion to the contents. For example, if the pressure is 1000 psi, the cylinder is half full. Adjust the flow meter to provide oxygen appropriate to the device used and the condition of the patient. Follow local protocol.

Safety Precautions. Observe the following safety precautions when you handle oxygen cylinders:

- Never allow combustible materials, such as oil or grease, to touch the cylinder, regulator, fittings, valves, or hoses.
- Never smoke or allow others to smoke in any area where oxygen cylinders are in use or on standby.
- Store the cylinders below 125° Fahrenheit.
- Never use an oxygen cylinder without a safe, properly fitting regulator valve.

- Never use a valve made for another gas, even if it has been modified.
- Keep all valves closed when the oxygen cylinder is not in use, even when a tank is empty.
- Keep oxygen cylinders secure to prevent them from toppling over. In transit, they should be in a carrier rack.
- Never place any part of your body over the cylinder valve. A loosely fitting regulator can be blown off with sufficient force to amputate a head.
- Never stand an oxygen tank upright near the patient. If the tank is not in a commercial pack, lie it on its side by the patient.

Using the Cylinders. Prepare the tank if it is not used every day by following these steps (Figure 6–26):

1. Place the cylinder securely upright, and place yourself to the side. Then identify the cylinder as oxygen and remove the protective seal.
2. "Crack" the tank with the wrench supplied. Slowly open and rapidly close the cylinder valve to clear it of debris.
3. Inspect the regulator valve to be certain that it is the right type of oxygen cylinder. Be sure it has an intact washer. Place the yoke of the regulator over the cylinder valve and align the pins.
4. Hand-tighten the T-screw on the regulator.
5. Open the main cylinder valve to check the pressure. Make one-half turn beyond the point where the regulator valve becomes pressurized. Read the gauge to be sure that the tank has an adequate amount of oxygen. Most tanks will not function with less than 200 psi. Many organizations have a policy to replace or refill oxygen tanks that get below 500 psi.
6. Attach the oxygen-delivery device to the regulator.
7. Adjust the flow meter to the appropriate liter flow.
8. Apply the oxygen delivery device to the patient.

When you are ready to stop oxygen therapy, detach the mask from the patient. Then shut off the control valve until the liter flow is at zero.

OXYGEN ADMINISTRATION

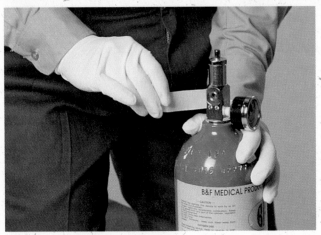

Figure 6-26a   Identify the cylinder as oxygen and remove the protective seal.

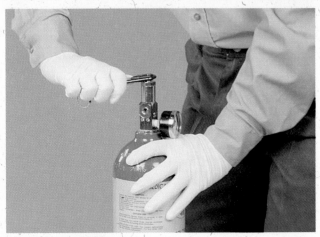

Figure 6-26b   Crack the main cylinder for one second to remove dust and debris.

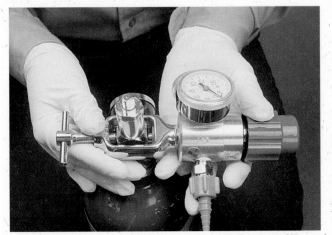

Figure 6-26c   Place the yoke of the regulator over the cylinder valve and align the pins.

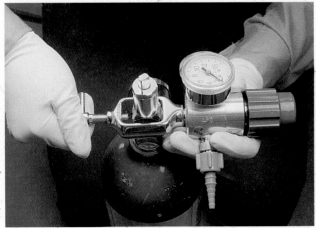

Figure 6-26d   Hand-tighten the T-screw on the regulator.   *(Continued)*

Shut off the main cylinder valve. Then bleed the valves by leaving the control valve open until the needle or ball indicator returns to zero. Shut the control valve on all tanks you carry.

It should be part of your daily routine to check the oxygen tank carried in your vehicle. You should open the main cylinder valve and check the pressure remaining on the cylinder. It is very discouraging, not to mention negligent, to arrive at the scene of a crash with lights, sirens, and other fanfare only to find that you have an empty oxygen cylinder.

Always replace a cylinder when the pressure is low. Have backup portable oxygen cylinders in your vehicle. Note that oxygen itself does not burn. It does, however, feed and support

OXYGEN ADMINISTRATION (Continued)

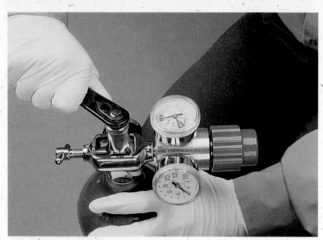

Figure 6-26e Open the main cylinder valve to check the pressure.

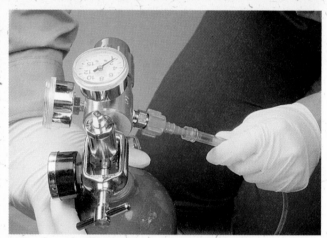

Figure 6-26f Attach the oxygen-delivery device to the regulator.

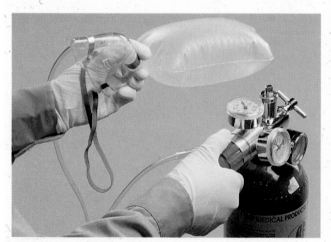

Figure 6-26g Adjust the flow meter to the appropriate liter flow.

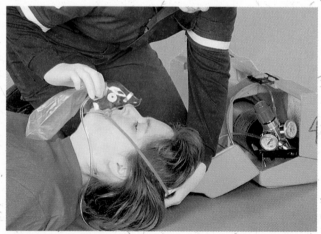

Figure 6-26h Apply the oxygen delivery device to the patient.

combustion, especially when the oxygen is pressurized. Make absolutely sure that there are no open flames in the area when you are using oxygen.

Oxygen Delivery Equipment

A variety of devices are available to deliver oxygen to the patient. Proper training in their use is essential. Follow all local protocols.

Oxygen equipment either delivers low- or high-flow oxygen. Use low-flow oxygen through a **nasal cannula.** Use high-flow oxygen through a **nonrebreather mask.** Note that the patient must be breathing in order for you to use either of these devices. If the patient is not breathing or is breathing inadequately, begin artificial ventilation with supplemental oxygen.

Nasal Cannula. One of the most common oxygen devices is the nasal cannula. Its two soft plastic tips are inserted a short distance into the nostrils. The tips are attached to the oxygen source with thin tubing. It is comfortable and convenient. Most patients are able to tolerate it with ease.

The nasal cannula provides safe, comfortable, low-flow oxygen in concentrations of 24% to 44% with a one- to six-liter flow. It should be used at low rates of less than six liters per minute. Higher flows can cause headaches, drying of the membranes in the nose, and nosebleeds.

The nasal cannula is good for patients who are anxious about a mask, for patients who are nauseated or vomiting, and in situations in which you need to communicate with the patient.

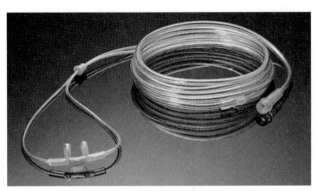

Figure 6-27a Nasal cannula.

To use a nasal cannula (Figure 6–27):

1. Set liter flow to the desired rate. Make sure oxygen flows from the cannula tips.
2. Insert the two tips into the nostrils with the tab facing out.
3. Position the tubing over and behind each ear. Gently secure it by sliding the adjuster underneath the chin.

Do not adjust the tubing too tightly. If an elastic strap is used, adjust it so that it is secure but comfortable. If the tubing causes irritation, pad the patient's cheeks and behind the ears with 2″ × 2″ gauze pads. Be sure to check placement often. The cannula can be dislodged easily.

Nonrebreather Mask. A nonrebreather mask has an oxygen reservoir bag and a one-way valve. The one-way valve allows the patient to inhale from the bag and exhale through the valve. Adjust the oxygen flow to prevent the bag from collapsing during inhalation, using about 10 to 15 liters per minute.

A nonrebreather mask requires a tight seal. If fitted properly to the face, it can deliver oxygen concentrations up to 90%. So it is ideally suited for patients who have severe hypoxemia, such as those with chest pain or injuries. Remember that flow rate must be adequate to keep the bag inflated as the patient breathes. If the bag collapses, the patient will not receive oxygen and

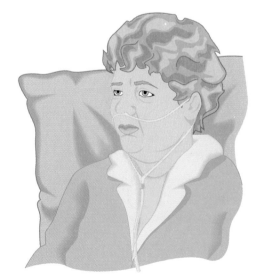

Figure 6-27b Nasal cannula applied to a patient.

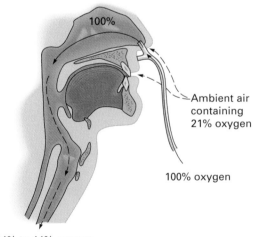

may suffocate. Be ready to remove the mask if the patient vomits. Note also that caution must be exercised when using this device on patients with some chronic lung diseases. (See "Special Considerations" below.)

To use the nonrebreather mask (Figure 6–28):

1. Select a mask with the oxygen supply tube preattached. The other end attaches to the oxygen source.

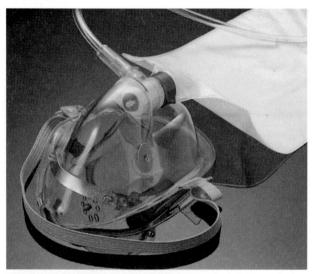

Figure 6-28a A nonrebreather mask.

2. Turn on the oxygen at 10 to 15 liters per minute to fill the bag. Then set the flow at the prescribed level. Make sure the bag is full before using it.
3. Gently place the mask over the patient's face. Slip the loosened elastic strap over the head so that it is positioned below or above the ears. Then pull the ends of the elastic until the mask fits the patient's face. Note that you should not lift the head of a trauma patient. Such movement may worsen a spine injury. Instead, gently tape the mask to the patient's cheeks. Then, monitor the airway.

Some masks have a thin piece of metal where the mask covers the bridge of the patient's nose. To ensure a good seal, that metal should be pinched so that the mask conforms to the shape of the nose.

Patients who have trouble breathing or who are in shock may get anxious when you try to place a mask on them. To these patients, it feels as if they are being suffocated. Try to convince them to accept the mask. Explain to the patient what the mask is and why you are using it. You might tell them that the mask can feel confining, but that it also provides the high concentration of oxygen they need. As a last resort, use a nasal cannula to provide some oxygen.

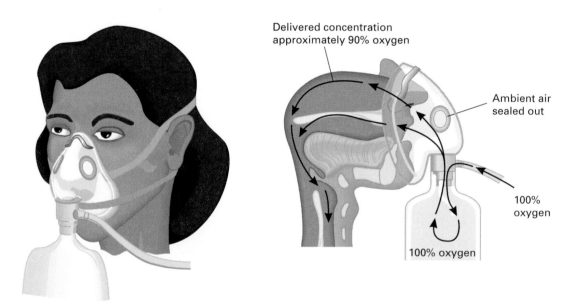

Figure 6-28b Nonrebreather mask applied to a patient.

Special Considerations

WARNING! The term "respiratory depression" refers to a slow breathing rate of less than 8 breaths per minute. It is sometimes the result when oxygen is applied to patients who have a chronic obstruction pulmonary disease (COPD) such as emphysema or chronic bronchitis. Beware of this rare complication.

Respiratory depression sometimes happens to patients with COPD. Their drive to breathe may come from the lack of oxygen (hypoxic drive). Very high oxygen levels may eliminate the COPD patient's drive in isolated cases.

COPD patients cannot eliminate carbon dioxide properly. Their breath centers have become used to high carbon dioxide and low oxygen levels. They are stimulated to breathe by oxygen receptors in the aorta and carotid arteries. So, oxygen therapy may supply high enough oxygen levels to stop the body's messages to breathe.

Be sure to ask your patient if there is a history of respiratory disease before beginning oxygen therapy. If patients suffer from COPD, closely monitor their breathing as you give oxygen. If a COPD patient's breathing rate becomes very slow or shallow, of if the patient begins to get groggy or sleepy, assist ventilations with a pocket face mask or bag-valve-mask device.

Although cautions must be used, oxygen should never be withheld from any patient who needs it. A COPD patient who has been injured in a car crash, for example, will most likely need high concentrations of oxygen. A COPD patient who complains of minor respiratory distress may not need such aggressive care.

FOREIGN BODY AIRWAY OBSTRUCTION (FBAO)

An upper airway obstruction is anything that blocks the nasal passages, the back of the mouth, or the throat. A lower airway obstruction can be caused by breathing in a foreign body or by severe spasm of the bronchial passages. *A foreign body airway obstruction (FBAO) is a true emergency.* It must be cleared from the airway before the patient can breathe and before you can give artificial ventilation.

Airway obstruction in a responsive patient can be the cause of cardiac arrest. The most common FBAO is food. If your patient was eating prior to collapsing, suspect he or she choked on food. Elderly people are at risk for choking because they have a weaker gag reflex. As a result, they are more frequently misdiagnosed as having heart disease if they collapse. Other common causes of airway obstruction in a responsive patient are bleeding into the airway and aspirated vomit.

Airway obstruction can also be the result of cardiac arrest. In an unresponsive patient, an FBAO may be caused by vomiting, loose or broken dentures or bridges, or injury to the face or jaw. The most common source of upper airway obstruction in an unresponsive patient is the tongue.

Other causes of airway obstruction include secretions, blood clots, cancerous conditions of the mouth or throat, enlarged tonsils, and acute epiglottitis.

Types of FBAO

There are two types of foreign body airway obstruction (FBAO)—partial and complete.

A partial FBAO means an object is caught in the throat but it does not totally occlude (block) breathing. Even if he or she has good air exchange, you should *never leave a patient with a partial airway obstruction.* The obstruction can shift and become complete.

A patient with a partial FBAO but with good air exchange may:

- Remain responsive.
- Be able to speak.
- Cough forcefully.
- Wheeze between coughs.

A patient with a partial FBAO and poor air exchange may have:

- Weak, ineffective cough.
- High-pitched noise when inhaling.
- Increased respiratory difficulty and may clutch at the throat.
- Cyanosis (bluish discoloration of the skin and mucous membranes).

In a complete FBAO, all air exchange has stopped because an object fully occludes the patient's airway. The patient may be either responsive or unresponsive, depending in part on how long the airway has been blocked.

A patient with a complete FBAO will be unable to breathe, cough, or speak. He or she may clutch at the neck with thumb and fingers (the universal signal for choking). The amount of oxygen in the blood will decrease rapidly when air cannot enter the lungs. This will result in unresponsiveness. Death also will occur rapidly if the obstruction is not relieved.

The way you manage an obstructed airway depends on whether the obstruction is partial or complete.

Partial FBAO with Good Air Exchange

A patient with a partial obstruction and good air exchange is responsive and able to cough forcefully. In this case:

- Do not interfere with the patient's own attempts to dislodge the obstruction by coughing.
- Encourage the patient to "cough up" the foreign body.
- Do not make any specific attempts to relieve the obstruction.
- Never leave the patient until you are certain the airway is clear and there are no other problems that threaten the airway.
- If the patient cannot dislodge the object on his own, even if good air exchange continues, activate the EMS system.
- Place the patient in a position of comfort, where it is easiest for him or her to breathe.

Partial FBAO with Poor Air Exchange or Complete Obstruction

The American Heart Association (AHA) recommends the **Heimlich maneuver** in cases of partial airway obstruction with poor air exchange and in cases of complete airway obstruction. Also called "subdiaphragmatic abdominal thrusts," or simply "abdominal thrusts," the Heimlich maneuver pushes the diaphragm quickly upward (Figure 6–29). This action forces enough air from the lungs to dislodge and expel the foreign object.

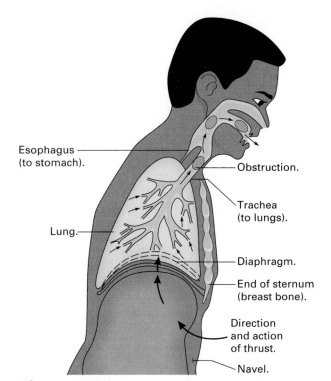

Esophagus (to stomach).

Obstruction.

Trachea (to lungs).

Lung.

Diaphragm.

End of sternum (breast bone).

Direction and action of thrust.

Navel.

Figure 6-29 Abdominal thrusts push the diaphragm up, forcing air to expel the foreign object.

The AHA recommends against the use of back blows in an adult.

Each individual abdominal thrust must be delivered with enough force and pressure to dislodge the foreign object. You must keep trying if the first thrust is unsuccessful. Deliver each thrust with the intent of relieving the obstruction. It may take as many as five or more thrusts to succeed.

Responsive Adult. If the patient is responsive, perform the Heimlich maneuver as follows (Figure 6–30):

1. *Get in position.* Stand behind the patient. Wrap your arms around his waist. Keep your elbows out, away from his ribs.
2. *Position your hands.* Make a fist with one hand. Place the thumb side of the fist on the middle of the abdomen slightly above the navel and well below the xiphoid process.

FOREIGN BODY AIRWAY OBSTRUCTION (FBAO)— RESPONSIVE ADULT

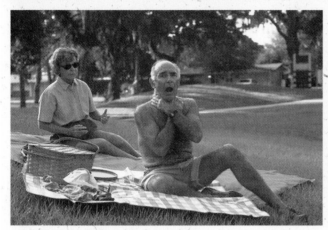

Figure 6-30a The universal sign of choking.

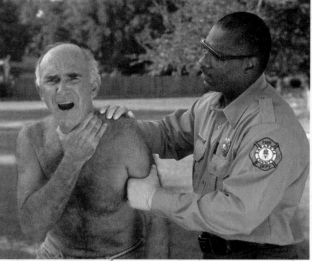

Figure 6-30b Determine if the patient can speak or cough by asking, "Are you choking?"

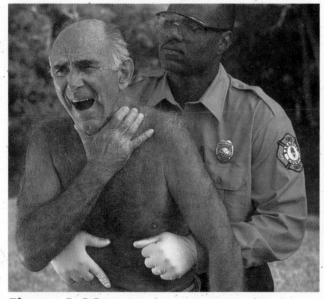

Figure 6-30c If so, perform the Heimlich maneuver to dislodge the object.

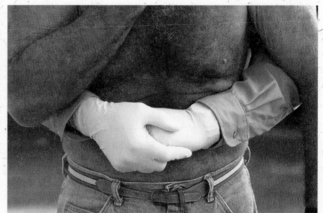

Figure 6-30d Hand position for Heimlich maneuver.

3. *Perform an abdominal thrust.* First, grasp your fist with your other hand, thumbs toward the patient. Then press your fist into the patient's abdomen with a quick inward and upward thrust.

4. *If the first thrust does not dislodge the foreign body*, make each new thrust separate and dis-tinct. Continue until the object is expelled or the patient becomes unresponsive.

Beware of certain dangers. First, if you are improperly positioned or if you perform the thrusts too rapidly or too forcefully, you can lose your balance and fall into the patient. If your hands are positioned too high, you could cause internal injury. Finally, the Heimlich maneuver can cause vomiting. Correct hand placement and use of appropriate force minimizes this risk.

Pregnant or Obese Responsive Adult. If the patient is in the advanced stages of pregnancy or is markedly obese, there may be no room between the rib cage and the abdomen to perform abdominal thrusts, or you may be unable to reach around the patient. In these cases, perform chest thrusts as follows (Figure 6–31):

1. *Get in position.* Stand behind the patient. Place your arms directly under the patient's armpits. Wrap your arms around the patient's chest.
2. *Position your hands.* Make a fist with one hand. Place the thumb of your fist on the middle of the patient's sternum. If you are near the margins of the rib cage, your hand is too low.
3. *Perform a chest thrust.* First, seize your fist firmly with your other hand. Then thrust backward sharply.
4. *If the first thrust does not dislodge the foreign body*, repeat thrusts until the object is expelled or the patient becomes unresponsive.

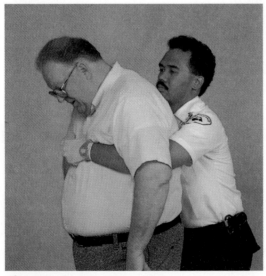

Figure 6-31 Chest thrusts on a standing obese patient with an FBAO.

Unresponsive Adult. If your patient is unresponsive when you find him, activate the EMS system. Then place the patient in a supine position and proceed with the following (Figure 6–32):

1. *Attempt to ventilate the patient.* First open the airway. Then try to ventilate using the mouth-to-mask, mouth-to-barrier device, or mouth-to-mouth technique.
2. *If ventilation is unsuccessful*, reposition the patient's head and try again. If ventilation is still unsuccessful, proceed with the following.
3. *Get in position.* Kneel astride the patient's thighs.
4. *Position your hands.* Place the heel of one hand on the midline of the patient's abdomen, slightly above the navel and well below the xiphoid process. Place your second hand on top of your first.
5. *Perform up to 5 abdominal thrusts.* Press into the abdomen with quick upward thrusts. If you are in the right position, the thrusts will stay in the center of the abdomen and will not veer to the left or right.
6. *Perform a tongue-jaw lift.* That is, grasp both the tongue and the lower jaw between your thumb and fingers and lift the jaw.
7. *Perform a finger sweep.* Use the hooked index finger of your gloved hand to sweep deeply into the mouth along the inner cheeks and to the base of the tongue. Use a hooking motion to dislodge the foreign object, move it to the mouth, and remove it. Remember, use this maneuver only on an unresponsive patient.
8. *If the foreign body is not dislodged*, repeat the sequence. That is, alternate these maneuvers in rapid sequence: attempted ventilation, repeated abdominal thrusts, and tongue-jaw lift with finger sweep. Continue until the foreign body is expelled and ventilation is successful or until you are relieved by other EMS personnel.

If a choking patient becomes unresponsive while you are attempting to dislodge an FBAO, then follow these steps.

1. *Perform a tongue-jaw lift.* This action will draw the tongue away from the back of the throat and from a foreign body that may be lodged

FOREIGN BODY AIRWAY OBSTRUCTION (FBAO)— UNRESPONSIVE ADULT

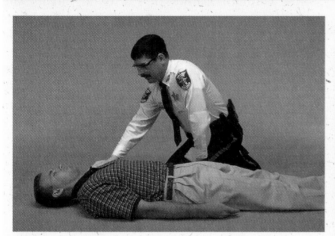

Figure 6-32a   If the patient is unresponsive, open the airway.

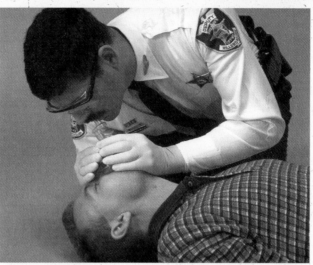

Figure 6-32b   Try to ventilate. If unsuccessful, reposition the head and try again.

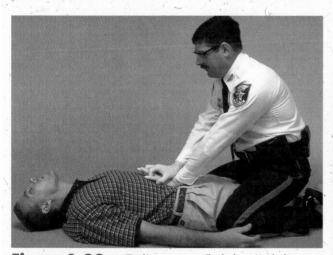

Figure 6-32c   Deliver up to 5 abdominal thrusts.

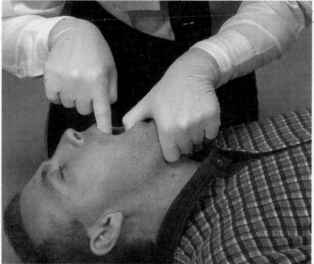

Figure 6-32d   Remove the object, or repeat attempted ventilation, abdominal thrusts, tongue-jaw lift, and finger sweep until effective.

there. In fact, the maneuver itself may partially relieve the obstruction.

2. *Perform a finger sweep* to remove the object.

3. If necessary, continue with airway care as outlined above for an unresponsive adult.

Pregnant or Obese Unresponsive Adult. If you find an unresponsive patient who is in the late stages of pregnancy or is markedly obese, attempt to ventilate. If you are unsuccessful, reposition the head and try again. If still unsuccessful, you must use chest thrusts (Figure 6–33). That is, kneel close to the patient's side. Place the heel of one hand directly over the lower half of the sternum, above the tip of the xiphoid process. Place your second hand on top of the first. Give distinct, separate thrusts downward.

If the first few thrusts do not dislodge the foreign body, repeat the sequence of attempted ventilation, repeated thrusts, tongue-jaw lift, and finger sweep in rapid sequence. Continue until the foreign body is expelled and ventilation is successful or until you are relieved by other EMS personnel.

FBAO in Infants and Children

Manage a complete airway obstruction in children older than eight years the same way you would for adults. Treatment for infants (birth to one year) and children (one to eight years) is different.

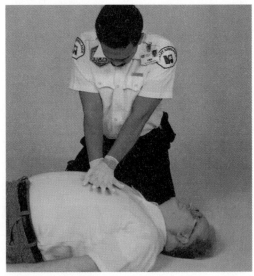

Figure 6-33 Chest thrusts on a supine obese patient with an FBAO.

More than 90% of childhood deaths for FBAO are in children younger than five years old. Nearly 65% of those who die are infants. The most common causes of FBAO in infants and small children are toys, balloons, small objects such as plastic lids, and food such as hot dogs, round candies, nuts, and grapes.

Airway obstruction in an infant or small child also can be caused by swelling and infection. Both narrow the airway. Croup and epiglottitis can cause complete blockage of the airway.

Suspect that obstruction is caused by infection instead of by a foreign object if you detect:

- Fever, especially if accompanied by congestion.
- Hoarseness.
- Drooling.
- Lethargy or limpness.
- Unexplained unresponsiveness in a normally healthy infant or small child.

If you suspect the obstruction is caused by infection, arrange for immediate transport to a medical facility.

An FBAO should be suspected in an infant or child who has sudden onset of respiratory distress associated with coughing, gagging, stridor, or wheezing, especially when food or small items are found near the child. You should try to clear only a complete airway obstruction or a partial airway obstruction with poor air exchange.

Never perform a blind finger sweep on an infant or child. In a child age one or older, perform a tongue-jaw lift, look into the airway, and use your finger to sweep the foreign body out *only* if you can actually see it.

Responsive Infant. If the infant has a partial airway obstruction but still has good air exchange, activate the EMS system. Let the infant try to expel the object by coughing. Place the patient in a position of comfort (in the parent's arms if possible) so that secretions and vomit will drain out of the mouth. The jaw will also fall forward, bringing the tongue and epiglottis away from the back of the throat.

If the infant has serious difficulty breathing, an ineffective cough, and no strong cry, he or she has a partial obstruction with poor air exchange.

According to the AHA, you should perform the following procedure *only* if the infant has a complete FBAO or a partial obstruction with poor air exchange and *only* if the obstruction is due to a witnessed or strongly suspected foreign object. Do not perform the following procedure if you suspect the obstruction is caused by infection. Instead, arrange for immediate transport to a medical facility.

If you are not able to dislodge the FBAO in an infant within *one minute* using the following procedure, then activate the EMS system.

To relieve an FBAO in a responsive infant:

1. *Get in position.* Straddle the infant over one of your arms, face down with his head lower than the rest of the body. Rest your arm on your thigh for support. Support the infant's head by firmly holding the jaw with your hand.
2. *Deliver up to 5 back blows.* Use the heel of your hand between the shoulder blades (Figure 6–34).
3. *If the FBAO is not expelled*, turn the infant face up. Support him on your arm, with his head lower than the rest of his body.
4. *Position your hand.* Place your middle and ring finger over the middle of the infant's

sternum. They should be just below an imaginary line drawn between the infant's nipples (Figure 6–35).
5. *Deliver up to 5 chest thrusts.* Use a quick downward motion.
6. *If the first set of thrusts do not dislodge the foreign body*, continue alternating sets of 5 back blows and 5 chest thrusts until the FBAO is expelled or the infant becomes unresponsive.

When an FBAO is expelled, a responsive infant will usually start to cry and make noise. An unresponsive infant may not make noise or breathe spontaneously. You will need to try to ventilate the infant to determine if air is reaching the lungs.

Unresponsive Infant. If you find an infant who is unresponsive:

1. *Call out "Help!"* When someone responds, have that person activate the EMS system. If you are alone, activate the EMS system within one minute, if you are unable to clear the airway.

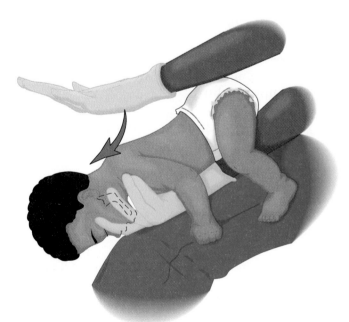

Figure 6-34 Back blows for an infant with an FBAO.

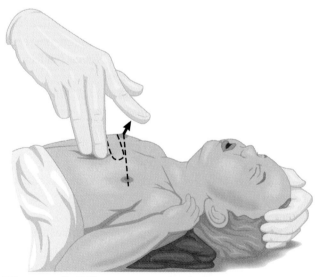

Figure 6-35 Locating the finger position for chest thrusts on an infant with an FBAO.

2. *Position the patient.* Place the infant on his back on a firm, hard surface. Support his head and neck. Note that the infant's head should be in a neutral position. Overextension of the infant's neck can obstruct the airway.

3. *Attempt to ventilate the patient.* First open the airway. Then seal your mouth over the infant's mouth and nose. Deliver breaths.

4. *If ventilation is unsuccessful,* reposition the infant's head and try again. If ventilation is still unsuccessful, proceed with the following.

5. *Get in position.* Straddle the infant over one of your arms, face down with his head lower than the rest of the body. Rest your arm on your thigh for support. Support the infant's head by firmly holding the jaw with your hand.

6. *Deliver up to 5 back blows.* Use the heel of your hand between the infant's shoulder blades.

7. *If the FBAO is not expelled,* turn the infant face up. Support him on your arm, with his head lower than the rest of his body.

8. *Position your hand.* Place your middle and ring fingers over the middle of the infant's sternum. They should be just below an imaginary line drawn between the infant's nipples.

9. *Deliver up to 5 chest thrusts.* Use a quick downward motion.

10. *Perform a tongue-jaw lift.* Look into the infant's mouth. If you see the object, perform a finger sweep to remove it. (Never perform a blind finger sweep in an infant.)

11. *If the first set of ventilations, back blows, and chest thrusts do not dislodge the foreign body,* repeat the procedure. Continue with alternating sets of attempts to ventilate, 5 back blows, 5 chest thrusts, and tongue-jaw lift until the FBAO is expelled or until you are relieved by another EMS worker.

If a choking infant becomes unresponsive while you are attempting to dislodge an FBAO, have a second person activate EMS. Perform a tongue-jaw lift and, if you can see the object, perform a finger sweep to remove it. If necessary, continue with airway care as described above for an unresponsive infant.

Once the foreign body is removed, check the infant for breathing and pulse. If there is no pulse, begin infant CPR as described in Chapter 7. If the infant is breathing and has a pulse, place him or her in a recovery position. Monitor breathing and pulse while you maintain an open airway.

Responsive Child. A patient one year to eight years old is considered a child. If a child has a partial obstruction with good air exchange, encourage him to expel it himself by coughing. If there is a partial obstruction with poor air exchange or a complete obstruction, then follow the steps outlined below (Figure 6–36):

1. *Get in position.* Stand behind the child. Wrap your arms around his waist. Keep your elbows out, away from his ribs.

2. *Position your hands.* Make a fist with one hand. Place the thumb side of the fist on the middle of the abdomen slightly above the navel and well below the xiphoid process. Never place your hands on the xiphoid process or on the lower edge of the ribs. Keep in mind a child's smaller size and proportions as you determine hand placement.

3. *Perform an abdominal thrust.* First, grasp your fist with your other hand, thumbs toward the patient. Then press your fist into the patient's abdomen with a quick inward and upward thrust.

4. *If the first thrust does not dislodge the foreign body,* make each new thrust separate and distinct. Continue until the object is expelled or the patient becomes unresponsive.

Unresponsive Child. If you find an unresponsive child, have a second person activate the EMS system. Then:

1. *Position the patient.* Place the child in a supine position.

2. *Attempt to ventilate the patient.* First open the airway. Then try to give several rescue breaths using the mouth-to-mask, mouth-to-barrier device, or mouth-to-mouth technique.

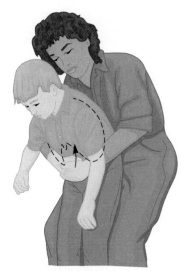

Figure 6-36 Performing the Heimlich on a standing or sitting responsive child with an FBAO.

3. *If ventilation is unsuccessful*, reposition the patient's head and try again. If ventilation is still unsuccessful, proceed with the following.

4. *Get in position.* Kneel astride the child's thighs.

5. *Position your hands.* Place the heel of one hand on the midline of the child's abdomen, slightly above the navel and well below the xiphoid process. Place your second hand on top of your first.

6. *Perform up to 5 abdominal thrusts.* Press into the abdomen with quick upward thrusts.

7. *Perform a tongue-jaw lift.* If you see the object, perform a finger sweep to remove it.

8. *If the first 5 thrusts and tongue-jaw lift do not dislodge the foreign body*, repeat the sequence. That is, alternate these maneuvers in rapid sequence: attempted ventilation, abdominal thrusts, and tongue-jaw lift. Continue until the foreign body is expelled and ventilation is successful. If you are not successful after one minute, activate the EMS if it has not already been done.

If a choking child becomes unresponsive while you are attempting to dislodge an FBAO, have a second person activate EMS. Perform a tongue-jaw lift and, if you can see the object, remove it with a finger sweep. Then, if necessary, continue with airway care as outlined above for an unresponsive child.

FIRST RESPONDER FOCUS

Without adequate respiration, we die. The body requires oxygen to live. These statements alone provide your focus. As a First Responder, you must evaluate respiration. Then do everything possible to make sure respirations continue adequately and without obstruction.

Consider this scenario. You come upon the scene of a motor vehicle crash. You find a patient who has been ejected from the vehicle. While he appears to have multiple injuries, you immediately notice bleeding from the mouth and nose. The patient is unresponsive and is making gurgling sounds from his airway.

After performing a scene size-up and taking BSI precautions, your first priority is the airway. The patient needs suctioning. Depending on the amount of bleeding, he may need frequent suctioning. If you leave the airway, even briefly to perform more of your assessment, the patient will lose his airway and die.

If all you do is take care of the airway, and you do it well, you have done everything possible to save a life. A nicely assessed and packaged patient who does not have an airway has not been properly cared for. In the ABCs and in the care you provide, the airway comes first. ■

CASE STUDY FOLLOW-UP

At the beginning of this chapter, you read that First Responders were called to help an unresponsive adult with snoring respirations. To see how chapter skills apply to this emergency, read the following. It describes how the call was completed.

INITIAL ASSESSMENT *(Continued)*
Since it was not possible to assess her airway while she was slumped in a chair, we quickly but carefully moved the patient to the floor. My partner, Pete, immediately performed a head-tilt/chin-lift maneuver. It eliminated the snoring sounds.

Pete suctioned the airway to remove the built up secretions. Mrs. Constantino didn't have a gag reflex. She accepted the oropharyngeal airway well.

Our assessment of her breathing revealed that there was minimal chest movement and slow respirations. She also was beginning to show signs of blue coloring around her lips.

Realizing that Mrs. Constantino was breathing inadequately and her pulse was rapid and weak, we ventilated her using a pocket face mask with one-way valve and supplemental oxygen.

PHYSICAL EXAMINATION
We believed that Mrs. Constantino had a medical problem rather than a traumatic condition. I did a quick physical examination while my partner continued to assist ventilations. There were no signs of injury on Mrs. Constantino's head, neck, chest, abdomen, or extremities. Her pulse was 96 and bounding. The respiratory rate was 8 and shallow.

PATIENT HISTORY
Mr. Constantino told us that his wife had a heart attack several years ago. She takes medications for her heart and high blood pressure. She had complained of a headache about an hour before she became unresponsive. She ate breakfast earlier. She has no allergies.

ONGOING ASSESSMENT
Our primary focus was on making sure Mrs. Constantino was ventilated properly. We made sure that we checked her pulse frequently. Her pulse on our second check was 104, bounding, and regular. Her respirations were about 6 and shallow, being assisted.

PATIENT HAND-OFF
We had the airway under control when the paramedics arrived. The patient's color had improved. Her pulse also had slowed a bit. Pete gave them the hand-off report:

"This is Mrs. Constantino. She is 74 years old. She had a headache about an hour ago. She was found by her husband slumped over in a chair. We moved her to the floor and found that she had inadequate ventilations. We began assisting with a pocket mask and oxygen. She will groan with loud verbal stimulus. Her respiratory rate was about 6, pulse 104 and bounding. She has a history of heart attack and high blood pressure. She ate breakfast. She has no allergies."

I saw Mr. Constantino in the grocery store recently. He told me that his wife had had a severe stroke. She remained in the hospital for some time and was eventually moved to a rehabilitation center. He thanked me again and told me that he hoped his wife would be home soon.

It has been said that the priorities in patient care are the airway, the airway, and the airway! Without a clear and open airway plus adequate ventilations, no patient can survive. So even as you approach your patient's side, the first questions in your mind should be "Is she breathing? Is she breathing adequately?" Remember, without an airway, there is no chance of survival.

REVIEW QUESTIONS

Page references where answers may be found or supported are provided at the end of each question.

Section 1

1. What are the nine major components of the respiratory system? (pp. 81–82)

Section 2

2. What are two maneuvers that you can use to open a patient's airway? Describe when you should use each one. (pp. 85–87)
3. What are two types of airway adjunct? Describe when you should use each one. (pp. 87–90)
4. How can you find out if a patient is breathing? (p. 94)
5. What are the signs of inadequate breathing? (pp. 94–95)

Section 3

6. What are the three techniques used by a First Responder to artificially ventilate a patient? Name them in order of preference. (p. 95)
7. How do you perform artificial ventilation? Briefly describe each step, including rates for infants, children, and adults. (pp. 96–103)
8. What are the signs that show your ventilations are adequate? (p. 95)
9. How do you relieve a foreign body airway obstruction in a responsive adult? Briefly describe each step. (pp. 110–112)
10. How do you relieve a foreign body airway obstruction in an unresponsive adult? Briefly describe each step. (pp. 112–114)

CHAPTER 7

CIRCULATION

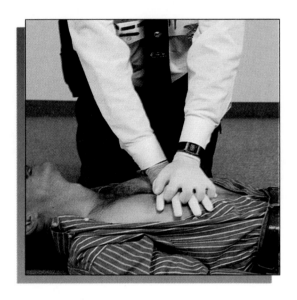

INTRODUCTION

Heart disease takes the lives of about 600,000 Americans each year, many before they ever reach a hospital. The patients who can be saved need immediate CPR followed by advanced medical care, including defibrillation, within 8 to 10 minutes of collapse.

But even with CPR, many patients will not live. They may have been without a pulse or oxygen for too long or the attack may have caused irreversible damage to the heart. Please do not let that discourage you. Emergency care in the field is still critical to saving many lives. And today's new hospital techniques often help to reverse the crippling effects of heart attack.

Note that several studies have shown that you can lose your CPR skills unless you have frequent practice and retraining. Retraining should occur often. Recertification should occur every one to two years.

Cognitive, affective, and psychomotor objectives are from the U.S. DOT's 1995 "First Responder: National Standard Curriculum." Enrichment objectives, if any, identify material that is supplemental to the DOT curriculum.

Cognitive

4-1.1 List the reasons for the heart to stop beating. (p. 123)

4-1.2 Define the components of cardiopulmonary resuscitation. (pp. 123–124)

4-1.3 Describe each link in the chain of survival and how it relates to the EMS system. (p. 123)

4-1.4 List the steps of one-rescuer adult CPR. (pp. 129–130)

4-1.5 Describe the technique of external chest compressions on an adult patient. (pp. 126–127, 129)

4-1.6 Describe the technique of external chest compressions on an infant. (pp. 135, 137)

4-1.7 Describe the technique of external chest compressions on a child. (pp. 135, 137)

4-1.8 Explain when the First Responder is able to stop CPR. (p. 124)

4-1.9 List the steps of two-rescuer adult CPR. (pp. 129–132)

4-1.10 List the steps of infant CPR. (pp. 135, 137)

4-1.11 List the steps of child CPR. (pp. 135, 137)

Affective

4-1.12 Respond to the feelings that the family of a patient may be having during a cardiac event. (pp. 124, 129)

4-1.13 Demonstrate a caring attitude towards patients with cardiac events who request emergency medical services. (p. 124)

4-1.14 Place the interests of the patient with a cardiac event as the foremost consideration when making any and all patient care decisions. (p. 124)

4-1.15 Communicate with empathy with family members and friends of the patient with a cardiac event. (pp. 124, 129)

Psychomotor

4-1.16 Demonstrate the proper technique of chest compressions on an adult. (pp. 126–127, 129)

4-1.17 Demonstrate the proper technique of chest compressions on a child. (pp. 135, 137)

4-1.18 Demonstrate the proper technique of chest compressions on an infant. (pp. 135, 137)

4-1.19 Demonstrate the steps of adult one rescuer CPR. (pp. 129–130)

4-1.20 Demonstrate the steps of adult two rescuer CPR. (pp. 129–132)

4-1.21 Demonstrate child CPR. (pp. 135, 137)

4-1.22 Demonstrate infant CPR. (pp. 135, 137)

SECTION 1: THE CIRCULATORY SYSTEM

The circulatory system is responsible for delivering oxygen and nutrients to the body's tissues. It also is responsible for removing waste from the tissues. Its basic components are the heart, arteries, veins, capillaries, and blood. (See Chapter 4 for an illustration.)

The heart is a hollow, muscular organ about the size of a fist. It lies in the lower left central region of the chest between the lungs. It is protected in the front by the ribs and sternum (breastbone). In the back it is protected by the spinal column. The heart contains four chambers. The two upper ones are the left and right atria. The two lower ones are the left and right ventricles. The septum (a wall) divides the right side of the heart from the left side. The heart also contains several one-way valves that keep blood flowing in the correct direction.

The circulatory system also contains blood vessels. These vessels transport blood throughout the body. You will recall from Chapter 4 that the arteries transport blood away from the heart. Veins carry blood back to the heart. The tiny capillaries allow for the exchange of gases and nutrients between the blood and the cells of the body.

HOW THE HEART WORKS

The heart is like a two-sided pump (Figure 7–1). The left side receives oxygenated blood from the lungs and pumps it to all parts of the

CASE STUDY

DISPATCH
Our engine company was dispatched for an EMS assist because the closest ambulance was unavailable. The call was for a cardiac patient. We knew that time would really count.

SCENE SIZE-UP
There were three of us on the pumper. I was the officer. I sized up the scene carefully from the cab before we got out. I reminded the others to remember their BSI equipment.

INITIAL ASSESSMENT
We observed a woman performing CPR on an older gentleman. The woman seemed to be doing pretty well but she was getting tired. My crew approached and took over. We rechecked the patient's ABCs (airway, breathing, and circulation), found no pulse or respirations, and continued CPR.

CPR is an important skill for the First Responder. Though needed in only a small percent of calls, when it is used, it is vitally important. In the scenario described above, the firefighters have begun CPR. How long do you think they should continue? Could CPR injure the patient? Will the patient live? Consider these questions as you read Chapter 7.

body. The right side receives blood from the body and then pumps it to the lungs to be reoxygenated.

The blood is kept under pressure and in constant circulation by the heart's pumping action. In a healthy adult at rest, the heart contracts between 60 and 80 times per minute. The pulse is a sign of the pressure exerted during each contraction of the heart. Every time the heart pumps, a wave of blood is sent through the arteries. That wave is felt as a pulse. It can be palpated most easily where a large artery lies over a bone close to the skin. Sites include: the carotid pulse in the neck, the brachial pulse in the upper arm, the radial pulse in the wrist, and the femoral pulse in the upper thigh.

The pulse is felt most easily over the carotid artery on either side of the neck. The carotid artery should be palpated (felt) first when a patient is unresponsive. The radial artery on the thumb side of the inner surface of the wrist is also easy to feel. It should be palpated first when the patient is responsive.

The heart, lungs, and brain work together closely to sustain life. The smooth functioning of each is critical to the others. When one organ cannot perform properly, the other two are handicapped. If one fails, the other two soon will follow.

WHEN THE HEART STOPS

Clinical death occurs when a patient is in **respiratory arrest** (not breathing) and **cardiac arrest** (the heart is not beating). Immediate CPR may

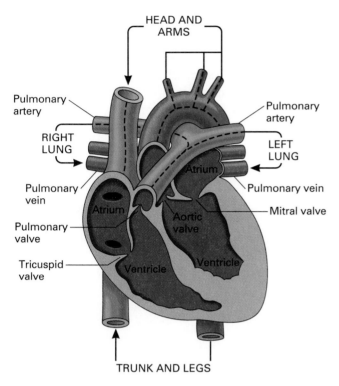

HEAD AND ARMS

Pulmonary artery

RIGHT LUNG

Pulmonary vein

Pulmonary valve

Tricuspid valve

Pulmonary artery

LEFT LUNG

Atrium

Pulmonary vein

Mitral valve

Aortic valve

Atrium

Ventricle

Ventricle

TRUNK AND LEGS

RIGHT HEART:
Receives blood from the body and pumps it through the pulmonary artery to the lungs where it picks up fresh oxygen.

LEFT HEART:
Receives oxygen-full blood from the lungs and pumps it through the aorta to the body.

Figure 7-1 The heart.

• *Early access.* Lay people must activate the EMS system immediately. The use of a universal access number (9-1-1, for example) helps to speed system access.
• *Early CPR.* Family members, citizens, and First Responders must be trained in CPR and begin as soon as possible. CPR will help to sustain life until the next step.
• *Early defibrillation.* Defibrillation is the process by which an electrical current is sent to the heart to correct fatal heart rhythms. The earlier defibrillation can be performed, the better.
• *Early advanced care.* Advanced care, or the administration of medications and other advanced therapies, must start as soon as possible. This can be done by paramedics at the scene or by prompt transportation to the emergency department.

As a First Responder, you have an important role. You can provide early CPR and, if permitted in your area, defibrillation.

The principle of CPR is to oxygenate and circulate the blood of the patient until defibrillation and advanced care can be given. Any delay in starting CPR increases the chances of nervous system damage and death. The faster the response, the better the patient's chances are. Survival rates improve when the time between arrest and the delivery of defibrillation and other advanced measures is short.

reverse that state and restore the patient without damage. However, if a patient is clinically dead for 4 to 6 minutes, brain cells begin to die. After 8 to 10 minutes without a pulse, irreversible damage occurs to the brain.

There are many reasons why a heart will stop. They include heart disease, stroke, allergic reaction, diabetes, prolonged seizures, and other medical conditions. The heart also may stop because of a serious injury. In infants and children, respiratory problems are the most common cause of cardiac arrest. This is why airway care is so important in young patients.

The patient in respiratory and cardiac arrest has the best chance of surviving if all of the links in the **chain of survival** come together. This "chain" as identified by the American Heart Association (AHA) contains four links:

SECTION 2: CARDIOPULMONARY RESUSCITATION (CPR)

According to the American Heart Association (AHA), proper assessment of the patient's airway, breathing, and circulation is critical to successful CPR. The AHA also states that no patient should undergo the intrusive procedures of CPR until need is clearly established.

You can establish the need for CPR by determining that the patient is unresponsive, breathless, and pulseless.

To provide CPR, you must maintain an open airway, provide artificial ventilation, and provide artificial circulation by means of chest compressions. (For a detailed discussion of airway maintenance and artificial ventilation, see Chapter 6.)

It was once thought that chest compressions work because they squeeze the heart between the sternum and backbone to force blood out. Newer evidence indicates that they produce pressure changes inside the chest cavity. This pressure may be responsible for increased circulation to the body. So, be sure to pay as much attention to the duration as to the rate of chest compressions. Be sure to stay current on new CPR developments.

CPR must begin as soon as possible and continue until:

STEPS PRECEDING CPR

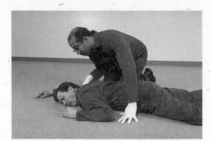

Figure 7-2a Determine unresponsiveness.

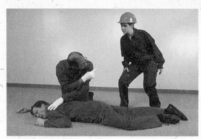

Figure 7-2b Activate the EMS system.

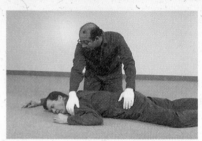

Figure 7-2c Position the patient on a firm, flat surface.

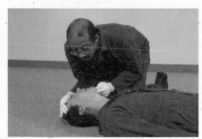

Figure 7-2d Open the airway.

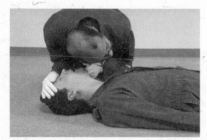

Figure 7-2e Determine breathlessness.

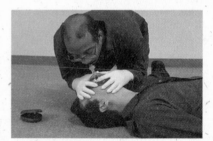

Figure 7-2f Perform artificial ventilation.

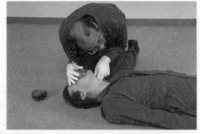

Figure 7-2g Determine pulselessness.

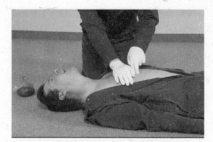

Figure 7-2h Begin CPR.

- The First Responder is exhausted and is unable to continue.
- The patient is turned over to another trained rescuer or the hospital staff.
- The patient is resuscitated.
- The patient has been declared dead by a proper authority.

A cardiac event is very serious. Without your interventions, the patient may not survive. So remember to place his or her interests first. And be sure to demonstrate a caring attitude. When possible, respond to the feelings of the patient's family and friends with empathy.

STEPS PRECEDING CPR

Before providing CPR to a patient, you must first (Figure 7–2):

- Determine unresponsiveness.
- Determine breathlessness.
- Determine pulselessness.

To determine unresponsiveness, tap or gently shake the patient and shout, "Are you okay?" If the patient does not respond, immediately activate the EMS system for an adult (after one minute of care for an infant or child). This increases the patient's chances of early defibrillation and early advanced care. Then continue with your assessment.

If, after opening the patient's airway, you determine breathlessness, provide artificial ventilation. (Follow the procedures described in Chapter 6.) Provide supplemental oxygen, if you are allowed, by attaching it to your pocket face mask. The oxygen should flow at 15 liters per minute.

To determine pulselessness, find the carotid artery pulse point (Figure 7–3):

1. Place two fingers on the larynx ("Adam's apple").
2. Slide your fingers to the side. Stop in the groove between the larynx and the large neck muscle.
3. Feel for the pulse. Press for 5 to 10 seconds, gently enough to avoid compressing the

artery. Do not use your thumb. Do not rest your hand across the patient's throat.

If the patient has a pulse—even a weak or irregular one, do not begin chest compressions. You could cause serious problems. If the patient has no pulse, assume that he or she is in cardiac arrest. Begin CPR immediately.

Note that to perform CPR correctly, your patient must be in a supine position on a firm, flat surface such as the floor.

You may wish to refer to the CPR summary, Figure 7–4, as you read the rest of this chapter.

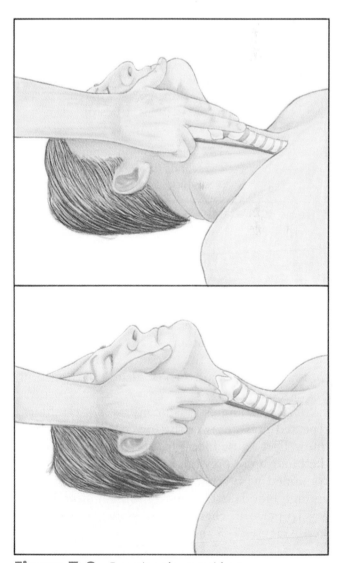

Figure 7-3 Locating the carotid artery.

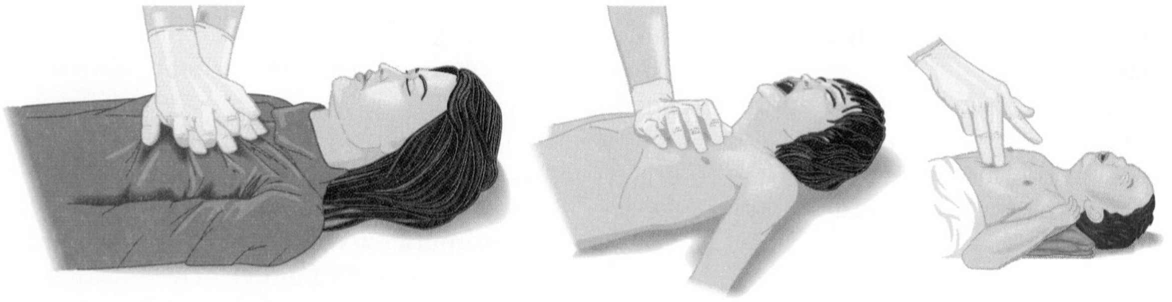

	Adult (over 8 years)	Child (1 to 8 years)	Infant (under 1 year)
Hand Position	Two hands on lower half of sternum	Heel of one hand on lower half of sternum	Two or three fingers on lower half of sternum (one finger width below nipple line)
Compressions	Approximately 1½ to 2 inches in depth	Approximately 1 to 1½ inches in depth (equal to ⅓ to ½ the total chest depth)	Approximately ½ to 1 inch in depth (equal to ⅓ to ½ the total chest depth)
Breaths	Slowly, until chest gently rises (about 1½ to 2 seconds per breath)	Slowly, until chest gently rises (about 1 to 1½ seconds per breath)	Slowly, until chest gently rises (about 1 to 1½ seconds per breath)
Cycle	15 compressions, 2 breaths (one rescuer) 5 compressions, 1 breath (two rescuers)	5 compressions, 1 breath	5 compressions, 1 breath
Rate	15 compressions in about 10 seconds or 80–100 per minute	5 compressions in about 3 seconds or 100 per minute	5 compressions in about 3 seconds or at least 100 per minute

Figure 7-4 CPR summary.

CPR FOR ADULTS

CPR involves a combination of skills. When a patient's heart has stopped, artificial ventilation alone cannot help the patient. Chest compressions also must be used to circulate the oxygen in the blood.

Chest compressions consist of rhythmic, repeated pressure over the lower half of the sternum. They cause blood to circulate as a result of the build-up of pressure in the chest cavity. When combined with artificial ventilation, they provide enough blood circulation to maintain life.

To perform chest compressions, follow these steps (Figures 7–5 and 7–6):

1. *Position the patient.* He or she must be supine on a firm, flat surface such as the floor.

2. *Uncover the chest.* Remove the patient's shirt or blouse. Do not waste time unbuttoning it. Rip it open or pull it up. Cut a woman's bra in two or slip it up to her neck.
3. *Get in position.* Kneel close to the patient's side. Have your knees about as wide as your shoulders.
4. *Locate the xiphoid process.* First feel the lower margin of the rib cage on the side nearest you. Use the middle and index fingers of your hand, the one closest to the patient's feet. Then run your fingers along the rib cage to the notch where the ribs meet the sternum in the center of the lower chest.
5. *Locate the compression site.* Place your middle finger on the xiphoid process (the notch). Put your index finger of the same hand on the lower end of the patient's sternum. Then

LOCATION OF XIPHOID

LOCATING XIPHOID

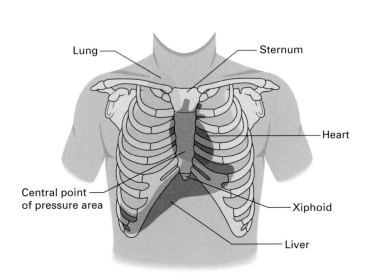

Lung — — Sternum

— Heart

Central point of pressure area —

— Xiphoid

— Liver

Posterior movement of xiphoid may lacerate liver. Lowest point of pressure on sternum must be above, not on, the xiphoid.

Figure 7-5 Locating proper hand placement for CPR.

place the heel of your other hand alongside your fingers. There should be two finger widths between the tip of the sternum and the place where you rest the heel of your hand. When you apply pressure at this point, the sternum is flexible enough to be compressed without breaking. (A fracture of the sternum or the ribs can cut the heart, lungs, or liver.)

6. *Position your hands.* Put your free hand on top of the hand that is on the sternum. Your hands should be parallel. Extend or interlace your fingers to hold them off the chest wall. If your fingers rest against the chest wall during compressions, you increase the chance of separating and injuring the patient's ribs. (An alternative position for large hands and hands or wrists with arthritis is to use your free hand to grasp the wrist of the hand on the patient's sternum.)

7. *Position your shoulders.* Put them directly over your hands.

8. *Perform chest compressions.* Keeping your arms straight and your elbows locked, thrust from

your shoulders. Apply firm, heavy pressure. Depress the sternum 1.5 to 2 inches on an adult. Be sure the thrust is straight down into the sternum. If it is not, the torso will roll and part of the force of the thrust will be lost.

Use the weight of your body as you deliver the compressions. If necessary, add force to the thrusts with your shoulders. Never add force with your arms—the force is too great and could fracture the sternum. Compressions should be 50% of the cycle. That is, the compression and release time should be about equal.

9. *Completely release pressure after each compression.* Let the sternum return to its normal position, and allow blood to flow back into the chest and heart. If you do not release all pressure, blood will not circulate properly. Do not lift or move your hands in any way. You could lose proper positioning. Avoid sudden jerky movements. Effective compressions provide only one-fourth to one-third of normal blood circulation. Anything less is ineffective.

CORRECT POSITIONING FOR CPR

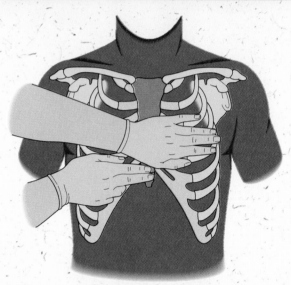

Figure 7-6a Place the heel of your hand on the patient's sternum.

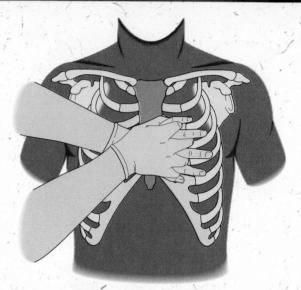

Figure 7-6b Interlace your fingers.

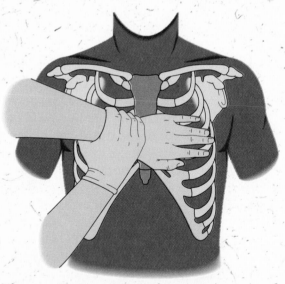

Figure 7-6c Alternative hand placement for CPR.

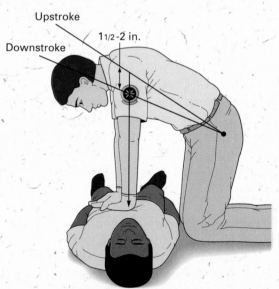

Figure 7-6d Position your shoulders, and then perform chest compressions.

10. *Count as you administer compressions.* You should be able to say (and do) the following in a bit less than 2 seconds:
    - One — push down.
    - and — let up.
    - Two — push down.
    - and — let up.

This procedure should let you administer 80 to 100 compressions per minute to an adult. Practice until you can perform 15 complete compressions in 9 to 11 seconds. Beware of becoming hyperventilated. If you find you are, continue breathing at a regular tempo, but not at the same rhythm you used before.

One-Rescuer CPR

To perform CPR alone, you must do the following: Determine unresponsiveness. Activate the EMS system. Open the airway, and determine breathlessness. Perform artificial ventilation, and remove foreign body airway obstructions as needed. If breathing is restored and the patient has a pulse, then place him or her in the recovery position. Do not begin CPR.

If the pulse is absent, begin CPR as follows (Figure 7–7):

1. *Get in position*, and locate the proper hand position (described earlier).
2. *Perform chest compressions.* Perform 15 chest compressions at a rate of 80 to 100 per minute. Either count out loud or use some other way to keep track of the number of compressions you deliver.
3. *Deliver two slow breaths.* After completing 15 compressions, open the airway. Then deliver two breaths, each lasting 1.5 to 2 seconds. Be sure you inhale deeply between breaths.
4. *Continue until you have completed four cycles of 15 compressions and 2 ventilations.*
5. *Then check the patient's pulse.* Check for three to five seconds at the carotid artery. If the pulse has returned, monitor the patient's pulse and breathing closely until the EMTs arrive. If the pulse has returned but the patient is not breathing, provide artificial ventilation at 10 to 12 breaths per minute. If there is still no pulse, resume CPR. Check again for pulse and breathing every two or three minutes.

If another First Responder trained in CPR arrives at the scene, he or she should do two things. First, the rescuer should verify that the EMS system has been activated and is responding. Have him activate the EMS system, if necessary. Second, the rescuer may take over CPR when the first rescuer gets tired.

To relieve the first rescuer with as little interruption as possible, follow these steps:

- If the first rescuer is currently performing chest compressions, the second rescuer should take a position at the patient's head. The second rescuer should then check the pulse while the first rescuer compresses the chest. Adequate CPR will usually create a carotid pulse. When the first rescuer completes the compressions, the second rescuer should provide two ventilations and check the pulse. The second rescuer can then resume CPR.
- If the first rescuer is performing ventilations when the second rescuer arrives, the second rescuer should prepare to perform compressions. After the first rescuer completes two ventilations and checks the pulse, the second rescuer should begin compressions.

There is no exact sequence to cover all situations. The examples above are efficient ways to change rescuers when performing CPR. The main objective is to minimize the amount of time the patient goes without CPR. It is usually convenient to incorporate pulse and breathing checks into the changes.

Any rescuers who are not currently performing CPR can help prepare the scene for the arrival of the ambulance. EMTs and paramedics require space for stretchers, equipment, and additional personnel. Moving furniture away from the patient may help to create extra space. Directing the ambulance crew to the patient is also valuable. If time permits, find out from family and bystanders the exact sequence of events leading to the time the patient's heart stopped.

Two-Rescuer CPR

All First Responders should learn both the one-rescuer and two-rescuer techniques. The two-rescuer coordinated technique is less tiring. When

ONE-RESCUER ADULT CPR

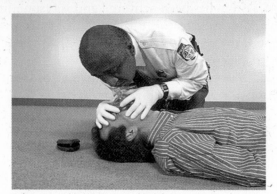

Figure 7-7a Determine the patient is unresponsive and breathless, and provide artificial ventilation.

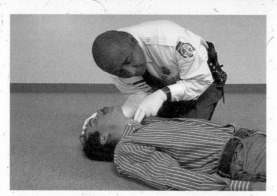

Figure 7-7b Determine pulselessness.

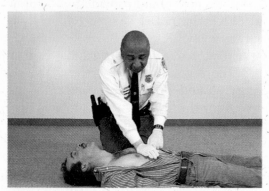

Figure 7-7c Locate proper hand position.

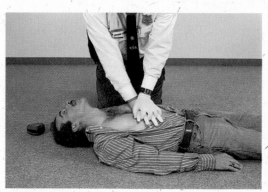

Figure 7-7d Perform chest compressions and ventilations at a ratio of 15:2 at a rate of 80 to 100 per minute.

possible, use an oral airway and a pocket face mask.

Before performing CPR, you and your partner must first determine that the patient is unresponsive, breathless, and pulseless. One rescuer may determine unresponsiveness, provide initial ventilations, and check the pulse. At the same time, the second rescuer can activate the EMS system and prepare to do compressions.

Note that in two-rescuer CPR, the ratio of compressions to ventilations is 5:1 (five compressions and then one ventilation). The ventilation should be delivered during a 1.5- to 2-second pause after every fifth chest compression.

If the patient remains unresponsive, breathless, and pulseless after your initial breaths, proceed as follows (Figure 7–8):

1. *Get in position.* The rescuers, if possible, should take position on opposite sides of the patient. One rescuer kneels by the patient's side for compressions. The other kneels at the patient's head and provides ventilations.

2. *Perform five chest compressions.* Perform five chest compressions at a rate of 80 to 100 per minute. The compression rescuer should count the sequence out loud. Use an audible count of "one and two and three and four

and five and pause," so that five compressions can be achieved every three to five seconds.

3. *Deliver one slow breath.* The ventilation rescuer should take a deep breath on "three and," get into position to ventilate on "four and," and begin breathing into the patient after "five." The compression rescuer pauses for 1.5 to 2 seconds so that the patient receives a slow, full breath. If you have the proper equipment and training, ventilate with 100% oxygen.

4. *After one minute of CPR, check the patient's pulse.* Check for three to five seconds at the carotid artery. If the pulse has returned, monitor the patient's pulse and breathing closely until the EMTs arrive. If the pulse has returned but the patient is not breathing, pro-

vide artificial ventilation at 10 to 12 breaths per minute. If there is still no pulse, resume CPR. Check again for pulse and breathing every two or three minutes.

When the compression rescuer gets tired, he or she should switch with the ventilation rescuer. Here is the 7-second method (Figure 7–9):

1. The compression rescuer should call for a switch at the beginning of the compression cycle by substituting "change" for "one." The audible count remains the same for the remaining four compressions. (Any mnemonic that satisfactorily accomplishes the change is acceptable. Another popular technique uses

TWO-RESCUER ADULT CPR

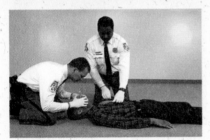

Figure 7-8a The ventilation rescuer provides artificial ventilation while the compression rescuer bares the patient's chest.

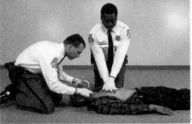

Figure 7-8b The ventilation rescuer determines pulselessness as the compression rescuer gets into position.

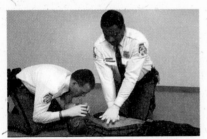

Figure 7-8c Perform compressions and ventilations at a ratio of 5:1 at a rate of 80 to 100 per minute.

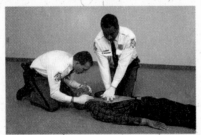

Figure 7-8d Stop CPR to assess the carotid pulse after the first minute and every few minutes thereafter.

"Change, on, the, next, breath.") A similar phrase can also be used to call for the move of the patient or for a pulse check. It simply involves substituting. For example:
- "1 and 2 and 3 and 4 and 5 and pause."
- "Change and 2 and 3 and 4 and 5 and pause."
- "Lift and 2 and 3 and 4 and 5 and pause."
- "Pulse and 2 and 3 and 4 and 5 and pause."
2. After the fifth compression, the ventilation rescuer should give a full breath. Then he or she should move to the chest, locate the xiphoid process, and get hands in position for compressions.

3. At the same time, the compression rescuer should move quickly to the patient's head. Then he or she checks the carotid pulse and breathing for a maximum of five seconds.
4. If no pulse is found, the rescuer at the head gives a breath and announces, "No pulse. Continue CPR."
5. The rescuer at the chest is in position and begins compression. If shortness of breath prevents the rescuer from giving a full count out loud, he or she should at least say the "four and five and" count so that the ventilation rescuer will know when to breathe.

CHANGING POSITIONS

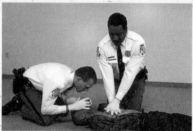

Figure 7-9a The tired compression rescuer calls for a switch.

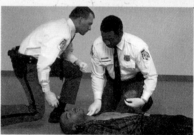

Figure 7-9b The ventilation rescuer delivers a breath as usual, then moves to the patient's side. The second rescuer moves to the patient's head.

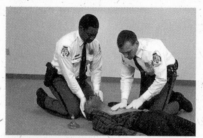

Figure 7-9c The rescuer at the head opens the airway and checks respirations and pulse for five seconds. The second rescuer prepares for compressions.

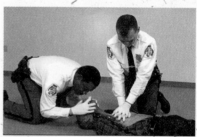

Figure 7-9d If the patient is still unresponsive, breathless, and pulseless, continue CPR.

Monitoring the Patient

The patient's condition needs to be monitored throughout CPR. This will ensure that rescue efforts are effective. It also lets you know when spontaneous breathing and the pulse returns.

In two-rescuer CPR, there is a ventilation rescuer and a compression rescuer. To monitor the effectiveness of chest compressions, the ventilation rescuer should feel for a pulse at the carotid artery during compressions. To determine if a spontaneous pulse has returned, the ventilation rescuer should check the carotid artery for three to five seconds at the end of the first minute of CPR and every few minutes thereafter. Note that the pulse must be checked when CPR is not in progress.

In general, CPR should not be interrupted for more than five seconds. One of the few exceptions to this rule applies to moving a patient. It may not be possible to perform CPR in a cramped bedroom or other small area. In this case, it is acceptable to move the patient so proper CPR can be performed. These actions must be kept as close to five seconds as possible.

Signs of Successful CPR

Signs of successful CPR include the following:

- Each time the sternum is compressed, you should feel a pulse in the carotid artery. It will feel like a flutter.
- The chest should rise and fall with each ventilation.
- The pupils may react or appear to be normal. (Pupils should constrict when exposed to light.)
- A heartbeat may return.
- A spontaneous gasp of breathing may occur.
- The patient's skin color may improve or return to normal.
- The patient may move his or her own arms or legs.
- The patient may try to swallow.

Remember that "successful" CPR does not mean that the patient lives. "Successful" only means that you performed CPR correctly.

Very few patients will survive if they do not receive **advanced cardiac life support (ACLS)**. The goal of CPR is to prevent the death of cells and organs for a few crucial moments. Hopefully, advanced providers will arrive in time.

Mistakes in Performing CPR

The most common ventilation mistakes are as follows:

- Failing to maintain an adequate head tilt.
- Failing to maintain an adequate seal around the patient's mouth, nose, or both with a pocket face mask or face shield. The seal should be released when the patient exhales.
- Completing a two-rescuer cycle in fewer than five seconds.
- Failing to watch and listen for exhalation.
- Not giving full breaths.
- Providing breaths too rapidly.

Some common chest compression mistakes include the following:

- Bending your elbows instead of keeping them straight.
- Not aligning your shoulders directly above the patient's sternum.
- Placing the heel of your bottom hand too low or not in line with the sternum (Figure 7–10).
- Not depressing the sternum to proper depth.
- Not extending the fingers of your hands, touching the patient's chest.
- Pivoting at the knees instead of at your hips.
- Compressing at an incorrect rate.
- Moving your hands from the compression site between compressions.

Complications Caused by CPR

Even properly performed, CPR may cause rib fractures in some patients. Other complications that can occur with proper CPR include:

- Fracture of the sternum.
- Pneumothorax (collapse of the lungs caused by air in the chest).
- Hemothorax (collapse of the lungs caused by bleeding in the chest).
- Cuts and bruises to the lungs.
- Lacerations (cuts) to the liver.

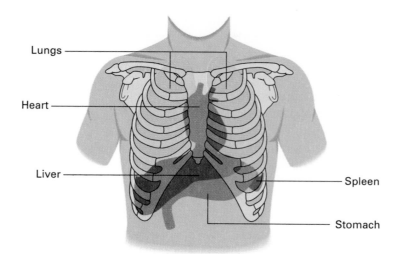

Lungs

Heart

Liver

Spleen

Stomach

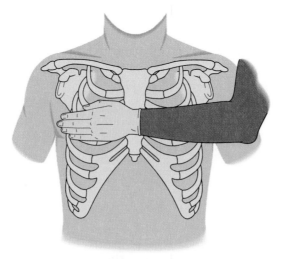

Too far right:
May fracture ribs and cause
lacerations to lung and liver.

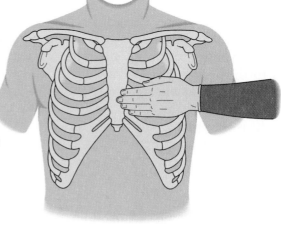

Too far left:
May fracture ribs and cause
lacerations to lung and heart.

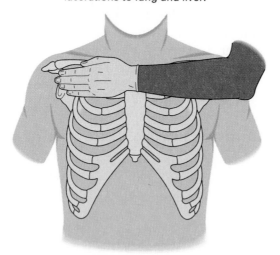

Too high:
May crack sternum.

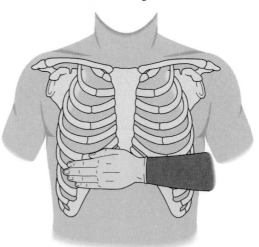

Too low:
May break off xiphoid process
and lacerate the liver.

Figure 7-10   Consequences of improper hand placement.

These complications are rare. However, you can help minimize the risk by giving careful attention to your performance. Remember that effective CPR is necessary, even if it results in complications. After all, the alternative is death.

In addition, the rib cartilage in elderly patients separates easily. You will hear it crunch as you compress. Be sure that your hand is positioned correctly and that you are compressing to the correct depth, but do not stop.

CPR FOR INFANTS AND CHILDREN

Infants (up to one year old) and children (one to eight years old) need slightly different care. Cardiac arrest in them is rarely caused by heart problems. The heart nearly always stops beating because of too little oxygen due to injuries, suffocation, smoke inhalation, **sudden infant death syndrome (SIDS),** or infection.

See Chapter 6 for how to determine if your infant or child patient is unresponsive and breathless. Follow the directions there, too, for caring for an infant or child who is not breathing. Remember that according to AHA guidelines, you should resuscitate an infant or child for one minute before you activate the EMS system.

Determining that your infant or child patient is pulseless is important. For an infant, check the brachial pulse on the inside of the upper arm between the elbow and shoulder. Press the artery gently with your index and middle fingers. Never use your thumb. In a child, check the pulse at the carotid artery.

It can be difficult to find a pulse in an infant or child. So, you should not spend too much time trying to locate one. According to the AHA, if the infant or child is not breathing, heart rate is probably inadequate and chest compressions are usually necessary.

Performing CPR

If the infant or child is breathless and pulseless, then begin CPR. Follow these guidelines to perform chest compressions (Figures 7–11 and 7–12):

1. *Position the patient.* Make sure the patient is lying on a firm, flat surface. If the patient is an infant, put him or her in your lap with head tilted back slightly. Use your palm to support the baby's back. Make sure his or her head is not higher than the rest of the body.

2. *Locate the compression site.* For an infant, it is one finger-width below an imaginary line between the nipples.

   For a child, locate the lower margin of the rib cage on the side next to you. Use your middle and index fingers, while your hand nearest the child's head maintains head tilt. Follow the rib cage to the xiphoid process, where the ribs and sternum meet. Then place your index finger next to the middle finger. While looking at the position of the index finger, lift that hand and place its heel next to where the index finger was.

3. *Perform chest compressions.* For an infant, use the flat part of your middle and ring fingers to compress the infant's sternum one-half to one inch, or one-third to one-half of the depth of the chest. The compression rate for an infant is at least 100 per minute.

   For a child, compress the sternum 1 inch to 1.5 inches, or one-third to one-half of the depth of the chest, with the heel of one hand. The compression rate for a child is 100 compressions per minute.

The ratio of compressions to ventilations in both infants and children is 5:1 (5 compressions and then one ventilation). In one-rescuer CPR for an infant or child, ventilate during a pause after each fifth compression. Count compressions at this rhythm:

- Infant — 1, 2, 3, 4, 5, breathe.
- Child — 1 and 2 and 3 and 4 and 5 and breathe.

After one minute, or 20 cycles, check for the return of a spontaneous pulse. If there is none, then activate the EMS system.

Signs of Successful CPR

The methods of checking for successful CPR in infants and children are almost the same as for adults.

INFANT AND CHILD CPR

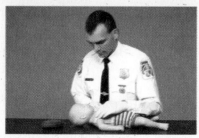

Figure 7-11a Determine unresponsiveness with a "shake and shout" method.

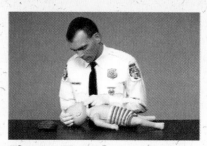

Figure 7-11b Gently open the airway.

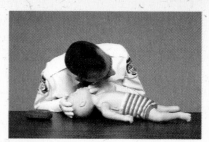

Figure 7-11c Determine breathlessness.

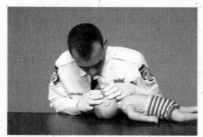

Figure 7-11d Cover the infant's mouth and nose with a pocket mask. Then ventilate.

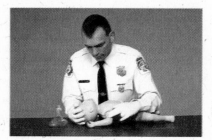

Figure 7-11e Determine pulselessness at the brachial artery.

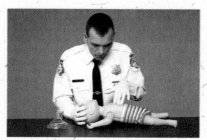

Figure 7-11f Locate the correct hand position.

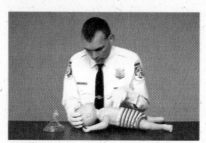

Figure 7-11g Compress the lower sternum at a rate of at least 100 per minute.

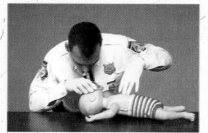

Figure 7-11h A gentle puff of air is given after every fifth compression.

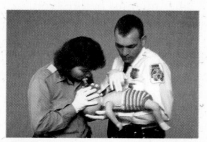

Figure 7-11i Performing CPR while carrying the baby.

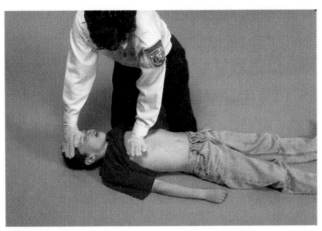
Figure 7-12 Chest compressions on a larger child.

- Check the patient's pulse periodically. In the infant, check the brachial pulse. In the child, check the carotid pulse.
- Check the pupils. CPR is successful if they are reacting normally or appear to be normal.
- Watch for a spontaneous heartbeat, spontaneous breathing, and responsiveness.

Complications of CPR

One of the most common complications with injury and sudden illness in children is hypothermia (a below-normal body temperature). So keep the infant or child warm.

FIRST RESPONDER FOCUS

Circulation, like respiration, is essential to life. If a patient's heart fails to beat, he or she will surely die unless actions are taken to restore the heartbeat. As a First Responder, you will help to take these actions.

Cardiopulmonary resuscitation (CPR) is the first step in saving the life of a patient whose heart has stopped beating. The sooner CPR is started, the better. Permanent damage may occur after as few as four minutes.

Over the years, scientists have discovered that CPR has limitations. It is not nearly as effective as the patient's own heartbeat. This is why CPR pro-

cedure calls for you to activate EMS before beginning CPR. This allows other members of the EMS system to respond while you perform CPR.

The next chapter covers automated external defibrillation. The AED is a device that applies an electric shock to the patient's chest, which can restore a heartbeat. You will recall that the chain of survival requires early access, early CPR, and early defibrillation together with advanced care for an optimal chance of survival.

Perform CPR in accordance with AHA standards when you are called to do so. Be sure you have a barrier device with you at all times. ■

CASE STUDY FOLLOW-UP

At the beginning of this chapter, you read that First Responders took over CPR from a bystander. To see how chapter skills apply to this emergency, read the following. It describes how the call was completed.

PHYSICAL EXAMINATION
Our first concern was providing good CPR. Two men in my crew were doing that. A thorough physical exam would have to wait. The patient

was on the grass and didn't appear to have any injuries from falling to the ground.

PATIENT HISTORY
I talked to a bystander, who told me that the patient had been mowing the lawn when he collapsed. He wasn't sure how long his neighbor had been down, but he thought it was less than five minutes.

The patient's wife told me that her husband was 71 and had bypass surgery two years ago

CASE STUDY FOLLOW-UP *(Continued)*

after a heart attack. He was on medication for his heart and high blood pressure. She went to get it, as I radioed the incoming EMS units with an update.

ONGOING ASSESSMENT
All we could do at this point was monitor the success of the CPR. We checked the carotid pulse during chest compressions, and the chest rise and fall during ventilations.

PATIENT HAND-OFF
When the EMTs arrived, I told them that the patient was a 71-year-old male. He was found in cardiac arrest by his wife, who began CPR. The patient was unresponsive with no pulse or respirations when CPR was continued by our crew. I told them I didn't believe the patient had any injuries. He had a history of bypass surgery and high blood pressure, and took medication. I gave them the patient's medication vials.

The EMTs continued emergency care as we watched. It took three shocks from the AED to get the patient's heart started again. But he still had no respirations. So one of them continued to ventilate the patient while the others put the patient on a backboard. The backboard would give them a hard surface to compress against in case they had to start CPR again.

Later, the EMTs told me that the patient had improved slightly in the ambulance, and was transferred to the cardiac unit at the hospital. Not all patient's survive. I was happy we helped one who did.

> Heart disease is still the number one killer in the U.S. Be prepared to provide CPR to any patient who needs it. And remember to take refresher courses frequently and get recertified as per local protocol or every one or two years.

REVIEW QUESTIONS

Page references where answers may be found or supported are provided at the end of each question.

Section 1

1. What is the name and location of each of the four chambers of the heart? (p. 121)
2. What are the links in the "chain of survival"? (p. 123)
3. What is the pulse? Where can you best palpate it? (p. 122)

Section 2

4. Before performing CPR on your patient, what must your assessment of his or her condition reveal? (pp. 124–125)

5. How can you find the correct CPR compression site on an infant, child, and adult? (pp. 126, 135)
6. What are the appropriate compression depths for an infant, child, and adult? (pp. 127, 135)
7. Why is it essential to perform CPR in spite of the problems it may cause? (p. 135)
8. When should you activate EMS if your patient is an unresponsive adult? An unresponsive infant? (p. 125)

CHAPTER 8

AUTOMATED EXTERNAL DEFIBRILLATION

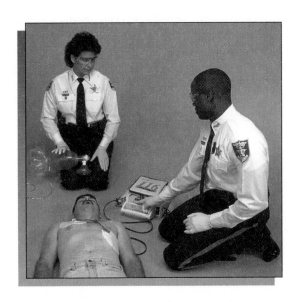

INTRODUCTION

As you will recall from Chapter 7, early defibrillation is part of the "chain of survival." In order to get defibrillation to patients early enough, as many trained people as possible—not just physicians and paramedics—must be able to perform this life-saving skill.

Automated external defibrillators have made that possible. Now First Responders, EMT-Basics, and even members of the public are able to defibrillate a patient when it is needed.

Cognitive, affective, and psychomotor objectives are from the U.S. DOT's 1995 "First Responder: National Standard Curriculum." Enrichment objectives, if any, identify material that is supplemental to the DOT curriculum.

Cognitive

No objectives are identified.

Affective

No objectives are identified.

Psychomotor

No objectives are identified.

Enrichment

* List the indications and contraindications for automated external defibrillation. (pp. 142–144)
* Differentiate between fully automated and the semi-automated external defibrillators. (pp. 140, 142)
* List the steps in the operation of an automated external defibrillator. (pp. 144–145, 147)
* Describe the care for a patient whose pulse has returned after automated external defibrillation. (p. 147)
* Discuss the need to complete the automated defibrillator operator's shift checklist. (p. 147)
* Explain the role medical direction plays in the use of automated external defibrillation. (p. 147)
* Describe the maintenance of an automated external defibrillator. (pp. 147, 149)

SECTION 1: ABOUT DEFIBRILLATORS

Defibrillation is the application of an electric shock to the chest of a patient who is in cardiac arrest—a nonbreathing and pulseless patient. It has been used for many years by physicians and paramedics. Most of them use *manual* defibrillation. This means they interpret the information the machine reports, decide if shocks are indicated, and then apply the shocks themselves with "paddles" to the patient chest.

The **automated external defibrillator (AED)** can perform all those tasks. The AED has a microprocessor that actually interprets the heart rhythm, just as a physician would. When necessary, shocks are then delivered by the device directly to the patient.

The actual shocks are delivered to the chest through adhesive pads. These pads are connected to the AED through cables, which can transmit a shock to the chest that is powerful enough to correct a lethal heart rhythm. The pads make defibrillation safer since no one needs to touch the patient at all during analysis or shocks.

EMS systems that allow First Responders to use AEDs should have all of the following in place:

* All of the links of the "chain of survival." Without early access, early CPR, and early advanced care, the patient will not have the best chance of survival (Figure 8–1).
* *Medical direction.* A physician must issue standing orders for First Responders to use an AED.
* *Quality improvement programs* to monitor the use of AEDs in the field.
* *Mandatory continuing education.*

TYPES OF AEDS

There are two types of automated defibrillator—one that is fully automated and one that is semi-automated (Figure 8-2). The operator attaches a fully automated defibrillator to the patient, turns it on, and the device does the rest. The **semi-automated external defibrillator (SAED)** performs the same tasks, but the operator must push a button to analyze the patient's heart rhythm and to deliver the shock.

CASE STUDY

DISPATCH

Our engine company was sent on a call to an unresponsive woman at 326 Riverview Lane.

SCENE SIZE-UP

We approached the scene carefully and saw a man frantically waving to us. We were still alert to the possibility of danger as we pulled closer.

When we got to the house, the man said his neighbor, a nurse, was performing CPR. We saw her working on an elderly woman who was lying on the lawn. "My wife collapsed while she was carrying in the groceries," the man said. "Please help her. Please!"

There was only one patient. We decided to call for the medics right away. After putting on our gloves and grabbing a pocket face mask, we joined the nurse at CPR. She was doing a good job.

INITIAL ASSESSMENT

We checked the patient's pulse and respirations. There were none.

Cardiac arrest is literally a life-or-death situation. Some patients may be saved through the use of an automated external defibrillator. Consider this patient as you read Chapter 8. See if you can decide if she needs defibrillation. If she does, then how and when would you apply it? And when should you stop?

Chain of Survival

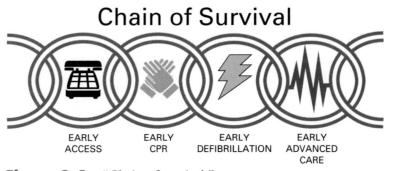

EARLY ACCESS   EARLY CPR   EARLY DEFIBRILLATION   EARLY ADVANCED CARE

Figure 8-1 "Chain of survival."

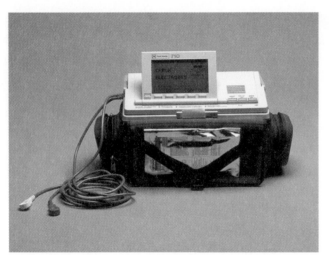

Figure 8-2a Example of a fully automated defibrillator.

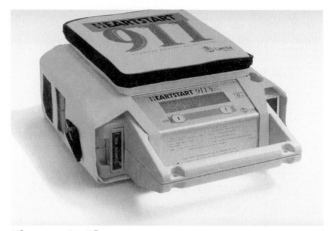

Figure 8-2b Example of a semi-automated defibrillator.

There are many brands of AED. Many of them include:

- *On/off button.* This button controls power to the AED.
- *Analyze button.* Press this button to instruct the AED to analyze heart rhythm.
- *Shock button.* Depress this button to deliver an electric shock to the patient.
- *Voice synthesizer.* Some units have an electronic voice that prompts you to perform specific actions. The "voice" may direct you to "analyze rhythm" or "push to shock" at the appropriate time.
- *Tape recorder.* Some units have a built-in microphone and tape recorder that tape the events of a cardiac arrest. The recording can then be used for training or quality improvement at a later date.
- *EKG screen or light.* Even though First Responders do not analyze heart rhythms, some AEDs have a built-in screen or light that shows the electrical activity of the heart.

SECTION 2: OPERATING A DEFIBRILLATOR

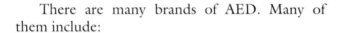

AEDs are very safe and accurate. Even so, you must follow operation guidelines carefully. They will assure safe and proper use of the defibrillator:

- Become familiar with the AED you are using.
- Make sure the AED batteries are fully charged. Carry extra fully charged batteries.
- Carefully follow your local protocols regarding AED use in your area.
- Make sure no one touches the patient while the AED is analyzing the heart rhythm or while a shock is being delivered. If someone is in contact, the shock may be transferred to that person. Touching the patient or cables also may cause interference with the accuracy of the AED.
- Do not apply the AED to a patient with a pulse. The shock could cause the heart to stop.

In addition, AEDs must not be used on patients less than 12 years of age or those who weigh less than 90 pounds. Many EMS systems also do not allow an AED to be used with patients who have cardiac arrest due to injury or hypothermia (low body temperature).

HEART RHYTHMS

The normal electrical impulses of the heart occur in an orderly, rhythmic fashion. When you place an AED on a patient, it evaluates your patient's heart rhythm (Figure 8–3).

There are two specific rhythms that require an AED shock. They are:

HEART RHYTHMS

Chaotic electrical discharge as occurs
in heart muscle wall.

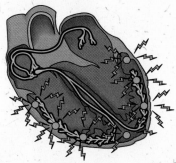

Chaotic electrical discharge as seen on an ECG tracing.

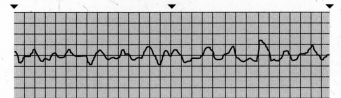

Figure 8-3a Ventricular fibrillation.

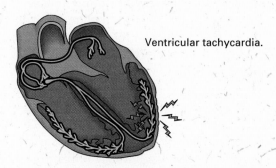

Ventricular tachycardia.

ECG tracing of ventricular tachycardia.

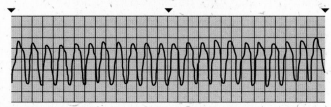

Figure 8-3b Ventricular tachycardia.

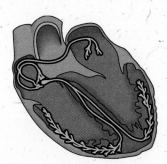

Asystole

ECG tracing of asystole

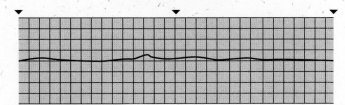

Figure 8-3c Asystole.

- *Ventricular fibrillation.* This is a chaotic, unorganized heart rhythm. It cannot create a pulse or circulate blood to sustain life.
- *Ventricular tachycardia.* This is a rhythm that is more organized but very rapid and inefficient. It is capable of producing a pulse. (Note that AED shocks must only be delivered to patients without a pulse.)

Heart rhythms that do not require an AED shock are:

- *Pulseless electrical activity (PEA).* If you were to look at an electrocardiogram (EKG) displaying this rhythm, you might think nothing was wrong. You would find electrical activity on the display, but you would not find a pulse.
- *Asystole.* Also known as "flatline," this is a condition where there are no electrical impulses present and, therefore, no pulse. The EKG shows a flat line.

A saying common to paramedics and doctors applies to First Responders who use AEDs: "Treat the patient, not the machine." For example, if the AED, reads a "flatline," it may only mean that one of the electrodes or cables has become detached from the patient. Other times an AED might read "normal" electrical activity. If you were only to pay attention to a machine's monitor screen, you would not realize that a PEA patient needs CPR immediately. Remember, the AED only analyzes heart rhythms. It does not check pulse.

Always follow your local protocols when determining a candidate for defibrillation. If you have questions, contact medical direction. Also be sure to practice AED procedures frequently and attend continuing education sessions.

OPERATION GUIDELINES

Automated defibrillation is easy to learn. An AED may be applied and the patient defibrillated in less than a minute. A sequence of shocks may be delivered in about 90 seconds.

Be sure that you are familiar with AED application and operation. Always remember that it is a definitive step toward returning the heart to a normal rhythm and function. CPR is vital, but its main

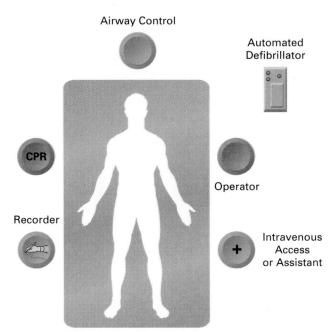

Figure 8-4 Ideal positioning. (Alternatives may be needed.)

purpose is to prolong life until defibrillation can be performed. When there is a pulseless patient and a defibrillator ready to go, use the defibrillator first!

(See ideal positioning in Figure 8–4.)

Applying Adhesive Pads

It is through the adhesive pads that the AED monitors heart rhythm and delivers shocks. So, the pads must be placed in very specific locations (Figure 8–5). Remember, all directions refer to the *patient's* right and left, not yours.

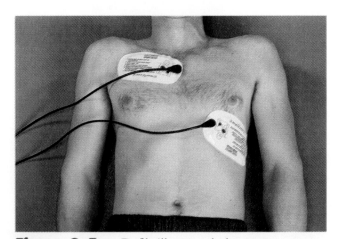

Figure 8-5a Defibrillator pad placement.

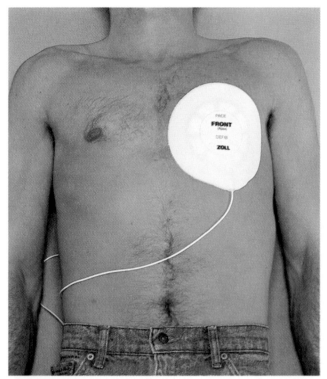

Figure 8-5b Alternative pad placement, front view.

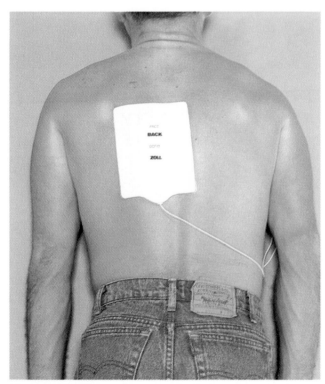

Figure 8-5c Alternative pad placement, back view.

Place one pad just below the patient's right clavicle and to the right of the sternum. Then attach the cable with the white tip to it. Place the other pad over the patient's left lower ribs, and attach the red electrode to it. The mnemonic "white to right, red to ribs" may help you remember where the pads and cables are to be placed.

Occasionally, you will find patients who have nitroglycerin patches on their chests. Do not place pads on or near them. Arcing or burning of the patient's skin could occur. Instead, remove the patches and use a towel to wipe off any paste that remains.

Be sure the AED's adhesive pads are not positioned over a pacemaker. It is possible to observe or feel a pacemaker once you bare the patient's chest. You also may be told by a family member that the patient has one. Place the AED's adhesive pads so they are not touching the pacemaker.

Adhesive pads should be securely applied to the chest. This may not be possible if the patient is extremely hairy. Be sure to carry a razor with your AED. Use it to quickly but safely shave the areas where the pads are to adhere.

Procedure for Unresponsive Patients and Those with CPR in Progress

After sizing up the scene and taking BSI precautions, perform an initial assessment. Stop CPR, if it is in progress, to check the patient's pulse and respirations (Figure 8–6). Then:

1. If the patient is pulseless, attach the AED. If there will be a delay in administering a shock, resume CPR.
2. Turn on the AED power.
3. Stop CPR, and instruct everyone to clear the patient.
4. Press the "analyze" button.

If the AED advises to administer a shock, then make sure everyone is still clear and:

1. Deliver the shock.
2. The AED will then reanalyze the heart rhythm.
3. If you are advised by the AED, deliver a second shock.
4. Again the AED will reanalyze the heart rhythm.

USING A SEMI-AUTOMATED DEFIBRILLATOR

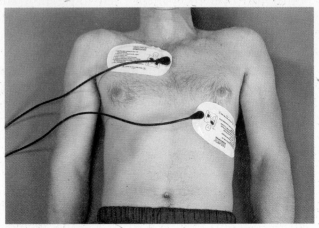

Figure 8-6a Determine the patient is breathless and pulseless.

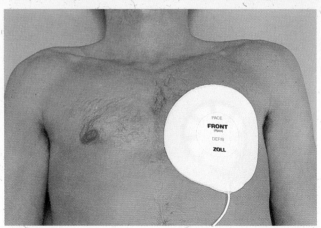

Figure 8-6b One rescuer initiates CPR, while the other prepares the AED.

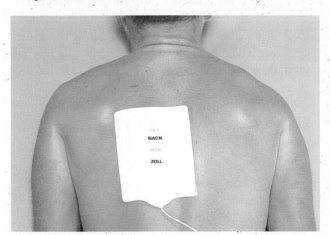

Figure 8-6c Place electrodes on the patient's chest.

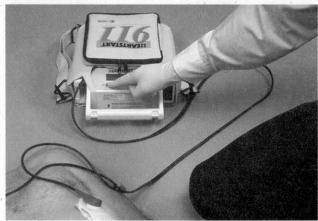

Figure 8-6d Turn on the AED.

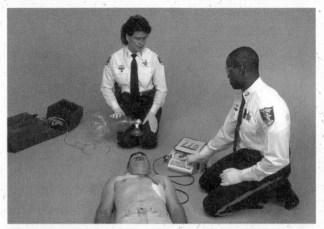

Figure 8-6e Stop CPR and get clear of the AED as it analyzes heart rhythm.

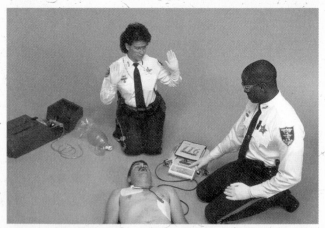

Figure 8-6f If a shock is advised, clear all others from the patient and deliver the shock.

5. If you are advised by the AED, deliver a third shock.
6. After the third shock, check the patient's pulse. Note that it is not necessary to check the pulse between shocks, unless the AED prompts you to do so. It can waste valuable time.
7. If a pulse is present, check respirations. Remember, the patient most likely will have inadequate breathing at this point if he or she is breathing at all.

   If there is no pulse, begin CPR for one minute. After one minute, repeat the cycle described above of up to three shocks.
8. Transportation should occur after two sets of three shocks.

If the AED advises NOT to administer a shock, then:

1. Recheck the patient's pulse.
2. If a pulse is present, check respirations. If breathing is inadequate, assist with ventilations. If the pulse is not present, perform CPR for one minute and reanalyze the heart rhythm.

If you are alone and find an unresponsive patient, then:

1. Assess the patient's breathing and pulse. If these are absent *and* your AED is immediately available, proceed with the following.
2. Apply the AED, and analyze the heart rhythm immediately. Do not begin CPR first. Defibrillation is more important at this point and more beneficial to the patient.
3. Follow the instructions outlined above in response to the AED prompts.

POST-RESUSCITATION CARE

In some, but not all cases, your patient will regain a pulse. This is exciting, but there is much more to be done. Your patient is still in serious condition. Remember the following points when caring for a patient whose pulse has returned:

• Monitor the pulse carefully. It may disappear.
• Many patients will not breathe, even though a pulse has returned. This is common. Ventilate the patient or assist ventilations as necessary.

• If your patient has regained pulse and adequate respirations—and has not been injured, place him or her in a recovery position.
• Apply high concentration oxygen, if you are trained and allowed by local protocol.
• Keep the AED attached to the patient. EMS personnel who take over care will want it attached during transport.
• Your assessment of the patient should be ongoing until you turn over care.

It will help the patient if advanced care is also available. Arrange for the paramedics to respond to the scene, if you have not done so already. Whether the advanced care is performed by them or by physicians, advanced care includes medications and other interventions that will help stabilize the patient and prevent another cardiac arrest. If the paramedics cannot respond in a reasonable amount of time, an ambulance should transport the patient promptly to the nearest hospital emergency department.

CALL REVIEW

After using an AED, the call should be reviewed by a quality improvement committee. (Your medical director will be involved.) The committee reviews all AED calls to determine if protocols were followed. This review uses the run report and, if your AED was equipped, the tape recording of the call.

While the call review looks for problem areas, it is not designed to get people "into trouble." If needed, the committee may recommend further training for some or all rescuers who use AEDs. The goal of the review is to have trained First Responders providing quality care to patients.

AED MAINTENANCE

The AED is a vital piece of equipment. It would be devastating to arrive at the side of a patient in cardiac arrest with a non-working machine. It may also be a cause of liability against you and your agency.

AUTOMATED DEFIBRILLATORS: OPERATOR'S SHIFT CHECKLIST

Date: _____ Shift: _____ Location: _____

Mfr/Model No.: _____ Serial No. or Facility ID No.: _____

At the beginning of each shift, inspect the unit. Indicate whether all requirements have been met. Note any corrective actions taken. Sign the form.

	Okay as found	Corrective Action/Remarks
1. Defibrillator Unit Clean no spills, clear of objects on top, casing intact		
2. Cables/Connectors a. Inspect for cracks, broken wire, or damage b. Connectors engage securely		
3. Supplies a. Two sets of pads in sealed packages, within expiration date b. Hand towel c. Scissors d. Razor * e. Alcohol wipes * f. Monitoring electrodes *g. Spare charged battery *h. Adequate ECG paper *i. Manual override module, key or card *j. Cassette tape, memory module, and/or event card plus spares		

4. Power Supply
 	
a. Battery-powered units
  (1) Verify fully charged battery in place
  (2) Spare charged battery available
  (3) Follow appropriate battery rotation schedule per manufacturer's recommendations
b. AC/Battery backup units
  (1) Plugged into live outlet to maintain battery charge
  (2) Test on battery power and reconnect to line power		

5. Indicators/*ECG Display * a. Remove cassette tape, memory module, and/or event card b. Power on display c. Self-test ok * d. Monitor display functional *e. "Service" message display off *f. Battery charging; low battery light off g. Correct time displayed — set with dispatch center		
6. ECG Recorder a. Adequate ECG paper b. Recorder prints		
7. Charge/Display Cycle * a. Disconnect AC plug — battery backup units b. Attach to simulator c. Detects, charges and delivers shock for "VF" d. Responds correctly to non-shockable rhythms *e. Manual override functional f. Detach from simulator *g. Replace cassette tape, module, and/or memory card		
8. *Pacemaker a. Pacer output cable intact b. Pacer pads present (set of two) c. Inspect per manufacturer's operational guidelines		

☐ **Major problem(s) identified**   **(OUT OF SERVICE)**

*Applicable only if the unit has this supply or capability

Signature: _____

Figure 8-7 Operator's shift checklist for AEDs, courtesy of Laerdal.

Complete the AED operator's shift checklist at the beginning of every shift (Figure 8–7). Make sure that the AED battery—and a spare—are fully charged and ready. Make sure the leads are with the unit and there are several sets of adhesive pads available. Always treat the AED carefully. Do not expose it to unnecessary jarring or other rough moves. Finally, follow the manufacturer's guidelines for maintenance.

FIRST RESPONDER FOCUS

Automated external defibrillation saves lives. It is a skill that the American Heart Association (AHA) believes should be taught to every First Responder.

Remember that CPR will sustain life for a period of time until more advanced care can be provided. An automated defibrillator can actually shock certain abnormal heart rhythms back to normal. Never delay defibrillation. If you have a choice between CPR and defibrillation, chose defibrillation. The earlier the shock is applied, the better chance you have of restoring normal heart patterns in your patient.

Finally, when you are called to the scene of a patient in cardiac arrest, there will be considerable stress, especially if you have not been on many such calls. The old adage "practice makes perfect" applies here. If you practice with your AED frequently and if you are familiar with protocols, you will perform better under the stress of the situation. ■

CASE STUDY FOLLOW-UP

At the beginning of this chapter, you read that First Responders were at the scene of a patient in respiratory and cardiac arrest. To see how chapter skills apply to this emergency, read the following. It describes how the call was completed.

INITIAL ASSESSMENT *(Continued)*
I had the AED. It took only a few seconds to hook up the electrodes and cables while CPR continued. I turned on the AED and instructed everyone to clear the patient while it analyzed the heart rhythm. The machine advised me to press the shock button.

After making sure everyone was clear, I shocked the patient. The machine automatically went back to "analyze" mode. It instructed me to shock again. Everyone was clear, and I shocked again. The AED analyzed. It then told me to check the pulse. I couldn't believe it. There was a pulse.

We immediately checked the patient's respirations. There were none. We hooked oxygen into the pocket face mask and ventilated her.

PATIENT HISTORY
Among the facts the patient's husband, Mr. Jones, told us was that his wife was in good health. She hadn't been to a doctor in years. She took no medications. She had no complaints before she went down. They had sandwiches for dinner two hours ago. She had no allergies. "She was always so healthy. I just don't understand," he said.

PHYSICAL EXAMINATION
We checked quickly for any obvious signs of injury and found none.

ONGOING ASSESSMENT
We never got to the ongoing assessment. The medics were already on scene.

PATIENT HAND-OFF
The hand-off report to the medics was as follows:

"This is Georgia Jones. She is 66 and was carrying groceries into the house when she collapsed on the grass. A nurse who lives next door started

CASE STUDY FOLLOW-UP *(Continued)*

CPR. She was doing a good job. We hooked up the AED and gave two shocks, which caused the pulse to return, but no respirations. We ventilated the patient and monitored her pulse until you arrived. Georgia hasn't been to the doctor recently, has no meds, and no allergies. Her husband says she is in good health, and there were no problems before she collapsed. There appear to be no injuries from the fall. She had a sandwich two hours ago for dinner."

The medics began their advanced life support. They started intravenous lines (IVs), put in airway adjuncts, and gave medications. The patient went back into cardiac arrest once while they were caring for her. They used their manual defibrillator and got her pulse back with one shock. Georgia made it to the hospital with a pulse, but the doctors said her heart and brain had suffered too much damage to survive.

After a day in the cardiac unit, Georgia passed away. We were sad to hear it and disappointed. We realized that we had done the best we could. Many patients don't live. I know that. The next time maybe we'll get to shake the hand of the person we help when they walk out of the hospital.

> SPECIAL NOTE: The AED is a device that has tremendous potential to save lives. But there are some patients who will not be saved. Some will have been "down" too long or suffered heart damage so great that they could not be saved even if they were in a hospital. Do your best for all patients. If a patient does not survive, even with your best efforts, it is not your fault.
>
> Losing a patient is a difficult experience. Focus on the good you have done for prior patients and the good you will do for future ones. Also seek out experienced members of your agency. They undoubtedly have felt the same at some point in their career. If necessary, speak to your medical director about the call.

REVIEW QUESTIONS

Page references where answers may be found or supported are provided at the end of each question.

Section 1

1. What is the difference between an automated and semi-automated defibrillator? (pp. 140, 142)

Section 2

2. What role does medical direction play in the use of an AED? (pp. 140, 144, 147)

3. When should the AED not be used? (p. 142)
4. Why is it so important to make sure no one is touching the patient while the AED analyzes or shocks the patient? (p. 142)
5. If given a choice between performing CPR and using an AED, which should be performed first? Explain your answer. (p. 144)
6. Where are the AED's adhesive pads placed on the patient? (pp. 144–145)
7. When should the patient's pulse be checked— before or after the first shock? When should it be checked again? (pp. 145, 147)

CHAPTER 9

SCENE SIZE-UP

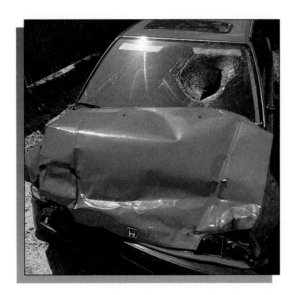

INTRODUCTION

The purpose of scene size-up is to assure the safety of people at the scene, to identify the mechanism of injury or nature of illness, and to determine the necessary additional resources. Most likely you will not have contact with your patient during scene size-up. Even so, your observations, decisions, and actions set the foundation for the success of the entire call.

Cognitive, affective, and psychomotor objectives are from the U.S. DOT's 1995 "First Responder: National Standard Curriculum." Enrichment objectives, if any, identify material that is supplemental to the DOT curriculum.

Cognitive

3-1.1 Discuss the components of scene size-up. (pp. 151, 152, 155, 164)

3-1.2 Describe common hazards found at the scene of a trauma and a medical patient. (p. 152)

3-1.3 Determine if the scene is safe to enter. (pp. 153–154)

3-1.4 Discuss common mechanisms of injury/nature of illness. (pp. 155–163)

3-1.5 Discuss the reason for identifying the total number of patients at the scene. (p. 164)

3-1.6 Explain the reason for identifying the need for additional help or assistance. (pp. 164–165)

Affective

3-1.22 Explain the rationale for crew members to evaluate scene safety prior to entering. (pp. 153–154)

3-1.23 Serve as a model for others by explaining how patient situations affect your evaluation of the mechanism of injury or illness. (pp. 155–163)

Psychomotor

3-1.33 Demonstrate the ability to differentiate various scenarios and identify potential hazards. (pp. 152–154, 164–165)

SECTION 1: ASSURING PERSONAL SAFETY

PERSONAL PROTECTIVE EQUIPMENT

Body substance isolation (BSI) precautions must be taken on every call. See Chapter 2 for a full discussion. What follows is a brief review.

Personal protective equipment (PPE) includes:

- *Gloves.* Wear them when there is any chance of coming in contact with a patient's blood or body fluids.
- *Eye protection.* Wear it when there is any chance of blood or body fluids spraying or splashing into your eyes.
- *Mask.* Wear one when there is any chance of blood or body fluids spraying or splashing into your nose or mouth.
- *Gown.* Wear one when there is any chance of clothing becoming soiled with blood or other body fluids.

Remember that you should always have personal protective equipment available. When you approach the scene, anticipate which items may be needed and then put them on. Waiting too long may cause you to become so involved in patient care that you forget to protect yourself.

Nothing is more important at the emergency scene than your safety. Hazards may include obvious situations such as violence, downed power lines, or hazardous materials. Do not overlook the dangers at other scenes such as car crashes, unstable vehicles, unstable surfaces (slopes, ice, etc.), and dangerous pets. Place your safety first. If you do not, you may become a patient yourself and quite possibly prevent others from caring for the patient you were sent to help.

The vast majority of calls go by uneventfully. When there is danger, three words sum up the actions required to respond appropriately: *plan, observe,* and *react* (Figure 9–1).

PLAN

Many First Responders work together to prevent danger and know what do to when danger strikes. However, scene safety begins long before the actual emergency. For example, you should:

- *Wear safe clothing.* Nonslip shoes and other practical clothing will help you to respond to danger without restriction.

CASE STUDY

DISPATCH

I am a First Responder for the Fire Department. My partner and I were dispatched to a car crash at the corner of Central and Devine. The caller indicated that the crash seemed "pretty bad."

SCENE SIZE-UP

When we approached the scene, we saw the caller was correct. It was a head-on into a telephone pole.

> The scene size-up on this call will be very important. As you read Chapter 9, consider what the First Responders should do to size up the scene, as well as handle other parts of the call.

- *Prepare your equipment properly.* Make sure it is not cumbersome. Remember that you will be carrying it into emergencies. If your first response kit is too heavy or large, it will distract your attention from where it should be—observing the scene.
- *Carry a portable radio.* A radio allows you to call for help if you are separated from your vehicle.
- *Plan safety roles.* If there will be more than one rescuer on any call, tasks can be split. For example, one rescuer can care for the patient, while the other observes for safety. The "observer" could look for nearby weapons or other threats, for example, and for clues to the patient's condition, such as prescription medications.

OBSERVE

Remember that it is always better to prevent danger than it is to deal with it. Observation and awareness are the best ways to accomplish this goal.

Observation begins early in the call. As you approach the scene, turn off your lights and sirens to avoid broadcasting your arrival and attracting a crowd. Observe the neighborhood as you look for house numbers. If possible, do not park directly in front of the call. This provides two benefits. First, you may be able to approach the scene unnoticed, which allows you to size it up without distraction. Second, since many first response units do not transport, the area directly in front of the call is left open for the ambulance.

As you approach an emergency scene, look for the following signs of potential danger:

- *Violence.* Any indication that violence has or may take place is significant. These signs include arguing, threats, or other violent behavior. Also notice any broken glass, overturned furniture, or the like.
- *Weapons of any kind.* If a weapon is on scene, it is a serious potential danger.
- *Signs of intoxication or drug use.* When people are under the influence of alcohol or drugs, their behavior is unpredictable. In addition,

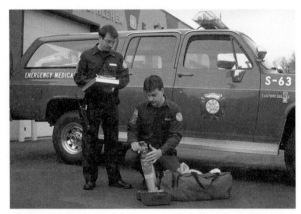

Figure 9-1a   Plan for the possibility of a dangerous scene.

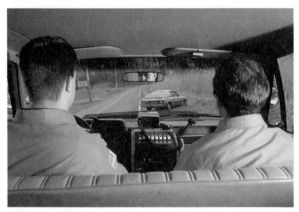

Figure 9-1b   Observe the scene for signs of potential danger.

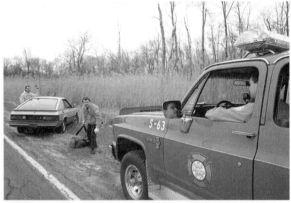

Figure 9-1c   React to danger appropriately—retreat, radio, and reevaluate.

even though you see yourself as there to help, other people may not. You may be mistaken for the police, because you are in uniform and you drove up in a vehicle with lights and sirens.

• *Anything unusual.* Even an awkward silence should cause you to be wary. Emergencies are usually very active events. In situations where you observe an unusual silence, a certain amount of caution is advisable.

Note that nothing in this textbook is meant to create fear or unwarranted suspicion. Remember that the vast majority of EMS calls will go by uneventfully. Some calls, however, do pose a threat. Those calls usually provide subtle clues that may be picked up *before* the danger strikes. Use your observation skills on every call to determine important safety information.

Remember, the general rule is: *If the scene is unsafe, make it safe if you are trained to do so. If not,* do not enter *and call for the appropriate teams to handle the situation.*

REACT

If you find danger at the scene, there are three "Rs" of reacting: *retreat, radio,* and *reevaluate.*

Retreat

With the exception of the police who train with this textbook, it is not a First Responder's responsibility to subdue violent persons or wrestle weapons away. A clear and justified course is to retreat from danger.

There are safer ways to retreat than others. When leaving the scene of danger, remember the following points:

• *Flee far enough away that danger will not threaten you again.* Retreating only a short distance keeps you in danger. In addition, when fleeing a scene of danger, place two major obstacles between you and it. If a dangerous person moves in your direction and gets through one obstacle, the second obstacle acts as a built-in buffer.
• *Take cover.* Cover and concealment are important. Find a position that hides your body and protects it from projectiles (getting behind a brick wall, for example). This is preferred over concealment, which only hides your body but offers no protection (like getting behind a shrub). When fleeing danger, moving a consid-

erable distance from the scene and taking cover are usually the best options.

• *Discard your equipment.* Do not get bogged down. The equipment you carry can be thrown at the subject's feet to give you additional time to retreat.

Radio

The portable radio is an important piece of safety equipment. Its main function is to call for police assistance and to warn other rescuers of impending danger. When using the radio, speak clearly and slowly. Advise the dispatcher of the exact nature and location of the problem. Specify how many people are involved and whether or not weapons were observed.

Remember that the information you have must be shared as soon as possible to prevent others from coming up against the same danger.

Reevaluate

Do not reenter the scene until it has been secured by the police. Even then, keep in mind that violence may begin again. Emergencies are situations packed with stress for families, victims, rescuers, and bystanders. Maintain a level of observation throughout the call. Occasionally, weapons or illegal drugs are found while you are assessing your patient. Notify the police immediately.

After the call, document the situation on your run report. Occasionally, the danger may cause delays in reaching the patient. Courts have held this acceptable, provided that there has been a real and documented danger.

SECTION 2: MECHANISM OF INJURY OR NATURE OF ILLNESS

During scene size-up, you must determine the nature of the patient's problem. You may already have some idea from dispatch whether your patient is a **medical patient** (ill) or a **trauma patient** (injured). So when you scan the scene for safety factors, also try to determine if the patient is ill or injured.

A medical patient's condition is caused by some internal factor such as a heart or breathing problem. There is nothing at the scene that suggests injury. In this case, speak to the patient, family, or bystanders to determine why EMS was called and what the **nature of illness** might be.

When you scan the trauma scene, note the **mechanism of injury** (forces that caused the injury). For example, if your patient fell from a ladder, it would be important to note how far the patient fell. The greater the distance, the more serious and extensive the injuries may be.

Occasionally, a patient may have a combination of illness and injury. Consider the patient who fell from a ladder, for instance. What if he passed out from a medical problem and then fell to the ground? As you approach the scene, the mechanism of injury may be obvious. The illness may not be. It will be your examination of the scene, as well as the eventual patient history, that will make a difference. (See Chapter 10 for instructions on how to gather a patient history.)

KINEMATICS OF TRAUMA

Trauma is the leading cause of death for people between the ages of 14 and 40. It also is the third leading cause of death overall—behind only heart disease and cancer.

Emergency medical treatment of trauma depends on the extent of the injuries. However, it is not quite so simple. Too often hidden injuries prove to be fatal. In order to understand how seriously a patient may be injured, you must determine the mechanism of injury. It will tell you what injuries or patterns of injury the patient may be suffering.

The science of analyzing the mechanism of injury is called the *kinematics of trauma.* The process is based on physical laws such as an object (mass) in motion contains energy, and energy is influenced by the interaction of velocity (speed) and mass.

Kinetic energy is the total amount of energy contained by an object in motion. When the weight of that object is doubled, its energy also is doubled. In other words, it is twice as damaging to be hit by a two-pound baseball than by a one-pound baseball.

Velocity is the speed at which an object moves. According to physical laws, velocity is more important than weight in producing kinetic energy. The higher the speed of an object, the more energy it has. The rate at which an object changes speed (its acceleration and deceleration) is also significant. As you know, the faster a car travels, the longer it takes to stop.

The process of gaining and losing velocity occurs with each impact in a crash. The number of impacts varies, but there are three basic ones (Figure 9–2). First, the car impacts the object. Then, the occupant impacts the interior of the car. Finally, the occupant's organs impact on the surfaces inside the body.

Each impact in a crash has the potential of causing harm. The amount of kinetic energy that is absorbed on impact, however, depends on how much energy is absorbed by other things first. For example, a person who falls on freshly plowed soil will not be injured as severely as the person who falls the same distance onto cement pavement.

Remember that the mechanism of injury is an important part of your assessment of a trauma patient. It can suggest which body parts are injured and how severe the injuries might be. Whenever you care for a trauma patient, maintain a high index of suspicion and take note of:

- The body position at the time of impact.
- The part of the body impacted.
- The object that penetrated the body, or the surface the body landed on.
- The distance involved, if any.

Common mechanisms of injury are falls, vehicular crashes, fire, explosions, and penetrating objects such as bullets and knives.

CAR CRASHES

There are five basic types of car crashes: head-on impact, rear impact, side impact, rotational impact, and rollover. Each one has its own predictable pattern of injury.

Head-on Impact

A head-on impact occurs when a car hits an immovable object, such as a tree (Figure 9–3). The greater the car's speed, the greater the energy, the greater the damage. When the car stops, its occupants continue to travel forward. They take one of two possible pathways of motion—up-and-over or down-and-under (Figure 9–4). Each pathway has a distinctive pattern of injury, which can be affected by the use of a seatbelt.

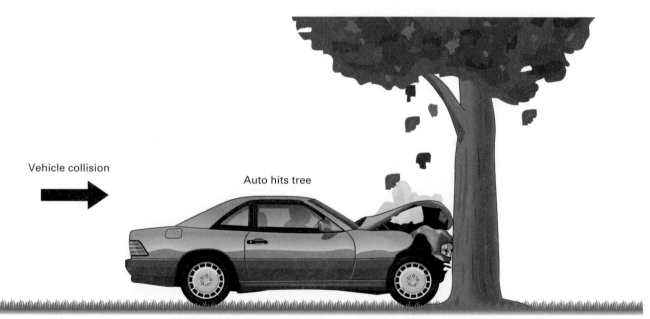

Figure 9-2a   Impact #1—the vehicle strikes an object.

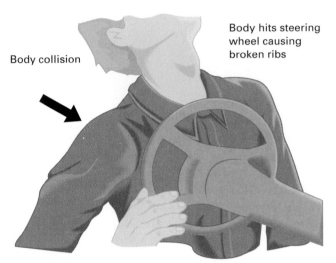

Figure 9-2b Impact #2—the occupant continues to move forward and collides with the steering wheel.

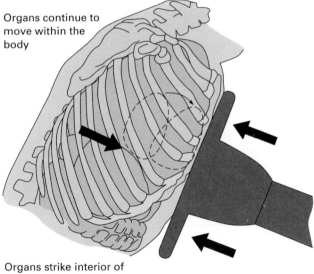

Figure 9-2c Impact #3—the internal organs continue to move forward and collide with the inside of the chest and other organs.

In the up-and-over pathway, the torso may be thrown over the steering wheel. The face, head, and neck then strike the windshield. The chest and abdomen may then strike the steering wheel. Note the following patterns of injury:

• *Face, head, and neck injuries.* Look for obvious clues like hair, tissue, or blood on the wind-

shield or rear-view mirror. The windshield also may bulge out in a classic bull's-eye or spider-web pattern.

The face can sustain extensive soft-tissue damage. However, bleeding from its rich supply of blood vessels may not be as serious as it looks. Watch for airway problems if there is bleeding from the mouth, nose, or face.

Skull fracture may occur. Almost all head injuries have the potential to cause damage to the brain. Brain tissue can compress, rebound against opposite sides of the skull, and bruise. Brain tissue also can be cut or bruised on the floor of the skull, which is very rough or jagged.

Energy can travel down the neck, causing the potential for cervical-spine injury. The neck may be flexed or extended too far, resulting in whiplash injuries or fractures. An impact at the top of the head can cause compression fractures of the cervical spine. The anterior neck also can be injured by hitting the steering wheel or dashboard. Cartilage rings in the trachea (windpipe) can be separated, which would impair breathing.

• *Chest injuries.* When the chest strikes the steering wheel, the ribs and sternum may break. The heart may be compressed and bruised, making it unable to pump blood effectively. The aorta may be torn, resulting in life-threatening bleeding. As the lungs are compressed, they can be bruised or ruptured. Remember that broken ribs can also injure the lungs and heart.

• *Abdominal injuries.* When the abdomen strikes the steering wheel, the liver, spleen, and other organs are compressed. Sometimes they are cut. The liver may be cut in half as it is forced against the ligament that holds it in place. The spleen may be torn from its attachment, resulting in severe internal bleeding.

In the down-and-under pathway of motion, a body slides under the steering wheel. The knees strike the dashboard. Energy travels up the legs. The abdomen and then the chest strike the steering wheel. Classic injuries include dislocated hip and broken patella (kneecap), femur (thigh bone), and pelvis.

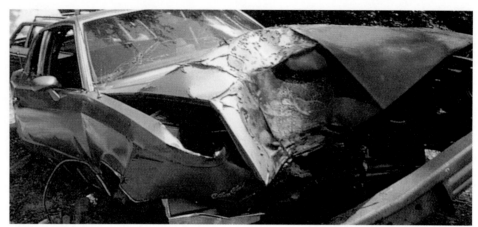

Figure 9-3 Head-on impact.

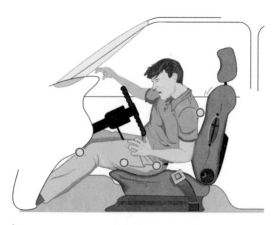

a.

b.

Figure 9-4 In a head-on impact, the patient is either forced (a) up and over or (b) down and under.

Rear Impact

Rear impact occurs when a car is struck from behind by another vehicle traveling at greater speed (Figure 9–5). The car that is hit accelerates suddenly, and the occupant's body is slammed backward and then forward (Figure 9–6). Suspect the same kinds of injuries as discussed for head-on collisions. If positioned properly, a headrest will prevent the head from whipping back. If the headrest is not in place, suspect soft-tissue injury to the neck, compression of the cervical spine, and cervical-spine fractures.

Side Impact

The side impact is often called a "broadside" or "T-bone" collision. The person closest to the impact absorbs more energy than a person on the opposite side. As the energy of the impact is absorbed, the body is pushed sideways and the head moves in the opposite direction. The following injuries commonly occur:

- *Head and neck injuries.* The head often impacts the door post. This can result in skull injury, brain injury, and tears in neck muscles and ligaments. Cervical-spine fractures are common, since the vertebrae are not designed for extreme lateral movement.
- *Chest injuries.* If the door slams against the shoulder, the clavicle will probably break. If the arm is caught between the door and the chest,

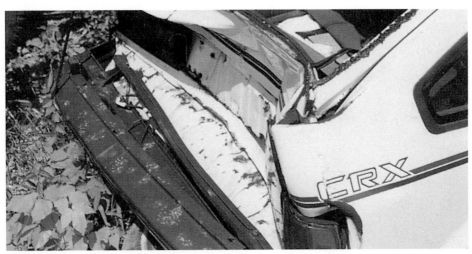

Figure 9-5 Rear impact.

or if the door impacts against the chest directly, suspect broken ribs and possible breathing problems. Fractures low in the rib cage can injure the liver and spleen.

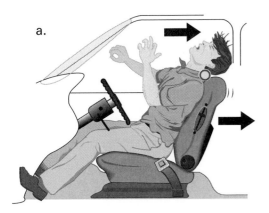

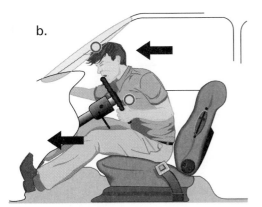

Figure 9-6 Rear impact forces the patient (a) back and then (b) forward.

• *Pelvis injuries.* Lateral impact to the pelvis often causes fractures of the pelvis and femur.

The person on the opposite side of the car is subject to similar kinds of head and neck injuries. In addition, if there is more than one person sitting on a seat, heads often collide.

Rotational Impact

A rotational impact is one that occurs off center. The car strikes an object and rotates around it until the car either loses speed or strikes another object. The sturdiest structures in the car (such as the steering wheel, dashboard, door posts, and windows) are the ones that cause the most serious injuries. A variety of injury patterns may occur due to the initial strike and subsequent striking of stationary objects. Look for the same kinds of injuries that occur with head-on and side impacts.

Rollover

During a rollover (Figure 9–7), car occupants change direction every time the car does (Figure 9–8). Every fixture inside the car becomes potentially lethal. A specific pattern of injury is impossible to predict, but rollovers almost always cause injuries to more than one body system.

If car occupants are not wearing seat belts, they have a much greater chance of being thrown from the car, either partially or fully. Common

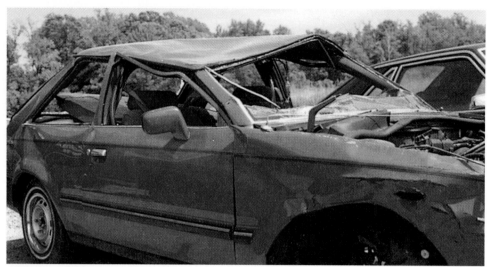

Figure 9-7 Rollover impact.

injuries include severe soft-tissue injuries, multiple broken bones, and crushing injuries resulting from the car rolling over the occupant.

Restraints

Restraints help to reduce the severity of injuries. However, occupants of a car can still be injured, especially if restraints are not used properly.

- *Lap belt*. When worn properly, a lap belt can prevent the occupant from being thrown out of the car. But it does not prevent the head, neck, and chest from striking the steering wheel or dashboard. When the torso is thrown forward, compression fractures of the lower back can occur. If the belt is worn across the upper abdomen instead of over the pelvis, the spleen, liver, intestines, or pancreas can be injured. There also may be enough pressure in the abdomen to injure the diaphragm and force abdominal contents into the chest cavity.

- *Lap-and-shoulder belt*. This type of restraint can prevent the occupant from striking the steering wheel or dashboard. A severe impact can cause the shoulder belt to break the clavicle. Even properly used, it does not prevent the head and neck from moving sideways or forward and back. If a headrest is not in place, suspect cervical-spine injury.

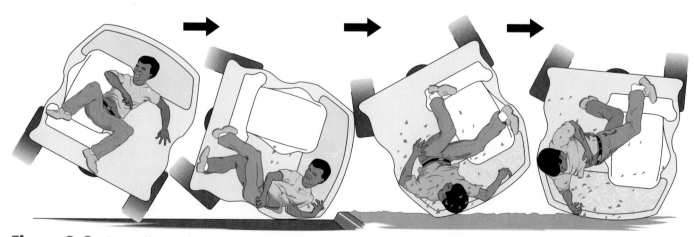

Figure 9-8 In a rollover, the unrestrained occupant changes direction every time the car does.

- *Air bag.* It cushions the occupant and absorbs energy in a head-on crash. Without a seat belt, however, it is not effective in rollovers, rear-end or side collisions, or collisions involving multiple vehicles and repeated impact. Serious, even fatal injuries have occurred in children in the passenger seat when airbags deploy.
- *Car seat.* An infant car seat that faces backwards in an upright position minimizes risk in a head-on collision. In a crash, all unrestrained parts of an infant's body continue to move forward. The greatest danger is to the neck. An infant's head is large for its body, and it tends to snap forward with great force. Suspect injury to the neck any time the mechanism of injury indicates it may be possible, even if the patient appears to be uninjured.

MOTORCYCLE CRASHES

Motorcycle crash injuries are greatly reduced when the rider wears a helmet. With no helmet, chances of severe head injury and death increase 340%. There are three types of impact in motorcycle accidents. They are head-on, angular, and ejection. "Laying the bike down," an evasive action, often prevents serious injuries but can cause extensive scrapes, bruises, and burns.

Head-on Impact

In a head-on impact, the rider generally impacts the handlebars at the same speed the bike was traveling. A variety of injuries can be expected. For example, if the rider's feet get caught, the thighs or pelvis will strike the handlebars, resulting in fractures.

Angular Impact

In this type of impact, the rider strikes an object at an angle. The object then usually collapses on the rider. Common objects are the edges of signs, outside mirrors on cars, or fence posts. Severe amputations can result.

Ejection

If the rider clears the handlebars, ejection occurs. The body is thrown until it hits a stationary object or the ground. The body may hit several objects or strike the ground many times before stopping. Expect severe head and facial injuries if the rider is not wearing a helmet. Fractures and internal injuries are likely. Expect severe soft-tissue damage if the rider is not wearing boots and leather clothing.

Laying the Bike Down

A rider who anticipates a crash may try to "lay the bike down." That is, the rider may turn the motorcycle sideways and drag a leg on the ground to lose enough speed to get off. If successful, the rider slides along the ground, clearing the bike and the object it hits. Expect severe abrasions (scrapes) from contact with the pavement. Many victims are also burned by contact with the motorcycle's hot exhaust pipe.

RECREATIONAL VEHICLE CRASHES

Injuries caused by recreational vehicle crashes are similar to those caused by motorcycles. However, since ATVs (all-terrain vehicles) are often used on fields and hilly terrain, patients can be harder to reach. One of the most dangerous ATV crashes occurs when a rider runs into an unseen wire fence. Cut neck vessels, severed windpipes, and even decapitations have resulted.

ATVs are prone to collision with other vehicles. Expect head, neck, and extremity injuries. The three-wheel ATV is especially unstable. A simple turn can cause a rollover, resulting in head and crush injuries. Unfortunately, many of those who ride ATVs are children. Their lesser body weights make ATVs even more unstable.

Another type of recreational vehicle is the snowmobile. It is often driven at high speed. When there is a crash, riders sustain severe head and neck injuries. Rollovers are also common.

FALLS

The most common mechanism of injury is a fall. Falls account for more than half of all trauma-related accidents. The severity of injury depends on the following:

- The distance of the fall.
- Anything that interrupts the fall.
- The body part that impacts first.
- The surface on which the victim lands.

Some experts say that the surface on which a victim lands is more important than the height of the fall. For example, diving into deep water from a high diving board is a recreational activity. Diving the same distance onto a concrete sidewalk is not.

Generally, a fall of two times a patient's height onto an unyielding surface is considered severe. (The U.S. DOT suggests that any fall of 15 feet or greater onto an unyielding surface is severe.) In either case, you should have a high degree of suspicion about internal injuries no matter how the patient looks.

Feet-First Fall

A feet-first landing causes energy to travel up the skeleton (Figure 9–9). If the knees are flexed when the person lands, injury to the bones will

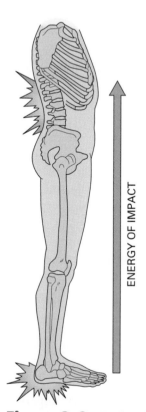

ENERGY OF IMPACT

Figure 9-9 In feet-first falls, the energy of impact is transmitted up the skeletal system.

be less severe. Common injuries include fractures of the spine, hip socket, femur, heel, and ankle. Head, back, and pelvis injuries are common if the victim falls backward. If the victim extends arms to break a forward fall, expect broken wrists. A broken shoulder and clavicle are common, too.

In falls of 15 feet or more, internal organs are likely to be severely injured from sudden deceleration. The liver may be sliced in two. The spleen or kidneys may be torn from their attachments. The heart may be torn from the aorta.

Head-First Fall

In head-first falls, the pattern of injury begins with the arms and extends up to the shoulders. Head and spine injuries are very common. There is usually extensive damage to the neck. When the body is falling, the torso and legs are thrown either forward or backward, commonly causing chest, lower spine, and pelvis injuries.

PENETRATING TRAUMA

This kind of injury occurs when an object penetrates the surface of the body. Hand-powered weapons, such as knives or arrows, generally cause low-velocity injuries. These are limited to the immediate site of impact. Projectiles powered by another source, such as bullets from a handgun, cause medium-velocity or high-velocity injuries. These affect tissues far from the site of impact.

When you encounter a scene of violence, it is absolutely essential that you make sure the scene is safe before you try to reach a patient. Follow local protocol.

Low-Velocity Injuries

Among the factors that help determine the severity of a low-velocity injury are the gender of the offender, the position of the victim when stabbed, and the length of the object used to penetrate the body.

The gender of the offender can give you important clues. Women generally have less upper-body strength. They usually stab overhand, or downward. Men have more upper-body strength, so they usually stab up and out. For example, if the victim was stabbed on the right side by a man, the most likely injuries would be to the liver, kidney, and intestine. If the victim was stabbed by a woman, the most likely injury would be to the lungs.

The length of the weapon also gives valuable clues. For example, a person stabbed in the chest with a three-inch paring knife would probably suffer a pneumothorax (collapse of the lungs due to air in the chest). The same stab wound inflicted by an eight-inch knife could cut the pulmonary veins, the aorta, and the heart muscle itself.

Medium- and High-Velocity Injuries

In general, medium-velocity weapons include shotguns and hand guns. High-velocity weapons include high-power rifles. Knowing a weapon's velocity helps to determine how severe an injury might be. Other factors include:

- Trajectory, or the path the bullet travels after it enters the body.
- Drag, or the factors that slow a bullet down.
- Impact point, or the bullet's point of entry into the body.
- Whether or not the bullet fragments, or breaks apart.
- The kind of pressure wave caused by the energy of the bullet as it travels through body tissue.

The injury can also be complicated by clothing, gun powder, bacteria, and other foreign matter that is pulled into the wound. A soft-nose, high-velocity bullet is especially destructive. It can cause a wave of energy through the body that is 30 times the diameter of the bullet (Figure 9–10).

As you care for a gunshot victim, remember that tissue damage can be much more widespread than the surface wound indicates. A bullet wound that bleeds very little can be accompanied by a devastating internal injury.

If all the energy of a bullet is absorbed by the body, the bullet will remain there. If all is not absorbed, the bullet will exit the body. You need to assess the victim carefully. Look for both an entry and an exit wound. Note that an exit wound can be much larger than the entrance wound.

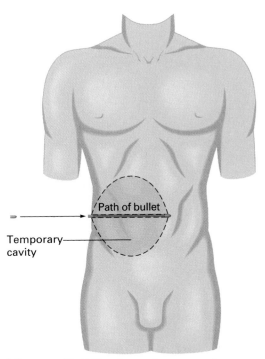

Figure 9-10   A gunshot wound can cause devastating damage, much more than a surface wound might indicate.

BLAST INJURIES

The most common explosions involve natural gas, gasoline, fireworks, or grain elevators. They occur in three phases, each with a typical pattern of injury (Figure 9–11):

- *Primary.* The pressure wave of an explosion affects gas-containing organs such as the lungs, stomach, intestines, inner ears, and sinuses. Blood vessels and membranes of the organs can be ruptured. Death can occur without any obvious external injury. Common primary blast injuries include pneumothorax, pulmonary contusion (bruising of the lungs), and perforation of the stomach and intestines.
- *Secondary.* Injuries result from flying debris created by the force of the blast. Unlike primary blast injuries, these are obvious. They most commonly include open wounds, impaled objects, and broken bones.
- *Tertiary.* Injuries in this phase occur when the victim is thrown away from the source of the explosion. They are basically the same as those of a victim who is ejected from a car during a collision.

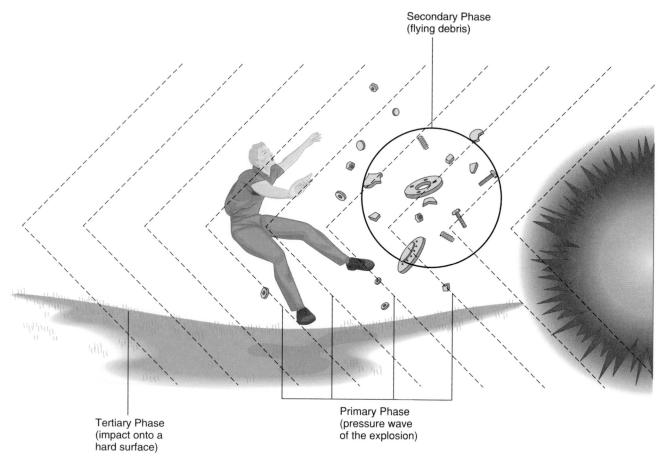

Secondary Phase
(flying debris)

Tertiary Phase
(impact onto a
hard surface)

Primary Phase
(pressure wave
of the explosion)

Figure 9-11 Blast forces.

SECTION 3: RESOURCE DETERMINATION

Once you have assured scene safety and determined the mechanism of injury or nature of illness, you must make sure you have the appropriate resources. For example, if the scene involves hazardous materials, you need to call a specialized hazmat team. If you have two or more patients, you may need to call for extra EMS personnel and ambulances.

If special teams or extra units will be required, call dispatch to request them. Do this before you begin patient care. Experience has shown that getting immersed in patient care can cause any First Responder to forget to call for additional help. Call first. It will help to prevent inefficiency and confusion later.

Never be too proud to ask for help when you need it! Situations in which you may need help include the following:

- When there are more patients than you can deal with in a multiple-casualty incident, call for additional personnel and ambulances. Until help arrives, you will need to make decisions about who must be treated first based on the severity of injuries. This is called "triage." (See Chapter 29 for details.)
- Hazardous materials can cause complicated emergencies. And they are everywhere. They are stored in homes and businesses. They are transported by ground, sea, and air. Hazmat incidents require specialized training to manage and decontaminate. Be alert and call for a hazmat team as soon as an incident is suspected. (See Chapter 28 for details.)

- It may be necessary to call for law enforcement if violence or the potential for violence exists. Situations such as problems with traffic, bystanders and crowds, or violations of the law will also require the police.

Other situations may require the fire service for fire or rescue, or the power company for downed wires. Confined-space rescue, high- and low-angle rescue, and helicopter rescue or evacuation also may be needed. Call for the resources you need immediately. If later you find they are not needed, they may be canceled. Time is of the essence.

FIRST RESPONDER FOCUS

The scene size-up is the first step of every call you go on. This is one of the few rules for which there are no exceptions. A proper scene size-up creates a proper foundation for a call.

The individual components of the scene size-up are scene safety, BSI precautions, resource determination, and observation of the mechanism of injury or nature of illness. Do not rush through them.

You may notice experienced First Responders who seem to respond to each emergency calmly. A calm, observant approach not only allows you to perform an optimal scene size-up, it also allows you to keep your wits about you. Some experienced EMS personnel who feel as if they are starting to rush will stop and count to three. This brief pause, usually not noticed even by crew members, returns the focus to a proper scene size-up and quality patient care. ∎

CASE STUDY FOLLOW-UP

At the beginning of this chapter, you read that First Responders were at the scene of an auto crash. To see how chapter skills apply to this emergency, read the following. It describes how the call was completed.

SCENE SIZE-UP (*Continued*)

We kept a safe distance from the car. We could see that the pole seemed intact, and there were no wires down. There were no gasoline leaks either. I saw that there was one patient in the car. He was responsive, so I told him not to move.

The patient had blood on his face. Looking at the mechanism of injury, I felt that he could be seriously injured. There was a lot of damage to the front of the car, and a large star in the windshield where the patient's head hit. So I called the dispatcher to make sure the EMT-paramedics were on the way. We also called for an extrication truck.

We put on turnout gear and eye protection. Over our latex gloves, we put on heavy duty gloves to protect ourselves from all the broken glass.

INITIAL ASSESSMENT

The car was stable and safe, so I climbed into the back seat and held the patient's head and neck in a neutral in-line position. I asked him some quick questions, and saw that he was alert.

The blood on the patient's face wasn't causing any airway problems. He was breathing deeply and at a good rate. This was a 30-year-old man who could be seriously injured due to the mechanism of injury.

My partner went to the window nearest the patient. She talked to him to calm him down. We saw no severe bleeding, and his pulse was good. My partner placed him on oxygen and then updated the incoming units.

CASE STUDY FOLLOW-UP *(Continued)*

PHYSICAL EXAMINATION

The man had cuts and bruises to his forehead, which was oozing blood. He admitted that he was not wearing a seat belt at the time of the crash. He complained of pain in his neck and chest. His neck was tender upon palpation. The left side of his chest was also tender, but there were no signs of broken ribs or open wounds. My partner listened to the patient's lungs. Air was moving in and out of both, she said. The man had no problems with his abdomen or hips. We could not get to his legs.

PATIENT HISTORY

We had not gotten far into the SAMPLE history when extrication started. It was more important to get the patient out of the car. And we could not hear or do much with the tools in operation anyway.

ONGOING ASSESSMENT

We continued to monitor the patient's breathing and pulse during extrication. We also protected him from flying debris.

PATIENT HAND-OFF

When the patient was extricated, the paramedics took over care. We told them what we had found so far: respiratory rate and pulse, the patient's complaints, our physical findings, and that we had him on oxygen.

We stuck around and helped with the back-boarding. Later we found out that the man got worse in the ambulance. He had a hemothorax, with blood accumulating in his left lung. Fortunately, the ambulance went to a trauma center where he was rushed into surgery. He was in the hospital for a while and recovered fully.

> As you can see, scene size-up is an important part of any call. It begins as you approach the scene, even before you see the patient. Scan for dangers, additional patients, and the mechanism of injury. Do not rush in. Determine right away whether or not you will need help and what kind. Then call for it.

REVIEW QUESTIONS

Page references where answers may be found or supported are provided at the end of each question.

Section 1

1. What are the components of scene size-up? (pp. 151, 152, 155, 164)
2. What are some signs of potential danger at an emergency scene? (pp. 153–154)
3. What is a general rule you can follow if you find a scene to be unsafe? (p. 154)

Section 2

4. What is the effect of mass (weight) and velocity (speed) on the severity of injuries? (p. 156)

5. What are three impacts that may occur in a crash? (p. 156)
6. What trauma can be expected from the "down-and-under" and "up-and-over" pathways of injury in a car crash? (pp. 156–157)
7. What factors affect the seriousness of the injuries caused by a fall? (pp. 161–162)

Section 3

8. In what emergency situations would you typically need to call for additional resources? (pp. 164–165)

CHAPTER 10

PATIENT ASSESSMENT

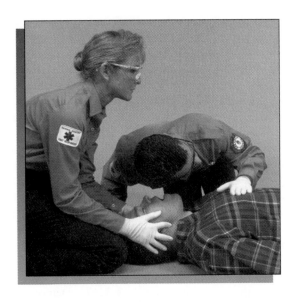

INTRODUCTION

First Responders must be able to assess a patient's condition quickly and accurately. This chapter will help you learn how. It presents a step-by-step routine used by many experienced emergency care providers. The routine includes a scene size-up, the initial assessment, a physical exam, patient history, ongoing assessment, and patient hand-off. (See Figure 10–1.)

As you already know from Chapter 9, scene size-up is always the first step. When the scene is safe to enter, the next step is to identify immediate threats to the patient's life. This is called the initial assessment. You will perform a more thorough physical exam and get a patient history afterwards. The ongoing assessment follows. It is an organized way of monitoring the patient's condition while you wait for help. Finally, there's the patient hand-off. It is a summary of the patient's condition, which you report to the EMTs when they take over patient care.

PATIENT ASSESSMENT PLAN

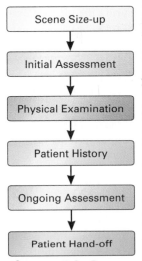

Figure 10–1
Patient assessment plan.

OBJECTIVES

Cognitive, affective, and psychomotor objectives are from the U.S. DOT's 1995 "First Responder: National Standard Curriculum." Enrichment objectives, if any, identify material that is supplemental to the DOT curriculum.

Cognitive

3-1.7 Summarize the reasons for forming a general impression of the patient. (pp. 170–171)

3-1.8 Discuss methods of assessing mental status. (pp. 171–172)

3-1.9 Differentiate between assessing mental status in the adult, child, and infant patient. (pp. 171–172)

3-1.10 Describe methods used for assessing if a patient is breathing. (pp. 172–173)

3-1.11 Differentiate between a patient with adequate and inadequate breathing. (p. 173)

3-1.12 Describe the methods used to assess circulation. (pp. 173–175)

3-1.13 Differentiate between obtaining a pulse in an adult, child, and infant patient. (pp. 174–175)

3-1.14 Discuss the need for assessing the patient for external bleeding. (pp. 173–175)

3-1.15 Explain the reason for prioritizing a patient for care and transport. (pp. 175–176)

3-1.16 Discuss the components of the physical exam. (pp. 176–189)

3-1.17 State the areas of the body that are evaluated during the physical exam. (pp. 178–189)

3-1.18 Explain what additional questioning may be asked during the physical exam. (pp. 188–189)

3-1.19 Explain the components of the SAMPLE history. (pp. 189–191)

3-1.20 Discuss the components of the on-going assessment. (p. 191)

3-1.21 Describe the information included in the First Responder "hand-off" report. (pp. 191–192)

Affective

3-1.24 Explain the importance of forming a general impression of the patient. (pp. 170–171)

3-1.25 Explain the value of an initial assessment. (pp. 169–176)

3-1.26 Explain the value of questioning the patient and family. (pp. 188–191)

3-1.27 Explain the value of the physical exam. (p. 176)

3-1.28 Explain the value of an on-going assessment. (p. 191)

3-1.29 Explain the rationale for the feelings that these patients might be experiencing. (pp. 177, 191)

3-1.30 Demonstrate a caring attitude when performing patient assessments. (pp. 177, 191)

3-1.31 Place the interests of the patient as the foremost consideration when making any and all patient care decisions during patient assessment. (pp. 177, 191)

3-1.32 Communicate with empathy during patient assessment to patients as well as with family members and friends of the patient. (pp. 177, 191)

Psychomotor

3-1.34 Demonstrate the techniques for assessing mental status. (pp. 171–172)

3-1.35 Demonstrate the techniques for assessing the airway. (pp. 172–173)

3-1.36 Demonstrate the techniques for assessing if the patient is breathing. (p. 173)

3-1.37 Demonstrate the techniques for assessing if the patient has a pulse. (pp. 174–175)

3-1.38 Demonstrate the techniques for assessing the patient for external bleeding. (p. 175)

3-1.39 Demonstrate the techniques for assessing the patient's skin color, temperature, condition, and capillary refill (infants and children only). (pp. 184–185)

3-1.40 Demonstrate questioning a patient to obtain a SAMPLE history. (pp. 189–191)

3-1.41 Demonstrate the skills involved in performing the physical exam. (pp. 176–189)

3-1.42 Demonstrate the on-going assessment. (p. 191)

Enrichment

* Describe when and how to manually stabilize a patient's head and neck. (pp. 171, 178)
* Identify the components of an assessment of vital signs. (pp. 182–188)
* Describe the methods used to obtain a breathing rate and a pulse rate. (pp. 183–185)
* Describe normal breathing rates and pulse rates. (pp. 182–184)
* Identify the terms that describe the quality of breathing and the quality pulse. (pp. 183–184)
* Describe the methods used to assess the pupils. (pp. 185–186)
* Describe the methods used to assess blood pressure. (pp. 186–188)
* Differentiate between a sign and a symptom. (pp. 189–190)
* State the importance of accurately reporting and recording the baseline vital signs. (p. 182)

CASE STUDY

DISPATCH

My partner and I were dispatched to a call for an "unresponsive man" at 46 Wilson Avenue. The dispatcher told us that the caller said she was unable to wake her husband after a nap.

SCENE SIZE-UP

We approached the scene carefully, as we always do. This call was in a quiet section of town but you never can tell. We realized that an unresponsive person could mean anything from a drunk to a cardiac arrest, so we had all our protective equipment ready.

A woman met us at the door, quite upset. She was about 60. We heard a dog in the yard, but the woman assured us that it couldn't get in the house. There was only one patient. The woman was sure her husband didn't fall or anything. We felt sure we had a medical problem on our hands.

INITIAL ASSESSMENT

We identified ourselves to the man, but received no response. As my partner assessed the patient's level of responsiveness, I took the pillows out from under his head and assessed his airway. I found some gurgling, so I suctioned him out, which helped. His respirations were slow and shallow. My partner found a pulse, which was rapid. There was no external bleeding visible. Our general impression was of a male unresponsive from unknown causes who required ventilation assistance.

Patient assessment is an important process for all levels of EMS responders. Here the First Responders performed a scene size-up and an initial assessment. Consider this patient as you read Chapter 10. What else may be done to assess and care for the patient's condition?

SECTION 1: INITIAL ASSESSMENT

The **initial assessment** may be the most important part of the patient assessment process. In it you must identify and treat conditions that cause an immediate threat to the patient's life. Life-threats usually involve breathing problems or severe bleeding.

The initial assessment includes getting a general impression of the patient; assessing responsiveness; assessing the **ABCs** (airway, breathing, and circulation); and updating incoming EMS units about the patient's condition. (See Figure 10–2.)

INITIAL ASSESSMENT

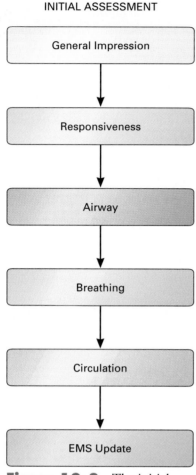

Figure 10-2 The initial assessment takes about a minute.

GENERAL IMPRESSION

Form a general impression as you approach the patient (Figure 10–3). It should include the patient's **chief complaint** and a brief immediate assessment of the environment in which the emergency has taken place.

The chief complaint is the reason that EMS was called. It is generally the response to the question "Can you tell me why you called EMS today?" Record the response on your forms in the patient's own words. "I fell down the stairs" or "My chest hurts" are examples of chief complaints. If the patient is unresponsive, get information from the person who called EMS.

The general impression is not designed to be the final word in the patient's condition. Rather,

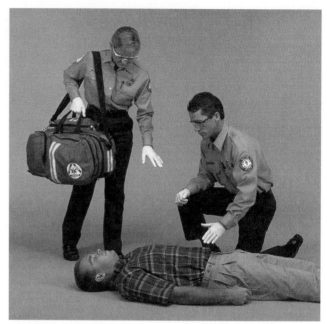

Figure 10-3 Form a general impression as you approach the patient.

it lets you get started on the right track with patient care. During this phase of the initial assessment, you are to determine if the situation is a trauma (injury) complaint or a medical (illness) complaint. Do this by listening to what the patient or bystanders tell you. Also look around the scene to gain a quick impression of the forces involved in an injury.

If your general impression is that you are facing a patient with a potentially serious injury or illness, you may wish to ask EMS dispatch for advanced life support or additional units to assist. (You may have already done this in the scene size-up.)

To complete your general impression, you must also determine the patient's age and sex.

Consider the following general impressions:

- A 12-year-old male patient, who was riding his bicycle, was struck by a dump truck. Your observation of the scene reveals that the boy's bicycle has been mangled by the truck. The boy appears to be unconscious.
- A 58-year-old woman is complaining of abdominal pain. She seems to be speaking normally, without a sign of strain. However, she is protecting her abdomen with one hand.

• A 26-year-old man is found on the floor of his bathroom, unconscious. No one is quite sure of what happened.

In the first case, the general impression leads you to believe the boy could be seriously injured. The second case appears to be a medical patient who is not in severe distress. The third case gives you little additional information on how to proceed. However, the mere fact that the man is unconscious can tell you that certain precautions must be taken.

RESPONSIVENESS

The next part of the initial assessment is determining the patient's **level of responsiveness.** This is important for many reasons. One of the most important is the patient who has an **altered mental status** (a change in his or her normal mental state). That patient will need airway care as well as other life-saving aid.

If the patient is confused, be sure to let him or her know who you are. Always make your identity clear as you approach a patient. State your name. Then explain that you are a First Responder and you are there to help.

If the mechanism of injury suggests possible spine or head injury, take **spinal precautions** at this time. This means hold the patient's head and neck stable and in a neutral position (Figure 10–4). If the spine-injured patient were to move, further injury could occur.

To stabilize a patient's head and neck, place your hands on either side of the head. Then spread your fingers apart. The object is to prevent movement. If the patient is responsive, explain what you are doing so he or she is not alarmed. Your hand position may reduce the patient's hearing. So be aware of the anxiety this may cause. (Spine injuries are covered in depth in Chapter 21.)

There are four levels of responsiveness that are commonly used to classify patients. They are *alert, verbal, painful,* and *unresponsive.* Together, these terms make up the mnemonic **AVPU.** The classifications, when applied to patients, are as follows (Figure 10–5):

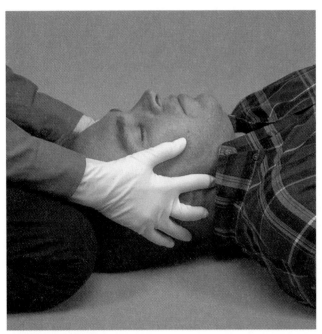

Figure 10-4 If there is possible spine or head injury, immediately stabilize the patient's head and neck.

A —Alert. A patient who is alert is responsive and oriented. That is, the patient is aware of his surroundings, the approximate time and date, and his name. This is commonly referred to as being "responsive to person, place, and date" (or "oriented × 3"). Each distinction is impor-

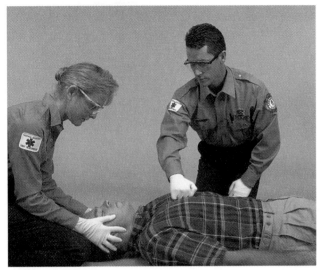

Figure 10-5 Assess the patient's level of responsiveness.

tant. Some patients may appear wide awake but in fact are not aware of the surroundings. A patient's mental status is important to determine because it can indicate injury or illness.

V—Verbal. This patient is disoriented but responds when spoken to. We say that he or she "responds to verbal stimulus." A patient who answers questions about place and date incorrectly is another example. He or she may be suffering from a medical condition such as seizures or diabetes or a traumatic condition such as shock.

P—Painful. The patient who responds only to a painful stimulus does not answer questions or open his eyes to any verbal commands. He or she only stirs or flinches. The stimulus may be a pinch or a careful but firm rub on the sternum in the absence of chest injuries. (Remember that you first check responsiveness by observation. If the patient is alert or verbal, there is no need to apply a painful stimulus.)

U—Unresponsive. This patient does not respond to any stimulus. He does not open his eyes, respond verbally, or even flinch when pain is applied. This patient is deeply unconscious, most likely in a critical condition and in definite need of airway and other supportive care.

Determining the level of responsiveness is different for infants and children and for elderly patients. For infants and young children, assess the response to the environment. They should recognize their parents, and they usually wish to go to them. Expect your assessment to cause tears, too. Children who do not recognize their parents or who are indifferent to your assessment and treatment may be very sick.

In the elderly there are common diseases and conditions, such as Alzheimer's, that cause changes in responsiveness. In cases such as these, try to find out from the family if there has been a change. That is, the patient may normally be somewhat confused, but has it worsened with this episode?

Some elderly patients live alone and have neither the means nor reason to keep track of the date and current events. If an elderly patient does not know the date or another piece of information, try other questions to determine orientation. You might ask about the immediate sur-

roundings, for example, or about what you are doing there.

AIRWAY

The patient's airway status is a foundation of patient care. No patient can survive without an adequate airway. So make sure the patient's airway is open and clear (Figure 10–6). The way you will assess the patient's airway depends on whether the patient is responsive or not.

- *The responsive patient.* When a patient can respond to your questions, notice if he can speak clearly. Gurgling or other sounds may indicate that something like teeth, blood, or other matter is in the airway. Also make sure the patient can speak full sentences.
- *The unresponsive patient.* A patient who is unresponsive needs aggressive airway maintenance. Immediately make sure the airway is open. If the patient is ill with no sign of trauma, use the head-tilt/chin-lift maneuver to open the airway. If trauma is suspected, use the jaw-thrust maneuver with great care to avoid tilting the head.

Inspect the airway for blood, vomit, or secretions. Also look for loose teeth or other foreign matter that could cause an obstruction. Clear the airway using suction or a gloved finger.

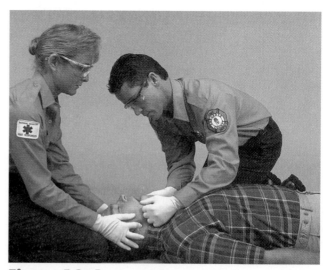

Figure 10-6   Open the patient's airway and make sure it is clear.

Remember that the airway check is not a one-time event. Some patients with serious trauma or unresponsive medical patients who are vomiting will need almost constant suctioning and airway maintenance.

BREATHING

After securing an open airway, look, listen, and feel for breathing (Figure 10–7). If there is breathing, determine if respirations are adequate. As you will recall from Chapter 6, breathing is not an all-or-nothing proposition. There will be times when a patient is breathing but not at a sufficient depth or rate to sustain life.

Adequate breathing is characterized by three factors: adequate rise and fall of the chest, ease of breathing (breathing should appear to be effortless), and adequate respiratory rate.

Inadequate breathing may be identified by (Figure 10–8):

- Inadequate rise and fall of the chest.
- Increased effort of breathing.
- Cyanosis (blue or gray color to the skin, lips, or nail beds).

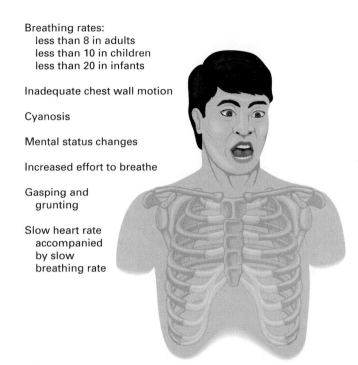

Breathing rates:
    less than 8 in adults
    less than 10 in children
    less than 20 in infants

Inadequate chest wall motion

Cyanosis

Mental status changes

Increased effort to breathe

Gasping and grunting

Slow heart rate accompanied by slow breathing rate

Figure 10-8   Signs of inadequate breathing.

- Mental status changes.
- Inadequate respiratory rate (less than 8 per minute in adults, less than 10 in children, and less than 20 in infants).

If the patient is breathing adequately, there may be no need to assist respiration in any way. However, during your assessment, you may determine that your patient would benefit from oxygen therapy. If you are trained and allowed, administer oxygen to these patients (Figure 10–9).

If you determine that the patient's respirations are absent or inadequate, you must begin ventilating immediately. Do not stop until you are relieved by another trained rescuer or until the patient regains adequate respirations. In most cases, you will continue ventilations until the EMTs arrive.

CIRCULATION

When you assess circulation, you are checking to see that the heart is pumping blood to all parts of the body. You also must be sure that the heart is pumping adequately and that there is no life-threatening external bleeding. To assess circulation (Figures 10–10 and 10–11):

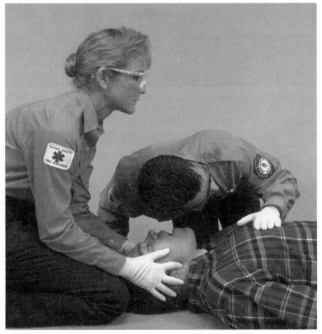

Figure 10-7   Look, listen, and feel for breathing.

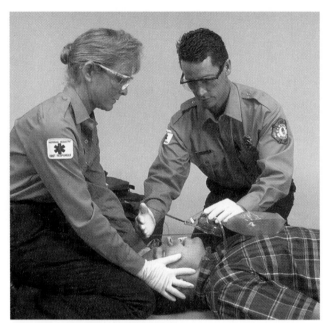

Figure 10-9 Apply oxygen if the patient needs it and if you are permitted to do so.

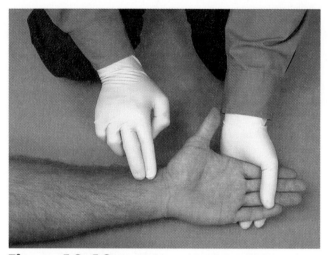

Figure 10-10a If the patient is responsive, assess the radial pulse.

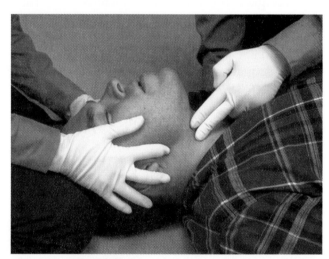

Figure 10-10b If the patient is unresponsive or if there is no radial pulse, assess the carotid pulse.

- *The responsive patient.* If the patient is a verbally responsive adult, use the radial pulse to assess circulation. Checking the carotid pulse may cause this patient undue anxiety. Always use the brachial pulse point for an infant. Use either the radial or brachial pulse point for the responsive child.

    When checking the pulse, note the approximate rate and rhythm. If the pulse is very

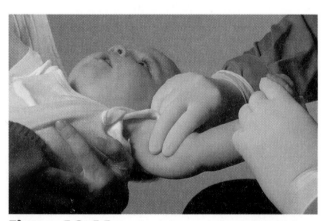

Figure 10-11a Assessing an infant's brachial pulse.

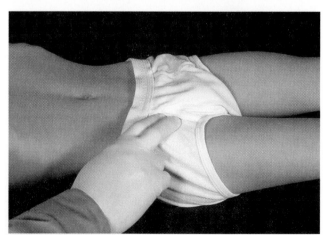

Figure 10-11b Assessing a child's femoral pulse.

irregular or feels extremely slow or fast, be on the lookout for serious conditions.

Also note the patient's skin at this time. Check the color and temperature (Figure 10–12). Skin that is pale, cool, and moist may indicate shock.

- *The unresponsive patient.* Check the pulse of an unresponsive adult at the carotid artery. Check the pulse of unresponsive children at the carotid or femoral arteries. Remember, the pulse check for all infants is done at the brachial artery. If the pulse is absent, begin CPR.

After checking the patient's pulse, check for serious external bleeding (Figure 10–13). Remember that the initial assessment is designed to identify and treat life-threatening problems. Be alert. Do not let minor wounds sidetrack you or keep you from caring for more serious injuries first.

Scan the patient for serious bleeding. Use your gloved hands to check areas that are hard to see, such as the small of the back and the buttocks. Remember that heavy clothes can absorb large quantities of blood. If serious bleeding is found, use the methods discussed in Chapter 17 to control the blood flow.

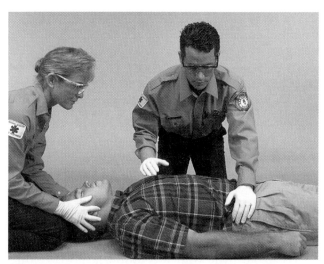

Figure 10-13 Assessing for major bleeding.

EMS UPDATE

At this point, you will know if your patient is barely breathing and requires ventilation (a high priority) or if your patient is stable with a minor complaint. In either case, the EMS units currently en route to the scene will be interested in an update. The information you provide will allow them to prepare for the patient and provide more efficient care.

If you have a phone or radio available (Figure 10–14), report the patient's:

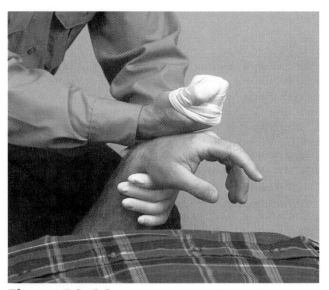

Figure 10-12 Assessing the patient's skin temperature.

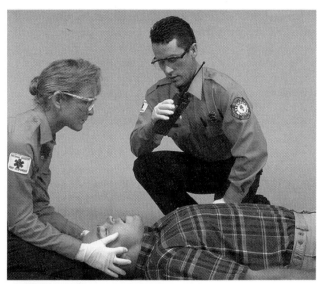

Figure 10-14 After the initial assessment, update incoming EMS units.

- Age and sex.
- Chief complaint.
- Level of responsiveness.
- Airway and breathing status.
- Circulation status.

Also ask the incoming EMS units to give you their estimated time of arrival (ETA), so you can continue patient care and prepare for their arrival.

The following is an example of a radio report. It might have been given by the First Responders in the "Case Study" that opened this chapter:

"Dispatcher, we have an approximately 60-year old male who was found responsive only to painful stimulus. His airway required suctioning, and we are assisting ventilations. The patient's pulse is rapid and weak."

After your report, the dispatcher will acknowledge your transmission and advise you of the ambulance's ETA.

SECTION 2: FIRST RESPONDER PHYSICAL EXAM

The initial assessment is designed to help you identify and treat life-threats. However, not all problems will be life-threatening. The First Responder physical exam is a survey of the patient's entire body. It is meant to reveal any signs of illness or injury. (See Figure 10–15.)

The physical exam is designed to be thorough. In some cases, you will have time to perform it. In others, you will only have time for an initial assessment before the EMTs arrive. When you have time and the patient does not need continued life-saving care, begin the physical exam.

The physical exam proceeds in a logical order, usually from head to toe. It will be slightly different for each patient. If a patient falls a considerable height from a ladder, for instance, he could have injuries anywhere on his body. This patient would require a full assessment. In the case of an isolated cut to a finger, a complete, hands-on examination would not be necessary.

THE PHYSICAL EXAM

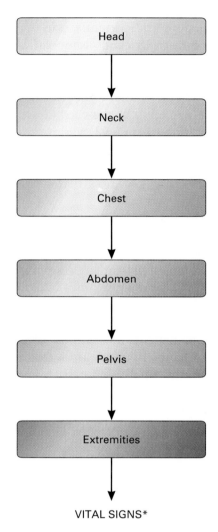

Figure 10–15 Components of the physical exam.

PRINCIPLES OF ASSESSMENT

Patient assessment is a skill. Like other skills, the more you practice it, the better you will be. If you do not practice regularly, the result could be poor performance and missed injuries.

Methods of Examination

The patient assessment process involves the use of your senses. There are three methods you will use during your patient assessment: **inspection** (looking), **auscultation** (listening), and **palpation** (feeling).

- *Inspection.* The first method is the easiest. Simply make an overall observation of the patient. Then observe the various parts of the body. What you see is very important throughout a call. As you approach a patient, even before you talk to him, you may observe that he is clutching his fist to his chest and appears to be uncomfortable. This could be your first indication of a heart problem.
- *Auscultation.* The most important listening you will do is for the sound of air entering and leaving the lungs. It will help you to determine the status of the patient's breathing. If you are required by your EMS system to perform this skill with a stethoscope, practice on your classmates. Become familiar with the sound of normal breathing.
- *Palpation.* Palpating, or feeling, with your fingertips is usually done last in the exam, because it can cause pain. The actual pressure you apply depends on the area you are palpating and the type of problem you suspect. For example, if you observe a swollen lower leg where the bone is normally near the surface, you only would need to palpate the area gently to determine if tenderness is present. Assessing the abdomen of an obese patient would require more pressure. Palpation will also identify areas where bones are rubbing together, abnormally rigid areas, skin temperature, and sweating.

Inspect and palpate each part of the body before you move on to the next area. Auscultate the chest. For example, observe the chest for rise and fall with breathing. Then auscultate for adequacy of breathing and palpate for tenderness or other sensations. After examining the chest, you would move to the abdomen where you would inspect and palpate as appropriate.

When conducting the exam, you will be looking for the following signs of injury:

- Deformities.
- Open injuries.
- Tenderness.
- Swelling.

Look at the first letters of each word listed above. The letters form the mnemonic **DOTS.** Use it to help you remember the signs you are looking for. Some signs will be obvious, such as a cut in the skin (open injury). Others, such as abdominal tenderness caused by internal injuries, will not be as obvious but are certainly serious.

As you proceed through the physical exam, be sure to listen to what your patient tells you. This may seem too simple to even mention, but you could be distracted by other activities at a busy emergency scene. Listening shows that you care. It gives you important information necessary to the proper treatment of the patient. If you have to ask a patient to repeat something three or four times, the patient will stop answering your questions and believe that you do not care.

Finally, remember that your patient will be anxious or scared. It is important to reassure him or her throughout the call. When the EMTs arrive, be sure to introduce your patient to them and relay special concerns or fears the patient may have discussed with you.

Medical vs. Trauma Patients

An examination of a trauma patient is different from an examination of a medical patient. It has been said that a trauma exam is 80% hands-on and 20% questioning, while a medical exam is 80% questions and 20% hands-on. For example, once you observe and examine an isolated injury, you do not need too much more information. The physical signs of injury can be observed and palpated.

Compare that to a patient who is having a heart problem. Chest pain is something you cannot observe or palpate. It can be felt only by the patient. So in order to provide the appropriate emergency care, you must use questions to encourage the patient to describe his symptoms to you.

THE PHYSICAL EXAMINATION

The following section details the examination of specific areas of the body. Use the DOTS mnemonic to guide your examination.

Examination of the Head

Assess all areas of the head, including the skull, face, and jaw (Figure 10–16). Also check pupils for size and responsiveness. Note that injuries to the head may be serious. Bleeding can be severe. Many areas are covered by hair and can hide injuries. Use DOTS to guide you:

D — *Deformities.* Examine the skull, face bones, and jaw for signs of deformity (depressions or indentations, for example). Also look for deformities such as loose teeth, which can create airway problems.

O — *Open injuries.* Open injuries to the head may bleed profusely. As such, they may have been treated in the initial assessment. Any injury that bleeds into the airway is of particular concern. Also look in the hair for injuries that may be hidden.

T — *Tenderness.* When you are palpating the head, the patient may complain of pain or tenderness where there is no obvious injury. Make a note of the locations of tenderness.

S — *Swelling.* Swelling frequently accompanies injuries to the head. It may be noted around injuries to the skull and to facial structures such as areas around the eyes, nose, and mouth.

Examination of the Neck

There are large blood vessels and major airway structures in the neck. Injuries can be quite serious. To examine the neck (Figure 10–17):

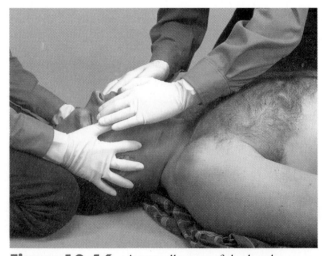

Figure 10-16 Assess all areas of the head.

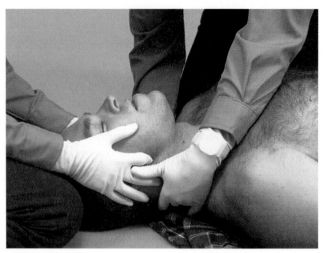

Figure 10-17 Examine both the front and back of the neck.

D — *Deformities.* Look to see that the trachea is not deformed or shifted. Either can indicate a critical condition such as excessive pressure in the chest cavity. Palpate the vertebrae in the posterior (back) of the neck.

O — *Open injuries.* Open injuries to the neck may result in serious blood loss. Bandage them immediately. Use an occlusive (airtight) dressing, which prevents air from entering the neck.

T — *Tenderness.* Palpate the soft tissues, trachea, and vertebrae for tenderness.

S — *Swelling.* Examine for swelling. The neck may accumulate blood. Also, air may escape from the trachea or other airway structure and cause a popping or crackling sound under the skin.

Whenever there is a possibility of spine injury, maintain manual stabilization of the head and neck until the patient can be completely immobilized. If you are equipped, trained, and allowed, apply a rigid cervical collar at this time (Figure 10–18). See Chapter 21 for a detailed discussion.

Examination of the Chest

Any injury to the chest may involve injury to the vital organs or to major blood vessels. Note, also include the shoulders in this exam.

If you are trained to do so, listen to the chest with a stethoscope. Determine if an adequate

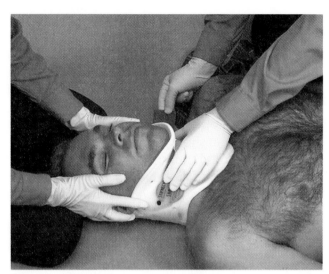

Figure 10-18 Apply a rigid cervical collar, if the patient needs it and if you are permitted to do so.

amount of air is entering the lungs. Compare both sides. The sounds you hear should be equal.

D — *Deformities.* Feel the rib cage for signs of deformity (Figure 10–19). Remember the ribs extend all the way back to the spine. Injuries to the back pose the same grave dangers as those to the front of the chest. Do not move the patient in order to examine the back until appropriate spinal precautions have been taken. Palpate the sternum. If the patient is responsive, ask him or her to take a deep breath. Determine if it causes pain.

O — *Open injuries.* Open injuries are of particular concern when they occur in the chest. If a wound extends into the chest cavity, air may enter the area around the lungs and cause a serious condition. Bandage open wounds to the chest immediately. Use an occlusive (airtight) dressing.

T — *Tenderness.* While palpating the chest, ask the patient if he or she feels any pain. Even times when there is no obvious injury, internal injuries may be present.

S — *Swelling.* Observe the chest for swelling. If there is swelling or any other sign of possible injury, assess for underlying breathing problems.

Examination of the Abdomen

As you will recall from Chapter 4, there are many organs within the abdominal cavity that can be injured. (Though the spine lies to the rear of the abdomen, it is not palpated in this location.) To examine the abdomen (Figure 10–20):

D — *Deformities.* Deformity of the abdomen usually refers to rigidity (hardness) or distention.

O — *Open injuries.* Open injuries to the abdomen include cuts and scrapes (lacerations and abrasions), penetrating wounds (from a knife or gunshot), or protruding organs (eviscerations). These wounds are severe because of the potential for bleeding and infection.

T — *Tenderness.* Tenderness is an important symptom because it may indicate underlying injury. Recall the abdominal quadrants from

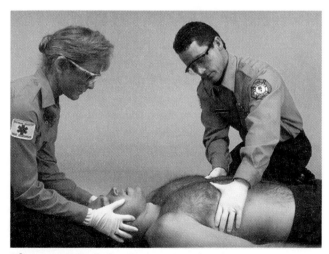

Figure 10-19 Examining the chest.

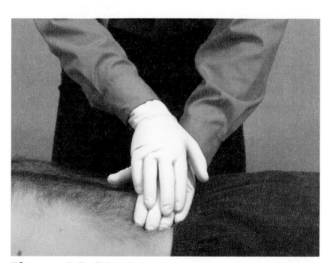

Figure 10-20 Palpating each quadrant of the abdomen.

Chapter 4. Palpate the quadrant where the patient complains of pain last. If you examine this area first, you could cause severe pain, making the examination of the other quadrants impossible or inaccurate.

S — *Swelling.* Swelling or discoloration of the skin is another indication of abdominal injury. Check the flanks (the lateral sides of the hips and buttocks) for pooling of blood.

Examination of the Back (Posterior)

While it is important to check the patient's back, you must also realize that moving a patient could result in making a neck or spinal injury worse. If there are enough rescuers present who are trained in moving or rolling the patient, you may wish to check the back.

If you suspect spine injury and a long backboard is available, you may wish to move it under the patient while the patient is being rolled. But do so only if you are trained in its use and have enough help to do so safely.

Check the patient's posterior as follows (Figure 10–21):

D — *Deformities.* Check for chest wall deformity, which may indicate broken ribs. Look for obvious deformity along the length of the spine.

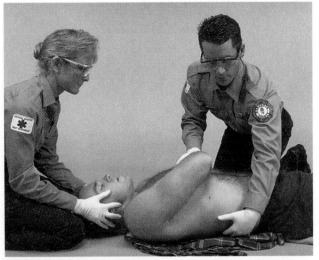

Figure 10-21 Examine the patient's back, keeping the head and neck in alignment at all times.

O — *Open injuries.* Injuries to the posterior chest can cause the same serious conditions that occur on the anterior chest. Look for open or sucking chest wounds (open chest wounds sometimes make a sucking sound with respiration). Observe for scrapes, cuts, and other open injuries. Look for both entry and exit gunshot wounds.

T — *Tenderness.* Tenderness may indicate a broken rib or an abdominal injury. Tenderness along the spine may indicate serious injury to the spinal cord.

S — *Swelling.* Look for blood accumulation in the flanks, which could indicate bleeding in the abdomen. Swelling anywhere indicates some type of injury.

Examination of the Pelvis

The pelvis is a large, bony structure. As you may recall, it is composed of a left and right ileum, ischium, and the pubis bone. Palpate each of these areas for injury. The pelvis, or hips, may be fractured, which could result in blood loss of 2 liters or more. This amount of blood loss is life-threatening. So be sure to identify any possibility of pelvic injury during the assessment process.

D — *Deformities.* Unlike the bones of the arms and legs, deformities of the pelvis are not always obvious. Palpate the bones to feel for deformity (Figure 10–22).

O — *Open injuries.* There may be open injuries to the pelvis, although this is not as common as in other areas of the body.

T — *Tenderness.* Assess for tenderness. Palpate with less force if the bones of the pelvis are close to the skin. Palpate with more force if the patient is obese with bones under a considerable amount of tissue. Though you may feel awkward assessing the pubis (groin) bone, be sure to check it.

S — *Swelling.* Look for swelling and discoloration around the hips.

Examination of the Extremities

The extremities are common sites of injury. So do not rush your examination. Be sure to inspect and palpate each one (Figure 10–23).

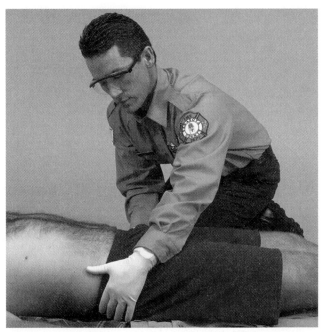

Figure 10–22 Examine the pelvis by applying gentle pressure.

D — *Deformities*. Because bones are close to the surface, deformities may be seen easily in the extremities. Check the entire length of each bone and all joints for deformity.

O — *Open injuries*. Look for open injuries, which are quite common in the extremities.

T — *Tenderness*. Just like in other areas of the body, there may be underlying injury without obvious deformity. So palpate each extremity for tenderness.

S — *Swelling*. Since injuries to the extremities are often close to the skin, swelling and discoloration may be evident. Any extremity that is painful, swollen, or deformed may be broken and should be manually stabilized until it can be splinted.

The extremities may also be checked by feeling for a pulse in each extremity (Figure 10–24). The radial pulse in each wrist will tell you if circulation in the entire arm is adequate. There are two pulses in the feet, either of which may be palpated to see if circulation is adequate in the lower extremities. They are the **dorsalis pedis pulse** and the **posterior tibial pulse.**

The ability to move an extremity, such as wiggling fingers or toes, is also an important sign to look for (Figure 10–25). Movement means that impulses from the nervous system can reach these points. If there is no movement, there may be a problem with a nerve. No movement on one side of the body or below a certain point could indicate problems with the central nervous system.

For the same reason, check to see that the patient has sensation in his or her limbs. Gently squeeze one extremity and then the other. As you

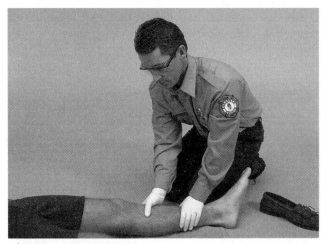

Figure 10–23 Visually inspect and palpate each extremity.

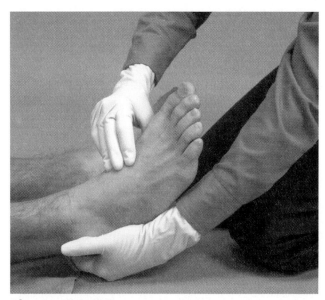

Figure 10–24 Also check the pulse in each extremity.

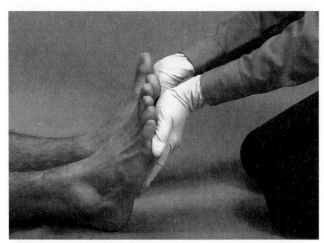

Figure 10-25   Check for sensation and the ability to move fingers and toes.

do, ask questions such as: Can you feel me touching your fingers? Can you feel me touching your toes?

VITAL SIGNS

Vital signs include the patient's respiration, pulse, skin, pupils, and blood pressure. (See Figure 10–26.) You can assess and monitor most vital signs by looking, listening, and feeling. However, it is best if you have the proper equipment:

- A wristwatch to count seconds.
- A pen light to examine pupils.
- A **stethoscope** to take a pulse, to listen to respiration, and to take blood pressure.
- A blood-pressure cuff, or **sphygmomanometer,** to take blood pressure.
- A pen and notebook to take notes.

More important than any one vital sign is change in vital signs over time. The vital signs taken by a First Responder are particularly important because they are taken early in the call. EMTs and hospital personnel will refer back to them to see if the patient has improved or gotten worse over time. For example, if you take a pulse and obtain a reading of 90 beats per minute, and later the pulse rises to 120, a serious condition may be developing. Without your early readings, this observation would not be possible.

VITAL SIGNS

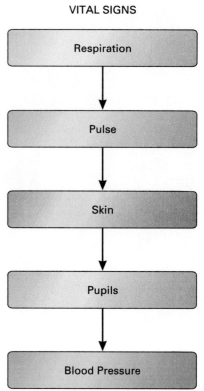

Figure 10-26   In some EMS systems, the First Responder may be required to assess a patient's vital signs.

Respiration

A respiration consists of one inhalation and one exhalation. The normal number of respirations per minute varies with gender and age. For an adult that number is between 12 and 20 times per minute (Table 10–1).

TABLE 10-1

NORMAL RESPIRATORY RATES

Patient	Respiratory Rate*
Infant	25-50
Child	15-30
Adult	12-20

* Approximate per minute at rest

Count your patient's respirations by doing the following (Figure 10–27):

1. Place your hand on the patient's chest or abdomen.
2. Count the number of times the chest (or abdomen) rises during a 30-second period. Then multiply that number by 2.

The depth of respiration gives a clue to the amount of air that is inhaled. You can gauge depth by placing your hand on the patient's chest and feeling for chest movement. Feel the abdomen to see if it is moving instead of the chest.

Normally, the work required by breathing is minimal. Some effort is required to inhale, but almost none is required to exhale. For this reason, normal inspiration takes slightly longer than normal exhalation. When exhaling is prolonged, the patient may have a chronic obstructive pulmonary disorder (COPD) such as emphysema.

Common signs and symptoms of respiratory distress include:

- Gasping for air.
- Breathing that is unusually fast, slow, deep, or shallow.
- Wheezing, gurgling, high-pitched shrill sounds, or other unusual noises.
- Unusually moist, flushed skin. Later, the skin may appear pale or bluish as the oxygen level in blood falls.

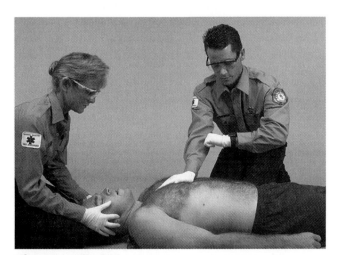

Figure 10-27 Assessing respirations.

- Difficulty speaking. Patient can say only a few words without catching his or her breath.
- Dizziness, anxiety.
- Chest pain and tingling in hands and feet.

Abnormal breathing conditions you should know about include:

- Shortness of breath or breathing difficulty.
- Abnormally slow breathing.
- Abnormally deep, rapid breathing.

If the patient is aware that you are assessing respiration, he may not breathe naturally. This can give a false reading. To get around this, take a pulse with the patient's arm draped over his chest or abdomen. Count the pulse for 15 seconds. Then, without moving the patient's arm, count respirations for the next 30 seconds. Readings are easily obtained by observing and feeling the chest rise and fall with your hand, which is already on the patient's torso.

Pulse

Each time the heart beats, the arteries expand and contract with the blood that rushes into them. The pulse is the pressure wave generated by the heartbeat. It directly reflects the rate, relative strength, and rhythm of the contractions of the heart.

When you take a pulse, note the following:

- Is the pulse rate slow or fast? (See Table 10–2 for normal rates).
- What is the strength of the pulse? A normal pulse is full and strong. A thready pulse is weak and rapid. A bounding pulse is unusually strong.

TABLE 10-2
NORMAL PULSE RATES

Patient	Pulse*
Infant	120 to 150
Child	80 to 150
Adult	60 to 80

* Approximate per minute at rest

• What is the rhythm of the pulse? A normal pulse has regular spaces between each beat. An irregular one is spaced irregularly. You can describe the pulse of a patient, for instance, as "72, strong, and regular." The rate, strength, and regularity of a pulse tell what the heart is doing at any given time.

The pulse can be felt at any point where an artery crosses over a bone or lies near the skin. First Responders often take a pulse at the wrist. This is where the radial artery crosses over the end of the forearm bone, the radius.

To take the radial pulse (Figure 10–28):

1. Have the patient lie down or sit.
2. Gently touch the pulse point with the tips of two or three fingers. (Avoid using your thumb. It has a prominent pulse of its own, which can be counted by mistake.)
3. Count the number of beats you feel for 15 seconds. Then multiply that number by 4. This will give you the number of beats per minute. If a pulse is irregular, slow, or difficult to obtain, count the beats for 30 seconds and multiply by 2 for a more accurate reading.
4. Write down the pulse and any other vital sign immediately. Never rely on your memory.

Other points where a pulse may be taken include the brachial artery in the upper arm, the carotid artery in the neck, the femoral artery in the groin, the dorsalis pedis on the top of the foot, the posterior tibial artery on the medial surface of the ankle, and the **apical pulse** under the patient's left breast (requires a stethoscope).

Checking pulses in several areas will help to determine how well the patient's entire circulatory system is working. The absence of a pulse in a single extremity may indicate a blocked artery. If left untreated, numbness, weakness, and tingling follow pain. The skin also gradually turns mottled, blue, and cold.

The Skin

Assessment of the skin temperature, color, and condition can tell you more about the patient's circulatory system.

Skin Temperature. Normal body temperature is 98.6°F (37°C). The most common way First Responders take temperature is by touching a patient's skin with the back of the hand. This is called **relative skin temperature.** It does not measure exact temperature, but you can tell if it is very high or low.

Changes in skin temperature can alert you to certain injuries and illnesses. A patient whose skin temperature is cool, for example, may be suffering from shock, heat exhaustion, or exposure to cold. A high temperature may be the result of fever or heat stroke. Body temperature also can change over a period of time, and it can be different in various parts of the body. Circulatory problems may be indicated by a cold arm or leg, for example. An isolated hot area could indicate a localized infection. Be alert to changes, and record them.

Skin Color. Skin color can tell you a lot about a patient's heart, lungs, and other problems as well. For example:

• Paleness may be caused by shock or heart attack. It also may be caused by fright, faintness, or emotional distress, as well as impaired blood flow.
• Redness (flushing) may be caused by high blood pressure, alcohol abuse, sunburn, heat stroke, fever, or an infectious disease.
• Blueness (cyanosis) is always a serious problem. It appears first in the fingertips and around the mouth. Generally, it is caused by reduced levels of oxygen as in shock, heart attack, or poisoning.

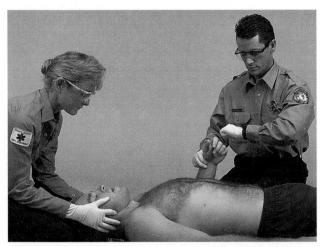

Figure 10-28 Assessing the pulse.

- Yellowish color may be caused by a liver disease.
- Black-and-blue mottling is the result of blood seeping under the skin. It is usually caused by a blow or severe infection.

If your patient has dark skin, be sure to check for color changes on the lips, nail beds, palms, earlobes, whites of the eyes, inner surface of the lower eyelid, gums, and tongue.

You may also wish to check the patient's nail beds. This is called assessing **capillary refill.** It is one way of checking for shock. Capillary refill is recommended only for children under 6 years of age. Research has proven that it is not always accurate in adults.

This procedure is performed by squeezing one of the patient's fingernails or toe nails (Figure 10–29). When squeezed, the tissue under the nail turns white. When you let go, the color returns to the tissue. To assess capillary refill, you have to measure the time it takes for the color to return under the nail. Two seconds or less is normal. If refill time is greater than two seconds, suspect shock or decreased blood flow to that extremity.

Measure capillary refill time by counting "one one-thousand, two two-thousand," and so on. Capillary refill may be checked on infants by squeezing the palm of the hand or sole of the foot and watching for color to return.

Note that when you recheck capillary refill in the ongoing assessment, be sure to do it at the same place. Different parts of the body may have different refill times.

Skin Condition. Normally, a person's skin is dry to the touch. When a patient's skin condition is wet or moist, it may indicate shock, a heat-related emergency, or a diabetic emergency. Skin that is abnormally dry may be a sign of spine injury or severe dehydration.

Pupils

Normally, pupils **constrict** (get smaller) when exposed to light and **dilate** (enlarge) when the level of light is reduced. Both pupils should be the same size unless a prior injury or condition changes this. (See Figure 10–30.)

With these normal responses in mind, assess a patient's pupils. Shine your penlight into one of the

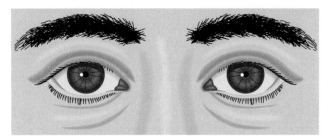

Constricted pupils

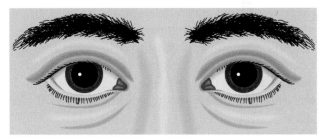

Dilated pupils

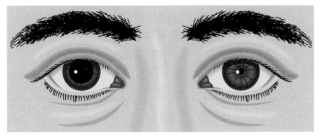

Unequal pupils

Figure 10–30 Check pupils for size, reactivity, and equality.

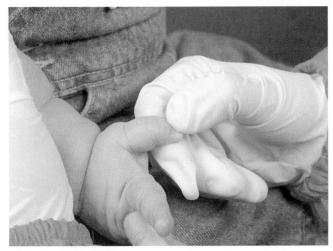

Figure 10–29 Assess capillary refill in children under 6 years of age.

patient's eyes and watch for the pupil to constrict in response to the light. If you are outdoors in bright light, cover the patient's eyes and observe for dilation of the pupils. Do not expose the patient's eyes to light for more than a few seconds as this can be very uncomfortable to the patient.

Abnormal findings for pupils include:

- Pupils that do not react to light.
- Pupils that remain constricted. (This may be caused by a drug overdose.)
- Pupils that are unequal. (This may be an indication of a serious head injury or stroke.)

Blood Pressure

Some First Responders are taught to assess blood pressure. Others are not. Be sure to follow all local protocols.

Blood pressure is the amount of pressure the surging blood exerts against the arterial walls. It is an important index of the efficiency of the whole circulatory system. In part, it tells how well the organs and tissues are getting the oxygen they need. The blood-pressure cuff is the instrument used to measure blood pressure.

The result of a contraction of the heart, which forces blood through the arteries, is called **systolic pressure.** The result of the relaxation of the heart between contractions is called **diastolic pressure.** With most diseases or injuries, these two pressures rise or fall together.

Blood pressure normally varies with the age, gender, and medical history of the patient. (See normal ranges in Table 10–3.) The usual guide for systolic pressure in the adult male is 100 plus the individual's age, up to 150 mmHg. Normal diastolic pressure in the male is 65 mmHg to 90 mmHg. Both the systolic and diastolic pressures are about 10 mmHg lower in the female than in the male. Blood pressure is reported as systolic over diastolic (for example, 120/80).

Measuring Blood Pressure. There are two methods of obtaining blood pressure with a blood pressure cuff. One is by *auscultation*, or by listening for the systolic and diastolic sounds through a stethoscope. The second method is by *palpation*, or by feeling for the return of the pulse as the cuff is deflated.

To assess blood pressure by auscultation, follow the steps described below (Figure 10–31):

1. Choose the proper size blood pressure cuff. It must be able to encircle the arm so that the Velcro on opposite ends meet and fasten securely. The cuff's bladder should cover half the circumference of the arm. If it covers less, it will not compress the blood vessels properly. If it covers more, it will suppress the pulse too quickly. The cuff should fit snugly with the lower edge at least an inch above the **antecubital space** (the hollow, or front, of the elbow) and the bladder centered over the brachial artery. It should not be too tight. You should be able to place one finger easily under its bottom edge. Some cuffs have markers for overlap placement, but they are not always in the correct location.

TABLE 10-3

NORMAL BLOOD PRESSURE RANGES

Patient	Systolic	Diastolic
Child	2 x patient's age + 80	50 to 80 mmHg
Adult	Patient's age + 100 (up to 150 mmHg)	65 to 90 mmHg

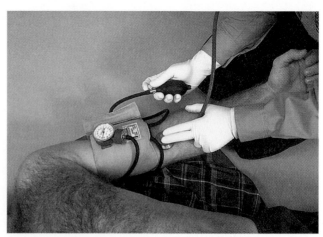

Figure 10-31   Taking blood pressure by auscultation.

2. Now inflate the cuff rapidly with the rubber bulb. At the same time, palpate the radial pulse until it can no longer be felt. Make a mental note of the reading. Without stopping, continue to inflate the cuff to 30 mm above the level where the pulse disappeared.

3. Apply the stethoscope. Place the diaphragm of the stethoscope over the brachial artery just above the hollow of the elbow. The diaphragm may be held with the thumb.

4. Deflate the cuff at approximately 2 mm per second (faster if skill permits). Watch the mercury column or needle indicator drop.

5. As soon as you hear two or more consecutive beats (clear tapping sounds of increasing intensity), record the pressure. This is the systolic pressure.

6. Continue releasing air from the bulb. At the point where you hear the last sound, record the diastolic pressure. Continue to deflate slowly for at least 10 mm. Remember that slow pulses require slower-than-normal rates of deflation. With children and some adults, you may hear sounds all the way to zero. In such cases, record the pressure when the sound changes from clear tapping to soft, muffled tapping.

7. Record the limb on which the blood pressure was taken. Record the position of the person when the blood pressure was taken, if other than supine. Record the size of the cuff if other than standard.

When it is too noisy for you to hear well enough to measure by auscultation, palpate the blood pressure. Follow these steps (Figure 10–32):

1. Inflate the cuff rapidly. As you do so, palpate the patient's radial pulse.

2. Make a mental note of the level at which you can no longer feel the pulse.

3. Without stopping, continue to inflate the cuff another 30 mmHg. Then slowly deflate it.

4. Note the pressure at which the radial pulse returns. This is the systolic pressure.

5. Record it as a palpated systolic pressure (for example, 120/P).

Take several blood pressure readings during the time the patient is in your care. Watch for changes, as this may indicate changes in the patient's condi-

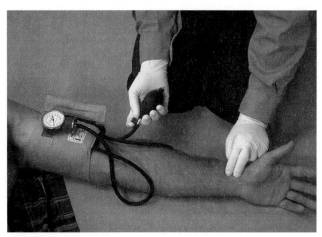

Figure 10–32 Taking blood pressure by palpation.

tion. Carefully record the blood pressure when you measure it, including the time it was taken.

It is not unusual for a patient's blood pressure to vary between the first reading on scene and the reading at the hospital emergency department. Record the pressure accurately so that the receiving physician can tell how much it has changed.

Blood pressure may be normal even if the patient is seriously injured. You will learn in Chapter 17 that by the time the blood pressure drops, the patient already is in serious condition. It is almost always necessary to treat for shock when injuries are present.

Standards for Adults. Blood pressures from person to person vary greatly. In general, systolic blood pressures above 180 and below 90 usually indicate problems. Diastolic blood pressures above 90 and below 60 also indicate problems. The most common blood pressure problem observed in the field is low blood pressure. However, if blood pressure increases dramatically, the patient may suffer a stroke.

In general, blood pressure changes occur late in an emergency. A person who has a blood pressure of 132/82 could actually be developing severe shock. On the other hand, an uninjured person may normally have a blood pressure of 92/62 and be perfectly healthy. Always consider the blood pressure reading as only one element of the patient's picture. Be sure to look at other vital signs, too.

Standards for Children. It is often difficult to take a child's blood pressure. Carrying a variety of cuff sizes is not always possible. But you must have a correctly fitting cuff if you are to get an accurate reading. Always try to get a complete set of vital signs. However, do not waste time attempting multiple blood pressure readings on a critical child if your first tries were unsuccessful. Note that a blood pressure reading is not recommended on children under three years of age.

Average blood pressures in children may be determined by the formula: 80 plus (2 times the age in years). This formula works until the child is about 12 years of age. From that point on, adult blood pressure values apply.

In children, adequate airway management is vital. Do *not* place blood pressure determination over assessment and treatment of life-threats. A child's blood pressure may not begin to drop until well over 40% of blood volume is lost. If the mechanism of injury suggests it, treat for shock regardless of vital signs.

Variable Factors. Factors that may increase blood pressure include conditions and substances that constrict blood vessels. They include:

- Cold environment.
- High altitude.
- Physical and emotional stress.
- Pain.
- Full bladder.
- Upper arm lower than heart level.
- Cigarette smoke.
- Caffeine (coffee, tea, cola, and some analgesic drugs).
- Decongestants.

Heart failure, trauma, and most types of shock can decrease blood pressure.

With the many possible variables that affect blood pressure, it is essential that you recognize the mistakes that can occur in taking a reading. The most critical of these possible errors are:

- The rescuer does not hear accurately due to noise, head cold, or distractions.
- Stethoscope ear pieces are improperly placed.
- Improper conditions exist, such as a cuff not at heart level or a patient not sitting or lying down.

- The systolic pressure is not palpated at the highest level.
- The cuff is the wrong size, either too wide or too narrow.
- The bladder is too wide.
- The cuff is deflated too fast.

SECTION 3: PATIENT HISTORY

The **patient history** is an important part of a thorough patient assessment. It involves gathering facts that you would not be able to gather otherwise. For example, the answer to a simple question such as "What happened?" can provide a good amount of information on the patient's condition and the events leading up to it.

Generally, you would ask the patient questions. If the patient is unresponsive, however, you would gather facts by observing the scene, looking for medical identification tags, and by questioning family members and bystanders (Figure 10–33).

Remember the differences between a trauma patient and a medical patient. In trauma patients,

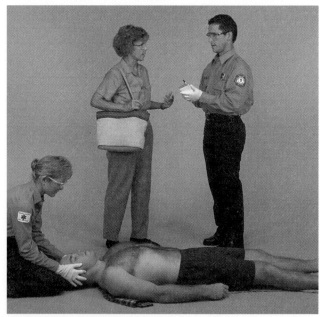

Figure 10-33 Gather facts from the patient or from family or bystanders.

you will most likely perform a physical exam first. For a medical patient, you may take a history first.

THE *SAMPLE* HISTORY

One way to remember the questions you need to ask is by using the mnemonic **SAMPLE.** Each letter identifies an important area of questioning (Figure 10–34):

S — Signs and symptoms.
A — Allergies.
M — Medications.
P — Pertinent past history.
L — Last oral intake.
E — Events.

Signs and Symptoms

Note a patient's signs and symptoms (Figure 10-35). A **sign** is something you can observe directly. That is, you can see, feel, or hear signs. Examples include deformities (see), skin temperature (feel), and wheezing (hear).

A **symptom** cannot be observed by anyone but the patient. In order for you to be aware of symptoms, they must be described by the patient.

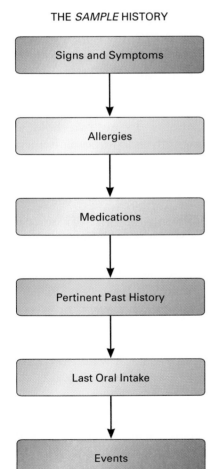

THE *SAMPLE* HISTORY

Signs and Symptoms
↓
Allergies
↓
Medications
↓
Pertinent Past History
↓
Last Oral Intake
↓
Events

Figure 10-34
Components of the SAMPLE history.

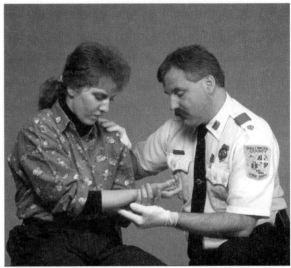

Figure 10-35a A *sign* is something one can observe—a deformed wrist, for example.

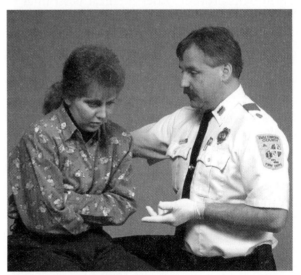

Figure 10-35b A *symptom* is something that the patient feels and describes, such as stomach pain.

Examples of symptoms include pain, tenderness, or difficulty breathing.

A good starting point to determine signs and symptoms is to ask the patient an open-ended question, such as "Why did you call today?" or "Describe how you feel." This technique allows patients to answer without restriction. They may even give you important information you may not have thought to ask about.

Responses to questions like "Do you have chest pain?" are restricted to yes-or-no answers. They can cause you to miss important information. Such questions might be better phrased as "What do you feel in your chest?" or "Tell me what you feel in your chest."

You will find signs and symptoms—as well as emergency care—for specific conditions in later chapters. Remember that you are not required to diagnose any medical condition. A First Responder's emergency care of a patient is based on assessment findings only.

Allergies

Determine if your patient is allergic to anything. This includes allergies to medications, foods, or substances in the environment. Being aware of an allergy can help to determine possible causes of the patient's condition. An allergic reaction can be very serious, in fact it can be life-threatening. Determining if a patient is allergic to a medication will help prevent other medical personnel in the field and in the hospital from administering it.

Medications

Identify all medications the patient is currently or has recently taken. This information may help to identify a medical condition. For example, a patient who takes insulin has diabetes. Other specific medications are used for seizures, cardiac conditions, and respiratory problems. Many EMS rescuers carry a pocket guide that lists common prescription medications and what they are used for.

Pertinent Past History

Most patients have had some type of medical condition in their lifetimes. Some of these may be pertinent to the emergency care you provide to the patient. What is pertinent depends on the type of emergency.

For example, if a patient has shortness of breath, the fact that they have a history of heart problems is pertinent. The fact that they had foot surgery many years ago is not. However, if the patient's present emergency involves dropping a bowling ball on a foot that once was operated on, then the surgery is pertinent.

Patients and family members who are in the middle of a medical crisis may not know what to tell you. Some people say very little. Others are willing to tell you everything there is to know. It is your job to guide them.

Sometimes you need to ask more than one question to guide a patient to an answer. For example, you may begin by asking a patient to tell you about any medical problems he may have. Your patient may answer "None," even though he has diabetes. This is because he may have understood his physician to say that he has "a little sugar problem," which is controlled by diet or pills.

So your next question might be, "Do you see a doctor for anything?" or "Have you ever been admitted to the hospital?" It may cause the patient to disclose the information you need.

Most patients do not withhold answers or answer incorrectly on purpose. Remember, they may be scared, confused, or both.

Last Oral Intake

You must find out the time of your patient's last oral intake. It may be pertinent to the patient who is unresponsive or confused. It also will be important if the patient needs immediate surgery.

Do not ask "When was your last meal?" People may not consider a snack or several drinks a "meal." Instead ask "When was the last time you had anything to eat or drink?" This may include anything from a glass of water to a large meal.

Events

Questions such as "What were you doing when this happened?" help to determine the events leading up to the incident. This information might not be as clear-cut as it seems.

Say a patient falls from a ladder. You arrive to find her complaining of a possible broken arm.

The patient is obviously a trauma patient, right? The answer is "yes," if the patient slipped on a broken rung of the ladder, for example. However, if she fell as a result of getting dizzy or losing consciousness, then she may also be a medical patient.

If a person is driving, has a heart attack, and passes out behind the wheel, he will surely crash. Upon your arrival at the scene you could assume that the patient has suffered serious trauma and is unresponsive from that trauma. It will be your assessment of the events that would help you determine what really happened. A passenger might tell you that he saw the driver clutch his chest before the crash, or a medical information tag may alert you to the heart condition.

As you can see, the SAMPLE history is an important part of the patient assessment process where information vital to patient care is obtained.

SECTION 4: ONGOING ASSESSMENT

Some patients are stable, others are not. So your patient assessment process must be ongoing. Continually reassess your patient until he or she is turned over to the EMTs. (See Figure 10–36.)

Complete the following every 5 minutes for an unstable patient and every 15 minutes for a stable one:

- Reassess level of responsiveness (AVPU).
- Reassess and correct any airway problems.
- Reassess breathing for rate and quality. Ventilate if necessary.
- Reassess pulse for rate and quality.
- Reassess skin temperature, color, and condition.
- Repeat any portions of the physical exam that might be necessary.
- Reassess your interventions (treatment) to see if they are effective.
- Continue to calm and reassure the patient.

Remember that the patients you come across as a First Responder are in crisis. They may be uncomfortable, confused, and possibly afraid that they will

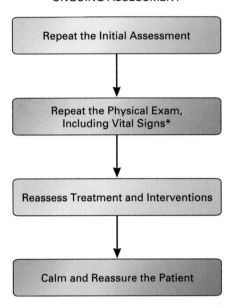

ONGOING ASSESSMENT

Repeat the Initial Assessment

Repeat the Physical Exam, Including Vital Signs*

Reassess Treatment and Interventions

Calm and Reassure the Patient

*Note that some EMS systems do not require First Responders to assess vital signs.

Figure 10–36 Components of ongoing assessment.

die. It is important for you to have a professional, calm, and caring attitude. Try to address the patient's concerns. For example, if you can protect the patient's modesty, do so. Do not leave the patient alone. If the patient feels cold, even if you are not, turn up the heat or provide another blanket.

The kindness and compassion you show will help to calm the patient. It also will be remembered for a long time to come.

SECTION 5: HAND-OFF REPORT

When the EMTs arrive, you must be prepared to tell them appropriate information about your patient and the care you have given. This is called your **hand-off report.**

The hand-off report contains (Figure 10–37):

- Age and sex of the patient.
- Chief complaint.

HAND-OFF REPORT

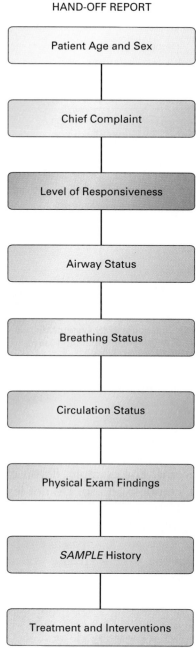

Patient Age and Sex

Chief Complaint

Level of Responsiveness

Airway Status

Breathing Status

Circulation Status

Physical Exam Findings

SAMPLE History

Treatment and Interventions

Figure 10-37 Information included in the hand-off report.

- Level of responsiveness (AVPU).
- Airway and breathing status.
- Circulation status.
- Physical exam findings.
- SAMPLE history.
- Treatment, interventions, and the patient's response to them.

The hand-off report is designed to give the transporting EMTs an up-to-the-minute account of the condition of the patient, what treatments have been performed, and other information that you feel is important. If you must complete a written report, many agencies require that you provide one copy to the EMTs at the scene.

FIRST RESPONDER FOCUS

Even after you have memorized the steps of the assessment process, you still may be amazed at the ease in which experienced First Responders and EMTs perform that complicated task. If you were to ask, many of them would tell you that patient assessment is an art.

You will see throughout the remaining chapters of this text that there are countless injuries and illnesses from which patients can suffer. In every condition the patient assessment finds injuries, signs and symptoms, and histories of past illnesses, all of which are important to patient care.

One experienced First Responder said it like this: "Patient assessment is like a puzzle. It is important to find all the pieces—the examination, the history—and put them together so that they make sense."

A proper patient assessment and history help you to make sense of the patient's condition and provide quality patient care. ■

CASE STUDY FOLLOW-UP

At the beginning of this chapter, you read that First Responders were on scene with an unresponsive male patient. To see how chapter skills apply to this emergency, read the following. It describes how the call was completed.

PATIENT HISTORY

Since the patient was unresponsive, we asked his wife if he had any problems before he went to sleep. She didn't know of any. In response to further questioning, she told us that he had no allergies and that he took insulin for his diabetes. He had taken his insulin in the morning but had been working in the yard all morning after a small breakfast. His wife added that he had a similar episode last year.

PHYSICAL EXAMINATION

Although it seemed like we had a medical problem, you never can be too sure, especially with a patient who cannot talk. I continued to assist ventilations and monitored the airway while my partner did a quick head-to-toe exam to check for injuries that may have been hidden. There were none. My partner then took a set of vital signs.

ONGOING ASSESSMENT

The patient required ventilation the entire time we were at the scene. I suctioned him one more time when I felt his secretions were building up. We continued to monitor the patient's mental status, and spoke to him by name just in case he could hear. His wife was quite upset, so we tried to reassure her and keep her calm.

PATIENT HAND-OFF

When the EMTs arrived, one of them performed an initial assessment. "Good job," he said after assessing the patient's airway. My partner gave them the hand-off report:

"This is George Jeffers. He is 62 and his wife could not wake him up from a nap. He responds only to painful stimulus. We had to suction him and assist ventilations. The physical exam did not turn up anything, but his wife says he has diabetes. He took his insulin, had a small meal, then worked all morning in the yard. His wife says this has happened before. His vitals were pulse 110 and weak, respirations 10 and shallow, blood pressure 110/68. Pupils were equal and reactive, skin cool and moist."

The EMTs thanked us and took over care. We were then dispatched pretty quickly to another run. A few days later I saw one of the EMTs. He told me that the hospital gave Mr. Jeffers glucose through an IV and he began to come around. By the time they left the hospital, he was sitting up and talking.

Patient assessment is performed on all patients you come in contact with. The procedure may vary depending on whether your patient is suffering from a medical problem or trauma and whether the patient has minor injuries or serious ones. It is important to be thorough and work in a logical order. Practice your patient assessment skills frequently and become proficient.

REVIEW QUESTIONS

Page references where answers may be found or supported are provided at the end of each question.

Section 1

1. What are the components of the patient assessment process? (p. 168)
2. What are the components of the initial assessment? (p. 169)
3. Why would you apply manual stabilization to your patient's head and neck? (p. 171)
4. What are the components of the EMS update? (p. 176)

Section 2

5. What are the three basic methods of performing a physical exam? (pp. 176–177)
6. What mnemonic helps you to recall the conditions to look for in the physical exam? What does each letter in the mnemonic stand for? (p. 177)
7. In what patients is capillary refill used? (p. 185)

Section 3

8. What mnemonic can help you to recall the parts of a patient history? What does each letter in the mnemonic stand for? (p. 189)

Section 4

9. What are the components of ongoing assessment? (p. 191)

Section 5

10. What information should be included in the patient hand-off report? (pp. 191–192)

CHAPTER 11

COMMUNICATION AND DOCUMENTATION

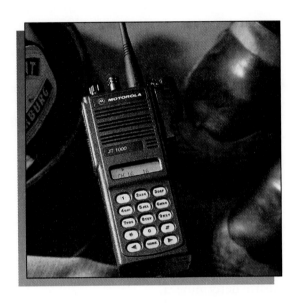

INTRODUCTION

When the stress and confusion of an emergency arise, a First Responder must be able to communicate effectively and precisely. You must be able to do so with the patient, family, bystanders, and other EMS personnel—by radio, in person, and in writing.

Cognitive, affective, and psychomotor objectives are from the U.S. DOT's 1995 "First Responder: National Standard Curriculum." Enrichment objectives, if any, identify material that is supplemental to the DOT curriculum.

Cognitive

No objectives are identified.

Affective

No objectives are identified.

Psychomotor

No objectives are identified.

Enrichment

* Explain the importance of effective verbal communication of patient information. (p. 196)
* Identify typical components of an EMS radio system. (pp. 196, 198)
* List correct radio procedures. (p. 198)
* Identify the essential components of a call to medical direction. (p. 199)
* Discuss the communication skills that should be used to interact with the patient. (pp. 199–200)
* List the components of the written report. (pp. 200, 202)
* Describe the legal implications associated with the written report. (p. 202)
* Review the special considerations concerning patient refusal. (p. 202)
* List special EMS reporting situations. (p. 202)

SECTION 1: COMMUNICATION

A First Responder must be able to determine a chief complaint, obtain a medical history, and properly reassure and comfort the patient. You also must be able to update incoming EMS units on your patient's status, request help from dispatch, ask medical direction for advice, and provide a hand-off report to the EMTs who take over patient care. All these tasks take skill, including communication skills.

You will have opportunities to communicate with other EMS personnel on the radio or phone as well as in person. In these situations it is important for you to be accurate and to speak slowly and clearly. Providing inaccurate information, omitting key information, or speaking in any way other than clearly could result in harm to your patient.

RADIO COMMUNICATION

Radios operate on frequencies that are regulated and licensed by the Federal Communication Commission (FCC). The FCC makes sure that unauthorized persons do not disrupt emergency radio traffic.

There are many components to a radio system. They usually include:

* *A base station* (Figure 11–1). This is a stationary radio located in a dispatch center, station, or hospital.
* *Mobile radios* (Figure 11–2). These are radios mounted in vehicles.

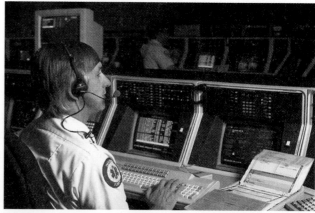

Figure 11-1   Example of an EMS communications center.

CASE STUDY

DISPATCH

Our first response unit was sent to the Bishop McGinn Senior Housing Center for an 80-year-old female patient who was "disoriented and behaving strangely."

SCENE SIZE-UP

The outside of the complex was quiet. We were met at the door by the resident aide, who told us that Mrs. Gherson was acting "in a most peculiar manner." She brought us up to the apartment. We stayed alert.

INITIAL ASSESSMENT

Mrs. Gherson was sitting at her kitchen table, wondering what all the fuss was about. Two neighbors stood beside her. They told us that Mrs. Gherson was wandering the halls, babbling incoherently just a short time ago. They were amazed that she had suddenly improved.

We found the patient to be alert. She had no problems with her airway and could speak in full sentences. Her respirations seemed normal. She had no bleeding. Her friends had not witnessed or heard of a fall.

PATIENT HISTORY

Mrs. Gherson had no idea why EMS was called. She didn't remember being out of her apartment. She denied having allergies. She took insulin for diabetes and a "heart pill" since her heart attack eight years ago. She had eaten dinner and taken her medications.

PHYSICAL EXAMINATION

Mrs. Gherson had no complaints. We began to do a physical exam, but she stopped us. She said that she really didn't want our help. She felt she was fine. We convinced her to let us take her pulse and respiration. She told us that she would not go to the hospital.

Patient refusals are challenging calls for any EMS provider. You must make sure you have tried your best to convince the patient to accept your care and that of the EMTs. Consider this patient as you read Chapter 11. How do communication and documentation affect this situation?

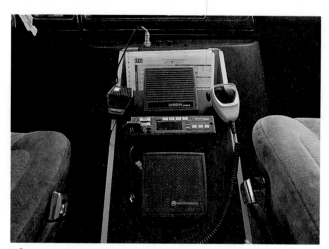

Figure 11-2 A mobile two-way radio.

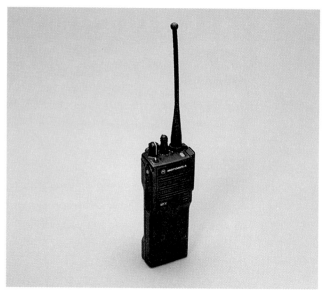

Figure 11-3 A portable hand-held radio.

- *Portable radios* (Figure 11–3). These are hand-held radios, which may be carried on your belt or elsewhere on your person.
- *Repeaters*. These devices receive a low-power radio transmission and rebroadcast it with increased power.
- *Cellular phones* (Figure 11–4). These phones may be used to contact medical direction or the dispatcher. They are often used where radio coverage is not available.

If your EMS system has a dispatch center and radios, you will need to advise the dispatcher of your activities during an emergency call. You must report when you:

- Are en route to a call.
- Arrive at the scene of a call.
- Require additional assistance or specialized personnel.
- Return to service and are available for the next call.

You also will use the radio when you update incoming EMS units or need to speak with medical direction.

Using a radio can cause some anxiety, especially the first few times. It is important to remember to speak slowly and clearly. Push the "push to talk" button one second before you begin to speak. Talk with your mouth two to

three inches away from the microphone. It is best to keep a transmission brief to allow others to use the frequency. Listen before you transmit, so you do not disrupt another conversation.

Remember that people with scanners are able to hear what you say over the radio. Never use a patient's name or say anything over the radio of a personal or confidential nature. Of course, you should never use profanities or speak in a less than professional tone of voice.

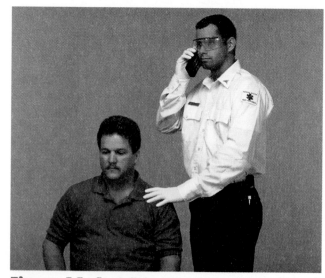

Figure 11-4 Cellular phones are commonly used in EMS.

COMMUNICATING WITH MEDICAL DIRECTION

Consulting with a physician while you are on scene can help you and your patient. If possible, consult medical direction whenever you have questions about a patient that cannot be resolved by protocols.

Since the physician may be many miles away, it is up to you to present information clearly and concisely. Be prepared to give a report that includes:

- Your unit identifier and the fact that you are a First Responder.
- Patient's age, gender, and chief complaint.
- Brief, pertinent history of the events leading to the injury or illness.
- Results of the patient's physical exam, including vital signs.
- Care given to the patient and the patient's response to that care.
- Specify why you are calling.

If the physician gives you orders, repeat the orders back to verify them. Be sure all orders or advice given to you by the physician are clear. If you have any questions, ask the physician for clarification.

INTERPERSONAL COMMUNICATION

Medical emergencies can be frightening to patients. So be sure to speak slowly and clearly. Use language patients and their families can understand. Avoid medical terms that will confuse them.

When speaking to patients, get down to their level, if possible, to avoid appearing threatening. Make eye contact (Figure 11–5). Use body language that makes you seem open and interested in what patients have to say. Also address patients by name whenever possible. Note, however, that if your patient is elderly, do not call him or her by a first name unless you are invited to do so.

Listen carefully to what patients tell you. Observe them when they talk. If a patient appears reluctant to speak about a topic, you may need to reassure him. Tell him that any information he

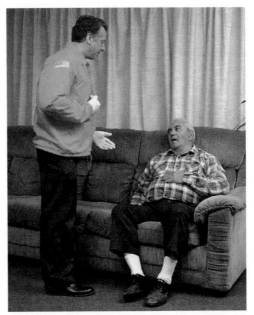

Figure 11-5a You can maintain an attitude of control and authority if you stand above the patient.

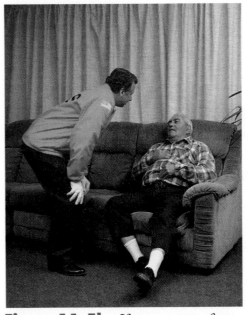

Figure 11-5b If you want to soften your approach, get down to the patient's level.

may have about the problem is important, even if it is upsetting to talk about.

Observe patients while they talk. It can help you to identify physical problems. If a patient can only speak a few words before catching a breath, for example, he may be in respiratory distress.

Find out why a patient is holding his stomach or clutching his chest. He may not even know he is doing it. A patient who winces with pain should be questioned about that pain.

Nothing is more annoying that not being listened to. Recall the last time you had to repeat information to someone several times. It is not a pleasant feeling. Listening lets a patient know that you believe he or she is important. If you ask a patient a question, listen for an answer. Make notes, if necessary, so you do not forget it. If you forget too often, the patient soon will stop answering your questions altogether.

Remember that all patients deserve equal care. One patient should be treated with the same respect and dignity afforded to any other. If you are called to a patient who does not speak a language you understand, call for someone who can translate. A family member or a neighbor, for example, may be able to speak both your language and the patient's.

There may be times when you are called to a patient who cannot hear. Persons with hearing problems may need you to speak up. Deaf patients may need someone who can use sign language. If that is not possible, try to write short messages back and forth.

If you are called to a blind patient, be sure to describe what is going on and what you are doing. Do not leave a patient who cannot see alone. You may find that talking or keeping a hand on his shoulder will help to reassure and calm him.

SECTION 2: DOCUMENTATION

Documentation should be considered an art. This is because it can "paint a picture" of the patient and his or her condition. A properly completed written report not only provides all the pertinent facts, it also provides them in a logical order.

PREHOSPITAL CARE REPORT

A prehospital care report is used for all of the following reasons:

- *To transfer patient information from one person to another.* Your report is turned over to the EMS personnel who transport your patient. They may turn it over to the hospital staff who use it to learn the patient's history, including the condition in which he was found, what emergency care was provided, and how the patient responded to that care.
- *To provide legal documentation.* A report prepared at the scene of an emergency is a legal record. If you provide care at the scene of an injury or act of violence, for example, your report may become evidence in the court proceedings.
- *To document the care you provided.* This is important for legal reasons, too. Unfortunately First Responders and other EMS professionals are sued by patients and their families. As you will recall from Chapter 3, accurate documentation can be one of your best defenses against lawsuits.
- *To improve your EMS system.* Research is performed in many different areas of your EMS system. It is used to improve such factors as response time and the effectiveness of certain procedures. Your accurate reports are vital to that research.

Description

A prehospital care report contains three parts (Figure 11–6). They include run data, patient information, and the narrative. For the run data you must fill in the date, time, unit involved, location of the call, and the names of the crew members.

Information on the patient is extensive. It includes the patient's name, address, date of birth, gender, chief complaint, physical exam including vital signs, patient history, changes in the patient's condition, and the care you gave. Some information can be written in specially designated areas of the form. Some can be recorded by way of check boxes. Some can be in narrative form.

It is important to fill out the report neatly and spell correctly. Do not draw conclusions or offer opinions. Simply state the facts. Avoid the use of radio codes or abbreviations that others might

REMO

First Responder Prehospital Care Report

M **D** **Y**	CALL REC'D
DATE AGENCY CODE RUN NO.	ENROUTE
	AT SCENE
NAME	
ADDRESS	
	VEH. ID.
	IN SERVICE
NEXT OF KIN	
PHYSICIAN	AGENCY NAME
AGE SEX M F Ph#	CALL LOCATION
CHIEF COMPLAINT	CALL TYPE

PAST MEDICAL HISTORY			TIME	RESP	PULSE	B.P.	CONS.
❑ HYPERTENSION	❑ STROKE	V I T A L S I G N S		RATE			
❑ SEIZURES	❑ DIABETES			❑ Regular	❑ Regular		
❑ COPD	❑ CARDIAC			❑ Shallow	❑ Irregular		
❑ ALLERGY	❑ OTHER			❑ Labored			
❑ MEDICATION	(LIST IN COMMENTS)			RATE			
				❑ Regular	❑ Regular		
				❑ Shallow	❑ Irregular		
				❑ Labored			

PHYSICAL EXAM FINDINGS

TREATMENT GIVEN

DISPOSITION	(SEE LIST)		DISP CODE	
C R E W	NAME NAME NAME			
	DRIVER ❑ EMT ❑ AEMT # ❑ EMT ❑ AEMT # ❑ EMT ❑ AEMT #			

Figure 11-6 A First Responder prehospital care report form. (Courtesy of the Regional Emergency Medical Organization, Albany, New York.)

not understand. Be sure to record your observations of the scene. Noting the mechanism of injury, for example, will help hospital personnel identify the extent of the patient's injuries.

If you must correct an error while you are filling out the report, draw a single horizontal line through the error. Then write the correct information beside it. If you try to totally cross out or otherwise deface a report, it will appear that you are trying to hide something.

If you realize that there is an error or that you omitted information after a report has been submitted, you may still be able to correct it. In general, you may cross out an error as described above. Write the correct information. Then mark your initials and date by the new information.

Confidentiality

In an emergency, you will observe the way a patient lives, the condition of the home, and his or her relationships with others. You also will be given a personal medical history. Whether the patient is a celebrity or private individual, you must respect their privacy. Everything you see, hear, and document at the scene is confidential. It cannot be disclosed to anyone except in very specific circumstances. (See Chapter 3.)

PATIENT REFUSAL

Patient refusal is a major cause of lawsuits against EMS providers. Remember, a competent adult has the right to refuse care and transportation. However, it is your responsibility to advise this patient of the risks associated with that refusal.

As described in detail in Chapter 3, before allowing a patient to refuse, take the following steps:

- Make sure the patient is competent and can make a rational, informed decision.
- Try to persuade the patient to accept EMS care and transportation.
- Advise the patient of the risks associated with refusing care.
- Consult medical direction as required by local protocol.

Document each of these points thoroughly. This includes the patient assessment you performed, that you offered care and transportation, and that you were willing to respond again at any time the patient desired. Some systems may expect you to have the patient sign a refusal or "release from liability" form. Other EMS systems prefer to have EMTs respond and speak to the patient. Follow all local protocols.

SPECIAL SITUATIONS

Special incident reports may be required for infectious disease exposure, injury to EMS personnel, conflicts between agencies, multiple-casualty incidents, and other reasons. Since these situations can be very stressful, be sure to stick to the facts when you fill out the reports. They must be accurate and objective accounts in order to serve their purposes well.

One such special situation is the multiple-casualty incident. When there are many patients present in an emergency, there may not be time to provide full documentation on each one. This does not mean that records can be ignored or prepared poorly. Most EMS systems have special tags that are used to record patient information. (See Chapter 29.) One copy of the tag remains with the patient, while another is kept for EMS records. Your local EMS plan for multiple-casualty incidents should explain the procedure for documentation.

FIRST RESPONDER FOCUS

Many of the patients you deal with will not be seriously ill or injured. They will, however, be frightened. This is where your communication skills will be important. Never forget the importance of calming and reassuring the patient. If

you have ever been a patient yourself, you will realize the importance of this concept.

Documentation is important for two reasons. First, the documentation you provide follows the patient. The information you note and pass on to the EMTs will be relayed to the hospital. Second, proper documentation is a form of legal survival. There is an old saying that is true today: "If you didn't write it, it didn't happen." This means that if you forget to document the care you gave to a patient, it will appear as if you never gave it. This not only looks bad, but it also could be used against you if you were ever called to court.

While communication and documentation may seem less important than other parts of a call, they are not. The way you communicate, both orally and in writing, puts forth an image of you. Make it an image to be proud of. ■

CASE STUDY FOLLOW-UP

At the beginning of this chapter, you read that First Responders were on scene with an elderly patient who refused emergency care. To see how chapter skills apply, read the following to see how the call was completed.

ONGOING ASSESSMENT
We observed Mrs. Gherson as we continued to try to get her to accept care. We were concerned that she had a serious condition. We felt she really needed to go to the hospital. Before we could change her mind, the ambulance arrived.

PATIENT HAND-OFF
When the EMTs arrived on scene, we reported Mrs. Gherson's behavior, pulse and respiration, medical history, and medications. Then we quickly planned how to explain to her the need to accept care and transportation.

I called Mrs. Gherson's friends away. This let the EMTs get close and allowed me to enlist their help in convincing Mrs. Gherson to accept transport. After a while one of the women, Mrs. Porter, went back in and explained how worried she was. "If you could have seen yourself, Ingrid," she said. She was very convincing. Mrs. Gherson agreed to go. We helped the EMTs and then carefully documented our actions.

We went back for a call a few weeks later. We saw Mrs. Porter, who told us that Mrs. Gherson had a "mini-stroke." She also said that the doctors were watching her more closely now.

> Communication and documentation are key elements in every call you make. Be sure you are aware of your EMS system's related rules and regulations.

REVIEW QUESTIONS

Page references where answers may be found or supported are provided at the end of each question.

Section 1

1. What are the components of a radio communication system? Describe each one briefly. (pp. 196, 198)
2. How can you make sure your radio transmissions are clear? (p. 198)
3. What are the basic components of a call to medical direction? (p. 199)

4. What are some ways you can improve interpersonal communication? (pp. 199–200)

Section 2

5. What are the purposes of the prehospital care report? (p. 200)
6. What three types of information does the prehospital care report include? (p. 200)
7. What are three situations in which you may be required to make a special incident report? (p. 202)

CHAPTER 12

CARDIAC AND RESPIRATORY EMERGENCIES

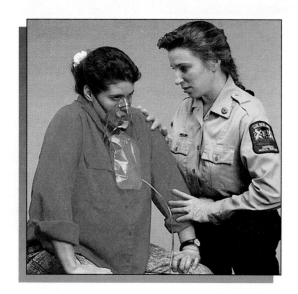

INTRODUCTION

Heart attacks and heart disease are the number-one killers in the U.S. today. Each year almost a half-million Americans die of the disease before they can reach a hospital. Almost 29 million more suffer from some form of it. About 1.5 million have heart attacks.

Illnesses that affect the respiratory system are also very common. Emphysema and chronic bronchitis alone affect more than 23 million people in the U.S. Asthma affects nearly 10 million.

Both types of problems—respiratory and cardiac—can be life-threatening. When they occur, patients can benefit from immediate life-saving care.

OBJECTIVES

Cognitive, affective, and psychomotor objectives are from the U.S. DOT's 1995 "First Responder: National Standard Curriculum." Enrichment objectives, if any, identify material that is supplemental to the DOT curriculum.

Cognitive

No objectives are identified.

Affective

5-1.16   Attend to the feelings of the patient and/or family when dealing with the patient with a specific medical complaint. (pp. 207, 213, 214, 216)

5-1.21   Demonstrate a caring attitude towards patients with a specific medical complaint who request emergency medical services. (pp. 207, 213)

5-1.22   Place the interests of the patient with a specific medical complaint as the foremost consideration when making any and all patient care decisions. (pp. 206, 213)

5-1.23   Communicate with empathy to patients with a specific medical complaint, as well as with family members and friends of the patient. (p. 207)

Psychomotor

No objectives are identified.

Enrichment

*   State the signs and symptoms of the patient experiencing chest pain or discomfort. (pp. 206–207)
*   Describe the emergency care of the patient experiencing chest pain or discomfort. (pp. 207, 209)
*   Discuss common causes of chest pain or discomfort, including angina pectoris and acute myocardial infarction. (pp. 209–211)
*   List the signs of adequate breathing. (pp. 211–212)
*   State the signs and symptoms of a patient in respiratory distress. (p. 212)
*   Describe the emergency care of the patient in respiratory distress. (pp. 212–213)
*   Discuss common causes of breathing difficulty, including chronic obstructive pulmonary disease, asthma, pneumonia, acute pulmonary edema, and hyperventilation. (pp. 213–216)

SECTION 1: CARDIAC EMERGENCIES

Cardiac emergencies can occur from abnormal heart rhythm patterns. They also occur when there is an interruption of oxygen to some part of the heart muscle. The reduction of oxygen causes chest pain or discomfort, one of the most common symptoms of a cardiac emergency.

Coronary artery disease affects the inner lining of the arteries that supply the heart with blood. People who have it usually suffer from arteriosclerosis, a condition that causes the walls of the arteries to become thick and hard.

In coronary artery disease, the opening of the coronary artery is narrowed. (See Figure 12–1.) This restricts the amount of blood that can reach and nourish the heart. The rough artery surfaces then cause a buildup of debris, further narrowing the artery. The more the artery narrows, the less oxygen gets to the heart. At some point, the patient may have chest pain. When the artery becomes blocked, the patient may suffer a heart attack that results in death of the heart muscle.

Researchers have identified a number of cardiac risk factors that predispose a person to heart attack. Obviously, some factors cannot be controlled. With awareness and determination, however, a person can change other factors and decrease his or her own risk.

The major risk factors are (Figure 12–2, p. 208):

*   Physical inactivity, a sedentary lifestyle.
*   Cigarette smoking.
*   Obesity.
*   High serum cholesterol and triglycerides.
*   Diabetes.

CASE STUDY

DISPATCH

I was working at the plant during my regular 4-12 shift. I also was assigned to the emergency response team (ERT), which is responsible for hazmat problems and medical emergencies. At about 6:30 p.m. I heard our team paged to respond. A man was having chest pain.

SCENE SIZE-UP

I approached the scene and looked around. Other than a few concerned coworkers, everything was quiet. It appeared that there was only one patient. I recognized the man, Harry Nowack, because I used to work with him. He told me that his chest hurt.

INITIAL ASSESSMENT

Harry was alert. His airway was clear. He could speak in full sentences, but his breathing was labored. He had no obvious external bleeding. Harry told me that he didn't fall or have any injuries. "My chest just hurts." I couldn't help but notice Harry's color. He looked ashen. It was definitely not normal.

I radioed my findings to the plant office, and told them to notify the 9-1-1 ambulance. I told them that my general impression was that of an alert 55-year-old man who had chest pain, poor color, and labored breathing. The ETA of the ambulance was 10 minutes.

> What do you think this patient's problem may be? What should be done to assess and treat his condition? Consider this patient as you read Chapter 12.

- Male gender.
- Age (incidence increases over 30 years of age).
- Hypertension (blood pressure above 140/90).
- Family history of coronary heart disease under age 60.
- Oral contraceptive use in women over 40.

There are many reasons a patient may develop a condition that leads to a cardiac emergency. However, you do not have to identify them. A First Responder's assessment and treatment of a patient with chest pain will be the same, no matter what the actual cause.

PATIENT ASSESSMENT

Signs and Symptoms

The general signs and symptoms of a cardiac emergency are as follows (Figure 12–3):

- Chest pain or discomfort described as heaviness or squeezing. The sensation also may radiate to the arms, shoulder, neck, or jaw.
- Difficulty breathing, shortness of breath.
- Unusual pulse (rapid, weak, slow, or irregular).
- Indigestion, nausea, vomiting.

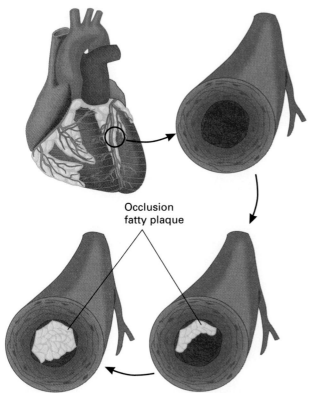

Figure 12-1 Fatty deposits build up in arteries, depriving the heart muscle of blood and oxygen.

- Sweating.
- Skin color, including mucous membranes, may be pale, gray, or cyanotic.
- A feeling of impending doom.

It is likely that when you gather a medical history the patient will tell you he or she has a history of heart problems or a previous similar experience.

Remember that a patient with chest pain will be very anxious. He may feel as if he was going to die. This requires compassion and reassurance. Be sure he understands that everything that can possibly be done is being done. Advise him and his family that further help is on the way and that he will be transported promptly to a medical facility.

Update incoming EMS units. Request advanced care if it is available in your area. Monitor the patient, because he or she may become unstable rapidly.

Chest Pain and Cardiac Patients

Continue to monitor the patient's airway and breathing during and after the initial assessment. Patients who experience chest pain may need airway maintenance and ventilation. Be alert for changes in the patient's mental status. These patients can lose consciousness rapidly. If the patient becomes unresponsive, be prepared to perform CPR and, if you are trained, to use an AED.

When you take a SAMPLE history, you may also want to use the **OPQRRRST** mnemonic to help you get a good description of the pain. Each letter identifies an important area of questioning:

O — *Onset.* When did the pain begin?
P — *Provocation.* Did anything cause or start the pain (exercise, an activity)?
Q — *Quality.* What is the pain like (crushing, stabbing, etc.)?
R — *Region.* Where is the pain?
R — *Radiation.* Does the pain begin in one place and then seem to travel somewhere else?
R — *Relief.* Does anything relieve the pain?
S — *Severity.* On a scale of 1–10, with 10 the worst, how bad is the pain?
T — *Time.* How long have you had the pain?

When you perform a physical exam, palpate the chest for DOTS. Make a note if your touch causes pain. If you are trained to do so, listen to the lungs to determine if air is moving in and out of both sides equally.

GENERAL GUIDELINES FOR EMERGENCY CARE

When the patient's chief complaint is chest pain, be prepared to provide CPR in case he or she becomes pulseless. If possible, you should perform CPR with supplemental oxygen by way of a pocket face mask, bag-valve-mask device, or resuscitator. (See Chapters 6–8 for details on basic life support techniques.)

To provide emergency care, first be sure you have taken BSI precautions. Then proceed as follows:

CARDIAC RISK FACTORS

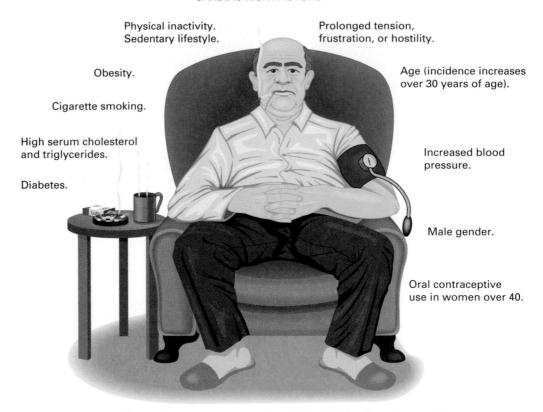

Physical inactivity. Sedentary lifestyle.

Prolonged tension, frustration, or hostility.

Obesity.

Age (incidence increases over 30 years of age).

Cigarette smoking.

High serum cholesterol and triglycerides.

Increased blood pressure.

Diabetes.

Male gender.

Oral contraceptive use in women over 40.

Family history of premature coronary heart disease (usually under age 60).

Figure 12-2 The risk for a patient with high cholesterol, high blood pressure, and heavy smoking is 10 times that of someone without those risk factors.

SIGNS AND SYMPTOMS OF A CARDIAC EMERGENCY

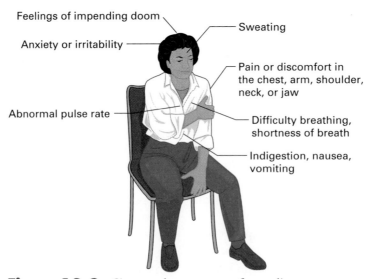

Feelings of impending doom

Sweating

Anxiety or irritability

Pain or discomfort in the chest, arm, shoulder, neck, or jaw

Abnormal pulse rate

Difficulty breathing, shortness of breath

Indigestion, nausea, vomiting

Figure 12-3 Signs and symptoms of a cardiac emergency.

1. Have the patient cease all movement.
2. Place the responsive patient in a position of comfort. This is usually a semi-reclining or sitting position.
3. Make sure that the airway is open. Administer high-flow oxygen with a nonrebreather mask. (Follow local protocol.) If needed, provide artificial ventilation or CPR.
4. Loosen tight clothing.
5. Maintain body temperature as close to normal as possible.
6. Comfort and reassure the patient.
7. If not done previously, activate the EMS system immediately.

Your patient may tell you that he or she has had heart surgery. Your patient also may tell you he or she has a pacemaker or an implanted defibrillator. (An implanted defibrillator delivers shocks to a patient but at much less power than an AED.) Treat these patients in the same way as described above. Note that a malfunctioning pacemaker may cause a slow heart rhythm. If this occurs, monitor the patient carefully. Provide oxygen and be prepared to administer CPR if necessary.

SPECIFIC CARDIAC CONDITIONS

Two problems are commonly caused by coronary artery disease. They are *angina pectoris,* sometimes called angina, and *myocardial infarction,* the medical term for heart attack.

The emergency care of patients with angina and myocardial infarction are the same. It is not necessary to differentiate between the two. Taking time to do so might even be harmful. Chest-pain patients need prompt care and constant monitoring. Early access to the EMS system and rapid transportation to a hospital can literally make the difference between life and death.

Angina Pectoris

The term *angina pectoris* literally means "pain in the chest." As you know, the heart relies on a constant supply of oxygen. If it does not get enough because of diseased or narrowed arteries, the patient experiences chest pain or discomfort.

Most often the pain of angina occurs as a result of physical activity beyond the patient's limit, emotional stress, or extreme hot or cold weather. Sometimes, though rarely, it has no apparent cause.

Angina is reversible. It does not cause permanent damage to the heart muscle. Generally, the pain is relieved by rest, usually within a few minutes after the patient stops the activity, calms down, moves indoors, or takes nitroglycerin as prescribed by a physician.

The pain of angina can change from a mild ache to a severe crushing pain. It can appear suddenly, but usually it is associated with physical exertion. It usually is in the chest, but it can radiate to the jaw, neck, left shoulder, left arm, or left hand. It often is mistaken for indigestion. Note that angina does not always manifest itself as pain. It may be a feeling of tightness, gripping, heaviness, squeezing, burning, or a dull constriction.

Other signs and symptoms include:

- Shortness of breath.
- Profuse sweating.
- Lightheadedness.
- Palpitations (a sensation of throbbing or fluttering of the heart).
- Nausea, vomiting.
- Pale, cool, moist skin.

It is impossible for you to tell the difference between the pain of angina and the pain of a heart attack. While angina usually leaves the heart undamaged, if it is left untreated, it may eventually cause a heart attack.

Acute Myocardial Infarction

Myocardial infarction means "death of the heart muscle." When blood to part of the heart is blocked off or greatly reduced, that part dies. Myocardial infarction is most commonly caused by blockage, the result of coronary artery disease.

Myocardial infarction, or heart attack, has four serious consequences. They are:

- *Sudden death.* Of the heart-attack patients who die before reaching a hospital, most die within two hours of the first signs and symptoms.

- *Shock.* If 40% or more of the left ventricle is damaged after an attack, the heart cannot pump the proper amount of blood to the body. Shock usually occurs within 24 hours, with a mortality rate of about 80%.
- *Congestive heart failure.* This condition may develop after a heart attack. It causes a buildup of fluid, which may accumulate in the lungs (pulmonary edema) and in other parts of the body. This is sometimes observed as swelling in the ankles. (See Figure 12–4.)
- *Cardiac dysrhythmias.* These are the abnormal heart rhythms that follow a heart attack. They are generally caused by injury to the electrical conduction system of the heart.

The most common symptom of heart attack is a sudden onset of chest pain. About 80% of all heart attack victims experience it. Many also have abnormal heart rhythms and may suffer nausea and vomiting. Note that 20% of all heart attack patients have no chest pain at all. (This is usually the elderly or patients with diabetes.) A heart attack without pain is called *silent* myocardial infarction.

Chest pain associated with heart attack ranges from mild discomfort to severe pain. The sensation felt by the patient may be described as pain, crushing, tightness, or numbness. It usually lasts longer than 30 minutes. Though the pain can be experienced in a number of ways, the common location is substernal, radiating to the neck, jaw, left shoulder, and left arm (Figure 12–5). It often includes the burning and bloating sensations of indigestion. It can be continuous. It might subside, but do not ignore it if it does. Any adult with pain or discomfort to the chest, neck, shoulder, arm, or jaw should be suspected of heart attack. Treat the patient accordingly.

Other signs and symptoms include:

- Sudden onset of weakness, nausea and vomiting, and profuse sweating without a clear cause.
- Pain not related to physical exertion and not relieved by rest.
- Abnormal pulse, which may be rapid (over 100), slow (below 60), or irregular.
- Difficulty breathing or rapid, shallow respirations.
- Cool, pale, moist skin, and possible cyanosis.
- Lightheadedness, loss of consciousness.
- Frightened appearance, anxiety, feelings of impending doom.

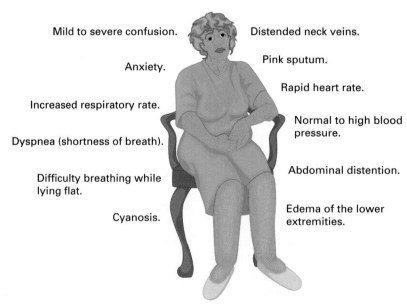

SIGNS AND SYMPTOMS OF
CONGESTIVE HEART FAILURE

Mild to severe confusion.

Anxiety.

Increased respiratory rate.

Dyspnea (shortness of breath).

Difficulty breathing while lying flat.

Cyanosis.

Distended neck veins.

Pink sputum.

Rapid heart rate.

Normal to high blood pressure.

Abdominal distention.

Edema of the lower extremities.

Figure 12-4 Signs and symptoms of congestive heart failure.

EARLY SIGNS OF HEART ATTACK

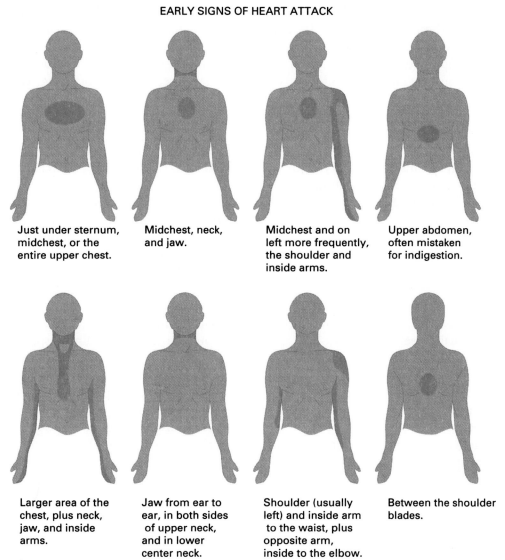

Just under sternum, midchest, or the entire upper chest.

Midchest, neck, and jaw.

Midchest and on left more frequently, the shoulder and inside arms.

Upper abdomen, often mistaken for indigestion.

Larger area of the chest, plus neck, jaw, and inside arms.

Jaw from ear to ear, in both sides of upper neck, and in lower center neck.

Shoulder (usually left) and inside arm to the waist, plus opposite arm, inside to the elbow.

Between the shoulder blades.

Figure 12-5 Pain or discomfort can occur in any one location or any combination of locations.

SECTION 2: RESPIRATORY EMERGENCIES

Without oxygen, cells such as those in the brain and heart can die within minutes. A variety of diseases and injuries can affect the body's ability to get enough oxygen. The need for rapid treatment in those cases is essential.

PATIENT ASSESSMENT

As you learned in Chapter 6, adequate breathing occurs at a normal rate. For adults, that is 12 to 20 breaths per minute. For children, it is 15 to 30 breaths per minute. For infants, it is 25 to 50 breaths per minute. Adequate breathing is regular in rhythm and free of unusual sounds, such as wheezing or whistling. The chest should expand adequately and equally with each breath. The depth of the breaths should be adequate, too. In addition, breathing should be effortless. That is, it should be accomplished without the use of accessory muscles in the neck, shoulders, or abdomen.

Respiratory distress is shortness of breath or a feeling of air hunger with labored breathing. It is one of the most common medical complaints. Two circumstances may cause respiratory distress. Either air cannot pass easily into the lungs or air cannot pass easily out of them. Signs and symptoms include (Figure 12–6):

- Inability to speak in full sentences without pausing to breathe.
- Noisy breathing.
- Use of accessory muscles to breathe. That includes neck muscles, muscles between the ribs, and abdominal muscles.
- **Tripod position.** In this position, the patient is sitting upright, leaning forward, fighting to breathe (Figure 12–7).
- Abnormal breathing rate and rhythm.
- Increased pulse rate.
- Skin color changes (pale, flushed, or cyanotic).
- Altered mental status.

Generally, breathing will be rapid and shallow. Patients may feel short of breath whether they are breathing rapidly or slowly. Remember, a certain amount of shortness of breath is normal following exercise, fatigue, coughing, or with the production of excess sputum.

GENERAL GUIDELINES FOR EMERGENCY CARE

Respiratory distress may be a symptom of an injury or an illness. It is not a disease in itself. Whatever the cause, the treatment is the same. To provide emergency care, first be sure you have taken BSI precautions. Then proceed as follows:

1. Carefully assess the patient's breathing to determine if it is adequate. Monitor it throughout the call. If you find respirations are inadequate, provide artificial ventilation immediately.
2. Place the responsive patient with adequate breathing in a position of comfort. This is usually a sitting position.
3. Administer oxygen, if you are trained and allowed to do so. Use a nonrebreather mask at 12–15 liters per minute.

SIGNS AND SYMPTOMS OF RESPIRATORY DISTRESS

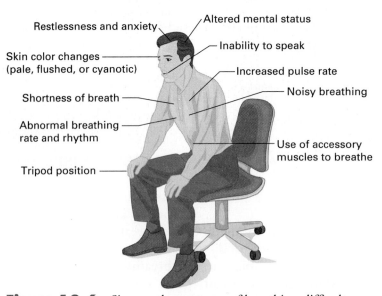

Restlessness and anxiety

Skin color changes (pale, flushed, or cyanotic)

Shortness of breath

Abnormal breathing rate and rhythm

Tripod position

Altered mental status

Inability to speak

Increased pulse rate

Noisy breathing

Use of accessory muscles to breathe

Figure 12-6 Signs and symptoms of breathing difficulty.

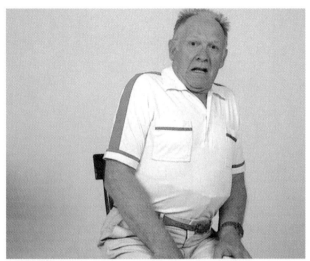

Figure 12-7 Patients with emphysema and chronic bronchitis often lean forward as they breathe.

4. Comfort and reassure the patient. There are few feelings as terrifying as not being able to breathe. Because of this fear, the patient may become agitated or even angry. Do not take it personally.
5. If not done previously, activate the EMS system immediately.

SPECIFIC RESPIRATORY CONDITIONS

The following conditions are among the breathing problems you will commonly see in the field. They include chronic obstructive pulmonary disease (COPD), asthma, pneumonia, acute pulmonary edema, and hyperventilation syndrome. Remember, though respiratory distress has a variety of causes, First Responder treatment is always the same.

Chronic Obstructive Pulmonary Disease (COPD)

Emphysema and chronic bronchitis are the most common chronic obstructive pulmonary diseases (COPDs). Together they affect more than 23 million people in the U.S.

In emphysema the alveoli lose elasticity, become distended with trapped air, and stop working. As the total number of alveoli decreases, breathing becomes more and more difficult.

Chronic bronchitis is characterized by inflammation, edema, and excessive mucus in the bronchial tree. It features a productive cough that has persisted for at least three months per year over two consecutive years. Patients who get medical help early can lead fairly normal lives with proper medication and a good exercise program.

The most important known factor to cause COPD is cigarette smoking. COPD is more common in men than in women. It also is more common among city dwellers than among rural populations. Urban air pollution also plays a role.

Victims of COPD usually get colds or flu often. They also become winded under conditions that do not tax most healthy people (such as walking on a level surface). Other signs and symptoms include:

- Shortness of breath, gasping for air.
- Tripod position (sitting upright, leaning forward, fighting to breathe).
- Bulging neck veins.
- Coarse rattling sounds in the lungs.
- Cyanosis.
- Prolonged exhaling through pursed lips.
- Barrel-shaped chest.
- Presence of home-oxygen systems, breathing treatments, medications, and inhalers (puffers).

Both emphysema and chronic bronchitis patients may develop a hypoxic drive to breathe. Healthy people get their drive to breathe from the amount of carbon dioxide in the blood. Patients who have emphysema or chronic bronchitis build up consistently high levels of carbon dioxide. Because of this, the body looks to the levels of oxygen, rather than carbon dioxide, to determine the need to breathe. If oxygen levels are low, the body breathes faster to get more oxygen.

Giving oxygen to a patient with hypoxic drive can be a problem. After oxygen is administered, its level in the blood increases. In the patient with a true hypoxic drive, increased levels of oxygen may signal the body to slow down or even stop breathing. However, this is rare in the field.

The general rule is to administer oxygen to all patients who need it. All patients with difficulty breathing, cyanosis, altered mental status, shock, or other signs of a serious condition should be given high-concentration oxygen by nonrebreather mask. All patients in respiratory or cardiac arrest should receive high concentrations of supplemental oxygen by pocket mask, bag-valve-mask, or resuscitator.

Asthma

Asthma affects approximately 3% of the people in the U.S., or about 10 million people. About 6000 of those die from it every year. It is most common among children and middle-aged women. Often, it is present in more than one member of the same family.

Typically, the person with asthma is free of symptoms between attacks. He or she often does not know what causes the attacks. Many times they occur while the patient is asleep.

The acute asthma attack varies in duration, intensity, and frequency. It reflects airway obstruction due to bronchospasm, swelling of mucous membranes in the bronchial walls, or plugging of the bronchi by thick mucus.

Signs and symptoms of an asthma attack include the following (Figure 12–8):

- Tripod position.
- Spasmodic, apparently unproductive cough.
- High-pitched wheezing during exhalation, which may also occur upon inhalation.
- Very little movement of air during breathing.
- Overinflated chest with air trapped in the lungs.
- Rapid, shallow respirations.
- Rapid pulse, often exceeding 120.
- Fatigue, confusion, agitation, lethargy.
- Inability to speak in full sentences without catching the breath.

Status asthmaticus is a severe, life-threatening, prolonged asthma attack. It is a dire medical emergency (Figure 12–9). The patient may begin shallow breathing or may stop breathing altogether. In these cases, the wheezing may stop, and it may appear that the patient has improved, but this is not true. Watch all asthma patients carefully for reduced respirations. Be prepared to provide artificial ventilation. Signs and symptoms include:

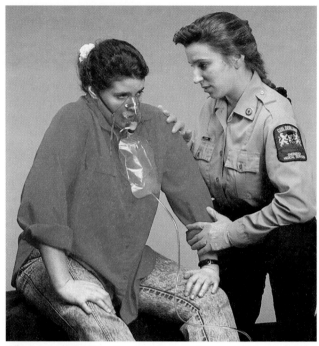

Figure 12-8   Reassure an asthma patient to help reduce stress and fear.

- Anxiety, exhaustion.
- Breathing through pursed lips.
- Wheezing at first, then inaudible breath sounds.
- Overinflated chest.
- Rapid heart rate.
- Tripod position.
- Extremely labored breathing.
- Cyanosis.
- Walking and talking only with great effort.

Caution: All that wheezes is not asthma. Many other diseases can cause wheezing, such as acute congestive heart failure, smoke inhalation, chronic bronchitis, anaphylaxis, and acute pulmonary embolism. All patients with wheezing should be treated with high-flow oxygen by nonrebreather mask if they are in respiratory distress.

Pneumonia

Pneumonia is a term used to describe a group of illnesses characterized by lung infection and fluid- or pus-filled alveoli. Both of these conditions lead to inadequately oxygenated blood. Pneumonia is most frequently caused by bacteria or a virus. It also may be caused by inhaled irritants such as smoke or aspirated materials such as vomit.

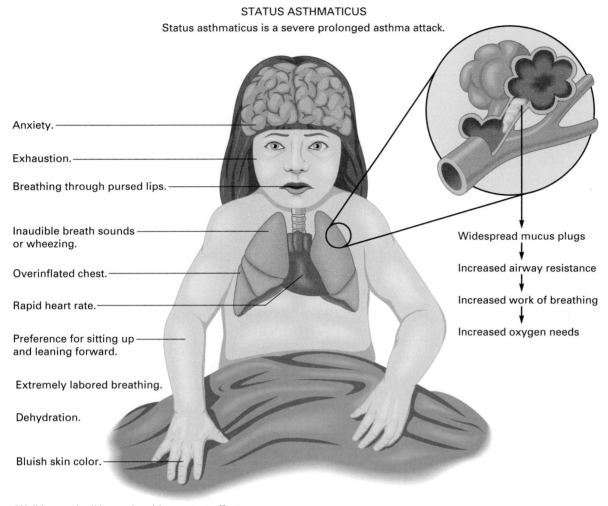

STATUS ASTHMATICUS
Status asthmaticus is a severe prolonged asthma attack.

Anxiety.

Exhaustion.

Breathing through pursed lips.

Inaudible breath sounds
or wheezing.

Overinflated chest.

Rapid heart rate.

Preference for sitting up
and leaning forward.

Extremely labored breathing.

Dehydration.

Bluish skin color.

Widespread mucus plugs

Increased airway resistance

Increased work of breathing

Increased oxygen needs

Walking and talking only with greatest effort.

Figure 12-9   Status asthmaticus is a dire medical emergency.

Pneumonia patients generally appear ill. Most complain of fever and chills "that shake the bed." Signs and symptoms may be influenced by the area of the lung that is affected. For example, pneumonia of the lower lobes of the lungs may not produce cough but may cause abdominal pain. In general, look for the following:

- Chest pain, usually made worse with breathing.
- Rapid breathing.
- Respiratory distress.
- Productive cough with pus in the sputum or mucus.
- Fever, usually exceeding 101°F.
- Chills.
- Hot, dry skin.

Acute Pulmonary Edema

Acute pulmonary edema can be caused by damage to the heart or lungs. It occurs when extra fluids build up in the tissues around the spaces of the lungs. So, if you know your patient has acute pulmonary edema and he or she is responsive and in a sitting position, let his or her legs dangle to encourage blood to pool in the legs. You also can support the back and shoulders with pillows.

Signs and symptoms of acute pulmonary edema include:

- Shortness of breath.
- Rapid, labored breathing.
- Cyanosis.
- Frothy pink, blood-tinged sputum (a late sign).

- Bulging neck veins.
- Rapid pulse.
- Cool, clammy skin.
- Restlessness.
- Anxiety.
- Exhaustion.

Note that oxygen therapy may be critical to this patient. So be sure to administer oxygen, if you are trained and allowed to do so. Also, monitor breathing and other vital signs carefully until medical help arrives.

Hyperventilation

Hyperventilation is a condition characterized by breathing too fast. It is normal for most people occasionally, such as when they are surprised. It remains normal as long as the rate of breathing quickly returns to normal.

Hyperventilation syndrome is an abnormal state in which rapid breathing persists. It is a common disorder usually associated with anxiety. As the patient becomes more anxious, he or she breathes more rapidly, which in turn makes the patient more anxious, and so on, creating a vicious cycle.

The syndrome is characterized by rapid, deep, or abnormal breathing. The lungs overinflate, and the patient blows off too much carbon dioxide. In prolonged cases, the patient may pass out. It typically occurs in young, anxious patients, most of whom are not aware that they are breathing too fast.

Signs and symptoms include:

- Air hunger, or "gulping" air.
- Deep, sighing, rapid breathing with rapid pulse.

- Sensation of choking.
- Dryness or bitterness of the mouth.
- Tightness or a "lump" in the throat.
- Marked anxiety escalating to panic and a feeling of impending doom.
- Dizziness, lightheadedness, fainting.
- Giddiness or unusual behavior.
- Drawing up the hands at the wrist and knuckles with the fingers flexed.
- Blurring of vision.
- Numbness or tingling of the hands and feet or around the mouth.
- Pounding of the heart with stabbing pains in the chest.
- Fatigue, great tiredness, or weakness.
- A feeling of being in a dream.

Note that not every patient who is breathing rapidly or deeply is hyperventilating. Several serious conditions may be the cause, including diabetes, asthma, or trauma. It also may have a medical origin, such as aspirin overdose. If you are certain that no life-threatening condition exists, then try to calm your patient. Be reassuring, and listen carefully to his or her concerns. Try to talk the patient into breathing slowly. If the patient does not respond immediately to your efforts, then administer oxygen. It will not make hyperventilation worse.

You may have heard that putting a paper bag over a patient's mouth is a cure for hyperventilation. This treatment is dangerous, especially if an underlying medical condition exists. As noted above, calming is a powerful benefit to the hyperventilating patient. Follow local protocol.

FIRST RESPONDER FOCUS

The condition of a patient with respiratory distress—or a patient with chest pain—can deteriorate rapidly. So make sure EMS has been notified and be prepared to provide basic life support as soon as it is needed. Also, remember that artificial ventilation is not only for patients in respiratory arrest. Be prepared to provide ventilations if your patient is breathing inadequately, too. You may want to review Chapters 6, 7, and 8 at this time.

Few things are more frightening than chest pain or not being able to breathe. A patient with either problem may be anxious, argumentative, and scared. Do your best to be calming and reassuring. If the patient yells or snaps at you, realize that he or she is reacting to the situation and not to you personally. ■

CASE STUDY FOLLOW-UP

At the beginning of this chapter, you read that a First Responder was caring for a patient with chest pain, labored breathing, and poor skin color. To see how chapter skills apply to this emergency, read the following. It describes how the call was completed.

PHYSICAL EXAMINATION
Two other members of the ERT arrived to help. They performed a head-to-toe exam, while I talked to Harry about his history.

PATIENT HISTORY
Harry told me that he was working at his bench when he started getting severe pain in his chest. He had never felt anything like it before, and I had never seen Harry that scared. I reassured him and asked a few questions, using the OPQRRRST mnemonic.

Harry was working when the pain came on. He told me it was crushing, like someone sitting right on the center of his chest. He held his fist there to show me. It didn't radiate. Nothing, he said, helped to relieve the pain. On a 1-to-10 scale, he said the pain was an "8." It started about 10 minutes ago.

Harry hadn't seen a doctor in years. He took no medications and had no medical problems or allergies. He ate a big spaghetti dinner during his break.

When I heard Harry's vital signs—pulse 92 and irregular, respirations 18 and adequate, blood pressure 146/96, with skin that was cool, gray, and moist, I began to wish our plant had an AED.

ONGOING ASSESSMENT
After helping to make Harry comfortable, I continued to talk and reassure him. We rechecked his ABCs, which remained okay. The chest pain did not diminish. A second assessment of vital signs revealed a pulse of 96 and irregular, and respirations 20 and still labored. Unfortunately, we didn't have oxygen to give him.

PATIENT HAND-OFF
The paramedics arrived a short time later. We immediately called their attention to Harry's chief complaint, poor color, labored breathing, and chest pain to let them know how serious I thought it was. They agreed. Then we filled them in on the rest:

> "This is Harry Nowack, 55 years old. His chest pain started while he was working. It is in the center of his chest and is crushing. It is an 8 out of 10 on the scale, and it doesn't radiate. He has no medical problems that he knows of, but he hasn't been to a doctor in years. He has no meds or allergies. He ate a big spaghetti dinner a short time ago. His pulse is 96 and irregular, respirations 20 and slightly labored, blood pressure 146/96."

The paramedics thanked us, and I helped them put the oxygen on Harry. He wanted me to come with him, and the paramedics didn't mind some help. I made sure that someone called Harry's wife.

Well, it turned out that Harry had a major heart attack. The word spread around the plant the next day. The way he looked was just like they described in the books. I always take chest pain seriously. I'm glad we did with Harry.

Problems with cardiac and respiratory systems are frequently the reasons why First Responders are summoned. Quickly recognizing these problems as potentially life-threatening and making sure the proper medical help is on the way can save your patient's life. Also keep in mind that these emergencies require compassionate emotional care as well as management of the patient's physical condition.

REVIEW QUESTIONS

Page references where answers may be found or supported are provided at the end of each question.

Section 1

1. What are the risk factors for heart disease? (pp. 205–206)
2. What are the signs and symptoms of a cardiac emergency? (pp. 206–207)
3. What is the emergency care for a chest-pain emergency? (pp. 207, 209)

Section 2

4. What are four signs and symptoms of respiratory distress in a patient? (p. 212)
5. What is the emergency medical care for respiratory distress? (pp. 212–213)
6. What is hypoxic drive? Describe how it works. (p. 213)
7. What two conditions are considered the most common types of chronic obstructive pulmonary disease (COPD)? (p. 213)

CHAPTER 13

OTHER COMMON MEDICAL COMPLAINTS

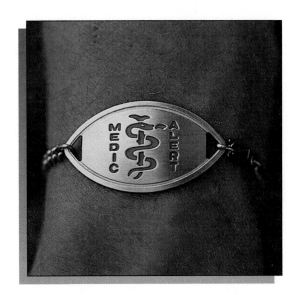

INTRODUCTION

A medical complaint is any chief complaint that is not caused by trauma. There will be many such calls in your career. They may involve abdominal pain, altered mental status, or even complaints such as "I don't feel well." As with any patient, your responsibility in the emergency care of a these patients is to follow your patient assessment plan from scene size-up to patient hand-off.

OBJECTIVES

Cognitive, affective, and psychomotor objectives are from the U.S. DOT's 1995 "First Responder: National Standard Curriculum." Enrichment objectives, if any, identify material that is supplemental to the DOT curriculum.

Cognitive

5-1.1 Identify the patient who presents with a general medical complaint. (pp. 221–222)
5-1.2 Explain the steps in providing emergency medical care to a patient with a general medical complaint. (pp. 221–222)
5-1.3 Identify the patient who presents with a specific medical complaint of altered mental status. (p. 222)
5-1.4 Explain the steps in providing emergency medical care to a patient with an altered mental status. (p. 222)
5-1.5 Identify the patient who presents with a specific medical complaint of seizures. (pp. 233–235)
5-1.6 Explain the steps in providing emergency medical care to a patient with seizures. (pp. 233–235)

Affective

5-1.15 Attend to the feelings of the patient and/or family when dealing with the patient with a general medical complaint. (p. 222)
5-1.16 Attend to the feelings of the patient and/or family when dealing with the patient with a specific medical complaint. (pp. 222, 233, 235)
5-1.18 Demonstrate a caring attitude towards patients with a general medical complaint who request emergency medical services. (p. 222)
5-1.19 Place the interests of the patient with a general medical complaint as the foremost consideration when making any and all patient care decisions. (pp. 219, 221–222)
5-1.20 Communicate with empathy to patients with a general medical complaint, as well as with family members and friends of the patient. (p. 222)
5-1.21 Demonstrate a caring attitude towards patients with a specific medical complaint who request emergency medical services. (pp. 222, 233, 235)
5-1.22 Place the interests of the patient with a specific medical complaint as the foremost consideration when making any and all patient care decisions. (p. 235)

5-1.23 Communicate with empathy to patients with a specific medical complaint, as well as with family members and friends of the patient. (pp. 222, 233)

Psychomotor

5-1.27 Demonstrate the steps in providing emergency medical care to a patient with a general medical complaint. (pp. 221–222)
5-1.28 Demonstrate the steps in providing emergency medical care to a patient with an altered mental status. (p. 222)
5-1.29 Demonstrate the steps in providing emergency medical care to a patient with seizures. (pp. 233–235)

Enrichment

* Establish the relationship between airway management and the patient with altered mental status. (p. 222)
* Describe the relationship between decreased oxygen levels (hypoxia) in the patient with an altered mental status and supplemental oxygen administration. (p. 222)
* Describe the assessment and emergency medical care of the patient with a diabetic emergency. (pp. 223–226)
* List various ways that poisons enter the body. (pp. 227–230)
* List signs and symptoms of poisoning. (pp. 227–230)
* Describe the assessment and emergency medical care of a patient with suspected poisoning. (pp. 227–230)
* Recognize the need for medical direction in caring for the patient with poisoning. (pp. 228, 230)
* Describe the assessment and emergency care of the patient with an altered mental status and a loss of speech, sensory, or motor function. (pp. 230–233)
* Recognize the common signs and symptoms of a generalized seizure. (p. 233)
* Explain the assessment and emergency care of a seizing patient. (pp. 233–235)
* Identify the signs and symptoms of abdominal pain or distress. (pp. 235–236)
* Describe the emergency medical care of a patient with abdominal pain or distress. (pp. 235–236)

CASE STUDY

DISPATCH

My partner and I were making rounds on the trails when a group of hikers stopped us. It seems that an older gentleman was suppose to have packed out that day. Several hikers remarked that he had looked sick. They asked us to check on him. We did.

SCENE SIZE-UP

As we approached the man's lean-to, we saw a supine body. We quickly did a scene size-up. There were no mechanisms of injury or obvious dangers, so we put on our gloves and approached the patient.

INITIAL ASSESSMENT

Our general impression was of an elderly male with a medical emergency. He was responsive to verbal stimuli, but his speech was slurred. His airway was patent. His breathing was adequate. Oxygen may have improved his altered mental status, but we don't carry it on the trail. The patient's radial pulse was slow, strong, and regular. There was no evidence of external bleeding, but he was very pale.

We were worried. We radioed our office to request immediate air medical evacuation.

> Consider this scenario as you read Chapter 13. What else may be done to assess and care for this patient?

SECTION 1: GENERAL MEDICAL COMPLAINTS

As a First Responder, you will be called to the scenes of patients with specific medical complaints, such as "my chest hurts" or "I can't breathe." Every once in a while, however, your medical patient will have a general complaint such as "I feel weak" or "I don't feel well."

Handle patients with a general medical complaint the same as you would any other. After your scene size-up, complete an initial assessment and treat any life-threatening conditions you observe. Perform a physical exam as needed, and be especially thorough gathering the patient's history. It could provide important clues to the underlying problem.

If you are unable to determine a more specific complaint or unable to obtain a pertinent history, do the following:

1. Monitor the airway and breathing. Be sure there is a patent airway with adequate breathing and circulation.
2. If the patient is responsive and there are no suspected spine injuries, allow the patient to get in a position of comfort.

3. Perform an ongoing assessment until the incoming EMTs take over patient care. Be sure to report any changes in the patient's condition.

These patients may be just as frightened and worried as patients with more specific problems. Consider their feelings as you assess and care for them. Be gentle and empathetic. If the family is present, they may be very concerned and ask you to tell them "what's wrong." Be truthful and kind. For example, you might tell them that though you do not know exactly what the problem is, you are doing all that is possible. Also reassure them that you have arranged for the patient to be transported to a hospital.

SECTION 2: SPECIFIC MEDICAL COMPLAINTS

ALTERED MENTAL STATUS

A change in a patient's normal level of responsiveness and understanding is called an **altered mental status.** It can occur quickly or slowly. It can range from disoriented to combative to unresponsive. There are many medical reasons for it. A few examples are:

- Hypoxia (decreased levels of oxygen in the blood).
- Hypoglycemia (low blood sugar).
- Stroke (loss of blood flow to part of the brain).
- Seizures.
- Fever, infections.
- Poisoning, including drug and alcohol poisoning.
- Head injury.
- Psychiatric conditions.

As a First Responder, you do not need to figure out why your patient has an altered mental status. Your job is to recognize it as soon as possible and to support the patient appropriately. So after assuring scene safety, proceed with patient

assessment. Gather an accurate patient history. Do so as soon as appropriate. A patient with altered mental status may deteriorate rapidly. If you wait too long, the history could be lost to the EMTs and hospital staff who take over care. A history of diabetes or seizures, for example, may be important to the EMTs and hospital personnel when they try to determine the cause of the altered mental status.

Emergency care of a patient with altered mental status is as follows:

1. *Assess and monitor the patient's airway and breathing closely.* These patients may not be able to protect their own airways. It is up to you to be aware of this danger. If the patient is unresponsive, secure the airway with an adjunct. Suction as needed.
2. *Position the patient.* If there is no reason to suspect head or spine injury, place the patient in a recovery position. Continue to monitor the patient's breathing closely.
3. *Administer high-flow oxygen.* One of the most common causes of altered mental status is hypoxia. So if the patient is breathing adequately, apply high-flow oxygen via nonrebreather mask. If the patient is not breathing adequately, assist with a bag-valve-mask device attached to an oxygen source. If you cannot provide oxygen, be prepared to assist ventilations.

Note that a patient with an altered mental status may be aware of his or her condition. This can be very frightening. If the patient has had a seizure, he or she could lose control of the bowels and bladder, which adds to embarrassment and anxiety. A caring attitude on your part, as well as helping the patient maintain some privacy, will help.

The patient's condition may be very upsetting to the family, too. Take time, if possible, to make sure they understand that you are caring for the patient and that an ambulance is on the way.

For your information, the following material will be presented in Section 2 of this chapter—hyperglycemia and hypoglycemia, poisoning, stroke, and seizures.

HYPERGLYCEMIA AND HYPOGLYCEMIA

The human body needs both oxygen and sugar to produce the energy that sustains it. When blood sugar is too low or too high, the body reacts. The most common reaction is altered mental status.

Hyperglycemia

Patients who have diabetes usually have increased blood sugar, or hyperglycemia. This condition is basically one of too little insulin and too much blood sugar. Common causes of hyperglycemia include:

- Infection, such as a respiratory infection.
- Failure of the patient to take insulin or to take a sufficient amount.

- Eating too much food that contains or produces sugar.
- Increased or prolonged stress.

Although a hyperglycemia emergency is sometimes called "diabetic coma," the patient is not usually found in a coma. Signs and symptoms may include (Figure 13–1):

- Sweet, fruity, or acetone-like breath.
- Flushed, dry, warm skin.
- Hunger and thirst.
- Rapid, weak pulse.
- Altered mental status.
- Intoxicated appearance, staggering, slurred speech.
- Frequent urination.
- Reports that the patient has not taken the prescribed diabetes medications.

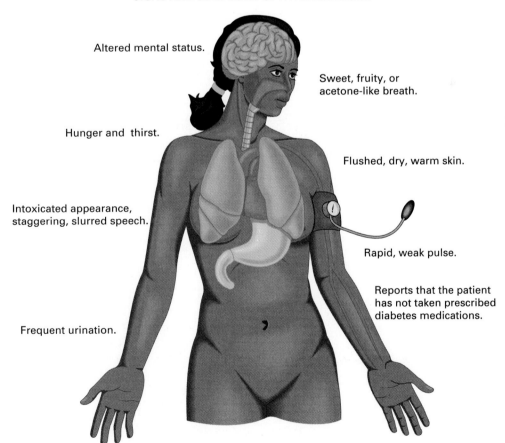

SIGNS AND SYMPTOMS OF HYPERGLYCEMIA

Altered mental status.

Sweet, fruity, or acetone-like breath.

Hunger and thirst.

Flushed, dry, warm skin.

Intoxicated appearance, staggering, slurred speech.

Rapid, weak pulse.

Reports that the patient has not taken prescribed diabetes medications.

Frequent urination.

Figure 13-1 Signs and symptoms of hyperglycemia.

The onset of severe hyperglycemia is gradual. In most cases it develops over a period of 12 to 48 hours. At first, the patient experiences excessive hunger, thirst, and urination. The patient appears extremely ill and becomes sicker and weaker as the condition progresses. If left untreated, the patient may die. With treatment, improvement is gradual, occurring 6 to 12 hours after insulin and intravenous fluid are administered.

Hypoglycemia

Low blood sugar, or hypoglycemia, is the result of two conditions. One is too much **insulin,** a drug used by people with diabetes. The other is too little sugar, such as occurs when a patient with diabetes does not eat properly. (See Figure 13–2.)

People with diabetes are not the only ones who can suffer from low blood sugar. So can alcoholics, people who have ingested certain poisons, and people who are ill. Some common causes of low blood sugar are:

- Skipped meals, particularly for a patient with diabetes.
- Vomiting, especially with illness.
- Strenuous exercise.
- Physical stress from extreme heat or cold.
- Emotional stress, such as at weddings or funerals.
- Accidental overdose of insulin.

The most recognized cause of hypoglycemia is the accidental overdose of insulin by a patient with diabetes. After a time, diabetes can inflict a degree of blindness in patients. This can make it

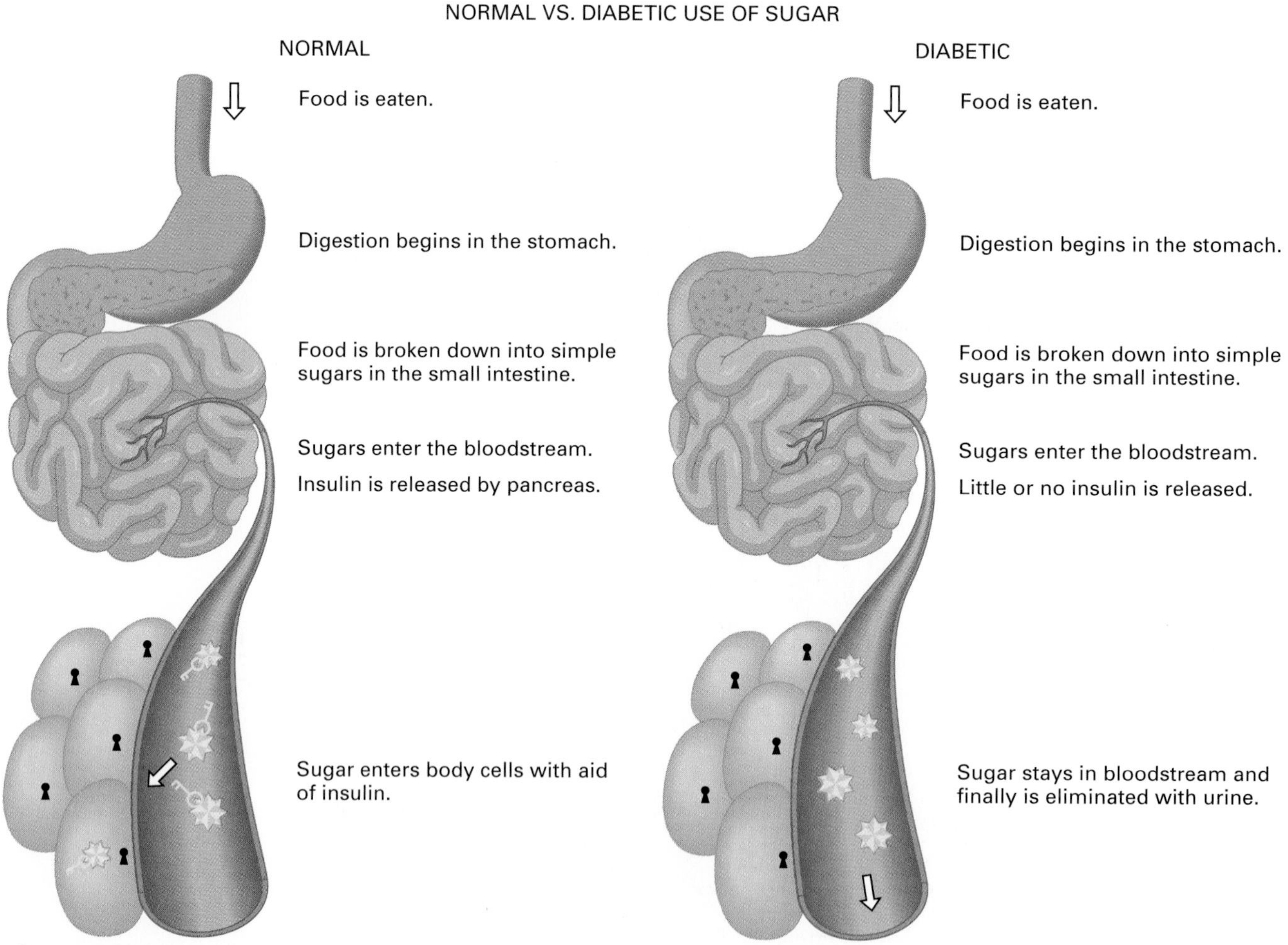

NORMAL VS. DIABETIC USE OF SUGAR

NORMAL

DIABETIC

Food is eaten.

Food is eaten.

Digestion begins in the stomach.

Digestion begins in the stomach.

Food is broken down into simple sugars in the small intestine.

Food is broken down into simple sugars in the small intestine.

Sugars enter the bloodstream.
Insulin is released by pancreas.

Sugars enter the bloodstream.
Little or no insulin is released.

Sugar enters body cells with aid of insulin.

Sugar stays in bloodstream and finally is eliminated with urine.

Figure 13-2 Diabetes has long been recognized as a serious disorder.

very hard for them to give themselves the proper amount of insulin. The result is an insulin overdose and hypoglycemia.

Signs and symptoms of hypoglycemia may include any of the following (Figure 13–3):

- Rapid onset of altered mental status.
- Intoxicated appearance, staggering, slurred speech.
- Rapid pulse rate.
- Cool, clammy skin.
- Hunger.
- Headache.
- Seizures.

Patient Assessment

When you gather the SAMPLE history, try to find out about the onset of the emergency. Be sure to ask, "Do you have diabetes?" If he or she says yes, ask: "Have you eaten today? Did you take your insulin?" Also ask about any current illness, stress, and problems with medications.

Look for a medical identification tag during the physical exam. If the police are present, ask them to check the patient's wallet, too. If the patient is at home, check the refrigerator for insulin. Also check around the house for needles and syringes. Special needle containers are often present in the house.

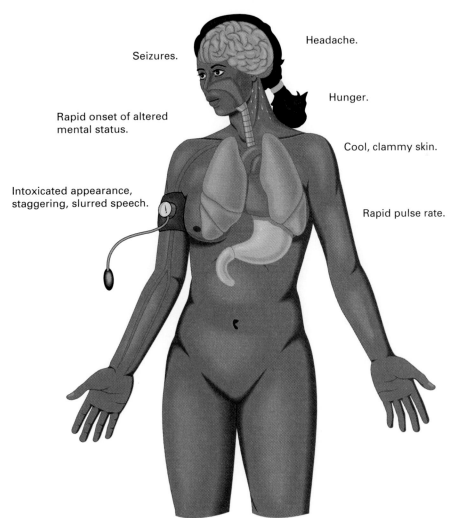

Figure 13-3 Signs and symptoms of hypoglycemia.

Emergency Care

Proceed with emergency care as you would for any patient with altered mental status. However, if you suspect hypoglycemia or hyperglycemia, alert the incoming EMS crew immediately. While waiting for them, monitor the airway closely. Note that this patient may suddenly have a seizure. Be prepared. (See "Seizures" later in this chapter.)

Remember, patients with diabetes can suffer from either hypoglycemia or hyperglycemia (Figure 13–4). *When in doubt, give sugar.* You will not harm a hyperglycemic patient with sugar, and you may save the life of a patient with hypoglycemia by this emergency treatment.

Your EMS system may permit you to help a patient take some sugar. To do so, the patient must be awake and able to control his or her own airway. Follow local protocols. The patient may benefit from one of the following:

- Dissolve some sugar in a glass of water.
- Pour a drink that is naturally rich in sugar such as orange juice.
- Squeeze a commercially prepared glucose paste onto a tongue depressor (Figure 13–5). Note that a tube of glucose should only be used for a single patient and then discarded.

Never give patients who cannot control their own airways anything to eat or drink. They could aspirate the substance into their lungs. This can have grave results, including death. If you are in doubt, call for medical direction. If sugar or glucose is administered, be sure to tell the EMTs who take over care. Also report any changes in mental status that occurred while the patient was in your care.

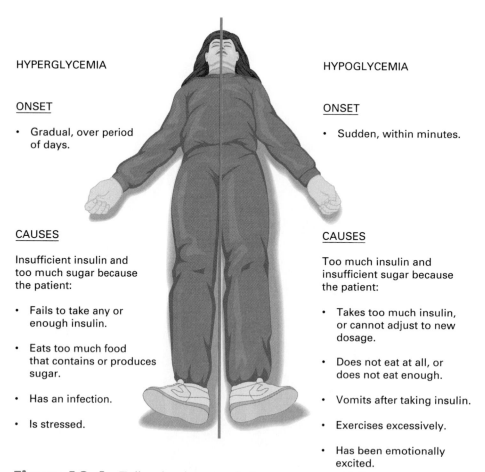

HYPERGLYCEMIA

ONSET

- Gradual, over period of days.

CAUSES

Insufficient insulin and too much sugar because the patient:

- Fails to take any or enough insulin.

- Eats too much food that contains or produces sugar.

- Has an infection.

- Is stressed.

HYPOGLYCEMIA

ONSET

- Sudden, within minutes.

CAUSES

Too much insulin and insufficient sugar because the patient:

- Takes too much insulin, or cannot adjust to new dosage.

- Does not eat at all, or does not eat enough.

- Vomits after taking insulin.

- Exercises excessively.

- Has been emotionally excited.

Figure 13-4 Follow local protocols for treatment guidelines.

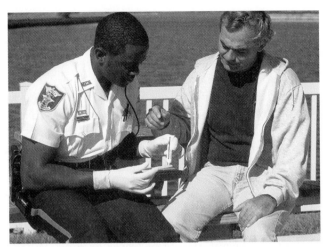

Figure 13-5 Your EMS system may allow you to help a patient self-administer oral glucose.

POISONING

A poison is a substance that can impair health if left untreated. Poisoning can occur in a variety of settings. However, many occur in the relative safety of the home (Figure 13–6).

Poisons may be inhaled, ingested, injected, or absorbed. So whenever you suspect a poisoning, try to answer these questions: What substance is involved? How much is involved? When did the poisoning occur? What has the patient done to relieve symptoms?

Ingested Poisons

An ingested poison is one that is introduced into the digestive tract by way of the mouth. Every year in the U.S. there are over eight million reported ingested poisonings. Drugs such as aspirin and alcohol are among the top offenders.

Patient Assessment. Be alert for clues when you size up the scene and after. A clue to a poisoning may be an overturned or empty pill box, scattered pills, chemical containers, household cleaners, empty alcohol bottles, or overturned plants.

Keep in mind as you do your initial assessment that patients who are poisoned often vomit. So be alert to airway obstruction and breathing difficulty. They can lead to hypoxia and death.

In addition to altered mental status, signs and symptoms may include:

- History of ingesting poisons.
- Burns around the mouth.
- Odd breath odors.
- Nausea, vomiting.
- Abdominal pain.
- Diarrhea.

Notice that the symptoms follow a path of ingestion. Start at the mouth. Look for chemical burns around the mouth or a chemical odor on the breath (Figure 13–7). Then notice if there is

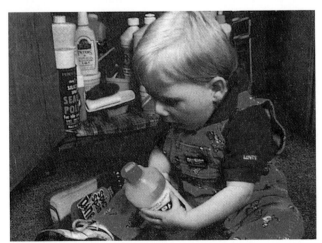

Figure 13-6 Poisoning is a leading cause of accidental death among children.

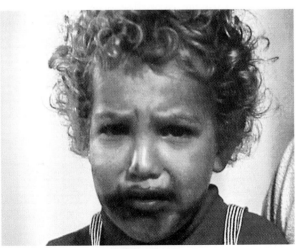

Figure 13-7 Burns or stains around the mouth may indicate poisoning.

or has been any nausea and vomiting. Finally, the patient may complain of abdominal cramps and diarrhea.

Often poisons will affect the central nervous system. You may see dilated or constricted pupils, or you may hear the patient complain of double vision. There may be excessive saliva or foaming at the mouth. There may be excessive tearing or sweating. Finally, the patient may become unresponsive or have seizures.

Emergency Care. Your top priority is the patient's airway. With that in mind, proceed as you would for any patient with altered mental status. To help limit the damage a poison can cause, make sure the EMS system is activated. If there will be a delay, call the poison control center in your area or medical oversight for instructions. Follow local protocols.

You may be instructed to give the patient **activated charcoal** (Figure 13–8). This is a finely ground charcoal that is very absorbent. It binds with the poisons in the stomach and then passes through the body harmlessly. It may be effective in reducing poisons for up to four hours after ingestion. Use it only by order of poison control or according to your local protocols.

Most activated charcoal is premixed with water. If it is dry, then you must mix two tablespoons of it in a glass of water to make a slurry. Be careful. It stains most clothing easily.

You may be ordered to induce vomiting in the patient. This is usually done with **syrup of ipecac.** Ipecac can have side effects. Use it only on the direct order of either poison control or medical oversight. In the field, it is never given with activated charcoal unless under direct medical orders. Follow all local protocols.

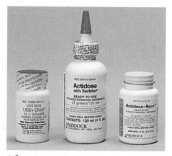

Figure 13-8 Activated charcoal.

Remember that you should never induce vomiting if the patient:

- Is unresponsive.
- Cannot maintain an airway.
- Has ingested an acid, a corrosive such as lye, or a petroleum product such as gasoline or furniture polish.
- Has a medical condition that could be complicated by vomiting, such as heart attack, seizures, and pregnancy.

If the patient swallows an acid, corrosive, or petroleum product, you may have to dilute it. Use either several glasses of water or milk. Whatever the situation, always follow local protocols. If that means calling poison control, do so and follow their instructions exactly.

Inhaled Poisons

A common source of poisonous gas is fire. The product of incomplete combustion, poison gas may contain carbon monoxide, the most common poison. It also may contain cyanide, a by-product of burning certain plastics.

Fire is not the only source of poison gas. Large amounts of carbon dioxide can come from sewage treatment plants or industrial sites. Even the chlorine gas in swimming pools can be lethal.

Patient Assessment. Remember, many poison gases are colorless, odorless, and tasteless. You may not know you are in danger until it is too late. Look out for hazardous materials. Pay constant attention to the nature of the incident and the dangers it might contain. Protect yourself! And keep others away from the scene.

It is imperative for you to give special attention to this patient's airway. Once in a safe location, open the airway. Then inspect the mouth and nose. Be careful to note the presence of soot, burns, or singed hair. Other signs and symptoms include:

- History of inhaling poisons.
- Breathing difficulty.
- Chest pain.
- Cough, hoarseness, burning sensation in the throat.
- Cyanosis (bluish discoloration of skin and mucous membranes).

- Dizziness, headache.
- Seizures, unresponsiveness (advanced stages).

Carbon monoxide is a poison gas that is especially lethal. Kerosene heaters, hot water heaters, and car exhaust fumes are some of the most common sources. Be particularly alert to carbon monoxide poisoning if several members of a household have the same signs and symptoms. Also suspect it if they say they are only sick when they are in a certain location. Be alert if the family pet seems sick as well.

Signs and symptoms of carbon monoxide poisoning include:

- Throbbing headache and agitation.
- Nausea, vomiting.
- Confusion, poor judgment.
- Diminished vision, blindness.
- Breathing difficulty with rapid pulse.
- Dizziness, fainting, unresponsiveness.
- Seizures.
- Paleness.
- Cherry red color to skin (very late sign).

Emergency Care.   The first rule of EMS is safety. You must protect yourself. Do not enter the scene of a poisonous gas. Call dispatch for specialized rescue teams who will have the appropriate safety equipment, including a self-contained breathing apparatus.

When it is safe to do so, quickly remove the patient from the source of the poison. Then proceed as you would for any patient with altered mental status. Verify that an ambulance is en route. Consider helicopter evacuation, if it would be quicker.

Note that all patients who are exposed to carbon monoxide need medical care, even those who seem to recover.

Absorbed Poisons

An absorbed poison is one that enters the body upon contact with the skin. Examples of natural sources include poison ivy, sumac, and oak (Figure 13–9). Other sources are corrosives, insecticides, herbicides, and cleaning products.

Patient Assessment.   An absorbed poison usually causes harm only to the point of contact. In general, signs and symptoms include:

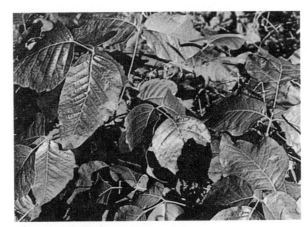

Figure 13-9a   Poison ivy.

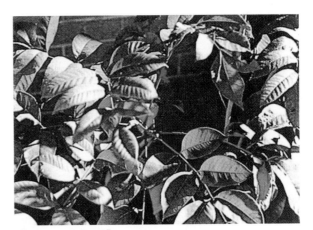

Figure 13-9b   Poison sumac.

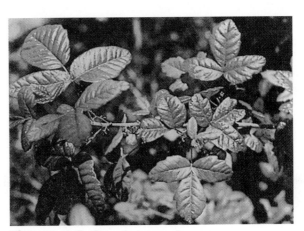

Figure 13-9c   Poison oak.

- History of exposures.
- Liquid or powder on the skin.
- Burns.
- Itching, irritation.
- Redness, rash, blisters (Figure 13–10).

Once a poison is identified, advise the incoming EMS units. If hazardous materials are suspected, follow local protocols. Note that an oil-based poison can spread easily from person to person. So protect yourself. Gloves are essential. Also consider a gown, mask, and eye protection.

Emergency Care. For emergency care of a patient who has been poisoned, contact poison control or medical direction. General guidelines for emergency care are as follows:

1. Remove the clothing that came in contact with the poison.
2. Then with a dry cloth blot the poison from the skin. If the poison is a dry powder, brush it off.
3. Flood the area with copious amounts of water. A shower or garden hose are ideal for this purpose. Continue until other EMS units arrive. Note that you may need to use alcohol or vegetable oil with some poisons. Follow instructions from poison control or medical direction.
4. Continually monitor the patient's vital signs. Be alert for sudden changes. Seizures and shock are not uncommon.

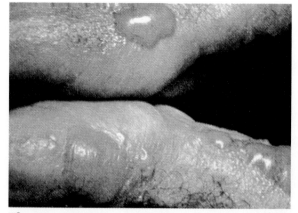

Figure 13-10 Blisters from poisonous plant contact.

The eyes are especially vulnerable to absorbed poisons. If ordered, flood the eyes with copious amounts of water. If only one eye is affected, be sure to avoid running contaminated water into the other eye. Advise incoming EMS units of the patient's condition. Follow local protocol.

Injected Poisons

An injected poison is one that enters the body by way of an object that pierces the skin. For example, an illegal drug may enter the body by way of a hypodermic needle. An overdose may be the result. For more information on overdose emergencies, please see Chapter 16.

Other causes of injected poisons include the bites and stings of insects, spiders, snakes, and marine animals. The venom of these creatures can cause serious allergic reactions, even death. For more information on this type of emergency, see Chapters 15 and 17.

STROKE

A patient may suffer a cerebral vascular accident (CVA) or stroke when an area of the brain is deprived of blood. This can occur when a blood clot (thrombus) blocks an artery, when matter (embolus) lodges in an artery, or when an artery bursts (aneurysm). (See Figures 13–11 and 13–12.)

The National Stroke Association refers to a stroke as a "brain attack." Strokes are the third leading cause of death in the U.S. and the leading cause of adult disability. They are more common in people over the age of 65 but can affect anyone.

Patients who are at risk for heart attack also may be in danger of having a stroke. They include patients with high blood pressure or diabetes, and patients who smoke tobacco.

Patient Assessment

The signs and symptoms of stroke are the result of several factors. Among them are the location and amount of brain damage. Signs and symptoms may be mild or life-threatening. Sometimes they are temporary. Temporary signs and symptoms indicate a "mini-stroke." Called transient

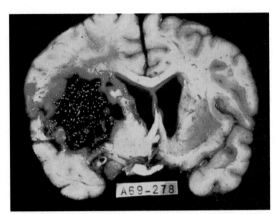

Figure 13-11a A cerebrovascular accident (CVA) or stroke from cerebral hemorrhage.

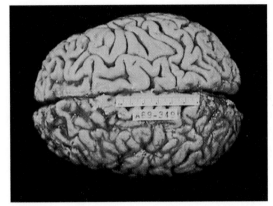

Figure 13-11b Brain damaged by stroke.

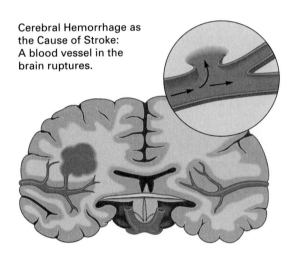

Cerebral Hemorrhage as the Cause of Stroke: A blood vessel in the brain ruptures.

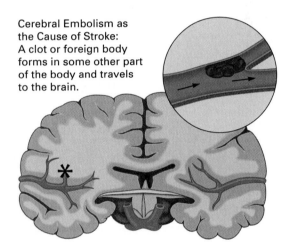

Cerebral Embolism as the Cause of Stroke: A clot or foreign body forms in some other part of the body and travels to the brain.

STROKE

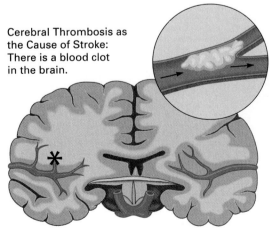

Cerebral Thrombosis as the Cause of Stroke: There is a blood clot in the brain.

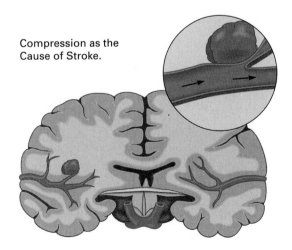

Compression as the Cause of Stroke.

Figure 13-12 Causes of stroke.

ischemic attacks (TIAs), these mini-strokes are warning signs of an impending larger stroke.

Signs and symptoms of stroke include (Figure 13–13):

- *Inability to communicate.* The patient may either fail to speak or fail to understand what is spoken.
- *Impairment in one part of the body.* For example, loss of muscle control on one side of the face or loss of movement on one entire side of the body.
- *Altered mental status.* This can range from a change in personality to seizures and unresponsiveness.

About 50% of stroke patients have an elevated blood pressure during a stroke. However, the combination of an elevated blood pressure, slow pulse, and rapid or irregular breathing is a sign of a major stroke. Be prepared if the patient should convulse suddenly.

Emergency Care

Proceed as you would for any patient with altered mental status. However, note that as pressure increases in the skull from swelling tissues and bleeding, the patient's breathing will be affected. Be especially alert to the airway of a patient who has difficulty speaking or slurred speech. Never give a suspected stroke patient anything to eat or drink. Be prepared to provide artificial ventilation.

If you suspect stroke in your patient, take a pulse at the carotid and radial pulse points on both sides of the body. Note if there is any difference between pulses. Following your initial assessment, try to gather a history from the patient,

GENERAL SIGNS AND SYMPTOMS OF STROKE

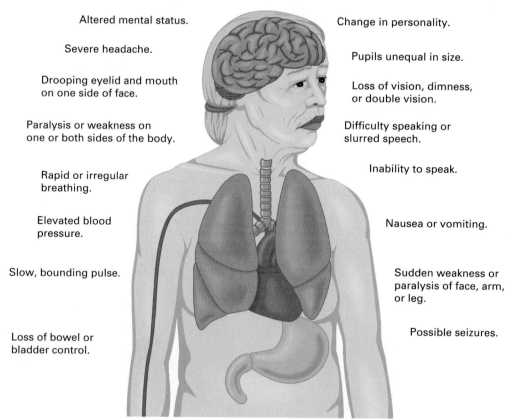

Altered mental status.

Severe headache.

Drooping eyelid and mouth on one side of face.

Paralysis or weakness on one or both sides of the body.

Rapid or irregular breathing.

Elevated blood pressure.

Slow, bounding pulse.

Loss of bowel or bladder control.

Change in personality.

Pupils unequal in size.

Loss of vision, dimness, or double vision.

Difficulty speaking or slurred speech.

Inability to speak.

Nausea or vomiting.

Sudden weakness or paralysis of face, arm, or leg.

Possible seizures.

Figure 13-13 One or more signs or symptoms may indicate a stroke.

family, and bystanders. Be sure to find out if there is a past medical history of stroke, high blood pressure, diabetes, or heart disease.

The loss of a mental or motor function is a frightening reality for stroke patients. Try to remain calm and never express surprise about abnormal physical findings. Instead, maintain a professional attitude. Reassure the patient. Do not make any statements about long-term disability.

Continue to talk to the patient even if he or she cannot speak. These patients often can hear very well. Explain to them what it is you are doing. Do not talk down to them or treat them like children.

Handle a patient's paralyzed limbs carefully. There may be no feeling in the limbs, so you could injure them without being aware of it. The patient also may unintentionally cause them to strike an object.

SEIZURES

There are many causes of seizures. Sometimes the cause is unknown. All of the conditions described in this chapter can lead to them. Common causes include:

- Chronic medical conditions.
- Epilepsy.
- Hypoglycemia.
- Poisoning, including alcohol and drug poisoning.
- Stroke.
- Fever (most common in children).
- Infection.
- Head injury or brain tumors.
- Hypoxia (decreased levels of oxygen in the blood).
- Complications of pregnancy.

A seizure is the result of a nervous system malfunction. It may last five minutes or it may be prolonged. Its symptoms can range from a twitch of a limb to whole body muscle contractions. Most patients become unresponsive. Many vomit during the attack. Typically, patients are tired and sleep afterwards. Seizures are rarely life-threatening, but they do indicate a very serious condition.

Patient Assessment

You will probably be called most often to a *grand mal*, or generalized seizure. There are four phases to this type of seizure. They are called in order (Figure 13–14):

- Aura phase.
- Tonic phase.
- Clonic phase.
- Postictal phase.

In the aura phase, the patient becomes aware that a seizure is coming on. The aura is often described as an unusual smell or a flash of light. It lasts a split second.

In the tonic phase, the patient becomes unresponsive and collapses to the ground. Then all of the muscles of the body contract. This often forces a scream out of the patient. It also can force out sputum, which can look like foam. During this phase the patient may stop breathing.

In the clonic phase, the patient's muscles alternate between contraction and relaxation. The patient may become **incontinent** of urine (unable to retain it). Because the patient may bite the tongue and cheek, there may be blood in the mouth.

In the postictal phase, the patient gradually regains responsiveness. At first the patient is confused and even combative. Gradually the patient becomes aware of his or her surroundings.

Note that a continuous seizure, or two or more seizures without a period of responsiveness, is called *status epilepticus*. This is a true medical emergency, which can be fatal. Complications include aspiration, hypoxia, hyperthermia (fever), and heart problems. If you suspect this type of seizure, advise responding EMS units. Transportation must not be delayed.

Emergency Care

During your scene size-up, ask yourself if the patient was injured when he or she fell to the ground. Pay careful attention to the potential for spine or head injury. When you arrive on scene, if the patient is still seizing, then:

1. Stay calm. Just wait. The seizure will be over in a few minutes.

STAGES OF A GENERALIZED SEIZURE

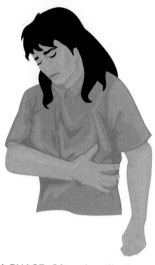

1. AURA PHASE. Often described as unusual smell or flash of light that lasts a split second.

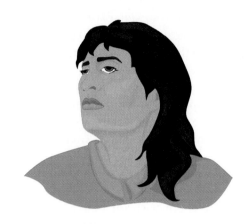

2. TONIC PHASE. 15 to 20 seconds of unresponsiveness followed by 5 to 15 seconds of extreme muscle rigidity.

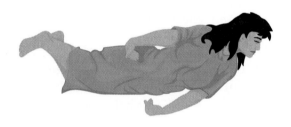

3. CLONIC PHASE. 1 to 5 minutes of seizures.

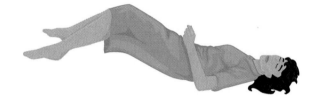

4. POSTICTAL PHASE. 5 to 30 minutes to several hours of deep sleep with gradual recovery.

Figure 13-14   Stages of a generalized seizure.

2. Prevent any further injury by moving objects away from the patient (Figure 13–15). If they cannot be moved, then put something between them and the patient. If needed, drag the patient a few feet away from the danger.

3. Place padding, such as a coat or blanket, under the patient's head. Remove the patient's eyeglasses. Do not force anything into the patient's mouth. Do not try to restrain the patient.

4. If you suspect status epilepticus, do your best to prevent aspiration. Position the patient on his or her side or suction if possible. Assist ventilations with a bag-valve-mask attached to 100% oxygen. Notify the incoming EMS unit immediately.

Most often you will arrive on scene when a seizure has passed or when the patient is in the last phase of seizing. When the seizure stops,

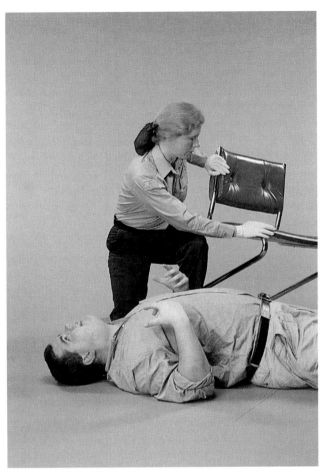

Figure 13-15 Move objects away from the seizure patient.

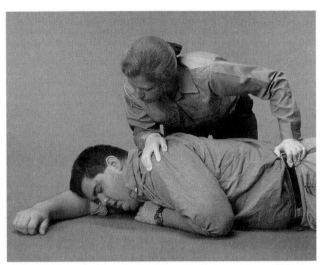

Figure 13-16 When the seizure stops, position the patient to allow drainage of saliva and vomit.

assess and monitor the patient's airway and breathing closely. If there is no reason to suspect head or spine injury, place the patient in the recovery position (Figure 13–16). If you are allowed, administer high-flow oxygen. If you suspect the patient was injured during a fall, use a jaw-thrust to open the airway. As the patient recovers, offer comfort and reassurance. Remember that they will have muscle soreness as well as fatigue.

While you wait for the EMTs to arrive on scene, consider the patient's feelings. Often he or she is embarrassed. Consider asking onlookers to move away to provide the patient with some privacy. Place a sheet or towel over the patient's body, if there was incontinence.

When you give your hand-off report to the EMTs, be sure to include a description of the seizure. It may be important in determining its cause.

ABDOMINAL PAIN AND DISTRESS

The abdominal cavity contains many different organs and blood vessels. Complaints of pain or discomfort could actually be caused by a number of problems or conditions. Abdominal pain may be located directly over a problem organ, or it may be in a totally different part of the body. This is called "referred pain."

Abdominal problems may cause referred pain to the shoulders and chest. Sometimes pain begins in the anterior abdomen and radiates to the back. Abdominal emergencies require aggressive care to prevent shock and to save lives. All abdominal pain should be taken seriously. Do not spend time trying to determine its cause. Rather, complete a thorough patient assessment and history.

Patient Assessment

Any severe abdominal pain should be considered an emergency. Any abdominal pain that is persistent or is significant enough for the patient or family to call for assistance should be considered

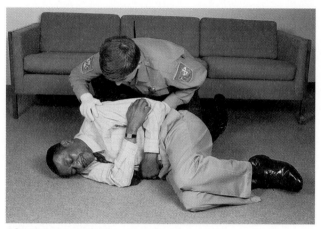

Figure 13-17   Guarding position.

an emergency. A patient with abdominal distress or pain appears to be very ill. Signs and symptoms include:

- Abdominal pain, local or diffuse.
- Colicky pain (cramps that occur in waves).
- Abdominal tenderness, local or diffuse.
- Anxiety, reluctance to move.
- Loss of appetite, nausea, vomiting.
- Fever.
- Rigid, tense, or distended abdomen.
- Signs of shock.
- Vomiting blood, bright red or like coffee grounds.
- Blood in the stool, bright red or tarry black.

A patient with acute abdominal distress often gets in a **guarding position** (Figure 13–17). In this position, the patient is on his or her side with knees drawn up toward the abdomen. This position reduces tension on the muscles of the abdomen, which in turn helps to reduce pain.

In assessing a patient with acute abdominal distress, the initial assessment is the first priority. Even after assuring the patient's ABCs, stay alert for signs of shock, which include a rapid thready pulse, restlessness, cold clammy skin, and falling blood pressure. Shock is common with internal bleeding and continued vomiting and diarrhea.

As with all medical patients, gather a good patient history. It may identify clues to the patient's condition, such as prior similar problems and factors that may have caused the pain.

During the physical exam, determine whether the patient is restless or quiet. Find out if movement causes pain. Check to see if the abdomen is distended, and ask the patient to confirm your observation. Note if the patient can relax the abdominal wall when asked to do so. Palpate the abdomen gently to determine if it is rigid or soft. If you know one area is causing pain, examine that area last.

Do not spend too much time on assessment before making sure the EMS system has been activated. Too much palpation can worsen the pain. It also can aggravate the medical condition that caused it.

Emergency Care

The goals of emergency care for acute abdominal distress are to prevent any possible life-threatening complications, to make the patient comfortable, and to arrange transport as quickly as possible. In addition:

1. *Maintain an open airway.* Be alert for vomiting and possible aspiration. If the patient is nauseated, position the patient on his or her left side if it does not cause too much pain.
2. *Administer oxygen* by way of a nonrebreather mask at 10 to 15 lpm, if you are trained and allowed to do so.
3. *Be alert for shock.* If vital signs and other observations point to it, position the patient on his or her back with legs elevated. If there are no signs of shock, then allow the patient to get into a position of comfort.

Protect the patient from any rough handling. Never give anything by mouth. Do not allow the patient to take any medications. Medications could mask symptoms and complicate the physician's diagnosis and treatment.

FIRST RESPONDER FOCUS

Medical complaints will be the most common type of emergency for most First Responders. The percentage of the population that is elderly is increasing dramatically. This means increased calls for medical problems in the future.

This chapter covered a wide range of medical problems—from stroke to diabetes to poisoning to generalized complaints. Remember that it is not ever necessary to diagnose a patient's medical problem. Sometimes diagnosis in the hospital is difficult, even with the tests and procedures available to physicians there. It is not practical for you to try to determine the cause of a patient's condition in the field.

There are many things you can do for your medical patients. You know you must treat any life-threatening problems in the initial assessment. A history is very important to a medical patient, too. It will provide the clues to the patient's condition, which will benefit you, the EMTs, and hospital personnel.

Finally, never jump to conclusions. In this chapter, for example, you learned that under certain conditions a patient who has diabetes may appear to be drunk. Consider all patients who are exhibiting an altered mental status or unusual behavior as having a medical problem. Never assume that the patient is drunk, drugged, or mentally ill. ■

CASE STUDY FOLLOW-UP

At the beginning of this chapter, you read that First Responders were on scene with a patient who was experiencing an altered mental status. To see how chapter skills apply to this emergency, read the following. It describes how the call was completed.

PATIENT HISTORY

As near as we could tell from the scene, the patient was probably eating breakfast when this all started. In response to questioning, he had no allergies and he was taking medication. We found high blood-pressure meds in his pack. He denied any other medical conditions. The patient also tried to describe the event. He indicated that his head hurt, then he passed out. When he woke, he found he could not move the right side of his body.

PHYSICAL EXAMINATION

We quickly performed a head-to-toe exam of the patient. He had definite weakness on the right side of his body. He had no deformities, no open injuries, no signs of tenderness or swelling. We realized quickly that we were very limited because the patient could not speak. We took a complete set of vital signs.

ONGOING ASSESSMENT

Our impression was that the patient had a stroke. Aware that he could get worse, we continued to perform the initial assessment as well as vital signs. Our patient appeared to be somewhat anxious. Who wouldn't be? So we tried to comfort and reassure him. We told him more help was on the way and that he would be in the hospital soon.

PATIENT HAND-OFF

When the Medflight team arrived, we gave them a quick hand-off report, including the physical findings and the history we were able to gather. The flight team took it from there. I have to say that this guy was lucky. If he had been left alone much longer, he might have died from exposure.

> Whether or not you know the cause of a medical emergency in your patient, your job is the same. Assess, care for, and monitor the airway until the EMTs arrive to take over. Be prepared to provide basic life support if needed. And try to get a complete patient history from the patient, the family, or bystanders.

REVIEW QUESTIONS

Page references where answers may be found or supported are provided at the end of each question.

Section 1

1. How would you treat a patient with a general medical complaint? (pp. 221–222)

Section 2

2. Why must you monitor the airway and breathing of all patients with altered mental status? (p. 222)
3. What are three common causes of an altered mental status in a patient? (p. 222)
4. What are three possible indicators of diabetes in a patient? (p. 225)
5. What are various ways a poison can enter the body? (pp. 227–230)

6. Why do inhaled poisons pose a risk for First Responders? (p. 228)
7. In addition to altered mental status, what are the signs and symptoms of an ingested poison? An inhaled poison? An absorbed poison? (pp. 227–230)
8. What are the characteristic signs of a stroke? (pp. 230, 232)
9. Why must you be careful with the limbs of a stroke patient? (pp. 232–233)
10. What can you do for a patient who is seizing? (pp. 233–235)
11. What can you do for a seizure patient when the seizure has stopped? (pp. 234–235)
12. What signs and symptoms are related to abdominal pain or distress? (pp. 235–236)
13. What are the goals of emergency care of a patient with acute abdominal distress? (p. 236)

CHAPTER 14

HEAT AND COLD EMERGENCIES

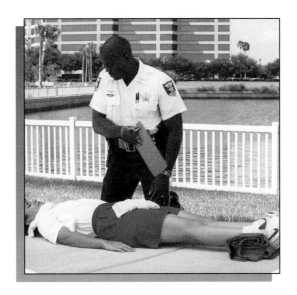

INTRODUCTION

A heat- or cold-related emergency can happen to anyone. Letter carriers, farmers, police officers, and countless others who work or play outdoors are at risk. People may be at risk indoors, too, especially the very young and the elderly. Some of these emergencies, such as frostbite, can be minor. Others, like heat stroke, can be life-threatening.

OBJECTIVES

Cognitive, affective, and psychomotor objectives are from the U.S. DOT's 1995 "First Responder: National Standard Curriculum." Enrichment objectives, if any, identify material that is supplemental to the DOT curriculum.

Cognitive

5-1.7 Identify the patient who presents with a specific medical complaint of exposure to cold. (pp. 243, 245–246)
5-1.8 Explain the steps in providing emergency medical care to a patient with an exposure to cold. (pp. 243, 245–246)
5-1.9 Identify the patient who presents with a specific medical compliant of exposure to heat. (pp. 248–249, 251)
5-1.10 Explain the steps in providing emergency medical care to a patient with an exposure to heat. (pp. 248–249, 251)

Affective

5-1.16 Attend to the feelings of the patient and/or family when dealing with the patient with a specific medical complaint. (pp. 243, 246)

5-1.21 Demonstrate a caring attitude towards patients with a specific medical complaint who request emergency medical services. (pp. 243, 246)
5-1.22 Place the interests of the patient with a specific medical compliant as the foremost consideration when making any and all patient care decisions. (pp. 243, 245)
5-1.23 Communicate with empathy to patients with a specific medical complaint, as well as with family members and friends of the patient. (p. 243)

Psychomotor

5-1.30 Demonstrate the steps in providing emergency medical care to a patient with an exposure to cold. (pp. 243, 245–246)
5-1.31 Demonstrate the steps in providing emergency medical care to a patient with an exposure to heat. (pp. 248–249)

Enrichment

* Describe the various ways that the body creates and loses heat. (pp. 240–241)
* Describe how to rewarm a patient with hypothermia and a patient with a local cold injury. (pp. 245–246)
* Describe how to cool a patient with hyperthermia. (pp. 249, 251)

SECTION 1: BODY TEMPERATURE

Heat and cold can produce a number of emergencies. To respond to them appropriately, you need a basic understanding of how people adjust to heat and cold.

The body produces and conserves heat mainly through the process of metabolism, including the digestion of food. In cold, the body holds onto its heat by constricting blood vessels near its surface. Hair also erects, thickening the layer of warm air trapped near the skin. The body can produce more heat, if needed, by shivering and by producing certain hormones such as epinephrine.

In general, the body loses heat in five ways (Figure 14–1):

* *Convection.* This occurs when moving air passes over the body and carries heat away. (See "wind chill index," Figure 14–2.)
* *Conduction.* This occurs when direct contact with an object carries heat away. For example, a swimmer is in direct contact with water. If it is cooler than the body, the water will take away the swimmer's body heat. It can do so 25 times faster than air.
* *Radiation.* This method involves the transfer of heat to an object without physical contact. Most loss is from the head and neck, areas rich in blood and blood vessels.

CASE STUDY

DISPATCH

It was 9 a.m. and we were on our way to 153 Western Avenue for a woman down. Rescue 3 was dispatched to assist with an ETA of 15 minutes.

SCENE SIZE-UP

The person who called EMS was there to greet us. "Mrs. Downe and I have tea every morning at 7 a.m.," she told us. "I just know something is wrong." We approached the neat little cottage. I knocked and then yelled through the door, "EMS. Can we help you?" We heard a faint voice from the back of the house.

We entered through the back door, and immediately saw the patient. She appeared to be about 80. She was lying supine on the kitchen floor, calling out weakly. The contents of a garbage bag were lying spilled on the floor. We could see dried blood in her hair and under her head.

INITIAL ASSESSMENT

My partner positioned himself and manually stabilized her head. I got down on my knees, introduced myself, and asked her what was wrong. She told us that last night at about 9 p.m. she tripped over her cat and fell. She was sore all over, but her hip hurt most. I was glad to note that she was awake and alert. Her airway was open, breathing was good, and all bleeding appeared to have stopped.

It appeared at first that Mrs. Downe was a trauma patient, the fall being her mechanism of injury. However, we found that her skin was ice cold and she was shivering. We reported to dispatch, and then continued the assessment.

> Consider this patient as you read Chapter 14. Might she have any problems other than an injured hip?

- *Evaporation.* The process by which sweat changes to vapor has a cooling effect on the body. Note that it stops when the relative humidity of the air reaches 75%.
- *Respiration.* This occurs when a person breathes in cold air and breathes out air that was warmed inside the body.

SECTION 2: COLD EMERGENCIES

Exposure to cold can cause two kinds of emergencies. One is a generalized cold emergency, or generalized **hypothermia.** It involves an overall

MECHANISMS OF HEAT LOSS

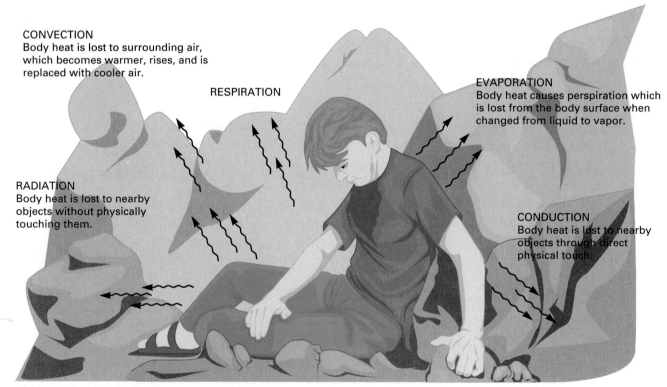

CONVECTION
Body heat is lost to surrounding air, which becomes warmer, rises, and is replaced with cooler air.

RESPIRATION

EVAPORATION
Body heat causes perspiration which is lost from the body surface when changed from liquid to vapor.

RADIATION
Body heat is lost to nearby objects without physically touching them.

CONDUCTION
Body heat is lost to nearby objects through direct physical touch.

Figure 14-1 Mechanisms of heat loss.

WIND CHILL INDEX

WIND SPEED (MPH)	WHAT THE THERMOMETER READS (degrees °F.)											
	50	40	30	20	10	0	–10	–20	–30	–40	–50	–60
	WHAT IT EQUALS IN ITS EFFECT ON EXPOSED FLESH											
CALM	50	40	30	20	10	0	–10	–20	–30	–40	–50	–60
5	48	37	27	16	6	–5	–15	–26	–36	–47	–57	–68
10	40	28	16	4	–9	–21	–33	–46	–58	–70	–83	–95
15	36	22	9	–5	–18	–36	–45	–58	–72	–85	–99	–112
20	32	18	4	–10	–25	–39	–53	–67	–82	–96	–110	–121
25	30	16	0	–15	–29	–44	–59	–74	–88	–104	–118	–133
30	28	13	–2	–18	–33	–48	–63	–79	–94	–109	–125	–140
35	27	11	–4	–20	–35	–49	–67	–82	–98	–113	–129	–145
40	26	10	–6	–21	–37	–53	–69	–85	–100	–116	–132	–148
	Little danger if properly clothed			Danger of freezing exposed flesh			Great danger of freezing exposed flesh					

Source: U.S. Army

Figure 14-2 Wind-chill index.

reduction of body temperature, which can be deadly. The other kind of emergency is called a **local cold injury,** or damage to body tissues in a specific (local) part of the body.

GENERALIZED HYPOTHERMIA

Exposure to extreme cold for a short time or moderate cold for a long time can cause hypothermia. There are several risk factors you should know about. They are:

- *Medical condition of the patient.* Any underlying problem—such as shock, head or spine injury, burns, infection, diabetes, and hypoglycemia—can weaken the body's responses to heat and cold.
- *Drugs, alcohol, and poisons.* These also impede the body's ability to maintain body temperature.
- *Age of the patient.* Very young or very old patients are especially at risk.

The anatomy of infants puts them at risk. The head is large in proportion to the body. The body surface is large compared to their mass. The result is that they lose more heat more rapidly than adults. Infants also have an immature nervous system, which means they cannot shiver well enough to warm themselves when needed.

Other people are at risk, too, especially the elderly. If they are on a fixed income, for example, they may not be able to afford to heat their homes properly. Sudden illness or injury can limit their ability to escape the cold. Impaired judgment due to a medication or limited mobility due to a medical condition also contribute to their risk.

Many outdoor clubs and organizations discourage or even ban the use of alcohol. The momentary flush of warmth felt after a drink actually increases heat loss. That along with impaired judgment can quickly turn a walk in the woods into a deadly excursion.

Patient Assessment

During scene size-up, notice the location of the patient. Ask yourself these questions: Does the environment suggest the possibility of hypothermia? How long has the patient been exposed to those conditions? If scene size-up suggests the possibility of a cold emergency, put your hand on the patient's abdomen during the physical exam. If it is cool or cold, treat for hypothermia.

Note that hypothermia is a progressive condition (Figure 14–3). At first the patient will shiver. When shivering stops, he may appear to be clumsy, confused, and forgetful. He may even appear to be intoxicated. Often witnesses will say that the patient had mood swings, one moment calm and the next animated or even combative.

Finally, the patient's level of responsiveness decreases. He becomes less communicative and is difficult to rouse. He may display poor judgment and do things like remove his clothing while still in the cold. There may be muscle stiffness, a rigid posture, and loss of sensation. The most ominous sign of a life-threatening condition is unresponsiveness. These patients are unstable and need immediate transport if they are to survive.

Signs and symptoms of hypothermia are summarized in Figure 14–4.

Emergency Care

After completing your scene size-up, initial assessment, and physical exam, there are several things you can do for your patient. To minimize further injury from cold (Figure 14–5):

1. *Remove the patient from the cold environment.* Move him to a shelter, away from the cold wind or water. If the patient is on the ground, get him off or put a blanket between him and the ground.
2. *Administer oxygen,* if you are allowed to do so. If possible, it should be warm and humidified.
3. *Remove all wet clothing, and cover the patient with a blanket.* A thin layer of dry clothing or even just a blanket is better than a thick layer of wet clothing.
4. *Handle the patient very gently.* Rough handling can make the patient's condition worse and even cause injuries. Do not massage the extremities. Do not allow the patient to walk or exert himself. Do not allow the patient to eat or drink stimulants.
5. *Comfort, calm, and reassure the patient.* Tell him that everything that can be done will be done. Communicate with empathy.

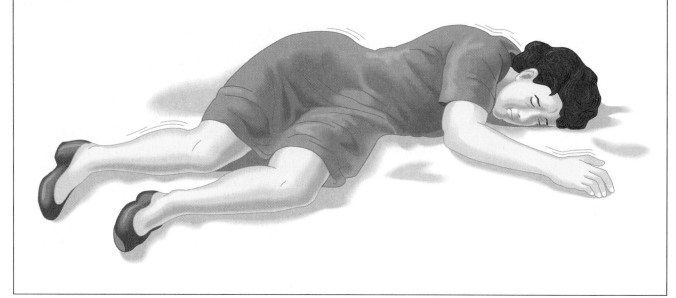

STAGES OF HYPOTHERMIA (Cold-Related Injury)

Stage 1: **Shivering** is a response by the body to generate heat. It does not occur below a body temperature of 90°F.

Stage 2: **Apathy and decreased muscle function**. First fine motor function is affected, then gross motor functions.

Stage 3: **Decreased level of responsiveness** is accompanied by a glassy stare and possible freezing of the extremities.

Stage 4: **Decreased vital signs**, including slow pulse and slow respiration rate.

Stage 5: **Death**.

Figure 14-3   Stages of hypothermia.

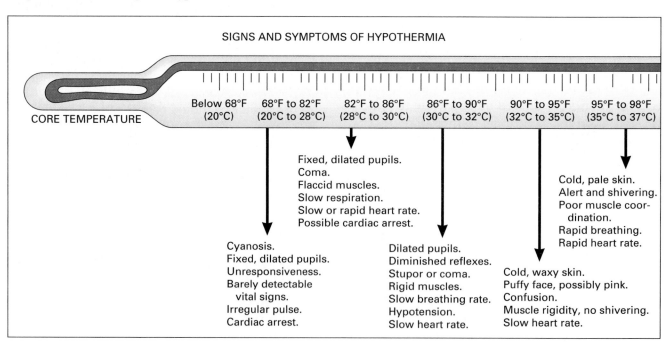

SIGNS AND SYMPTOMS OF HYPOTHERMIA

CORE TEMPERATURE

| Below 68°F (20°C) | 68°F to 82°F (20°C to 28°C) | 82°F to 86°F (28°C to 30°C) | 86°F to 90°F (30°C to 32°C) | 90°F to 95°F (32°C to 35°C) | 95°F to 98°F (35°C to 37°C) |

Fixed, dilated pupils.
Coma.
Flaccid muscles.
Slow respiration.
Slow or rapid heart rate.
Possible cardiac arrest.

Cold, pale skin.
Alert and shivering.
Poor muscle coor-
    dination.
Rapid breathing.
Rapid heart rate.

Cyanosis.
Fixed, dilated pupils.
Unresponsiveness.
Barely detectable
    vital signs.
Irregular pulse.
Cardiac arrest.

Dilated pupils.
Diminished reflexes.
Stupor or coma.
Rigid muscles.
Slow breathing rate.
Hypotension.
Slow heart rate.

Cold, waxy skin.
Puffy face, possibly pink.
Confusion.
Muscle rigidity, no shivering.
Slow heart rate.

Figure 14-4   Signs and symptoms of hypothermia.

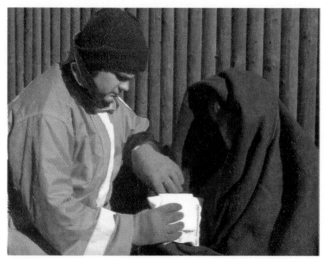

Figure 14-5 A patient with generalized hypothermia needs to be rewarmed.

Mild Hypothermia

The patient with mild hypothermia will present with cold skin and shivering and will still be alert and oriented. Signs and symptoms may include:

- Increased breathing rate.
- Increased pulse rate and blood pressure.
- Slow, thick speech.
- Staggering walk.
- Apathy, drowsiness, incoherence.
- Sluggish pupils.
- Uncontrollable shivering.

If the patient is alert and able, allow him to drink warm fluids. A good test of the patient's ability to protect the airway is to have him hold the cup. Do not allow the drink if there is a problem, such as he drops the cup or is unable to get it to his mouth. Never give a confused or lethargic patient anything to drink. The danger of aspiration is too great. Never give coffee, tea, or other caffeine drinks like cola. Do not allow the patient to smoke. Stimulants promote heat loss.

Cover the patient with a warm blanket. Remember that heat loss is greatest from the head and neck. So listen to an old sailor's saying, "When your feet are cold, put on a hat." Cover the patient's head, and wrap a blanket around him.

If heat packs are available, consider using them. (Be sure to follow local protocol.) Apply the packs to the patient's neck, armpits, and groin. Remember that the patient may have a decreased sense of touch. So check the skin beneath the heat packs periodically to be sure they are not burning it.

Severe Hypothermia

Patients with severe hypothermia may become unresponsive. This is a true medical emergency that can lead to death. Signs and symptoms may include:

- Extremely slow breathing rate.
- Extremely slow pulse rate.
- Unresponsiveness.
- Fixed and dilated pupils.
- Rigid extremities.
- Absence of shivering.

Consider using a nasopharyngeal airway to secure the airway of an unresponsive patient. Administer high concentration oxygen.

When assessing circulation, you may find no pulses in the patient's limbs. Remember that the body is a "metabolic icebox" at this stage. It does not need normal circulation to sustain life, because everything is slowed down. A slow pulse is not deadly and may actually be protective.

So, assess the carotid pulse for about one minute before starting CPR. If it is cold outside, remember that your sense of touch may be less than it should be. Consider putting your fingers in your armpits or your groin before taking a pulse. Remember to handle the patient gently. Any rough handling can induce ventricular fibrillation or sudden cardiac death.

If your patient is breathless and pulseless, begin CPR. Note that many of these patients have all the signs of death, including fixed pupils and stiff extremities. The rule of thumb in EMS is, "You're not dead until you're warm and dead." So even with these signs, start CPR.

Rewarming in the field is not recommended for patients with severe hypothermia. They need special attention in a hospital. So arrange for transport to the closest medical facility. Follow local protocols.

LOCAL COLD INJURIES

Patient Assessment

Frostbite, or local cold injury, is the freezing or near freezing of a body part. Usually the toes, fingers, face, nose, and ears are most at risk (Figure 14-6).

Frostbitten areas are usually easy to identify. With early or superficial frostbite, light skin will redden. Dark skin will turn pale. When the skin is depressed gently, it will blanch and then return to its normal color. The patient often will complain of loss of feeling and sensation in the injured area.

In the later stages of frostbite (called "late or deep cold injury"), the skin may appear to be waxy. It also may be firm to the touch. As freezing continues, it becomes mottled or blotchy. Finally, the area becomes swollen, blistered, and white.

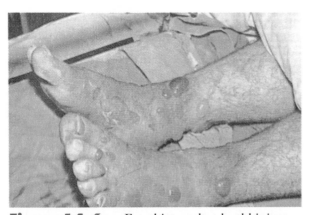

Figure 14-6a   Frostbite, or local cold injury.

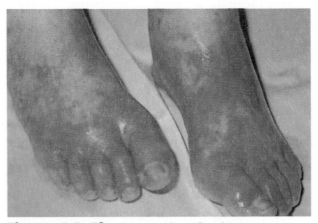

Figure 14-6b   Late or deep frostbite.

When the injured parts begin to thaw, skin color changes. It will appear to be flushed with areas of purple and blanching, or it may be mottled and cyanotic.

Emergency Care

Note that if you suspect hypothermia, treat it before you care for a frostbitten extremity. Emergency care for a local cold injury is as follows:

1. *Remove the patient from the cold environment.* Do not allow the patient to walk on a frostbitten limb.
2. *Administer oxygen,* if you are allowed to do so.
3. *Remove all wet clothing.*
4. *Protect the frostbite area from further injury.* If the injury is to an extremity, manually stabilize it. If the injury is superficial, cover it with a blanket. If it is late and deep, cover it with a dry cloth or dressings. Do not rub or massage the area. Ice crystals under the skin could damage the fragile capillaries and tissues, making the injury worse.
5. *Comfort, calm, and reassure the patient.* Tell him everything that can be done will be done.
6. *Monitor the patient for signs of hypothermia.*

Rewarming

If transport will be delayed, consider rewarming the affected area. Never rewarm an area with late or deep frostbite. Never rewarm a area if there is a chance that it may refreeze. The injury from the second freezing would be much worse than the original one.

Warm the entire frostbite area in tepid water (about 100°F to 105°F). The water should feel comfortable to the normal hand. Be sure to pick a container that permits the entire area to be immersed (Figure 14–7). Continue to support the injured limb during rewarming. Do not allow the injured area to touch the bottom or side of the container. If the water starts to cool, remove the patient. Then add more warm water. As the area rewarms, the patient may complain of tingling and shooting pains. In this case, some EMS systems allow First Responders to help an alert patient self-administer an analgesic such as Tylenol®. Follow local protocol.

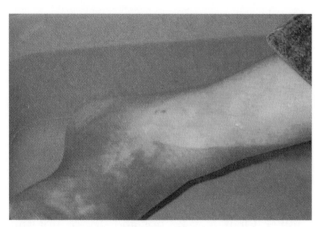

Figure 14-7 Active rewarming of a local cold injury.

When the injured area is rewarmed, the tissues will be fragile. To protect them, cover the injury with dry sterile gauze. If the injury is to the fingers or toes, place gauze between them too. Consider padding the entire area with a large bulky dressing.

SECTION 3: HEAT EMERGENCIES

When a person cannot lose excessive heat, he or she develops **hyperthermia.** Left untreated, hyperthermia can lead to organ damage and death. The stages of hyperthermia are commonly called "heat cramps," "heat exhaustion," and "heat stroke." Heat stroke, the most serious, is life-threatening.

CONTRIBUTING FACTORS

Factors that contribute to the risk of hyperthermia include the following:

- *Heat and humidity.* High air temperature can reduce the body's ability to lose heat by radiation. High humidity can reduce its ability to lose heat by way of evaporation. (See "Heat and Humidity Risk Scale," Figure 14–8.)

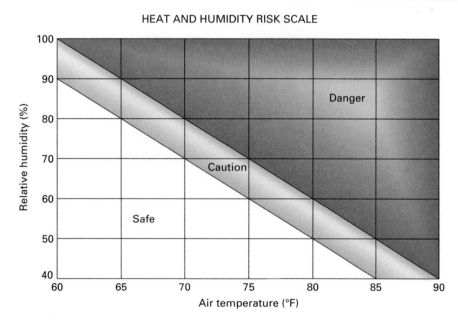

HEAT AND HUMIDITY RISK SCALE

Adapted with permission from William C. Brown Publishers, Dubuque, Iowa. Fox EL, Bowers RW, Foss ML: *The physiological basis of physical education and athletics*, ed. 4. Philadelphia, WB Saunders Co., 1988, p. 503.

Reproduced with permission from *Patient Care*, June 15, 1989. Copyright © 1989 Patient Care, Oradell, NJ. All rights reserved.

Figure 14-8 Heat and humidity risk scale.

- *Exercise and strenuous activity.* Each can cause a person to lose more than one liter of sweat (fluid and essential salts) per hour.
- *Age of the patient.* Very young and very old patients may be unable to respond to overheating effectively.
- *Medical condition of the patient.* Any number of conditions, such as heart or lung disease, diabetes, dehydration (fluid loss), obesity, fever, and fatigue can inhibit heat loss.
- *Certain drugs and medications.* Alcohol, cocaine, barbiturates, hallucinogens, and others can affect heat loss in many ways, including through side effects such as dehydration (fluid loss).

PATIENT ASSESSMENT

The general signs and symptoms of a heat emergency include the following:

- Muscle cramps.
- Weakness, exhaustion.
- Dizziness, faintness.
- Rapid pulse rate that is strong at first, but becomes weak as damage progresses.
- Headache.
- Seizures.
- Loss of appetite, nausea, vomiting.
- Altered mental status, possibly unresponsiveness.
- Skin may be moist, pale, and normal-to-cool in temperature ("heat cramps" or "heat exhaustion"). Or it may be hot and dry or hot and moist ("heat stroke").

"Heat cramps" involve acute spasms of the muscles of the legs, arms, or abdomen (Figure 14–9). This may be the result of losing too much salt during profuse sweating. Heat cramps usually follow hard work in a hot environment. Hard work in a hot, humid environment also can affect

SIGNS AND SYMPTOMS OF HEAT CRAMPS

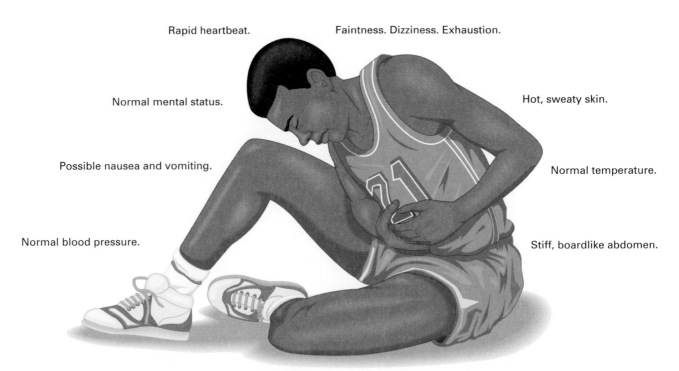

Rapid heartbeat.

Faintness. Dizziness. Exhaustion.

Normal mental status.

Hot, sweaty skin.

Possible nausea and vomiting.

Normal temperature.

Normal blood pressure.

Stiff, boardlike abdomen.

Severe muscular cramps and pain, especially of the arms, fingers, legs, calves, and abdomen.

Figure 14-9   Heat cramps are the most common but least serious heat emergency.

blood flow. This can result in a mild state of shock, or "heat exhaustion."

If the patient does not stop work, move to a cool environment, and replace lost fluid, his condition will get worse. The result can be "heat stroke," which is very serious and life-threatening. It occurs when the body becomes overheated and, in many patients, sweating stops. If left untreated, brain cells begin to die, causing permanent disability or death. (See Figures 14–10 and 14–11.)

Feel the abdomen to check the body temperature of a patient with a heat emergency. Remember that the chief characteristic of heat stroke is hot skin.

EMERGENCY CARE

For a patient with moist, pale, and normal-to-cool skin temperature, provide emergency care as follows (Figure 14–12):

1. *Remove the patient from the hot environment.* Place him in a cool one if possible. If the source of heat is the sun, place the patient in the shade.
2. *Administer oxygen*, if you are allowed to do so.
3. *Cool the patient.* Loosen or remove clothing. Then fan the surface of his body while applying a light mist of water. Be careful not to cool the patient so fast that he becomes chilled.

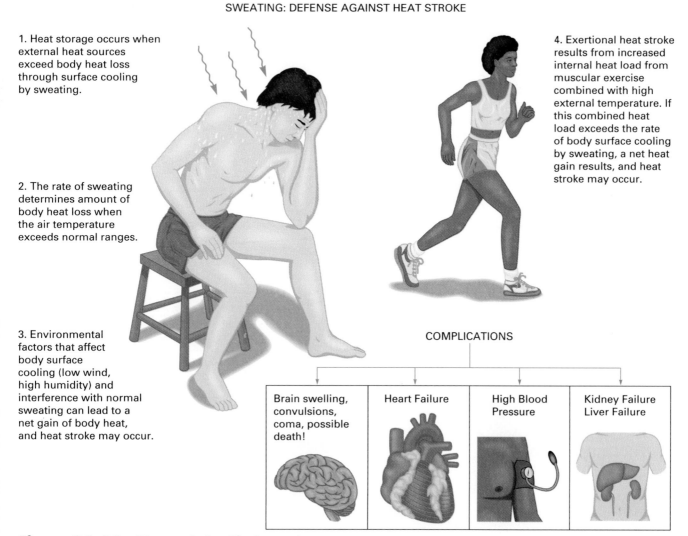

SWEATING: DEFENSE AGAINST HEAT STROKE

1. Heat storage occurs when external heat sources exceed body heat loss through surface cooling by sweating.

2. The rate of sweating determines amount of body heat loss when the air temperature exceeds normal ranges.

3. Environmental factors that affect body surface cooling (low wind, high humidity) and interference with normal sweating can lead to a net gain of body heat, and heat stroke may occur.

4. Exertional heat stroke results from increased internal heat load from muscular exercise combined with high external temperature. If this combined heat load exceeds the rate of body surface cooling by sweating, a net heat gain results, and heat stroke may occur.

COMPLICATIONS

Brain swelling, convulsions, coma, possible death!

Heart Failure

High Blood Pressure

Kidney Failure Liver Failure

Figure 14-10   Heat stroke is a life-threatening emergency.

SIGNS AND SYMPTOMS OF HEAT STROKE

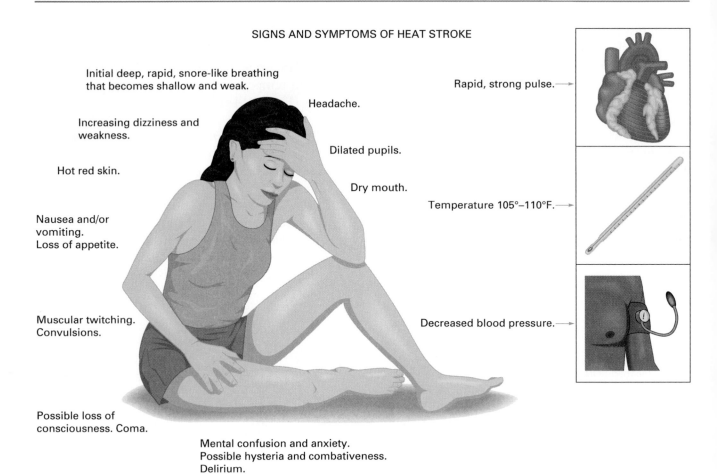

Initial deep, rapid, snore-like breathing that becomes shallow and weak.

Increasing dizziness and weakness.

Hot red skin.

Nausea and/or vomiting.
Loss of appetite.

Muscular twitching.
Convulsions.

Possible loss of consciousness. Coma.

Headache.

Dilated pupils.

Dry mouth.

Rapid, strong pulse.

Temperature 105°–110°F.

Decreased blood pressure.

Mental confusion and anxiety.
Possible hysteria and combativeness.
Delirium.

Figure 14-11 Signs and symptoms of heat stroke.

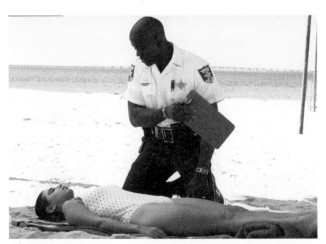

Figure 14-12 Cooling a patient with normal-to-cool skin temperature.

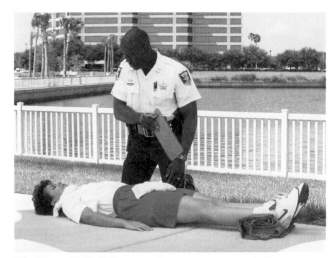

Figure 14-13 Cooling a patient with hot skin temperature.

4. *Position the patient.* Place him in a supine position with legs elevated 8 to 12 inches.
5. *Monitor the patient.* Take vital signs frequently. Advise incoming units or other EMS personnel on scene if the patient develops signs of shock.

If the patient is responsive and not nauseated, encourage him to drink about one-half glass of cool water every 15 minutes or so. Follow local protocol or consult medical direction.

A patient with hot and moist skin or hot and dry skin must be removed from the hot environment. Administer oxygen if possible. If the patient's breathing becomes shallow, assist it with a bag-valve-mask. Cool the patient with hot skin as follows (Figure 14–13):

1. Loosen or remove clothing.
2. Apply cold packs to neck, armpits, and groin.
3. Keep the skin wet by applying water with wet towels or a sponge.
4. Fan the patient aggressively. An effective way is to direct an electric fan over the patient's body while you wet his skin.
5. Continually monitor the patient as appropriate during your ongoing assessment.

FIRST RESPONDER FOCUS

Conditions resulting from extremes in heat and cold are common in most parts of the country. Even though many people are aware of the effects of these temperatures, they still fall victim.

Very young and old patients are at increased risk for heat and cold emergencies. Because their temperature control systems are not working optimally, it would not take bitter cold or extreme heat to cause an emergency. Patients who are exposed to moderate temperatures for long periods of time also may be striken. Patients with wet clothes in the cold and patients in heat who do not maintain their fluid levels will be overcome quickly. Patients may even suffer from these conditions indoors.

The most important concept in this chapter is that the First Responder can provide immediate life-saving help. Remove patients from extremes in temperature and begin to treat them. Be sure you do not become stricken by the same conditions yourself. ■

CASE STUDY FOLLOW-UP

At the beginning of this chapter, you read that First Responders were on scene with "a woman down." To see how chapter skills apply to this emergency, read the following. It describes how the call was completed.

PHYSICAL EXAMINATION
I performed a complete physical exam on Mrs. Downe. My findings included a swollen, painful deformity in her right hip, plus a number of bruises to her hips, knees, and ankles. I also noticed she had been incontinent of urine during the night. Her shivering continued.

Mrs. Downe had been lying on a cold, wet floor for nearly 12 hours. I suspected hypothermia. After completing the physical exam, we placed a warm blanket over her. We didn't want to move her because of her injuries and the ambulance was less than five minutes away.

PATIENT HISTORY
Mrs. Downe told us she had no allergies and that she took several medications including aspirin, digitalis, and insulin. She had a long history of circulatory problems. She had not eaten for 12 hours. Unable to get up from the floor, she had called out for help until she lost her voice.

ONGOING ASSESSMENT
We monitored Mrs. Downe's level of responsiveness and vital signs. We kept her head stabilized and tried to keep her as warm as possible.

CASE STUDY FOLLOW-UP (Continued)

PATIENT HAND-OFF

When the Rescue 3 team arrived, we told them:

"We have an 80-year-old female who fell 12 hours ago and remained down until we arrived. Her chief complaint is pain in her right hip. Her pulse is 100, respirations 18. We stabilized her head because of the blood we saw. We also felt that she could be hypothermic, so we warmed her with a blanket."

Later that week, I ran into Rescue 3's crew chief. He said that Mrs. Downe had suffered a broken hip and hypothermia. She was treated suc-cessfully at the hospital but would likely go to a nursing home after discharge.

Heat and cold emergencies often occur in isolated areas to such people as campers, hikers and skiers, and mountain climbers. But as you can see, they can also happen in our own neighborhoods. Always consider the environmental conditions as soon as you get your call. Early recognition and the appropriate care can save a life.

REVIEW QUESTIONS

Page references where answers may be found or sup-ported are provided at the end of each question.

Section 1

1. What are the five major mechanisms of heat loss? (pp. 240–241)
2. Which will take away a person's body heat faster, air or water? How much faster? (pp. 240–241)

Section 2

3. What factors contribute to the possibility that a patient may be at risk for hypothermia? (p. 243)
4. Is hypothermia a progressive condition? Whether your answer is yes or no, describe how a patient may present the signs of hypo-thermia. (pp. 243–245)

5. How can you minimize the injury your patient experiences from hypothermia? (p. 245)
6. If you find a hypothermic patient breathless and pulseless, and with signs of death, should you begin CPR? Explain your answer. (p. 245)
7. How can you identify a local cold injury? (p. 246)
8. What is the basic emergency care of a local cold injury? (p. 246)

Section 3

9. What factors contribute to the possibility that a patient may be at risk for hyperthermia? (pp. 247–248)
10. What are the signs and symptoms of a heat emergency? (pp. 248–249)
11. What is the appropriate emergency care for a patient with a heat emergency? (pp. 249, 251)

CHAPTER 15

BITES AND STINGS

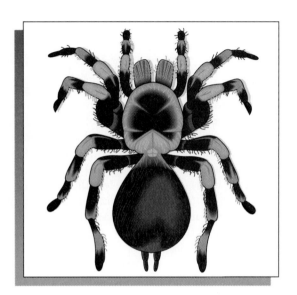

INTRODUCTION

Insect bites and stings are common and usually minor occurrences in the U.S. It is only when the insect is poisonous or when the patient has an allergic reaction that the situation becomes an emergency. Under those conditions, prompt emergency care can save lives and prevent permanent tissue damage.

Insects are not alone in posing a threat to human beings in the environment. Snakes and marine animals also can cause life-threatening problems. Every year in the U.S. 45,000 people are bitten by snakes. Though many different kinds of poisonous marine animals live in tropical waters, waders and swimmers have discovered they can be found in virtually all waters.

Cognitive, affective, and psychomotor objectives are from the U.S. DOT's 1995 "First Responder: National Standard Curriculum." Enrichment objectives, if any, identify material that is supplemental to the DOT curriculum.

Cognitive

No objectives are identified.

Affective

5-1.21 Demonstrate a caring attitude towards patients with a specific medical complaint who request emergency medical services. (p. 256)

5-1.22 Place the interests of the patient with a specific medical complaint as the foremost consideration when making any and all patient care decisions. (p. 256)

5-1.23 Communicate with empathy to patients with a specific medical complaint, as well as with family members and friends of the patient. (p. 256)

Psychomotor

No objectives are identified.

Enrichment

* Recognize the general signs and symptoms of bites or stings. (pp. 255–256)
* Recognize the signs and symptoms of allergic reactions to bites or stings. (pp. 255–256)
* Describe the guidelines for emergency care of patients with bites or stings, including those who have allergic reactions. (p. 256)
* Distinguish between poisonous and nonpoisonous snakes. (p. 257)
* Identify the signs and symptoms of poisonous snakebites. (p. 257)
* Identify the signs and symptoms of specific insect bites and stings, including those of spiders, scorpions, fire ants, mites, ticks, bees, wasps, and hornets. (pp. 259–264)
* Identify the signs and symptoms of poisoning by common marine life. (p. 264)
* Describe the proper method of applying a constricting band to an extremity. (pp. 257–258)
* Describe how to remove a stinger embedded in a patient's skin. (pp. 256, 264)

SECTION 1: GENERAL GUIDELINES FOR EMERGENCY CARE

For assessment and emergency medical care of a patient with a bite or a sting, follow the general guidelines described below.

PATIENT ASSESSMENT

As always, your priority during scene size-up is to protect yourself. If your patient has been bitten or stung, you could be bitten or stung. Exercise caution. Do not become a victim too. As you size up the scene, ask yourself: Is an insect nest visible in a nearby tree, under the eaves of a house, or in the ground nearby? Are there signs that the patient was engaged in activity such as clearing underbrush or gardening that might have disturbed snakes or insects? Was the patient working in a garage, basement, attic, or shed where spiders and other insects might nest? Are there dead insects on the ground near the patient? During your assessment of the patient, be alert to the possibility that insects may have become trapped in your patient's clothing.

Also keep in mind that some patients will have an allergic reaction to bites and stings. That reaction can lead to **anaphylactic shock,** an emergency that generally has a rapid life-threatening affect on the airway and breathing.

When you gather a patient history, be sure to ask the patient to identify any allergies he or she may have. Also, if possible and if it is safe to do so, try to identify what bit or stung your patient.

Signs and Symptoms

General signs and symptoms of bites and stings include:

CASE STUDY

DISPATCH

My first response unit was dispatched for a bee sting at a local campground.

SCENE SIZE-UP

Everything seemed safe when we arrived. A group was standing around a person who was sitting in a lawn chair. They were frantically waving to us. We put on gloves and approached.

INITIAL ASSESSMENT

The condition of the patient struck us immediately. Our general impression was of an adult female who was having an allergic reaction. The patient was wheezing, pale, and sweaty, but breathing adequately—for the moment. If the airway had constricted any more, we would have had to assist ventilations immediately. We were fortunate to have oxygen and applied it to the patient via nonrebreather mask. The patient's pulse was rapid. We notified dispatch to alert the paramedics of the patient's condition.

> Consider this patient as you read Chapter 15. What more may be done to assess and care for her condition?

- History of bites or stings.
- Bite mark or stinger embedded in the skin.
- Immediate pain that is severe or burning.
- Numbness at the site after a few hours.
- Redness or other discoloration of the skin around the bite or sting.
- Swelling around the site, sometimes spreading gradually.

If the patient has an allergic reaction, any combination of a range of signs and symptoms may develop. They include the following (Figure 15–1):

- Skin:
  - Warm, tingling feeling in the mouth, face, chest, feet, and hands.
  - Itching, hives, and flushing.
  - Swelling to the tongue, face, neck, hands, and feet.
- Respiratory system:
  - Tightness in the throat or chest.
  - Cough, hoarseness (losing the voice).
  - Rapid or labored breathing.
  - Noisy breathing, stridor, wheezing.
- Circulatory system:
  - Increased heart rate.
  - Decreased blood pressure.
- General findings:
  - Itchy, watery eyes.
  - Headache.
  - Runny nose.
  - Sense of impending doom.
  - Decreasing mental status.

If you suspect an allergic reaction, inform EMS dispatch immediately. Respiratory distress and shock can develop rapidly. (Read more about shock in Chapter 17.)

You may wish to note that allergic reactions are especially common following the stings of wasps, hornets, yellow jackets, and fire ants. Bites or stings from deer flies, gnats, horse flies, mosquitoes, cock-

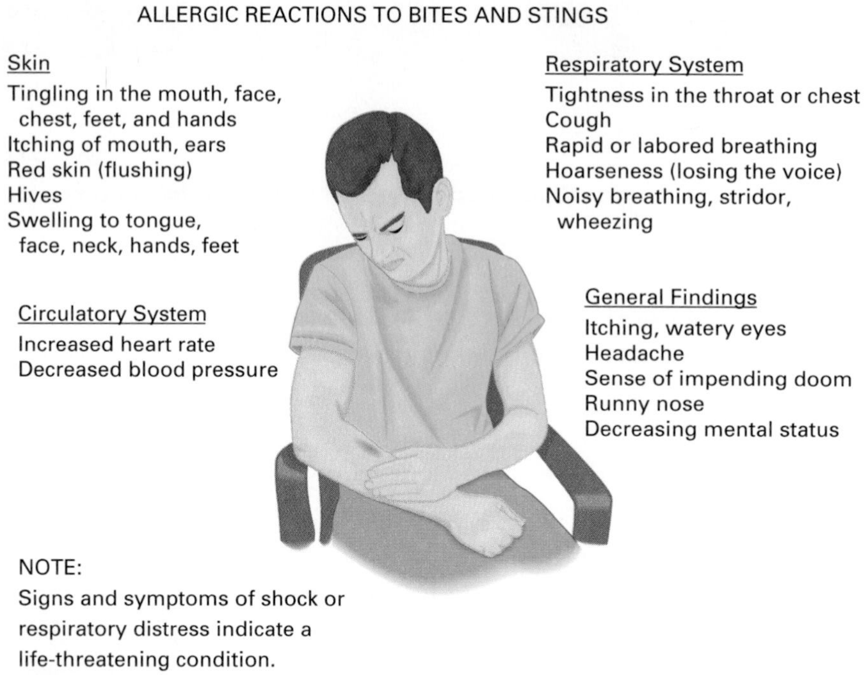

ALLERGIC REACTIONS TO BITES AND STINGS

<u>Skin</u>
Tingling in the mouth, face,
  chest, feet, and hands
Itching of mouth, ears
Red skin (flushing)
Hives
Swelling to tongue,
  face, neck, hands, feet

<u>Circulatory System</u>
Increased heart rate
Decreased blood pressure

<u>Respiratory System</u>
Tightness in the throat or chest
Cough
Rapid or labored breathing
Hoarseness (losing the voice)
Noisy breathing, stridor,
  wheezing

<u>General Findings</u>
Itching, watery eyes
Headache
Sense of impending doom
Runny nose
Decreasing mental status

NOTE:
Signs and symptoms of shock or
respiratory distress indicate a
life-threatening condition.

Figure 15-1 Possible allergic reactions to bites and stings.

roaches, and miller moths also can cause an allergic reaction. Venom from snakes and spiders can, too.

EMERGENCY MEDICAL CARE

General guidelines for emergency care of a patient with bites or stings includes the following. Remember to take all appropriate BSI precautions. Then follow these steps:

1. *Perform an initial assessment.* Treat all life-threats. If you suspect an allergic reaction, maintain the patient's airway. Insert an airway adjunct if appropriate. Suction as needed.
2. *Administer oxygen,* if you are equipped and allowed to do so. If breathing is adequate, deliver it by way of a nonrebreather mask. If the patient needs artificial ventilation, use supplemental oxygen.
3. *Position the site* of the bite or sting slightly below the level of the patient's heart. Manually stabilize a bitten or stung extremity until it can be immobilized.
4. *Remove any constricting objects* such as jewelry as soon as possible. Ideally this should happen before swelling begins.

5. *Inspect the bite or sting site.* If a stinger is present, remove it by scraping along the surface of the skin with the edge of a credit card or a knife. Make sure you remove the venom sac.
6. *Wash the area around the bite or sting.* Be very gentle. Use soap and water. Then irrigate with clean water. Follow local protocol.
7. *Apply a cold pack* (Figure 15–2). It will help relieve pain, itching, and swelling. Do not apply cold to snakebites or marine animal bites.
8. *Keep the patient calm, warm, and limit physical activity.*

During your ongoing assessment of the patient, monitor the ABCs continually. Be prepared to deliver basic life support if it is needed. If at any time during emergency care you suspect an allergic reaction, inform EMS dispatch immediately. (You can read more about emergency medical care of a patient in anaphylactic shock in Chapter 17.)

Demonstrate a caring attitude towards your patient. Place his or her interests first in any patient care decision. Remember to communicate with empathy with patients and their family members or friends.

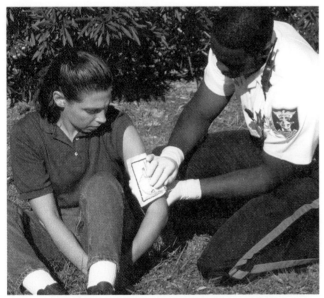

Figure 15-2 Apply a cold pack to an insect bite or sting to help relieve pain and swelling.

SECTION 2: SPECIFIC TYPES OF BITES AND STINGS

SNAKEBITE

About 20 of the 120 species of snake in the U.S. are poisonous. They include rattlesnakes, coral snakes, water moccasins or cottonmouths, and copperheads (Figure 15–3). Snake venom contains some of the most complex poisons known. It can affect the central nervous system, heart, kidneys, and blood. Simply stated, a snake's venom is its digestive enzyme. It "digests" any tissue into which it is injected.

Most poisonous snakes have the following characteristics:

- *Two large, hollow fangs* that work like a hypodermic needle. Nonpoisonous snakes (and the poisonous coral snake) have small teeth.
- *Elliptical pupils.* That is, the pupils look like vertical slits much like those of a cat. Nonpoisonous snakes (and the poisonous coral snake) have round pupils.
- *Presence of a pit.* Certain poisonous snakes have a telltale pit between the eye and the mouth. That is why they are called "pit vipers." That pit is a heat-sensing organ. It makes it possible

for the snake to strike a warm-blooded animal accurately, even if the snake cannot see.
- *Special markings.* Poisonous snakes are marked with shapes on a background of pink, yellow, tan, gray, or brown skin. The exception is the small coral snake, which is ringed with red, yellow, and black.
- *Triangular head,* which is larger than the neck.

Poisonous snakebites cause medical emergencies. However, only about one-third of all bites cause symptoms. When symptoms do develop, they usually occur immediately after a person is bitten.

Patient Assessment

Signs and symptoms of a poisonous snakebite include puncture wounds, swelling, discoloration, and severe pain and burning at the bite site. (See Figures 15–4 and 15–5.)

In addition, the venom of a coral snake affects the central nervous system. One to eight hours after the bite, the patient will experience symptoms that will get progressively worse. Signs and symptoms of coral-snake bite include:

- Blurred vision, drooping eyelids.
- Drowsiness, slurred speech.
- Increased salivation and sweating.
- Nausea, vomiting.
- Weakness, paralysis.
- Seizures, unresponsiveness.

Always make sure EMS has been activated if you suspect any kind of snakebite. When you gather a patient history, be sure to note how much physical activity the patient engaged in after the bite. (Activity helps to spread the venom.) Also find out when the patient last had a tetanus vaccine.

Emergency Care

For snakebite, follow the general emergency care guidelines for bites and stings described earlier in this chapter. However, if your EMS system allows, you also might want to apply a constricting band and suction the wound.

The use of constricting bands is controversial. Some say they should be used only within 30 minutes of the time of the bite. Others say a constrict-

COMMON POISONOUS SNAKES

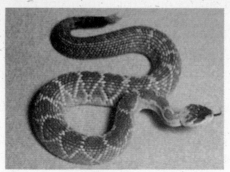

Figure 15-3a Rattlesnake.

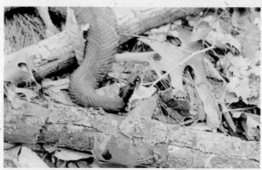

Figure 15-3b Water moccasin or cottonmouth.

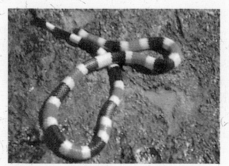

Figure 15-3c Coral snake.

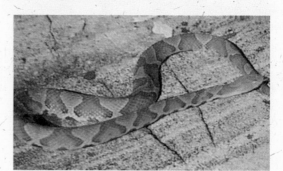

Figure 15-3d Copperhead.

ing band should not be used at all. Constricting bands are used only on extremities. Never place a constricting band around a joint or around the head, neck, or trunk. Follow local protocols.

In order to apply a constricting band, first find the fang marks. Then wrap a flat band that is about two to three inches wide around the extremity (Figure 15–6). Place it two to four inches above (proximal to) the fang marks between the bite and the patient's heart. The band should be snug, but not too tight. You should be able to slip two fingers between it and the patient's skin. You can adjust the constricting band as swelling occurs so that is does not become too tight. But leave it in place until a physician checks the patient.

The use of suction also is controversial. Some say it should be used only if the patient is at least two hours from medical help. Follow local protocols. Apply suction to the wound directly over the fang marks. An extractor from a snakebite kit is ideal. Never use your mouth to provide suction. Suction must be strong and must be applied within the first five minutes to be effective. After 30 minutes, the venom is diffused and cannot be removed by suction. Note, never suction a coral-snake bite.

INSECT BITES AND STINGS

For assessment and emergency care of insect bites and stings, follow the general guidelines described earlier in this chapter. The discussion below provides details on specific insects and spiders.

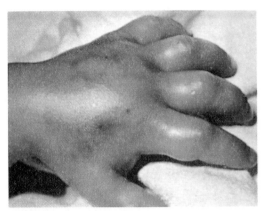

Figure 15-4 Snakebite to the hand.

Black Widow Spider

The black widow spider is characterized by a shiny black body, thin legs, and a crimson red mark on its abdomen the shape of an hourglass or two triangles. (See Figure 15–7.) Black-widow

bites are the leading cause of death in the U.S. from spiders. The venom—14 times more toxic than rattlesnake venom—results in pain and muscle spasms within 30 minutes to three hours. Severe bites cause respiratory failure and death. Those at highest risk for developing severe symptoms are children under 16 years old, people over the age of 60, people with chronic diseases, and anyone with hypertension (high blood pressure).

The most serious sign of a black-widow bite is high blood pressure. Other signs and symptoms, which last for 24 to 48 hours, include:

- A brief pinprick sensation at the bite site. It becomes a dull ache within 30 to 40 minutes. There is almost never a local reaction, although in some cases there may be some swelling or a wheal (a raised, round, red mark).
- Flushing, sweating, and grimacing of the face within 10 minutes to two hours.

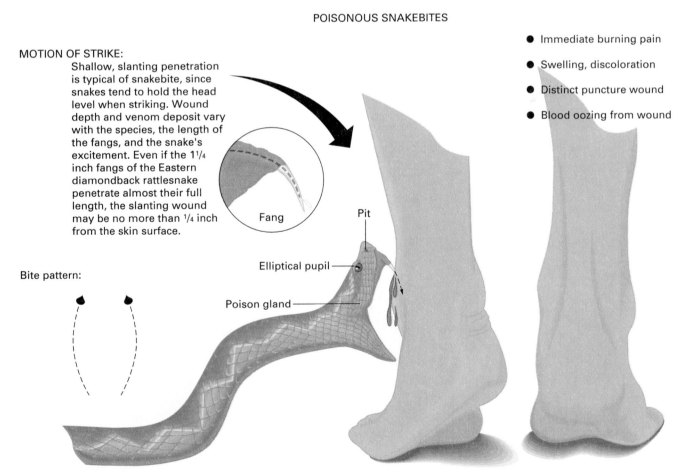

POISONOUS SNAKEBITES

MOTION OF STRIKE:
Shallow, slanting penetration is typical of snakebite, since snakes tend to hold the head level when striking. Wound depth and venom deposit vary with the species, the length of the fangs, and the snake's excitement. Even if the 1¼ inch fangs of the Eastern diamondback rattlesnake penetrate almost their full length, the slanting wound may be no more than ¼ inch from the skin surface.

Fang

Bite pattern:

Pit

Elliptical pupil

Poison gland

- Immediate burning pain
- Swelling, discoloration
- Distinct puncture wound
- Blood oozing from wound

Figure 15-5 Poisonous snakebites.

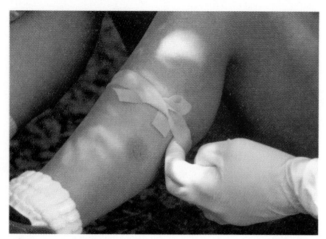

Figure 15-6 Follow local protocol regarding the use of a constricting band.

- Pain and spasms in the shoulders, back, chest, and abdominal muscles within 30 minutes to three hours. These gradually spread over the entire body within one to six hours.
- Rigid abdomen with cramping.
- Agitation, restlessness, anxiety.
- Lack of coordination.
- Weakness, headache, which may last for months.
- Profuse salivation, tearing, or sweating.
- Fever, rash.
- Nausea, vomiting.

The antivenom for the black-widow spider bite is generally used only for high-risk patients.

So if you can do so safely, find the spider. The patient's physician will be able to identify it, even if it is crushed, and will not have to guess about treatment.

Brown Recluse Spider

The brown recluse spider can range in color from yellow to dark chocolate brown. The characteristic marking is a brown, violin-shaped mark on the upper back. Its bite is not often serious. However, about 10% of the time, the bite does not heal and the patient needs a skin graft. A small percent of patients may develop kidney failure and die.

Brown-recluse bites are rare. They most often occur when spiders are trapped in clothing. Unfortunately, most victims are unaware that they have been bitten, since the bite often is at first painless. There may be a slight stinging sensation and itching. The most severe reactions are among children.

If the patient is going to react, the following signs and symptoms may occur:

- Within a few hours, the bite is surrounded by sunken tissue. There is a bluish area with white edges, gradually becoming surrounded by a red halo (a bulls-eye pattern). Two tiny puncture marks may be apparent.
- Within 72 hours, if there is a severe reaction, the bite becomes a large ulcer (Figure 15–8). The following also sometimes occur: a fever of 103°F, joint pain, nausea, vomiting, and chills.

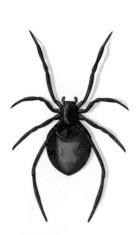

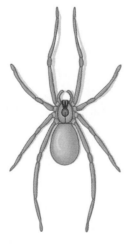

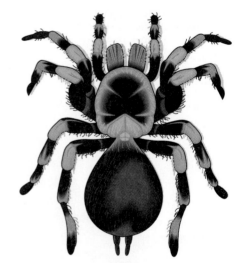

Black Widow   Brown Recluse   Tarantula

Figure 15-7 Poisonous spiders.

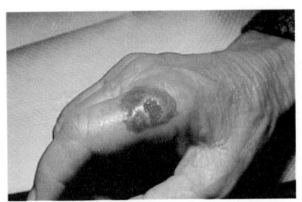

Figure 15-8 Bite mark of a brown recluse spider.

Again, it is important for you to identify the spider so that physicians may begin appropriate treatment as soon as possible.

Tarantula

Although the tarantula looks more menacing than the black widow and the brown recluse, its bite usually causes only moderate pain. Other symptoms from tarantula bites are rare.

Scorpion

In the U.S. there are three species of scorpion that sting and inject venom. Only one species can deliver a potentially fatal sting (Figure 15–9). Of all scorpion stings, 90% occur to the hands. In addition to the general signs and symptoms, those for scorpion bites include: nausea and vomiting, drooling, poor coordination, incontinence, and seizures.

If you are allowed, apply a flat constricting band to the extremity about two inches above the sting. The band should be snug, but not too tight. You should be able to slip two fingers between it and the patient's skin. Leave it in place until a physician checks the patient. Follow local protocols.

Fire Ants

Fire ants are most common in the southeastern U.S. They get their name not from their color (which ranges from red to black), but from the intense, fiery, burning pain their bites cause.

Fire ants bite and sting downward as they pivot. The result is a characteristic circular pattern of bites, which produce extremely painful vesicles

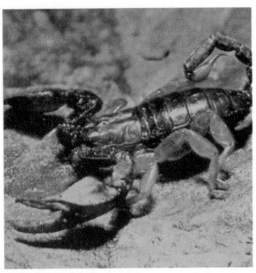

Figure 15-9 Scorpion.

(small blisters). At first the fluid in the vesicles is clear. Later it becomes cloudy. The bitten extremity usually becomes red, swollen, and painful. Within 24 hours, the bites develop pustules (raised areas filled with pus) on a red, swollen base (Figure 15–10).

Mites

Mites are most common in the southern part of the U.S. However, since they feed on tall grasses and grains, they are found in rural and agricultural areas throughout the country. There are many types of mites that bite humans. The most common are the scabies mite and chigger mite.

Mites embed themselves in the skin, generally without the patient realizing it. As soon as they are engorged with blood, the mites generally drop off or are brushed off. If the patient sees the mite at all, it is in the center of a red lesion. Most bites are on the legs and ankles or under tight-fitting clothing such as waistbands. Bite sites often enlarge into nodes that last for two to three weeks.

Ticks

Ticks can cause a serious problem because they can carry tick fever, Rocky Mountain spotted fever, Lyme disease, and other bacterial diseases. A prolonged attachment of a female tick can cause progressive paralysis.

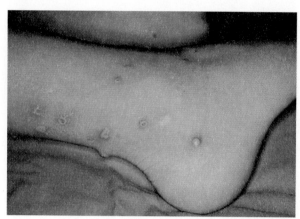

Figure 15-10 Fire-ant bites.

Tick bites are painless. The patient does not notice the bite until he or she finds an engorged tick, which can be as large as a pea (Figure 15-11). Ticks are visible after they have attached themselves to the skin. They often stay attached for more than 10 days. However, since they often choose warm, moist areas, you should carefully inspect the patient's scalp and other hairy areas such as the armpits, groin, and skin creases. If a tick is brushed off, the mouth parts may stay embedded in the skin, causing infection or an allergic reaction. Never pluck an embedded tick head out of the skin. You may force infected blood into the patient.

If you are providing emergency care in an isolated area, local protocol may permit you to remove a tick. If so, remove it as soon as you discover it. The longer the tick remains attached to the skin, the more likely it is that an infection will result. To remove a tick, first take BSI precautions. Then follow these guidelines:

1. Use tweezers, or cover your fingers with a tissue. If you touch the tick, you may contaminate yourself. If you do not have tweezers and cannot cover your fingers, do not wait to look for an appropriate implement.
2. Grasp the tick as closely as possible to the point where it is attached to the skin. Pull firmly and steadily until the tick is dislodged. Do not twist or jerk the tick, since that may result in incomplete removal. Avoid squashing an engorged tick during removal. Infected blood may spurt into your eyes, mouth, or cut on the surface of your skin.

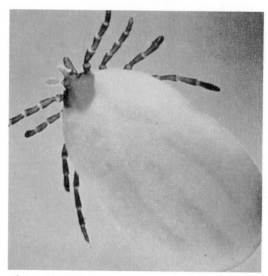

Figure 15-11 Engorged tick.

3. Once the tick is removed, wash your hands and the bite area thoroughly with soap and water. Apply an antiseptic to the area to prevent a bacterial infection.

Have the patient mark the date on a calendar. This will document the exact time of exposure and will serve as a reminder if he or she needs to seek medical care. If the patient develops fever with chills, headache, or muscle aches after being exposed to a tick, immediate treatment from a physician should be sought.

Bee, Wasp, or Hornet Stings

A patient with an insect sting should see a physician if the bite is on the face or if there are multiple stings, even if there seems to be no allergic reaction. If there is an allergic reaction, ensure an open airway and adequate breathing and arrange for the patient to be transported to a hospital immediately. (See Figure 15-12.)

Emergency care is the same as described for bites and stings at the beginning of this chapter. However, if you are allowed, proceed with the following:

1. Lower the affected part below the heart.
2. Apply a constricting band above the sting site if it is on an extremity. The band should be snug, but not too tight. You should be able to

WASPS, BEES, AND FIRE ANTS

The following members of this group commonly attack humans, causing local pain, redness, swelling, and subsequent itching. Always consider the possibility of anaphylaxis.

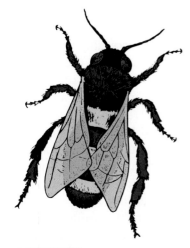

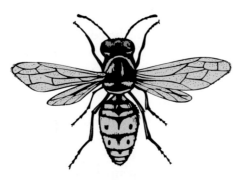

HONEYBEE: Found throughout the United States at anytime of year, except in colder temperatures when they remain in their hives. In the Northeast and Midwest, they are major insects causing sting reactions. Hives are usually found in hollowed out areas such as dead tree trunks. Honeybees principally ingest nectar of plants, so they are often seen in the vicinity of flowers. The honeybee with its barbed stinger will self-eviscerate after a sting, leaving the venom sac and stinger in place.

YELLOW JACKET: A principal insect causing sting reactions in the Northeast and Midwest. Yellow jackets tend to dominate in late summer and fall. Nests are located in the ground. Often seen in picnic areas, garbage cans, yellow jackets are ill-tempered and aggressive and can deliver multiple stings at one time. They will often sting without being provoked.

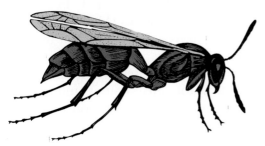

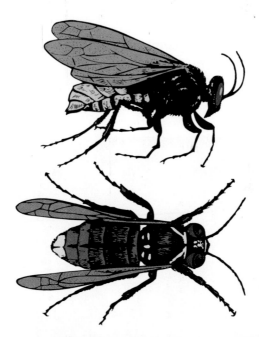

WASPS: The most likely insect to cause sting reactions in the Southeast and Southwest. Wasps tend to nest in small numbers under the eaves of houses and buildings. These are carnivores that are found in picnic areas, garbage cans, and food stands. Can deliver multiple stings at one time.

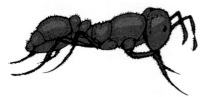

FIRE ANT: Can range from red to black and lives in loose dirt mounds. It is found throughout the southern states as far west as New Mexico. Fire ants may cause serious illness and/or anaphylaxis. The ant attaches itself to the skin by its strong jaws and swivels its tail-position stinger about, inflicting repeated stings.

YELLOW HORNET AND WHITE-FACED OR BALD-FACED HORNET: Seen mainly in the spring and early summer. Nests usually found in branches and bushes above ground. These are carnivores that are seen in picnic areas, garbage cans, and food stands. Can deliver multiple stings at one time.

Adapted with permission from: John W. Georgitis. "Insect Stings – Responding to the Gamut of Allergic Reactions," *Modern Medicine*

Figure 15-12 Wasps, bees, and fire ants.

slip two fingers between it and the patient's skin. Remember that the use of a constricting band is controversial. Follow local protocols.

3. If the stinger is still in the skin, remove it. Gently scrape against it with the edge of a knife or a credit card (Figure 15–13). Be careful not to squeeze the stinger. If you do, you could inject additional venom into the area. Make sure you remove the venom sac. It can continue to secrete venom for up to 20 minutes.

If you know the patient is allergic to stings, do not wait for signs or symptoms to develop. Delay can be fatal. If the patient has a history of severe allergic reactions and has an insect sting kit, assist in the administration of the kit's contents. *Follow all local protocols.*

MARINE LIFE POISONING

See Figure 15–14 for common sources of marine animal stings and wounds. If you are allowed, you also may wish to do the following (follow all local protocols):

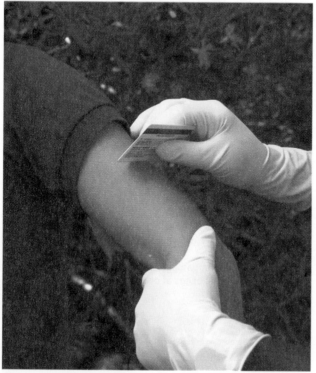

Figure 15-13 If the insect stinger is still present, remove it.

1. Use forceps to remove any material that sticks to the sting site on the surface of the patient's skin.
2. Irrigate the wound thoroughly with water.
3. If the skin is unbroken, wash the wound with an antibacterial agent. Do not scrub the area. Make sure that washings flow away from the body.
4. Remove stingers and barbs the same way you would remove a bee stinger. If you are unable to remove one without excessive force, then bandage it in place. Stabilize the area to keep the venom from spreading.
5. Apply heat. Maintain the injured area at a temperature of 110°F to 114°F for thirty minutes or until the EMTs take over care. Follow local protocol.
6. Activate the EMS system, if it has not already been done. Arrange for immediate transport of the patient.

Tentacle Stings

Tentacle stings can be inflicted by jellyfish, corals, hydras, and anemones (Figures 15–14 and 15–15). First, remove the patient from the water. With gloved hands, carefully remove dried tentacles if possible. Immediately rinse the wounds with sea water for 30 minutes until pain is relieved. If possible, pour vinegar on the affected area. Arrange for immediate transport of the patient to a hospital.

Puncture Wounds

To treat puncture wounds caused by stingray spines and spiny fish (Figure 15–16), first remove the patient from the water. If a spine is embedded in the skin, treat it as an impaled object and stabilize it in place. Stabilize the injured part to prevent movement. Apply a sterile dressing and bandage the area. Arrange for immediate transport of the patient to a hospital.

Large Bites

Bites from sharks or other marine life should be treated the same way you would treat any major injury. Perform an initial assessment, and treat life threats. Arrange for immediate transport of the patient to a hospital. If possible, try to identify the animal that caused the injury.

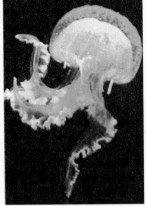

Figure 15-14a Jellyfish.

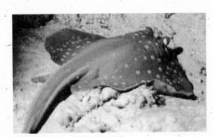

Figure 15-14b Stingray.

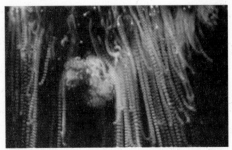

Figure 15-14c Tentacles of the Portuguese man-of-war.

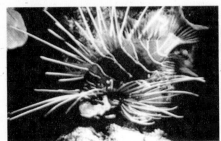

Figure 15-14d Lion fish.

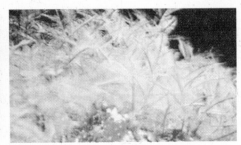

Figure 15-14e Feather hydroid.

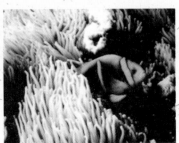

Figure 15-14f Sea anemone and clown fish.

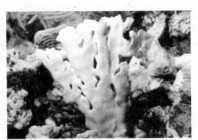

Figure 15-14g Fire coral.

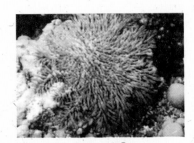

Figure 15-14h Crown-of-thorns starfish.

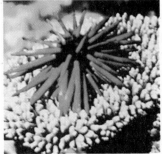

Figure 15-14i Sea urchin.

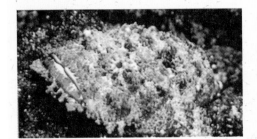

Figure 15-14j Scorpion fish.

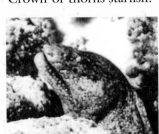

Figure 15-14k Moray eel.

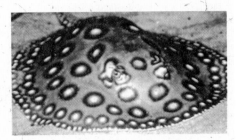

Figure 15-14l Stingray.

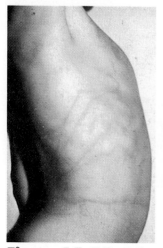

Figure 15-15 Jelly-fish sting.

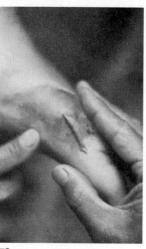

Figure 15-16 Stingray sting.

FIRST RESPONDER FOCUS

Bites and stings are a mere annoyance for most people. For others, however, these injuries can cause a severe allergic reaction. As a First Responder, you must be alert for the serious—and potentially fatal—reaction called *anaphylactic shock.*

Some snakebites and marine stings may be deadly to a patient, even without an allergic reaction. If you have poisonous snakes or other dangerous species in your area, be sure to become familiar with local protocols for assessment and treatment. Never forget scene safety. You do not want to be bitten or stung yourself! ■

CASE STUDY FOLLOW-UP

At the beginning of this chapter, you read that First Responders were on scene with a female patient who was having an allergic reaction to a bee sting. To see how chapter skills apply to this emergency, read the following. It describes how the call was completed.

PATIENT HISTORY
The patient's name was Socorro. The people with her told us that she was allergic to bee stings. She got a bee sting walking on a path to the lake. We found that she was allergic to nothing else. She had dinner an hour ago. She has a device that administers epinephrine when she is stung, but it was at home. She had no past medical history. I found the spot on her neck where she was stung. I didn't see a stinger in the wound.

PHYSICAL EXAMINATION
My partner spent most of his time trying to keep her calm. I checked her vital signs. Her pulse was 108 and weak. Her respirations were 20 and labored. Her blood pressure was 100/62. We took her out of the chair and placed her on the ground. She resisted lying flat.

ONGOING ASSESSMENT
We carefully monitored her respirations. It was getting harder for her to breathe. She was increasingly pale and getting sleepy. We decided to place her in a supine position. Then we assisted ventilations. Fortunately, the paramedics arrived quickly.

PATIENT HAND-OFF
We made our report quickly. We told the medics about the bee sting, her allergy, her declining condition, and vitals. They went to work immediately. They administered drugs that helped to reverse the allergic reaction and shock that developed. Socorro did fine, but it looked like it was a close one. The medics told us that she stabilized en route and they gave her their best advice. They made her promise never to leave the house without her medication again.

It is likely that a bite or sting will make your patient uncomfortable only for a few days. However, the chances that venom has been injected or that a patient may have an allergic reaction are real. So stay alert. Monitor vital signs continually. Be sure EMS has been activated, and be prepared to provide basic life support.

REVIEW QUESTIONS

Page references where answers may be found or supported are provided at the end of each question.

Section 1

1. What are the general signs and symptoms of bites and stings? (pp. 255–256)
2. What are the signs and symptoms of an allergic reaction in a patient with a bite or sting? Describe those related to the skin, respiratory system, and circulatory system, as well as general findings. (pp. 255–256)
3. What are the general guidelines for the emergency medical care of patients with bites and stings? Include care of a patient who may be having an allergic reaction. (p. 256)

Section 2

4. What is the proper method of applying an constricting band to an extremity? (pp. 257–258)
5. How would you remove an engorged tick from a patient's skin? (pp. 261–262)
6. What is the proper method of removing the barbed stinger of a bee from a patient's skin? (pp. 262, 264)

CHAPTER 16

PSYCHOLOGICAL EMERGENCIES AND CRISIS INTERVENTION

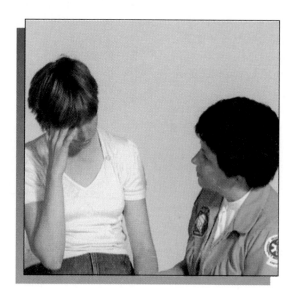

INTRODUCTION

In emergency care for physical problems you can see the wounds you care for.
You can assess, dress, and bandage them. Often, you also get to see the positive
results of your efforts.

Emergency care for behavioral emergencies is different. You cannot easily
see the comfort that your words or your presence provides to someone who is
panicked or depressed. But the care you give to patients in behavioral
emergencies can save lives too.

Cognitive, affective, and psychomotor objectives are from the U.S. DOT's 1995 "First Responder: National Standard Curriculum." Enrichment objectives, if any, identify material that is supplemental to the DOT curriculum.

Cognitive

5-1.11 Identify the patient who presents with a specific medical complaint of behavioral change. (pp. 270–271)

5-1.12 Explain the steps in providing emergency medical care to a patient with a behavioral change. (pp. 271–274)

5-1.13 Identify the patient who presents with a specific complaint of a psychological crisis. (pp. 271–274)

5-1.14 Explain the steps in providing emergency medical care to a patient with a psychological crisis. (pp. 271–274)

Affective

5-1.17 Explain the rationale for modifying your behavior toward the patient with a behavioral emergency. (pp. 270–271)

5-1.24 Demonstrate a caring attitude towards patients with a behavioral problem who request emergency medical services. (pp. 271–272)

5-1.25 Place the interests of the patient with a behavioral problem as the foremost consideration when making any and all patient care decisions. (p. 272)

5-1.26 Communicate with empathy to patients with a behavioral problem, as well as with family members and friends of the patient. (p. 272)

Psychomotor

5-1.32 Demonstrate the steps in providing emergency medical care to a patient with a behavioral change. (pp. 271–274)

5-1.33 Demonstrate the steps in providing emergency medical care to a patient with a psychological crisis. (pp. 271–274)

Enrichment

*   Discuss the guidelines for restraining patients with a behavioral emergency. (pp. 272–274)
*   List the legal considerations involved in providing emergency care to a patient with a behavioral emergency. (p. 274)
*   Identify the signs and symptoms of a patient with a drug or alcohol emergency. (pp. 274–276)
*   Describe management of a patient with a drug or alcohol emergency. (pp. 276–277)
*   Discuss the four general stages of rape trauma syndrome. (p. 278)
*   Describe the proper management of a rape scene. (p. 278)

SECTION 1:
BEHAVIORAL EMERGENCIES

▼

Behavior is the manner in which a person acts or performs. A **behavioral emergency** is a situation in which a patient exhibits "abnormal" behavior, or behavior that is unacceptable or intolerable to the patient, family, or community. Such an emergency may be due to extremes of emotion, a psychological condition such as a mental illness, or even a physical condition such as lack of oxygen or low blood sugar.

A number of factors can cause a change in a patient's behavior. They include:

*   Situational stresses.
*   Illness or injury, including head trauma, lack of oxygen, inadequate blood flow to the brain, low blood sugar in a person with diabetes, or excessive heat or cold.
*   Mind-altering substances, such as alcohol, depressants, stimulants, psychedelics, and narcotics.
*   Psychiatric problems, such as phobias (irrational fears of specific things), depression, paranoia, or schizophrenia.
*   Psychological crises, such as panic and bizarre thinking.

Patients with behavioral emergencies may act in unusual and unexpected ways. They can pose a

CASE STUDY

DISPATCH

I was driving home from my shift at the fire department when I saw a man running along the road. He was naked. He stopped every few hundred feet or so to throw punches in the air.

SCENE SIZE-UP

I realized this person might be dangerous. So I called the police on my cell phone from my car. I stayed there until they arrived.

INITIAL ASSESSMENT

After the man was restrained by the police, I offered my help. They were careful not to restrict the man's breathing. They also covered him with an emergency blanket to keep him warm. He was screaming at the police officers, so I knew he had adequate breathing. There were no indications of airway problems or external bleeding.

My general impression was that of a patient with an altered mental status, possibly from a psychiatric emergency, alcohol, or drugs. We called for an ambulance.

> Consider this patient as you read Chapter 16. What else may be done to assess and treat his condition?

danger to themselves through suicide or self-inflicted injuries. They also can pose a danger to others through violence or actions they are not able to understand.

PATIENT ASSESSMENT

Consider the need for law enforcement during your scene size-up and throughout the call. If you suspect that the patient may threaten him- or herself or others, arrange for backup law enforcement at the scene.

The following guidelines may help you determine if your patient is likely to become violent:

- During scene size-up, look around. Locate the patient before approaching (Figure 16–1). Check to see if there are any weapons or items that could be used as weapons such as a knife or blunt object. If there are, assume that the patient may use them to hurt you or himself. Overturned furniture or other signs of chaos also can indicate violent behavior.
- If the patient's family members, friends, or bystanders are at the scene, ask if the patient has a history of being aggressive or combative. Also find out if the patient has been violent or has threatened violence at the scene.
- Expect violence if the patient is standing or sitting in a way that threatens anyone (including him- or herself). Clenched fists, even when the patient is holding them at his or her side, may be a sign.
- Listen to the patient. Expect violence if he or she is yelling, cursing, arguing, or verbally threatening to hurt him- or herself or others.

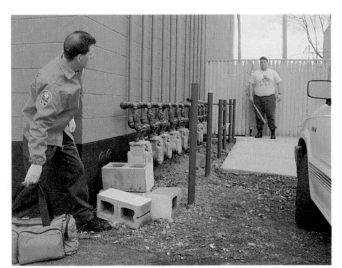

Figure 16-1 Locate the patient before approaching. Check to see if there are any weapons.

- Signs of possible violence in a patient include moving toward you, carrying a heavy or threatening object, making quick or irregular movements, and muscle tension.

Keep the following basic principles in mind whenever you are on the scene of a behavioral emergency.

- Identify yourself. Let the patient know you are there to help.
- Inform the patient of exactly what you are doing. Uncertainty will make the patient more anxious and fearful.
- Ask questions in a calm, reassuring voice. Speak directly to the patient. Stay polite. Use good manners. Show respect. Make no unsupported assumptions.
- Without being judgmental, allow the patient to tell you what happened.
- Show you are listening by rephrasing or repeating part of what is said. Ask questions to show you are paying attention. Also use gestures such as a nod of the head or verbal responses such as "I see" or "Go on."
- Acknowledge the patient's feelings. Use phrases like, "I can see that you are very depressed" or "I am not surprised that you feel frightened."
- Assess the patient's mental status by asking specific questions. Try to determine whether or not the patient is oriented to time, person, and place. Watch the patient's appearance, level of activity, and speech patterns.

GENERAL EMERGENCY CARE

While caring for a patient who has a behavioral emergency, be sure to comfort, calm, and reassure the patient as you proceed.

Never leave the patient alone. All such patients are escape risks, and violence is a real possibility. Once you have responded to a behavioral emergency, the patient's safety is legally your responsibility until someone with more training arrives on scene. Even if the patient pleads to be alone for just a few minutes, do not do it. Firmly explain that you could get in trouble if you did.

If you suspect the patient may have overdosed, provide emergency medical care as described in Chapter 13 for a poisoning patient. Give any medications or drugs you find on scene to the transporting EMS personnel.

Methods to Calm Patients with Behavioral Emergencies

The situations presented by behaviorally disturbed patients are often difficult. However, a number of techniques can help:

- Acknowledge that the patient seems upset, and restate that you are there to help.
- Inform the patient of exactly who you are and what you are going to do to help (Figure 16–2).
- Ask questions in a calm, reassuring voice. Speak directly to the patient.
- Maintain a comfortable distance between you and the patient. Many patients are threatened by physical contact. Unwanted touching could set off a violent response. After you have established some rapport with the patient, get his or her permission before moving in any closer (Figure 16–3).
- Encourage the patient to tell you what is troubling him or her. Ask the patient to explain the problem.

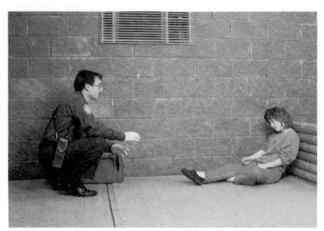

Figure 16-2 Explain who you are and that you are trying to help.

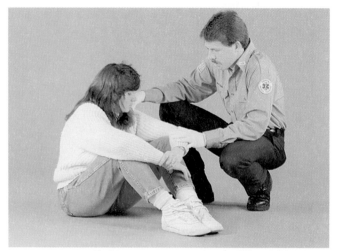

Figure 16-3 With the patient's consent, touch may be comforting.

- Never assume that it is impossible to communicate with the patient until you have tried, even if others insist it cannot be done.
- Do not make any quick movements. Act quietly and slowly. Let the patient see that you are not going to make any sudden moves.
- Respond honestly to the patient's questions. Instead of saying, for example, "You have nothing to worry about," say something like "Even with all your problems, you seem to have lots of people around who really care about you."
- Never threaten, challenge, belittle, or argue with disturbed patients. Remember that the patient is ill. His or her comments are not about you personally.
- Always tell the truth. Never lie to a patient.
- Do not "play along" with a patient's visual or auditory disturbances. Instead, reassure the patient that they are temporary and can clear up with treatment.
- Involve the patient's family members or friends when you can. Some patients are calmed and reassured by their presence. However, others may be upset or embarrassed. Let the patient decide.
- Be prepared to stay at the scene for a long time.
- Avoid unnecessary physical contact. Enlist the help of law enforcement if you are unable to maintain control on your own.
- Maintain good eye contact with the patient. It communicates your control and confidence. Also, the patient's eyes can reflect his emotions. They may tell you if the patient is terri-

fied, confused, struggling, or in pain. The eyes can telegraph intentions, too. If a patient is about to reach for a weapon or make a dash, the eyes may alert you.

Just as with any other patient, place the interests of the patient with a behavioral problem first in all patient care decisions. Communicate with empathy with the patient, as well as with his or her family and friends.

Restraining Patients

Restraint should be avoided unless the patient poses a danger to him- or herself or others. Restraints may require police authorization in your EMS system. Seek medical direction and follow local protocol. If you are not authorized by state law to use restraints, wait for someone with the authority. If you are authorized to use restraints, work in conjunction with other EMS providers and police. (See Figure 16-4.)

Be aware that a violent physical struggle usually is brief. However, after a struggle, some apparently calm patients may cause unexpected and sudden injury to themselves and others.

Avoid using unreasonable force. Never inflict pain or use unnecessary force in restraining a patient. Use only as much force as needed for restraint. **Reasonable force** depends on the amount of force needed to keep a patient from injuring himself or someone else. It depends on:

THE COMBATIVE PATIENT

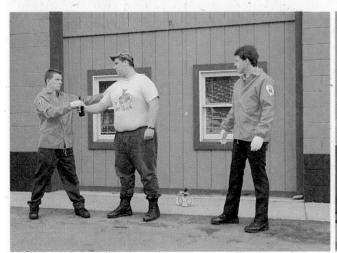

Figure 16-4a If asked to assist other EMS providers, stay beyond the range of the patient's arms and legs.

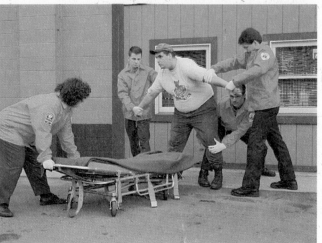

Figure 16-4b If restraints are needed, work in conjunction with an adequate number of other EMS providers.

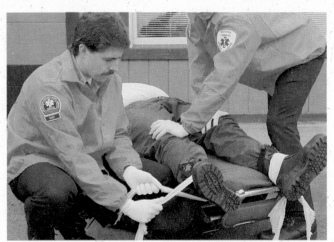

Figure 16-4c You also may be asked to assist the EMTs when they apply the ankle and wrist restraints.

- *The size and strength of the patient.* What may seem reasonable force on a 275-pound athlete may not be reasonable on a 150-pound homemaker.
- *The type of abnormal behavior the patient is exhibiting.* You would not expect to use the same kind of force against a frightened patient who is huddling quietly in a corner as you would against an angry patient who is loudly threatening to kill you.
- *The mental state of the patient.* It may be reasonable to use more force on a patient who is loud and threatening than on a patient who is quiet and subdued.

- *The method of restraint you are using.* Soft leather or cloth straps are called "humane restraints." They are generally considered reasonable. Metal cuffs are not.

In any case the best way to protect yourself legally is to involve your chain of command. A good rule of thumb is to seek medical direction before you restrain a patient. Follow local protocols.

Remember that law enforcement personnel also should be involved when you need to restrain a patient, when you need to give care without consent, and when there is any threat of violence. Law enforcement personnel can help protect you from injury, and they can serve as credible witnesses if a legal case arises.

The best way to protect yourself against false accusations by a patient is to carefully and completely document everything that happens during the call. In most jurisdictions anything you document during the call is legally admissible evidence. Anything that is not documented is considered hearsay (not legally admissible).

Another source of protection is witnesses, preferably throughout the entire course of treatment. It is common for emotionally disturbed patients to accuse medical personnel of sexual misconduct. To protect yourself against such allegations:

- Involve other EMS responders who can testify that there was no misconduct.
- Use EMS responders who are the same gender as the patient.
- Involve third-party witnesses whenever possible.

Legal Considerations

Your legal problems are greatly reduced if an emotionally disturbed patient consents to care. However, such patients commonly refuse treatment—especially patients who are intoxicated or who have taken a drug overdose. They may even threaten you or others.

Unless the patient is considered mentally incompetent, legally he or she must provide consent before you can treat. Remember, the patient—not concerned family members—must consent to care.

Generally, you may provide care against a patient's will only if the patient threatens to hurt him- or herself or others and only if you can demonstrate reason to believe that the patient's threats are real. A good rule of thumb to follow is to consult with medical direction and involve law enforcement.

SECTION 2: DRUG AND ALCOHOL EMERGENCIES

Drug abuse is the self-administration of one or more drugs in a way that is not in accord with approved medical or social practice. An **overdose** is an emergency that involves poisoning by drugs or alcohol. The term **withdrawal** refers to the effects on the body that occur after a period of abstinence from the drugs or alcohol to which the body has become accustomed. Note that withdrawal—especially from alcohol—can be as serious as an overdose emergency.

Most drug overdoses involve drug abuse by long-time drug users. (See Figure 16–5.) However, a drug overdose also can be the result of miscalculation, confusion, use of more than one drug, or a suicide attempt.

Various drugs can cause changes in respiration, heart rate, blood pressure, and central nervous system function. In addition, several major medical problems can result from a drug or alcohol overdose or from sudden withdrawal (Figure 16–6). Among them are:

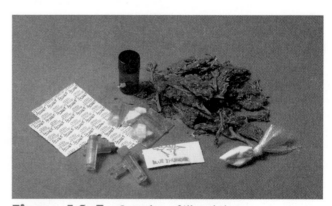

Figure 16-5 Samples of illegal drugs.

EFFECTS OF ALCOHOL AND DRUG ABUSE

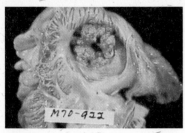

Figure 16-6a Fungal-damaged heart related to drug injections.

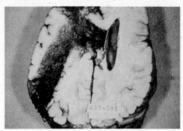

Figure 16-6b Bullet wound to the brain, alcohol-related.

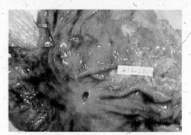

Figure 16-6c Chronic gastric ulcer from alcohol abuse.

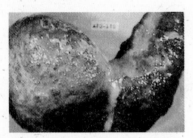

Figure 16-6d Alcoholic cirrhosis of the liver.

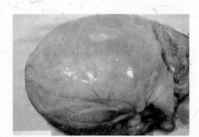

Figure 16-6e Enlarged weak heart, alcohol-related.

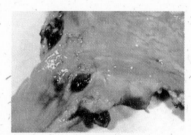

Figure 16-6f Ruptured vein in esophagus, alcohol-induced.

- Respiratory problems.
- Internal injuries.
- Seizures.
- Cardiac arrest.
- Hypothermia or hyperthermia.

PATIENT ASSESSMENT

Signs and symptoms that indicate a life-threatening emergency include (Figure 16–7):

- Unresponsiveness.
- Breathing difficulties or inability to maintain an open airway.
- Abnormal or irregular pulse.
- Fever.
- Vomiting with an altered mental status or without a gag reflex.
- Seizures.

If these signs and symptoms are present, your patient is a high priority for transport. Report to dispatch immediately. Additional signs and symptoms will vary widely. They may include:

- Altered mental status.
- Extremely low or high blood pressure.
- Sweating, tremors, and hallucinations (with alcohol withdrawal).
- Digestive problems, including abdominal pain and bleeding.
- Visual disturbances, slurred speech, uncoordinated muscle movement.
- Disinterested behavior, loss of memory.
- Combativeness.
- Paranoia.

If your patient is unresponsive and you suspect a drug or alcohol emergency, after your initial assessment proceed with the following:

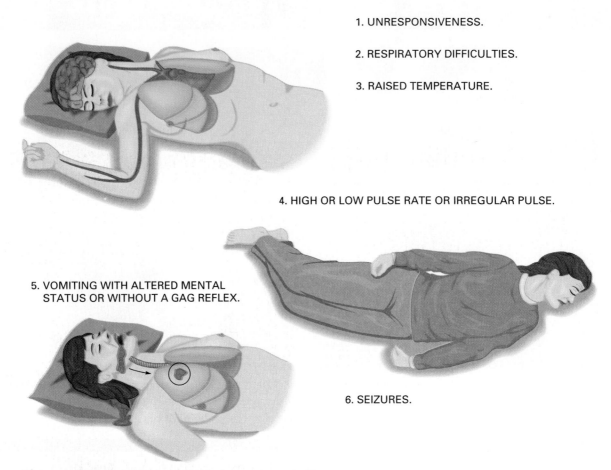

DRUG AND ALCOHOL EMERGENCY INDICATORS

1. UNRESPONSIVENESS.

2. RESPIRATORY DIFFICULTIES.

3. RAISED TEMPERATURE.

4. HIGH OR LOW PULSE RATE OR IRREGULAR PULSE.

5. VOMITING WITH ALTERED MENTAL STATUS OR WITHOUT A GAG REFLEX.

6. SEIZURES.

Figure 16-7 Drug and alcohol emergency indicators.

- With a gloved hand, check the patient's mouth for partially dissolved pills or tablets. If you find any, remove them so they cannot block the patient's airway.
- Smell the patient's breath for traces of alcohol. Do not confuse the smell of alcohol with a musky, fruity, or acetone odor. Those three can indicate an emergency related to diabetes.
- Ask the patient's friends or family members what they know about the incident.

Because signs and symptoms vary so widely and are so similar to many medical conditions, the most reliable indications of a drug- or alcohol-related emergency are likely to come from the scene and the patient history.

GENERAL EMERGENCY CARE

Your immediate goals are to protect your own safety, maintain the patient's airway, and manage life-threatening conditions (Figure 16–8). If you believe the patient has overdosed, follow emergency care directions offered below and in Chapter 13 for poisoning.

After taking BSI precautions, follow these steps:

1. *Establish and maintain an open airway.* Remove anything from the patient's throat or mouth that might obstruct the airway, including false teeth, blood, or mucus. In case of vomiting, turn the patient's head to the side for drainage (unless trauma is suspected).

ALCOHOL EMERGENCIES

CAUTION: Do not immediately decide that a patient with apparent alcohol on the breath is drunk. The signs may indicate an illness or injury such as epilepsy, diabetes, or head injury.

SIGNS OF INTOXICATION
• Odor of alcohol on the breath.
• Swaying and unsteadiness.
• Slurred speech.
• Nausea and vomiting.
• Flushed face.
• Drowsiness.
• Violent, destructive, or erratic behavior.
• Self-injury, usually without realizing it.

EFFECTS
• Alcohol is a depressant. It affects judgment, vision, reaction time, and coordination.
• When taken with other depressants, the result can be greater than the combined effects of the two drugs.
• In very large quantities, alcohol can paralyze the respiratory center of the brain and cause death.

MANAGEMENT
• Give the same attention as you would to any patient with an illness or injury.
• Monitor the patient's vital signs constantly. Provide life support when necessary.
• Position the patient to avoid aspiration of vomit.
• Protect the patient from hurting him or herself.

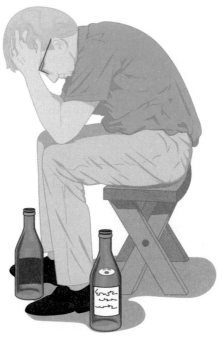

Figure 16-8 Alcohol emergencies.

2. *Monitor the patient's mental status and vital signs frequently.* Overdose patients can be alert one minute and unresponsive the next. Be prepared to provide basic life support if needed.
3. *Maintain the patient's body temperature.* If the patient is cold, cover him or her with blankets. If the patient is abnormally hot, sponge him with tepid water.
4. *Take measures to prevent shock,* which can result from vomiting, profuse sweating, or inadequate fluid intake. Be alert for allergic reactions.
5. *Care for any behavioral problem.* Follow the guidelines given earlier in this chapter for managing behavioral emergencies.
6. *Support the patient.* Comfort, calm, and reassure him or her while waiting for additional EMS personnel to arrive.

If the patient is responsive, try to get him to sit or lie down. Do not restrain a patient unless he poses a risk to safety—his, yours, or that of others.

If you suspect trauma in an unresponsive patient, begin emergency care by immediately stabilizing the patient's head and neck. If there is vomiting, roll the patient as a unit to facilitate drainage.

SECTION 3: RAPE AND SEXUAL ASSAULT

Rape is one of the most devastating crises that can occur in a person's life. It involves both emotional and physical trauma. Legally, **rape** is defined as sexual intercourse that is performed without consent and by compulsion through force, threat, or fraud. **Sexual assault** is defined as any touch that the victim did not initiate or agree to and that is imposed by coercion, threat, deception, or threats of physical violence.

Such crimes often are committed by someone the victim knows, such as a relative, friend or classmate, date, neighbor, or a friend of the parents.

RAPE TRAUMA SYNDROME

An intensely personal experience under forced or terrifying circumstances can destroy a person's inner defenses. Most rape victims go into acute emotional shock during or shortly after the attack. Common physical reactions to rape include:

- Struggling and screaming to avoid penetration.
- Physical and psychological paralysis.
- Pain and shock from penetration or physical abuse.
- Choking, gagging, nausea, vomiting.
- Urinating.
- Hyperventilating.
- Dazed state, unresponsiveness.

Following rape, most patients experience a great deal of disorganization in their lives. This emotional trauma follows a pattern described as **rape trauma syndrome.** It involves four general stages:

- Acute (impact) reaction, which takes effect immediately after the rape and continues for several days.
- Outward adjustment, which lasts for weeks or months after the rape.
- Depression, which is recurring for days and months after the rape.
- Acceptance and resolution, which takes months or years.

Rape is a difficult and complex problem. It involves physical and emotional trauma, as well as significant legal issues. Supporting the patient is of critical importance, especially during the acute reaction stage. So when you care for such a patient, remember that his or her coping system has already been stressed to the limit by the attack.

Note that too often the seriousness of rape is equated with physical damage alone. This is a mistake. Even if there are no external visible injuries, the rape victim will suffer profound emotional trauma.

MANAGING THE RAPE SCENE

Keep the following considerations in mind:

- Be sure EMS has been activated.
- Your immediate reaction to the patient is important. Do not impose your own feelings. Instead, try to find out the patient's emotional state.
- Action can minimize the helplessness the patient may be feeling. Tell the patient what can and should be done immediately.
- The patient might be comforted by a rescuer of his or her own sex (Figure 16–9).
- Perform patient assessment and care as you would for any patient. Treat all life-threats. Check for trauma, especially around the thighs, lower abdomen, and buttocks. If vaginal bleeding is significant, give appropriate care.
- Do not clean the patient. Keep him or her from showering or bathing, brushing teeth, gargling, douching, or urinating. Cleaning could destroy important evidence.
- Once you have cared for the patient's injuries, check the scene for evidence. Bag each piece separately and transport them with the patient. Follow local protocols.

Note that your documentation of the call should include the patient's chief complaint, information about the incident that relates to your care or injuries, and your objective observations and physical findings. Your notes may be used later as evidence in court.

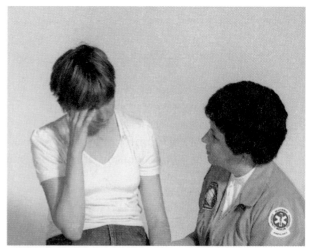

Figure 16-9   It may be best for a First Responder of the same sex to assist the rape patient.

FIRST RESPONDER FOCUS

A psychological crisis can be difficult for any EMS professional to deal with. Medical and trauma emergencies have specific sets of signs and symptoms. Psychological emergencies do not. This can make a psychological emergency awkward for both the patient and the First Responder.

So always assure your personal safety first. Not all patients with psychological emergencies will want to harm you, but you must be cautious. Second, the best way to care for this patient is to use good "people skills." Be empathetic. Listen. Use body language. Usually, if you convey the message that you care about the patient and his or her problems, you have the best chance for successful patient care. Finally, always keep in mind that there are many medical causes for unusual behavior. Never assume the problem is psychological or alcohol-related until medical conditions such as diabetes have been ruled out. ■

CASE STUDY FOLLOW-UP

At the beginning of this chapter, you read that a male patient was having a behavioral emergency. To see how chapter skills apply, read the following. It describes how the call was completed.

PHYSICAL EXAMINATION

I spoke to the patient. He was beginning to calm down a little. He denied any injuries. Knowing that head injuries or other conditions could affect mental status, I did a head-to-toe exam. It had to be quick, since the patient was still quite agitated. Pulse was 88 and bounding. His respirations were 20 and deep.

PATIENT HISTORY

When the patient was quieter, I tried to gather a history. He was talking in a very confused manner. One minute he said he was a god. The next he was crying like a baby. He didn't have any medical identification tags on him. Since he had no clothes, he certainly didn't have a wallet I could check.

One of the officers said he thought he knew the patient's name from a prior call. The dispatcher checked the police computer and found that the man had done this several times before. He was a frequent patient at the psychiatric center in the next county.

ONGOING ASSESSMENT

While the dispatcher's information answered some questions, I still felt that I should monitor the patient in case there was an underlying medical problem. However, the patient soon became agitated again, so I couldn't recheck vitals. There was really no other change that I could see.

PATIENT HAND-OFF

I told the EMTs what I saw and why I called the police. I told them about the possible psychiatric history, the vitals, and that there were no apparent physical injuries. The EMTs asked the police to ride along with them to the hospital.

I later found out that the local hospital transferred the patient back to the psychiatric center. It seemed that whenever he stopped taking his medications, incidents like this would occur.

Your patient's well being is your responsibility as a First Responder. However, your well being is important, too. Call for law enforcement and for additional EMS resources whenever they are needed at the scene. Remember, too, that a patient with a psychological emergency may have a medical problem such as diabetes or overdose. Monitor these patients carefully.

REVIEW QUESTIONS

Page references where answers may be found or supported are provided at the end of each question.

Section 1

1. How can you recognize a patient with a behavioral emergency? (pp. 269–271)
2. How can you know if a patient in a behavioral emergency will be violent? (p. 271)
3. What is the general emergency care of a patient with a behavioral emergency? (pp. 271–274)
4. What are some techniques that can help calm a patient with a behavioral emergency? List at least five. (pp. 271–272)
5. What is the definition of "reasonable force"? What factors would it depend on? (pp. 272–273)

6. Under what conditions would an EMS responder consider using restraints on a patient? (pp. 272–274)

Section 2

7. What are six signs and symptoms that indicate a life-threatening emergency in a drug or alcohol overdose patient? (pp. 274–275)
8. What are the general guidelines for First Responder care of a patient with an alcohol- or drug-related emergency? (pp. 276–277)

Section 3

9. What is the basic management of a scene in which a rape has occurred? (pp. 277–278)

CHAPTER 17

BLEEDING AND SHOCK

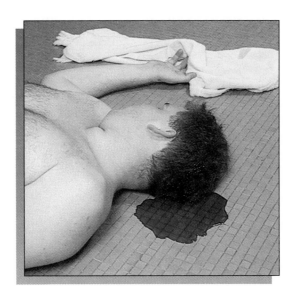

INTRODUCTION

Bleeding associated with trauma can be a significant, life-threatening emergency. If bleeding is left untreated, your patient could deteriorate rapidly, go into shock, and die. Control of severe external bleeding is performed during the initial assessment. Only airway and breathing have a higher priority. Internal bleeding is more difficult to detect and may even be more deadly than external bleeding. Both internal bleeding and shock are treated immediately following the initial assessment.

Cognitive, affective, and psychomotor objectives are from the U.S. DOT's 1995 "First Responder: National Standard Curriculum." Enrichment objectives, if any, identify material that is supplemental to the DOT curriculum.

Cognitive

5-2.1 Differentiate between arterial, venous, and capillary bleeding. (p. 285)

5-2.2 State the emergency medical care for external bleeding. (pp. 285–291)

5-2.3 Establish the relationship between body substance isolation and bleeding. (pp. 282–283)

5-2.4 List the signs of internal bleeding. (p. 291)

5-2.5 List the steps in the emergency medical care of the patient with signs and symptoms of internal bleeding. (p. 291)

Affective

5-2.15 Explain the rationale for body substance isolation when dealing with bleeding and soft tissue injuries. (pp. 282–283)

5-2.16 Attend to the feelings of the patient with a soft tissue injury or bleeding. (pp. 286, 291, 294)

5-2.17 Demonstrate a caring attitude towards patients with a soft tissue injury or bleeding who request emergency medical services. (pp. 286, 291, 294)

5-2.18 Place the interests of the patient with a soft tissue injury or bleeding as the foremost consideration when making any and all patient care decisions. (p. 286)

5-2.19 Communicate with empathy to patients with a soft tissue injury or bleeding, as well as with family members and friends of the patient. (pp. 286, 291, 294)

Psychomotor

5-2.20 Demonstrate direct pressure as a method of emergency medical care for external bleeding. (p. 286)

5-2.21 Demonstrate the use of diffuse pressure as a method of emergency medical care for external bleeding. (p. 286)

5-2.22 Demonstrate the use of pressure points as a method of emergency medical care for external bleeding. (p. 286)

5-2.23 Demonstrate the care of the patient exhibiting signs and symptoms of internal bleeding. (p. 291)

Enrichment

*   Discuss the use of splints and tourniquets as methods of controlling bleeding. (pp. 286–290)
*   Describe emergency medical care of a patient with a nosebleed. (pp. 290–291)
*   List the causes of shock. (pp. 291–292)
*   Describe the compensatory, decompensated, and irreversible stages of shock. (pp. 292–293)
*   Identify the signs and symptoms of shock. (pp. 292–293)
*   Describe the emergency medical care of a patient in shock. (pp. 293–297)
*   Identify the signs and symptoms of anaphylactic shock. (p. 295)
*   Describe the emergency medical care of a patient in anaphylactic shock. (pp. 295–297)

SECTION 1: BLEEDING

PROTECTING AGAINST INFECTION

Always take steps to protect yourself from diseases that can be transmitted by way of blood and body fluids. This is especially urgent when your patient has external bleeding. Body substance isolation (BSI) precautions are your best defense.

This may be a good time to review Chapter 2, "The Well-Being of the First Responder." Briefly, BSI precautions include:

• Keep a barrier between you and the patient's blood and body fluids. At a minimum, wear a pair of protective latex gloves. Also use a face mask with a one-way valve if you must provide ventilations.
• Wear approved goggles, mask, and gown if there is spurting or splashing blood or the potential for it.
• Never touch your mouth, nose, or eyes or handle food while you are giving emergency care.
• Keep all of the patient's open wounds covered with dressings.

CASE STUDY

DISPATCH
Our first response unit was dispatched to a call for a laceration.

SCENE SIZE-UP
When we arrived on scene, we parked at the curb. A woman opened the door of the house and approached our vehicle. She told us that she had been installing linoleum in her kitchen. She slipped with a knife and was bleeding badly from her arm. There were no dangers or hazards we could see, so we exited our vehicle. We put on our gloves and goggles right away.

INITIAL ASSESSMENT
We saw that the woman was holding a blood-soaked towel to her arm. She appeared to be alert and oriented. She had no airway problems and was breathing adequately. Blood was still flowing from beneath the towel.

> What steps would you perform to control this woman's bleeding? How much blood has she lost? At what point could her bleeding become critical? Consider this patient as you read Chapter 17.

• Wash your hands properly as soon as you have finished treating the patient.
• Decontaminate or properly dispose of any item that has been in contact with the patient's blood or body fluids. Follow local protocol.

HOW THE BODY RESPONDS TO BLOOD LOSS

Blood is part of the body's circulatory system (Figure 17–1). The natural response of the body to bleeding—external or internal—is blood vessel constriction and blood clotting. When a serious injury prevents that response, uncontrolled bleeding may be the result.

The sudden loss of one liter (1000 cc) of blood in an adult is serious. About one-half liter

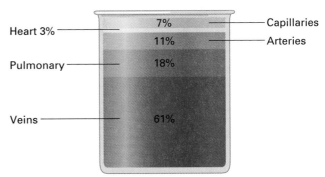

DISTRIBUTION OF BLOOD IN THE BODY

Heart 3% — 7% — Capillaries
11% — Arteries
Pulmonary — 18%
Veins — 61%

Figure 17-1 Blood is part of the circulatory system.

(500 cc) of blood loss is serious in a child. In an infant 100 cc to 200 cc blood loss can be serious. (See Figure 17–2.)

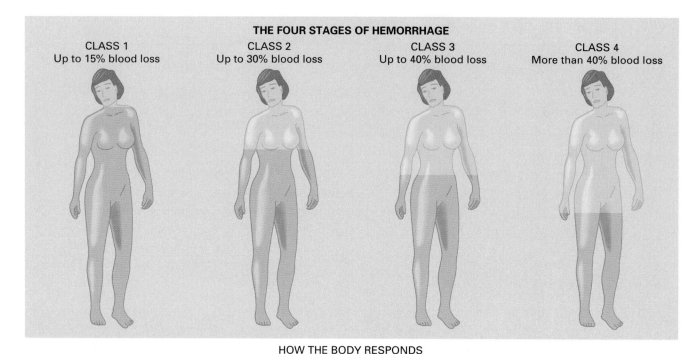

THE FOUR STAGES OF HEMORRHAGE

CLASS 1	CLASS 2	CLASS 3	CLASS 4
Up to 15% blood loss	Up to 30% blood loss	Up to 40% blood loss	More than 40% blood loss

HOW THE BODY RESPONDS

The body compensates for blood loss by constricting blood vessels (vasoconstriction) in an effort to maintain blood pressure and delivery of oxygen to all organs of the body.

EFFECT ON PATIENT

• Patient remains alert.
• Blood pressure stays within normal limits.
• Pulse stays within normal limits or increases slightly; pulse quality remains strong.
• Respiratory rate and depth, skin color and temperature all remain normal.

*The average adult has 5 liters (1 liter = approximately 1 quart) of circulating blood; 15% is 750 ml (or about 3 cups). With internal bleeding 750 ml will occupy enough space in a limb to cause swelling and pain. With bleeding into the body cavities, however, the blood will spread throughout the cavity, causing little, if any initial discomfort.

• Vasoconstriction continues to maintain adequate blood pressure, but with some difficulty now.
• Blood flow is shunted to vital organs, with decreased flow to intestines, kidneys, and skin.

EFFECT ON PATIENT

• Patient may become confused and restless.
• Skin turns pale, cool, and dry because of shunting of blood to vital organs.
• Diastolic pressure may rise or fall. It's more likely to rise (because of vasoconstriction) or stay the same in otherwise healthy patients with no underlying cardio-vascular problems.
• Pulse pressure (difference between systolic and diastolic pressures) narrows.
• Sympathetic responses also cause rapid heart rate (over 100 beats per minute). Pulse quality weakens.
• Respiratory rate increases because of sympathetic stimulation.
• Delayed capillary refill.

• Compensatory mechanisms become overtaxed. Vaso-constriction, for example, can no longer sustain blood pressure, which now begins to fall.
• Cardiac output and tissue perfusion continue to decrease, becoming potentially life threatening. (Even at this stage, however, the patient can still recover with prompt treatment.)

EFFECT ON PATIENT

• Patient becomes more confused, restless, and anxious.
• Classic signs of shock appear—rapid heart rate, decreased blood pressure, rapid respiration and cool, clammy extremities.

• Compensatory vasoconstriction now becomes a complicating factor in itself, further impairing tissue perfusion and cellular oxygenation.

EFFECT ON PATIENT

• Patient becomes lethargic, drowsy, or stuporous.
• Signs of shock become more pronounced. Blood pressure continues to fall.
• Lack of blood flow to the brain and other vital organs ultimately leads to organ failure and death.

Figure 17-2 The four stages of blood loss.

Just how severe bleeding is depends on a number of factors:

- The size of the blood vessel and how fast it is bleeding.
- Whether the blood is flowing from an artery or a vein. (Bleeding from an artery is faster and more profuse.)
- Whether the bleeding is external or internal.
- Whether or not the bleeding is a threat to respiration. (If bleeding is in the patient's airway, it could compromise breathing.)
- The patient's age, weight, and general physical condition.

In general, bleeding is considered severe when the patient's pulse quickens, level of responsiveness falls, breathing rate increases, and blood pressure drops. Uncontrolled bleeding or significant blood loss can lead to shock and, possibly, to death. (Read about shock later in this chapter.)

EXTERNAL BLEEDING

There are three types of external bleeding—**arterial**, **venous**, and **capillary.** Each type can be life-threatening. Each has its own characteristics (Figure 17–3):

- *Arterial bleeding*—Bright red blood spurting from a wound usually indicates a severed or dam-

aged artery. The blood is bright red because it is rich in oxygen. Spurting generally coincides with the patient's pulse or contractions of the heart. Because blood in the arteries is under high pressure, this type of bleeding can be more difficult to control than any other. As the patient's blood pressure drops, the arterial spurting also may decrease (a late sign of shock).

- *Venous bleeding*—Dark red blood that flows steadily from a wound usually indicates a severed or damaged vein. The blood is dark red because it holds little or no oxygen. It flows steadily because it is under less pressure than blood in the arteries. Venous bleeding may be profuse but it is usually easier to control than arterial bleeding.
- *Capillary bleeding*—Dark red blood that oozes slowly from a wound usually indicates damaged capillaries. In most cases, this type of bleeding clots spontaneously and is controlled easily. However, if the body surface involved is large, bleeding may be profuse and threat of infection may be great.

For emergency medical care of a patient with a bleeding wound, follow the general guidelines described below.

Emergency Medical Care

Remember that management of life-threatening bleeding must occur during the initial assessment. Only emergency care of a patient's airway and

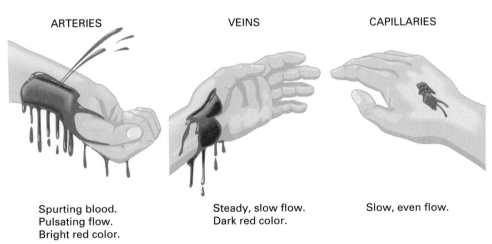

ARTERIES	VEINS	CAPILLARIES
Spurting blood. Pulsating flow. Bright red color.	Steady, slow flow. Dark red color.	Slow, even flow.

Figure 17-3   Types of external bleeding.

breathing takes precedence. In some cases, you may need to care for a patient's airway and breathing at the same time you control bleeding. So, for a patient with external bleeding (Figure 17–4), take BSI precautions and follow these steps (Figure 17–5):

1. *Apply direct pressure to the wound.* If profuse bleeding is discovered during the initial assessment, apply pressure to the bleeding site with your gloved hand until dressings can be applied. Then as soon as possible place a sterile gauze pad or dressing over the bleeding wound. If it is small, apply pressure directly over the point of bleeding using the flat part of your fingertips. If the wound is large and gaping, pack it with sterile gauze and apply direct hand pressure.
2. *Elevate the bleeding extremity.* As you apply direct pressure, lift the bleeding arm or leg above the level of the heart. This should slow the flow of blood and aid in clotting. Note, if you suspect a possible bone or joint injury, do *not* elevate the extremity.
3. *Assess bleeding.* If the wound has bled through the dressing, apply another dressing on top of it. Reapply direct pressure.
4. *Use pressure points.* If the bleeding in an extremity persists, apply pressure to the arterial pulse point to help reduce blood flow (Figures 17–6 and 17–7, pp. 288 and 289, respectively).

- For bleeding in the arm, find the brachial pulse point. Then use the flat surfaces of your fingers to compress the artery against the bone.
- For bleeding in the leg, find the femoral pulse point. Use the heel of one hand to compress it.

Because a number of arteries supply each extremity, you may need to use a pressure point at the same time you apply direct pressure to the wound. Always reassess bleeding immediately after using a pressure point to make sure that it has been controlled.

Be sure to support your patient while you wait for additional EMS personnel to arrive. Communicate with empathy. Comfort, calm, and reassure him or her. Keep safety and patient care your main priorities.

NOTE: In some EMS systems, bleeding control procedures are slightly different. After you find that direct pressure and elevation do not work to stop bleeding, in those systems you are required to remove the first dressing to assess the bleeding point. If it is still bleeding or if there is more than one bleeding point, then you are to apply more pressure directly to the point or points. If this still does not control bleeding, you are to use pressure points as described above. This is a controversial technique. Be sure to follow your own local protocols.

Other Methods of Bleeding Control

Two other methods of bleeding control are the use of splints and the use of a **tourniquet**. Be sure to follow local protocols.

Splints. Bleeding can be life-threatening in an open wound to an extremity that also has a bone or joint injury. If left unsplinted, the bone ends or bone fragments can move, damaging soft tissues and blood vessels and causing more bleeding. Immobilizing the extremity with a splint can help to avoid these problems. (For information on how to apply a splint, see Chapter 24.)

A special splint is used in some EMS systems. An air splint (also called a "pressure splint") can exert pressure to an extremity to help provide additional bleeding control. It may be effective

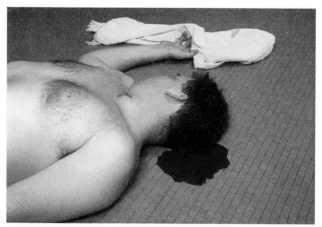

Figure 17-4 Control life-threatening bleeding during the initial assessment of your patient.

METHOD OF BLEEDING CONTROL

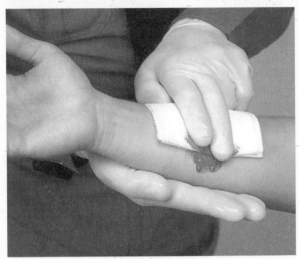

Figure 17-5a Apply direct pressure.

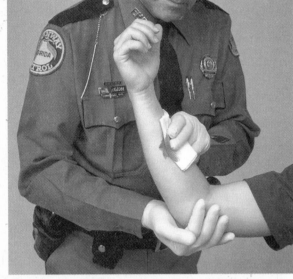

Figure 17-5b Elevate the extremity.

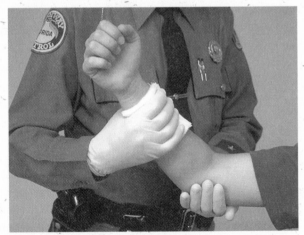

Figure 17-5c Assess bleeding, and apply additional pressure if needed.

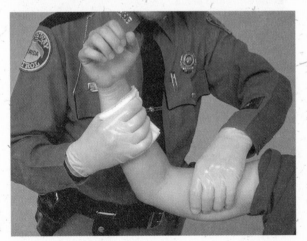

Figure 17-5d If bleeding persists, use a pressure point.

over a wound larger than your hand, which would be difficult to control with direct pressure. Note that an air splint will not provide enough pressure to control arterial bleeding or other types of severe bleeding.

To apply pressure to a bleeding wound with an air splint, be sure the wound is dressed and bandaged first. (See Chapter 24 for information on how to apply an air splint.)

Tourniquets. A tourniquet should be used only as a last resort to control life-threatening bleeding when all other methods have failed. Because it can stop all blood flow to an extremity, use a

ARTERIAL PULSE POINTS

Arterial pulse points are places where an artery lies close to the skin or passes over a bony prominence. When an artery is so located, it can be palpated, or felt with gentle fingertip pressure. Since most body parts are supplied by more than one artery, the use of arterial pressure points alone rarely controls hemorrhage. However, compression of arterial pulse points *in addition to direct pressure* can sometimes help to control severe bleeding. Major arterial pulse points include:

- **Carotid arteries** are located on each side of the neck next to the larynx. These two arteries supply blood to the head. *Do not exert pressure on the carotid pulse points.*

- **Maxillary arteries** supply much of the blood to the face. One can be palpated on each side of the face on the inner surface of the lower jaw.

- **Temporal arteries** supply part of the blood supply to the scalp. One can be palpated on each side of the face just above the upper portion of the ear.

- **Brachial arteries**, located on the inner arms just above the elbows, supply blood to the arms.

- **Radial** and **ulnar arteries**, located in the wrist, also supply blood to the arms and hands.

- **Femoral arteries**, which pass through the groin, supply blood to the legs.

- **Posterior tibial artery**, which passes through the ankle, and the **dorsalis pedis artery**, on the front surface of the foot, can determine circulation to the feet.

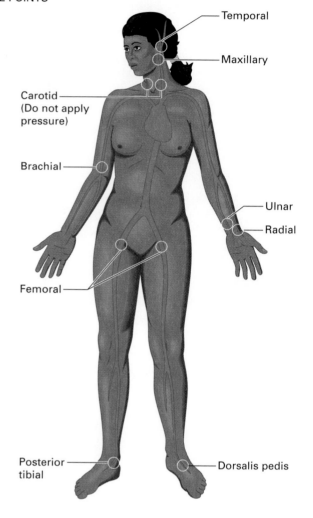

Figure 17-6 Arterial pulse points.

tourniquet only as a last resort. A tourniquet can cause permanent damage to nerves, muscles, and blood vessels, and it can result in the loss of the affected extremity. Always seek medical direction before using a tourniquet and follow local protocols.

To apply a tourniquet (Figure 17–8):

1. Select a bandage 4 inches wide and six to eight layers deep.
2. Wrap it around the extremity twice at a point above but as close to the wound as possible.
3. Tie a knot in the bandage material. Then place a stick or rod on top of it. Tie the ends of the bandage again in a square knot over the stick.
4. Twist the stick until the bleeding stops. Then secure the stick or rod in position.

5. Note the time.
6. Notify the EMTs who take over patient care that you have applied a tourniquet.

In some cases an inflated blood pressure cuff may be used as a tourniquet until bleeding stops. If you choose to do this, you need to monitor the cuff continuously to make sure pressure is maintained.

When using any type of tourniquet, take the following precautions:

- Always use a wide bandage and secure it tightly. Never use a wire, belt, or any other material that could cut the skin or underlying soft tissues.
- Once applied, never loosen or remove a tourniquet unless you are directed to do so by medical direction.

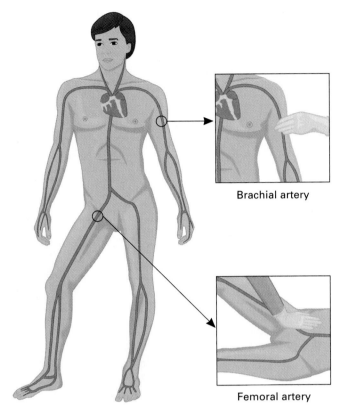

Figure 17-7 Pressure points in the extremities.

Brachial artery

Femoral artery

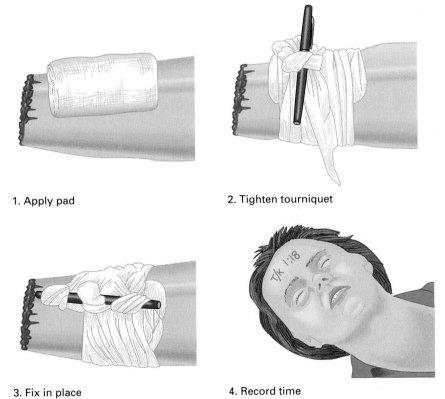

1. Apply pad

2. Tighten tourniquet

3. Fix in place

4. Record time

Figure 17-8 Apply a tourniquet only as a last resort.

- Never apply a tourniquet directly over a joint.
- Always make sure the tourniquet is in open view. A tourniquet that is covered by clothing or bandages may be overlooked, resulting in permanent tissue damage.

Nosebleeds

Nosebleeds are a relatively common source of bleeding. They can result from an injury, disease, activity, the environment, or other causes. Generally, they are more annoying than serious. However, enough blood can be lost to cause shock. In an unresponsive patient, a nosebleed also can be a serious threat to respiration (Figure 17–9).

In most cases a nosebleed may be treated as follows (Figure 17–10):

1. Keep the patient still and calm. Have him or her sit leaning forward in order to prevent aspiration of blood into the lungs. (Do not let the patient lean so far forward that his head is below his heart.) If sitting is impossible because of other injuries, then have the patient lie down with head and shoulders elevated.

2. Apply pressure by pinching the nostrils together. But do so only if you do not suspect a nasal fracture.

3. Apply cold compresses to the nose and face.

4. Instruct the patient to avoid blowing his or her nose for several hours. It could dislodge the clot and restart bleeding.

5. If bleeding continues and is severe enough, activate the EMS system if it has not already been done.

Note that if a fractured skull is suspected, do not try to stop a nosebleed. To do so might increase pressure on the brain. Cover the nasal

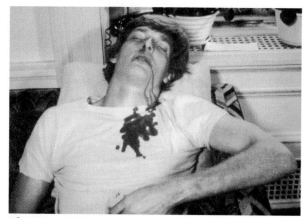

Figure 17-9   A nosebleed in an unresponsive patient can be a serious threat to respiration.

METHOD OF NOSEBLEED CONTROL

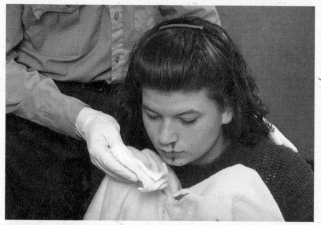

Figure 17-10a   Keep the patient quiet and leaning forward in a sitting position.

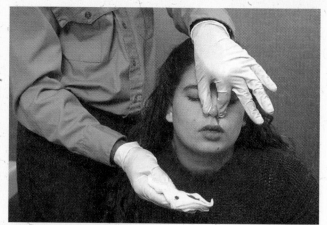

Figure 17-10b   Apply pressure by pinching the nostrils. Also apply cold compresses if needed.

opening loosely instead. Use dry, sterile dressings. Do not apply pressure. Treat the patient for skull fracture as outlined in Chapter 22.

INTERNAL BLEEDING

When internal organs are injured or damaged, they may bleed. This type of bleeding, which is concealed inside the body, is called **internal bleeding.** It may result from a variety of causes including blunt trauma, abnormal clotting, rupture of a blood vessel, or as a result of a fracture (especially a pelvic fracture). Because it is not visible, internal bleeding can result in severe blood loss with rapid progression to shock and death—all in a matter of minutes.

Patient Assessment

The two most common sources of internal bleeding are injured or damaged internal organs and fractured extremities (especially fractures of the femur and pelvis). The severity of internal bleeding depends on the patient's overall condition, age, and the source of the bleeding.

Suspect internal bleeding if the mechanism of injury suggests it and if there is evidence of scrapes and bruises, swelling, deformity, or impact marks. Always suspect it if there are penetrating wounds to the skull, chest, or abdomen. Always suspect it in cases of unexplained shock.

The signs and symptoms of internal bleeding are:

- Discolored, tender, swollen, or hard tissue.
- Increased respiratory and pulse rates.
- Pale, cool, clammy skin.
- Nausea and vomiting bright red blood or blood the color of dark coffee grounds.
- Thirst.
- Changes in mental status including anxiety, restlessness, or combativeness.
- Dark, tarry stools or stools that contain bright red blood.
- Tender, rigid, or distended abdomen.
- Weakness, faintness, or dizziness.

Emergency Medical Care

If you suspect internal bleeding in your patient, update the incoming EMS personnel. This patient is a priority for immediate transport. To care for a patient with internal bleeding, be sure you have taken BSI precautions and follow these steps:

1. Maintain an open airway and adequate breathing. Apply high concentration oxygen by way of a nonrebreather mask, if allowed. Provide artificial ventilation if needed.
2. Control any external bleeding with direct pressure, elevation, and pressure points when necessary.
3. Keep the patient warm, but be careful not to overheat him or her.
4. Treat for shock as described in the next section.

Always support, comfort, calm, and reassure the patient.

SECTION 2: SHOCK

Perfusion refers to the circulation of blood throughout a body organ or structure. Perfusion delivers oxygen and other nutrients to the body's cells and removes waste products.

When the cells of the body do not receive the oxygen and other nutrients they need, they begin to fail and die. **Shock,** or **hypoperfusion,** is a condition that results from the inadequate delivery of oxygenated blood. If the condition persists, cell failure, organ failure, and death will follow. It is therefore imperative to survival for shock to be recognized and treated promptly.

CAUSES OF SHOCK

Shock (hypoperfusion) can be caused by failure of the heart, abnormal dilation of blood vessels, or blood volume loss.

- *Failure of the heart*—Conditions that cause the heart to fail to provide oxygenated blood to the body include heart attack, coronary artery disease, heart-valve disease, pulmonary embolism (a blood clot), tension pneumothorax (air leaking from a lung into the chest cavity), and cardiac tamponade (fluid leaking into the sac around the heart).

HYPOVOLEMIC SHOCK

Watch for shock in all trauma patients. They can lose fluids not only externally through hemorrhage, vomiting, or burns, but also internally through crush injuries and organ punctures.

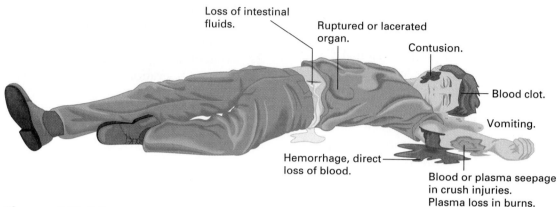

Loss of intestinal fluids.

Ruptured or lacerated organ.

Contusion.

Blood clot.

Vomiting.

Hemorrhage, direct loss of blood.

Blood or plasma seepage in crush injuries. Plasma loss in burns.

Figure 17-11 Loss of body fluids can be both external and internal.

- *Abnormal dilation of the blood vessels*—This is usually the result of a spine or head injury that causes the nervous system to lose control over the blood vessels. The blood vessels dilate (enlarge), causing blood pressure to drop and blood to pool in the outer areas of the body, away from vital organs.
- *Blood volume loss*—This is caused either by external or internal bleeding. It also may result from a profound fluid loss that occurs during illness or injury (Figure 17–11). One example is plasma loss due to burns. Another is dehydration due to diarrhea, vomiting, or excessive urination.

STAGES OF SHOCK

Shock passes through three stages: compensatory, decompensated, and irreversible. As shock progresses, the body works hard to make sure oxygen reaches its cells. (See Figure 17–12.) However, if shock is severe or prolonged, it may become irreversible and end in death.

Compensatory Shock

In the first stage of shock, the body uses its defenses to try to maintain normal function. If the injury does not get worse, the body could overcome the condition. The signs and symptoms of shock at this stage are very subtle. They include:

- Pale skin.
- Slightly rapid heart rate.
- Blood pressure in the normal range.
- Restlessness or anxiety.
- Delayed capillary refill in the infant or child.

Even though it is difficult to identify at this stage, it is vital that you recognize and treat shock early. You must prevent progression to the next more serious stage.

Decompensated Shock

At the decompensated stage, the body can no longer make up for reduced perfusion. Without medical intervention, further decline occurs. The body tries to keep vital organs perfused with oxygenated blood. It shunts blood away from arms, legs, and abdomen and directs it to the brain, heart, and lungs. As a result, tissues in the extremities and abdomen produce toxic by-products. Signs and symptoms include:

- Extreme thirst.
- Rapid heart rate.
- Decreased blood pressure.
- Cool and moist skin that is pale, gray, or bluish and mottled. (See Figure 17–13.)
- Major changes in the patient's mental status.

DEVELOPING SHOCK

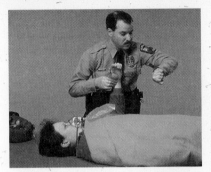

Figure 17-12a Compensatory shock: slight increase in pulse.

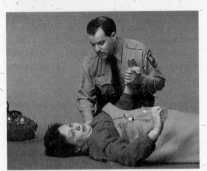

Figure 17-12b Compensatory shock: restlessness or anxiety.

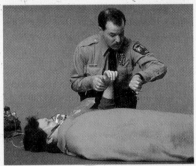

Figure 17-12c Decompensated shock: rapid, weak pulse.

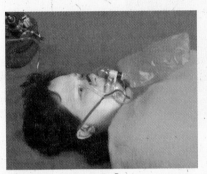

Figure 17-12d Decompensated shock: skin color changes and sweating.

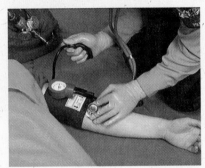

Figure 17-12e Decompensated shock: decreasing blood pressure.

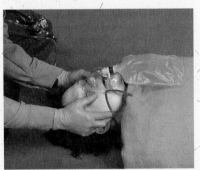

Figure 17-12f Decompensated shock: unresponsiveness.

Decreased blood pressure is a very late sign of shock. Note that infants and children can maintain their blood pressure until blood volume is cut almost in half. Then their condition suddenly and rapidly deteriorates. Dropping blood pressure in an infant or child is an ominous sign.

Irreversible Shock

In the irreversible stage of shock, blood flow is so low that body cells are dying. The main signs are very low blood pressure and extremely rapid pulse. At this stage, blood is shunted away from the liver and kidneys to the heart and brain. The liver and kidneys then die. Blood vessels are no longer able to sustain pressure. So blood begins to pool away from vital organs.

Even with treatment, damage to vital organs is permanent. The inevitable result of irreversible shock is death.

EMERGENCY MEDICAL CARE

Trauma is a major cause of shock in patients. The "Golden Hour" refers to the urgency with which care must be given. It marks the time that elapses from injury until the patient is actually in the operating room.

SIGNS OF SHOCK IN A DARK-SKINNED PATIENT

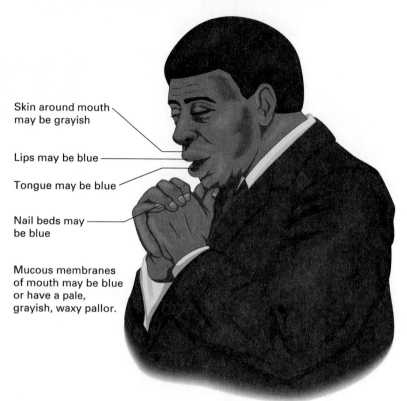

Skin around mouth may be grayish

Lips may be blue

Tongue may be blue

Nail beds may be blue

Mucous membranes of mouth may be blue or have a pale, grayish, waxy pallor.

Figure 17-13   Signs of shock in a dark-skinned patient.

Your role as a First Responder is vital. The general rule is for an ambulance to remain on scene no longer than 10 minutes. You can help keep time to a minimum by identifying serious trauma patients, performing initial assessments and treatment, and preparing patients for transport.

To provide emergency medical care, make sure you have taken BSI precautions and then follow these steps:

1. *Maintain an open airway.* If breathing is adequate, administer oxygen by way of nonrebreather mask at 15 lpm (Figure 17–14). Be prepared to provide artificial ventilation, if needed.
2. *Prevent further blood loss.* Control external bleeding through direct pressure, elevation, and pressure points if necessary.
3. *Elevate the lower extremities* about 8 to 12 inches (Figure 17–15). If there are serious injuries to the head, neck, spine, chest, abdomen, pelvis, or lower extremities, keep the patient supine.
4. *Keep the patient warm,* but do not overheat him or her. Try to maintain normal body temperature. Use a blanket over and under the patient, if necessary, to help prevent loss of body heat.
5. *Provide care for specific injuries* while waiting for EMS crews to arrive.

Be sure to comfort, calm, and reassure the patient while you wait for the EMTs to arrive on scene. Never give anything to the patient to eat or drink. During the ongoing assessment, assess the patient's vital signs every 5 minutes and monitor for changes in mental status. Report your observations to the EMS crew when they take over patient care.

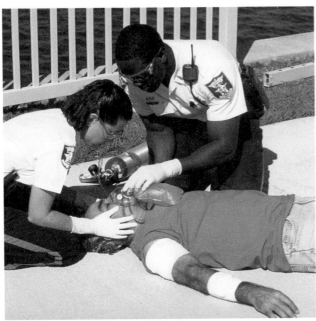

Figure 17-14 Patients in shock have a reduced ability to deliver oxygen to the body. Administer oxygen, if you are allowed.

ANAPHYLACTIC SHOCK

Anaphylactic shock results from a severe allergic reaction to a foreign protein. It can be caused by an insect sting, food, medicine, pollen, or some other inhaled, ingested, or injected substance. The most common causes of anaphylactic shock are drugs and bee stings (Figure 17–16). At least 1% of the general population is at risk for developing anaphylactic shock from bee stings alone.

Anaphylactic shock is a life-threatening medical emergency. A reaction can occur within seconds after a sting or other exposure. Immediate treatment is required to prevent death. Note that the shorter the time between exposure and the appearance of signs and symptoms, the greater the risk of a fatal reaction.

Anaphylactic shock may result in any combination of the following signs and symptoms:

- Skin:
  - Warm, tingling feeling in the mouth, face, chest, feet, and hands.
  - Itching, hives, and flushing.
  - Swelling of the tongue, face, neck, hands, and feet.

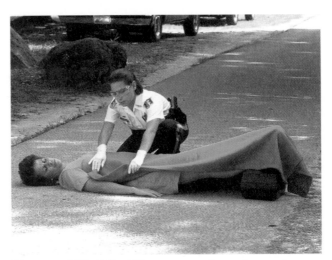

Figure 17-15 When appropriate, elevate the shock patient's feet 8 to 12 inches. Also be sure to keep the patient warm.

  - Cyanosis.
  - Paleness.
- Respiratory system:
  - Swelling of the mouth, tongue, or throat leading to airway obstruction.
  - Painful, squeezing sensation in the chest.
  - Cough, hoarseness (losing the voice).
  - Rapid or labored breathing.
  - Noisy breathing, stridor, wheezing.
- Circulatory system:
  - Increased heart rate.
  - Decreased blood pressure.
  - Dizziness.
  - Restlessness.
- General findings:
  - Itchy, watery eyes.
  - Headache.
  - Runny nose.
  - Sense of impending doom.
  - Decreasing mental status.

General guidelines for emergency care of a patient in anaphylactic shock is described below. Be sure EMS has been activated. The patient needs to be transported rapidly for further life-saving treatment. Arrange for advanced life support (ALS) care, if it is available. Then follow these steps:

1. Perform an initial assessment. Treat all life-threats. Be prepared to provide basic life support if it is needed.

ANAPHYLACTIC SHOCK

A grave medical emergency.
Anaphylactic shock is a severe allergic reaction to an injected, inhaled or ingested foreign protein. Onset can occur within minutes, even seconds.

Early signs and symptoms.
• Flushing, itching. Skin rash
• Sneezing. Watery eyes and nose.
• Airway swelling.
• Cough. "Tickle" or "lump" in the throat that cannot be cleared.
• Gastrointestinal complaints.

The signs and symptoms of anaphylactic shock may swiftly lead to:

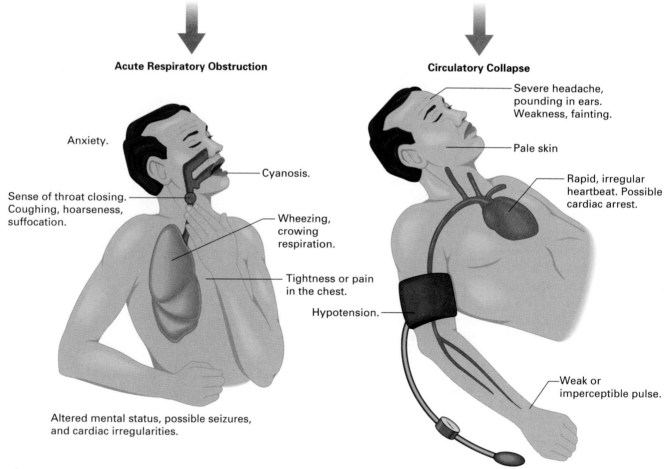

Acute Respiratory Obstruction

Anxiety.

Cyanosis.

Sense of throat closing. Coughing, hoarseness, suffocation.

Wheezing, crowing respiration.

Tightness or pain in the chest.

Altered mental status, possible seizures, and cardiac irregularities.

Circulatory Collapse

Severe headache, pounding in ears. Weakness, fainting.

Pale skin

Rapid, irregular heartbeat. Possible cardiac arrest.

Hypotension.

Weak or imperceptible pulse.

Figure 17-16 The most common causes of anaphylactic shock are drugs and bee stings.

2. Administer 100% high-flow oxygen, if you are equipped and allowed to do so. If breathing is adequate, deliver it by way of a nonrebreather mask. If the patient needs artificial ventilation, use supplemental oxygen.

3. Assist the patient with his or her medications, if local protocol allows. Medications may include an epinephrine auto-injector or antihistamines.

If the reaction is due to an insect sting or injection, local protocol may direct you to place a constricting band between the injection site and the heart. (See Chapter 15 for more specific directions.)

During your ongoing assessment of the patient, monitor the patient's ABCs continually. Be prepared to deliver basic life support if it is needed.

FIRST RESPONDER FOCUS

Severe bleeding is controlled during initial assessment and treatment. The only other problems that take priority concern the airway and breathing. Be assured, however, that even severe bleeding can be controlled by the simple methods described in this chapter—direct pressure, elevation, and pressure points. Experienced First Responders and EMTs will tell you that these methods work. Use them appropriately and confidently. ■

CASE STUDY FOLLOW-UP

At the beginning of this chapter, you read that First Responders were on scene with a woman who was bleeding from an arm. To see how chapter skills apply to this emergency, read the following. It describes how the call was completed.

INITIAL ASSESSMENT (*Continued*)

I saw blood flowing steadily from beneath the towel. This, combined with the amount of blood at the scene, indicated severe bleeding. I removed the towel, applied a sterile dressing, and direct pressure to the wound. The bleeding stopped in two or three minutes. I kept up the pressure for a bit longer to make sure the bleeding stayed under control. Lian, my partner, updated the EMTs.

PHYSICAL EXAMINATION

The patient claimed to have slipped with her knife. She denied injuring any other part of her body. My partner scanned the patient and revealed that this appeared to be true. The patient did not fall or lose consciousness. There was no need to do a further assessment. My partner took vitals. Pulse was 92, strong and regular. Respirations were 16 and adequate. Blood pressure was 118/84. The patient's skin was cool and dry.

PATIENT HISTORY

The patient claimed to be in good health. She took no medications, had no medical problems she knew of, and had a physical examination last year. She denied any allergies. She had Chinese food for lunch about two hours ago.

ONGOING ASSESSMENT

We took another set of vitals. Pulse was 88, strong and regular. Respirations were 16 and adequate. Blood pressure was 120/78. Her skin was cool and dry.

We rechecked the status of our bleeding control. The blood had been stopped for several minutes. We applied a pressure bandage to maintain pressure over the wound. We were careful not to cut off the patient's circulation. The EMTs arrived shortly after.

CASE STUDY FOLLOW-UP *(Continued)*

PATIENT HAND-OFF

We advised the EMTS that the bleeding was under control and reported:

"This is Jill Romano, a 27-year-old homemaker, who slipped with her knife while installing linoleum. The knife caused about a four-inch laceration to her left arm. The bleeding was steadily flowing on our arrival but was quickly brought under control by direct pressure. She did not lose consciousness or suffer any further injuries. Jill has no past medical history, no meds, no allergies. Her vitals are pulse 88 strong and regular, respirations 16, blood pressure 120/78, skin cool and dry. Jill had Chinese food for lunch about two hours ago. We applied a pressure bandage. The bleeding is controlled and there is good circulation distal to the bandage."

The EMTs took over care and applied oxygen to the patient. They transported her to the hospital. It was one of the worst cases of bleeding I had seen. I was glad to get it under control. We saw the EMTs later. They told us that the patient's wound took a lot of stitches. They also told us she had sliced open her leg on another home repair project three months ago. She was considering another hobby.

> A patient's blood can be an unnerving sight, especially if bleeding is profuse. One way to stay clear-headed is to stick to your patient assessment plan. Always start with scene size-up. Move to initial assessment and treatment. And continue, if you can, with a physical exam, a patient history, ongoing assessment, and patient hand-off. Remember, your patient's well-being depends on it.

REVIEW QUESTIONS

Page references where answers may be found or supported are provided at the end of each question.

Section 1

1. How could you identify arterial, venous, and capillary bleeding? (p. 285)
2. What is the emergency medical care for external bleeding? Describe each step briefly. (pp. 285–286)
3. What are the two most common sources of internal bleeding? (p. 291)

4. What is the emergency medical care of a patient with internal bleeding? (p. 291)

Section 2

5. What are the signs and symptoms of shock (hypoperfusion)? (pp. 292–293)
6. How should you care for a patient in shock? (pp. 293–294)

CHAPTER 18

SOFT-TISSUE INJURIES

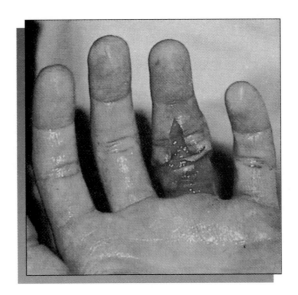

INTRODUCTION

Injuries to a patient's skin, muscles, nerves, and blood vessels are among the most common you will care for. Some will be minor cuts, scrapes, and bruises. Others may be life-threatening. Whatever your patient's soft-tissue injuries may be, your priorities will include controlling bleeding, preventing further injury, and reducing the risk of infection.

OBJECTIVES

Cognitive, affective, and psychomotor objectives are from the U.S. DOT's 1995 "First Responder: National Standard Curriculum." Enrichment objectives, if any, identify material that is supplemental to the DOT curriculum.

Cognitive

5-2.6 Establish the relationship between body substance isolation (BSI) and soft tissue injuries. (pp. 303, 305)

5-2.7 State the types of open soft tissue injuries. (pp. 303, 305)

5-2.8 Describe the emergency medical care of the patient with a soft tissue injury. (pp. 305–306)

5-2.9 Discuss the emergency medical care considerations for a patient with a penetrating chest injury. (pp. 306–307)

5-2.10 State the emergency medical care considerations for a patient with an open wound to the abdomen. (pp. 308–309)

5-2.11 Describe the emergency medical care for an impaled object. (p. 307)

5-2.12 State the emergency medical care for an amputation. (pp. 309–310)

5-2.14 List the functions of dressing and bandaging. (pp. 312–313)

Affective

5-2.15 Explain the rationale for body substance isolation when dealing with bleeding and soft tissue injuries. (pp. 303, 305)

5-2.16 Attend to the feelings of the patient with a soft tissue injury or bleeding. (pp. 305–306)

5-2.17 Demonstrate a caring attitude towards patients with a soft tissue injury or bleeding who request emergency medical services. (pp. 305–306)

5-2.18 Place the interests of the patient with a soft tissue injury or bleeding as the foremost consideration when making any and all patient care decisions. (pp. 305–306)

5-2.19 Communicate with empathy to patients with a soft tissue injury or bleeding, as well as with family members and friends of the patient. (pp. 305–306)

Psychomotor

5-2.24 Demonstrate the steps in the emergency medical care of open soft tissue injuries. (pp. 305–306)

5-2.25 Demonstrate the steps in the emergency medical care of a patient with an open chest wound. (pp. 306–307)

5-2.26 Demonstrate the steps in the emergency medical care of a patient with open abdominal wounds. (pp. 308–309)

5-2.27 Demonstrate the steps in the emergency medical care of a patient with an impaled object. (p. 307)

5-2.28 Demonstrate the steps in the emergency medical care of a patient with an amputation. (pp. 309–310)

5-2.29 Demonstrate the steps in the emergency medical care of an amputated part. (p. 309)

Enrichment

* Describe the emergency medical care for a patient with a large open neck wound. (p. 308)
* State the general principles of dressing and bandaging soft-tissue injuries. (pp. 314–317)

SECTION 1: SOFT-TISSUE INJURIES

Soft-tissue injuries are injuries to the skin, muscles, nerves, and blood vessels. They are often dramatic, but they are rarely life-threatening. They can be serious, however, if they lead to airway or breathing problems, uncontrolled bleeding, or shock.

A soft-tissue injury is commonly referred to as a **wound.** Wounds may be classified as open or closed, single or multiple. They also are classified by location (head wounds or chest wounds, for example).

In general, emergency medical care focuses on controlling bleeding, preventing further injury,

CASE STUDY

DISPATCH

I work as a lathe operator at the mill. I'm also a First Responder. One day the emergency signal broke into the noise of the machines. I called in and was told to report to Building B.

SCENE SIZE-UP

My partner and I arrived at the main entrance, where a guard directed us to the injury site. He advised us that there were no dangers. A worker had a piece of wood impaled in one hand. We put on protective gloves and glasses and approached the scene.

INITIAL ASSESSMENT

The patient was standing near a workbench. We saw that mental status, airway, and breathing were okay because she was swearing quite loudly about her injury. We approached and identified ourselves. There was surprisingly little bleeding coming from the wound. We calmed the woman down and asked her to sit while we assessed the injury.

We reported the patient's status and the nature of the injury to the incoming EMTs. Their ETA was 10 minutes.

> Consider this patient as you read Chapter 18.
> What may be done to treat her condition?

and reducing the risk of infection. Unless a life-threat, a soft-tissue injury is usually cared for after the initial assessment.

CLOSED WOUNDS

In a **closed wound,** soft tissues beneath the skin are damaged (Figure 18–1). The skin itself is not broken. There are three general types of closed wounds. They are a **contusion,** or bruise, a **clamping injury,** and a **crushing injury.**

Generally, contusions are characterized by swelling and pain at the injury site. If small blood vessels have been broken, the patient also will have **ecchymosis** (black and blue discoloration). If large blood vessels have been torn, a **hematoma** (a collection of blood beneath the skin) is evident as a lump with bluish discoloration.

A clamping injury usually involves a finger or limb stuck in an area smaller than itself. This type of injury occurs when a patient reaches into a space and is stuck there. The body part can swell rapidly, making the condition worse. Another type of clamping injury occurs when an object, such as a ring, strangles a body part that was previously injured.

Blunt trauma is caused by a sudden blow or force that has a crushing impact. A crushing injury may be open or closed. Either way, it can be treacherous. Blunt trauma can cause serious internal injuries, including organ rupture, with few external signs. A patient may look fine at first and then very quickly slip into shock. The result

CLOSED WOUNDS

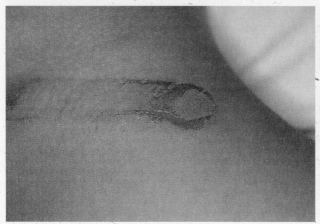
Figure 18-1a Contusions.

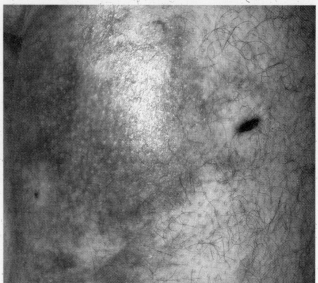
Figure 18-1b Hematoma.

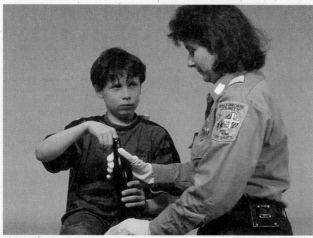
Figure 18-1c Clamping injury.

can be decompensated shock and death. For this reason, always suspect internal damage in patients with injuries involving blunt force.

General Guidelines for Emergency Care

Small contusions generally do not need treatment. Cold compresses help to relieve pain and reduce swelling in larger contusions.

For a clamping injury, a lubricant such as green soap may help to free the body part. If not, then it may need to be removed at the hospital. Apply a cold pack to help reduce swelling. Since circulation to the body part may be reduced, do not cool it for longer than 15 to 30 minutes at a time. Elevate the injured part above the level of the heart. Keep it well supported.

Large areas of discoloration of the skin can indicate serious internal bleeding. A bruise the size of a fist, for example, could mean a 10% blood loss. If the patient has a large contusion, or if the mechanism of injury suggests a crushing injury caused by blunt trauma, treat the patient for internal bleeding. Be sure to assess carefully for broken bones, especially when swelling or deformity is present.

If you are ever in doubt about the seriousness of a closed wound, treat the patient for internal bleeding.

NOTE: Always take BSI precautions when there is any possibility that you will come in contact with a patient's blood or other body fluids. When caring for a patient with closed wounds, at a minimum wear protective latex gloves.

OPEN WOUNDS

When skin breaks as a result of a blow, the wound is referred to as an **open injury.** (See Figure 18–2.) Open injuries place the patient at

risk for contamination, which can lead to infection. An open injury also may be the first indicator of a deeper, more serious injury such as a fracture.

Abrasions

An **abrasion** is an open wound caused by scraping, rubbing, or shearing away of the epidermis (outermost layer of skin). Even though an abrasion is considered a superficial injury, it is often very painful because of exposed nerve ends. Though there may be no bleeding at all from an abrasion, in most cases, there is capillary bleeding.

Small abrasions usually are not life-threatening. Large ones, however, may be cause for concern. For example, a motorcycle rider who is thrown and slides across the pavement will sustain head-to-toe abrasions ("road rash"). Bleeding in such a case may not be serious, but contamina-

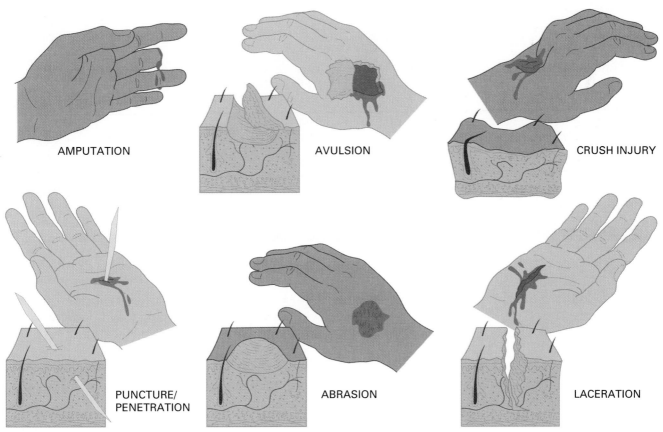

AMPUTATION

AVULSION

CRUSH INJURY

PUNCTURE/
PENETRATION

ABRASION

LACERATION

Figure 18-2 Open wounds.

ABRASIONS AND LACERATIONS

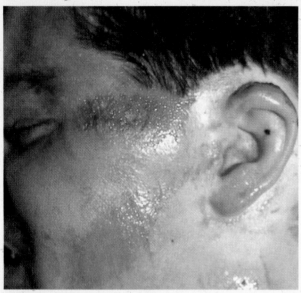

Figure 18-3a Abrasions.

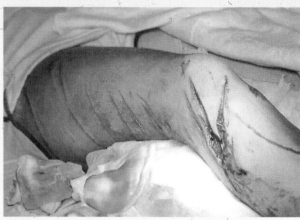

Figure 18-3b Lacerations.

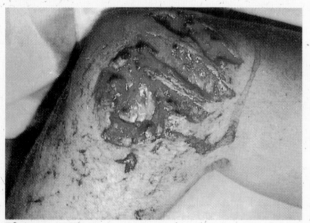

Figure 18-3c Deep abrasions and lacerations.

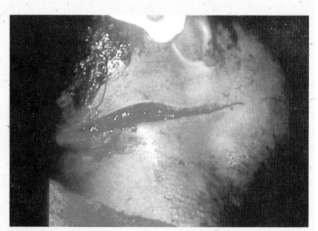

Figure 18-3d Laceration.

tion, infection, and the potential for underlying injuries may be.

Lacerations

A **laceration** is a break of varying depth in the skin. It may occur in isolation. It also may occur with other types of soft-tissue injuries (Figure 18–3). Lacerations are caused by forceful impact with a sharp object. Bleeding may be severe, especially if an artery is involved.

The edges of a laceration may be regular or irregular. Regular lacerations are usually caused by a knife or razor. They may heal better because their edges are smoother. Irregular lacerations are commonly caused by a blunt object, serrated knife, or broken bottle. The edges of the wound are jagged, and healing is usually prolonged.

Penetration/Puncture Wounds

A **penetration/puncture wound** is usually the result of a sharp, pointed object being pushed or driven into soft tissues. This type of injury may have both an entry wound and an exit wound.

The entry wound may be small, and there may be little or no external bleeding (Figure 18–4). However, such injuries may be deep, damaging, and cause severe internal bleeding. A gunshot injury is a good example (Figure 18–5). The entry wound in many cases is smaller than the exit wound. If the patient was shot at close range, the entry wound may be surrounded by powder burns. The larger exit wound generally bleeds more profusely.

The overall severity of a penetration or puncture wound depends on the following factors:

* The location of the injury.
* The size of the penetrating object.
* The forces involved in creating the injury.

It can be difficult to determine the extent of these injuries based only on external signs. So treat penetration or puncture wounds with great caution.

General Guidelines for Emergency Care

Since it is likely that you will be exposed to your patient's blood and body fluids, take all appropriate BSI precautions. Wear protective latex gloves. Protect your face and eyes, and wear a disposable gown, as necessary. After patient care, wash your hands—even if you wore gloves. Handwashing is still the single most important thing you can do to prevent the spread of infection.

To care for a patient with an open soft-tissue injury, follow the guidelines outlined below.

1. *Assess and treat all life-threats.* Maintain a patent airway and adequate breathing. Administer oxygen by way of a nonrebreather mask. If the patient's breathing is inadequate, provide ventilations with supplemental oxygen, if allowed.
2. *Expose the entire injury site.* Cut away clothing, if needed. Then clear the area of blood and debris with sterile gauze or the cleanest material available. Remember to look for additional wounds or injuries, especially in the case of a gunshot wound. (Often multiple gunshots wounds are involved.)
3. *Control bleeding.* Begin with direct pressure and elevation. If bleeding still is not controlled, then use a pressure point.
4. *Prevent further contamination.* Keep the wound as clean as possible. If there are loose particles of foreign matter around the wound, wipe them away from the wound, never toward it. Never try to pick embedded particles or debris out of the wound.
5. *Dress and bandage the wound.* Apply a dry sterile dressing. Then secure it with a bandage. Check distal pulses both before and after applying the bandage to make sure it is not cutting off circulation.

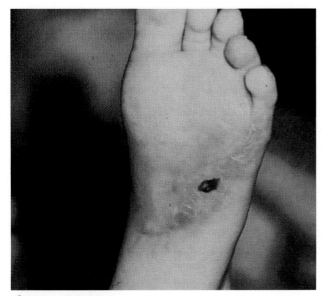

Figure 18-4 Puncture wound to the foot.

As you care for a patient's soft-tissue injuries—especially when there are open, bleeding ones, be careful what you say and do. Do not alarm the

GUNSHOT WOUNDS

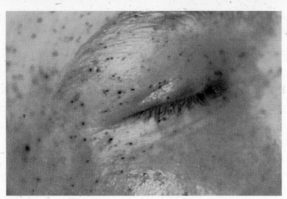

Figure 18-5a Powder burns from a gunshot.

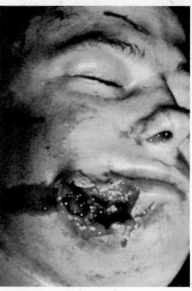

Figure 18-5b Gunshot wound to the chin.

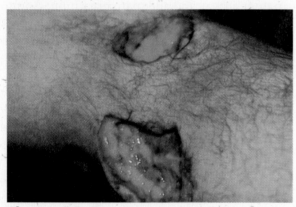

Figure 18-5c Entrance and exit gunshot wounds.

patient by your reaction to the wounds. In fact, it will help the patient significantly if you would do your best to be comforting, calming, and reassuring. If possible, also keep the patient's family members who are on scene informed and reassured.

SPECIAL CONSIDERATIONS

Some open wounds need special consideration. Basic emergency medical care is the same as for all other open wounds, but there are certain excep-

tions, which are described below. In all of these cases, administer oxygen by way of a nonrebreather mask or, if breathing is inadequate, provide ventilations with supplemental oxygen.

Chest Injuries

A penetrating chest wound can prevent a patient from breathing adequately. In this case, apply an **occlusive dressing.** (This is a special type of dressing used to form an air-tight seal.)

Secure the dressing with tape on three sides (Figure 18–6). Leave one side untaped to allow air to escape as the patient exhales. This will help

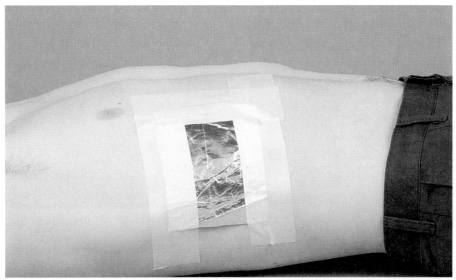

Figure 18-6 Occlusive dressing taped on three sides for a chest injury.

to prevent a condition called *tension pneumothorax*, a severe build-up of air that compresses the lungs and heart toward the uninjured side of the chest.

Let the patient assume a position of comfort, if you do not suspect spinal injury. Generally, the patient will favor the position that allows for the greatest chest expansion. Assume spinal injury if there is any significant mechanism of injury to the chest, including a gunshot wound.

Impaled Objects

An **impaled object** is an object that is embedded in an open wound. It should never be removed in the field unless it is through the patient's cheek or it interferes with airway management or CPR. To provide emergency care to a patient with an impaled object, follow these guidelines:

1. Manually secure the object to prevent any motion. Motion could cause further damage and bleeding.
2. Expose the wound area. Remove clothing from around it, but remember to take care not to move the object at all.
3. Control bleeding. Apply direct pressure to the edges of the wound. Avoid putting pressure directly on the impaled object.
4. Use a bulky dressing to help stabilize the object (Figure 18–7). Surround the entire

object with dressings. Pack them around the object, and tape it securely in place. A ring or doughnut pad may be used to stabilize it (Figure 18–8).

When an object is impaled in a patient's cheek, bleeding can interfere with breathing. If this is the case, then remove the object as follows (Figure 18–9):

1. While maintaining an open airway, feel inside the patient's mouth with gloved fingers. Find out if the object has penetrated completely.
2. Remove the object in the direction in which it entered.

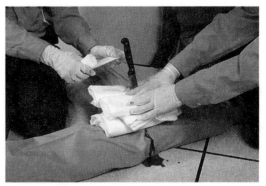

Figure 18-7 Bulky dressings can help to stabilize an impaled object.

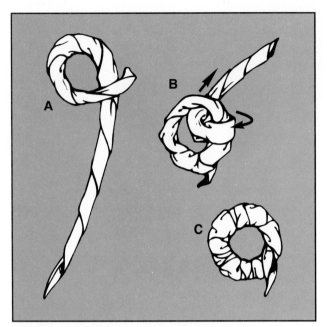

Figure 18-8 An alternative is to use a doughnut-type ring pad to stabilize an impaled object.

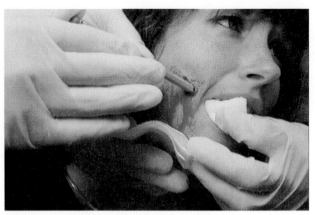

Figure 18-9 An impaled object in the cheek.

3. Control bleeding from the outside of the cheek. Then dress the wound.
4. If the object penetrated the cheek completely, pack sterile gauze between the cheek wall and the teeth.
5. Continue to monitor the airway. Suction when necessary.

You may encounter resistance when you try to remove the object from the cheek. If so, maintain an open airway and suction as needed. Stabilize the object while you wait for the EMTs to arrive on scene. Position the patient on his or her side for drainage.

Large Open Neck Wounds

Severe bleeding from a wound involving a major blood vessel of the neck is a serious emergency. In addition to the possible loss of a great deal of blood, there is danger of air being sucked into a neck vein and carried to the heart. This can be lethal. Also suspect spine injury with any significant injury to the neck.

In this case, control of bleeding and prevention of an air embolism (air bubble) are your major goals. Follow these steps:

1. Immediately place a gloved hand over the wound to control bleeding.
2. Apply an occlusive dressing. Make sure it extends beyond the wound on all sides to prevent it from being sucked in. Tape the dressing on all four sides.
3. Cover the occlusive dressing with a regular one. Then apply enough pressure to control the bleeding. Compress the carotid artery only if it is severed.
4. Once bleeding is controlled, apply a pressure dressing. Do not restrict air flow or compress major blood vessels. Do not apply a dressing that circles the neck.

Eviscerations

An **evisceration** occurs when internal organs protrude from an open wound. This most commonly occurs with abdominal wounds.

When you care for a patient with an evisceration, never try to replace protruding organs and never touch them. You could cause further damage and contaminate both the organs and the cavity from which they protrude.

Cover the exposed organs with a thick, moist, sterile dressing. You can moisten the dressing with sterile water or saline. The dressing should be large enough to cover all protruding organs. Sterile gauze is preferred. Never use absorbent materials such as toilet tissue or paper towels, which can shred and cling to the organs. Loosely cover the moistened dressing with an occlusive (airtight) dressing. (See Figure 18–10.)

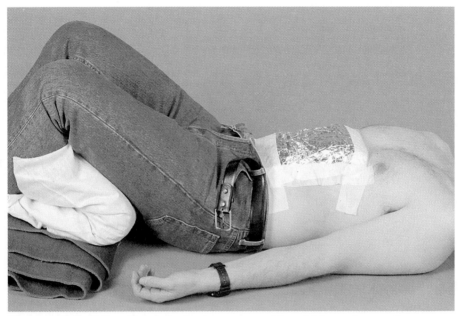

Figure 18-10 Abdominal evisceration with a thick, moist, sterile dressing and an occlusive covering.

Maintain the temperature of the wound area by covering the dressing with layers of a more bulky dressing such as a particle-free bath blanket or towel. The dressings may be held loosely in place with a bandage or clean sheet.

Amputations

In an **amputation,** a body part has been completely severed from the body (Figure 18–11). This is the result of ripping or tearing forces, often from an industrial accident or motor vehicle crash. Massive bleeding usually is present. In some cases, however, the elasticity of the blood vessels helps them to contract and bleeding is minimal. Care for an amputation in the same way you care for all open injuries.

With amputations, you also must care for the amputated part. First provide emergency care to the patient. Do not spend time looking for the amputated body part. If possible, have other First Responders or support personnel search for it. Once the body part is found, follow these guidelines (Figure 18–12):

1. Wrap the amputated part in sterile gauze that is moistened with sterile saline.

2. Place the amputated part in a plastic bag. Label the bag with the patient's name and the date and time the part was bagged. Never immerse the part in water.

3. Keep the amputated part cool. Place the bagged part in a larger bag or container of ice and water. Do not use ice alone. Never use dry ice. Never place the part directly on ice. Mark the container with the patient's name, date, and body part.

4. Give the packed part to arriving EMS personnel, so they can transport it with the patient to the hospital.

Note that if the amputation is partial, never complete it. Care for the injury as you would any other soft-tissue injury. Make sure that the partially amputated part is not twisted or constricted.

Avulsions

An **avulsion** is a torn flap of skin or soft tissue that has been torn loose or pulled off completely. (See Figure 18–13.) Healing generally is prolonged and scarring may be extensive.

AMPUTATIONS

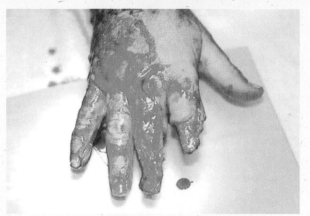

Figure 18-11a Finger amputation.

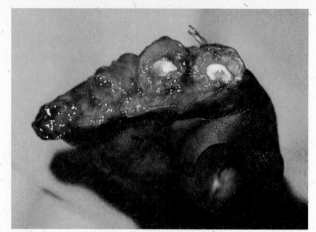

Figure 18-11b Finger amputation.

Avulsions are most commonly the result of accidents with industrial or home machinery and motor vehicles. They commonly involve the fingers, toes, hands, feet, forearms, legs, ears, and nose. The seriousness of the injury depends on how well blood can circulate to the avulsed skin. If it is still attached and the flap is folded back, circulation may be compromised severely. If this is the case, emergency care includes making sure the flap is lying flat and aligned in its normal position.

Bites

Bite wounds can be quite serious (Figure 18–14). Even when they look minor, soft tissues may be badly lacerated and the threat of infection is usually high. During emergency care, wash a bite wound with plenty of warm, soapy water. Check it for any teeth fragments, too.

Note that you should not kill the animal who bit your patient unless absolutely necessary to stop an attack. If you do kill the animal, call an animal control officer and request that the corpse

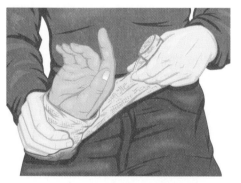

(1) Wrap completely in saline-moistened sterile dressings.

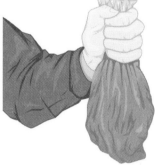

(2) Place in plastic bag and seal shut.

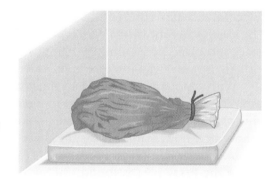

(3) Place sealed bag on top of a cold pack or another sealed bag of ice. Do not allow the tissue to freeze.

Figure 18-12 Emergency care for an amputated part.

AVULSIONS

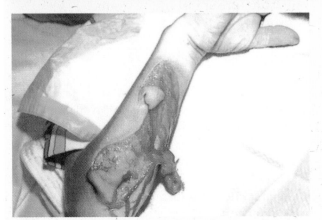

Figure 18-13a Avulsion to the forearm.

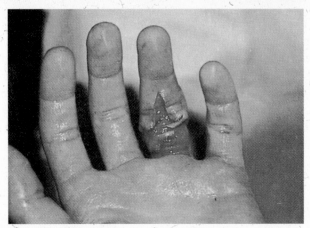

Figure 18-13b Ring avulsion.

be examined for *rabies*, a viral infection that affects the nervous system. If you do not kill the animal, try to trap it in some kind of enclosure so that it can be examined for rabies. Take care not to injure the animal's head. Remember to protect yourself from any danger.

If the animal is not present, find out where it can be located. If getting an address is not possible, obtain a description of it, where it was encountered, and whether or not the attack might have been provoked. Follow local protocols on reporting requirements.

BITES

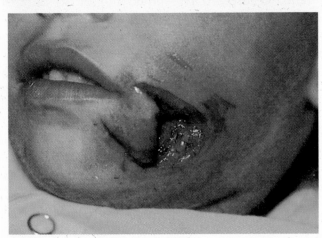

Figure 18-14a Horse bite.

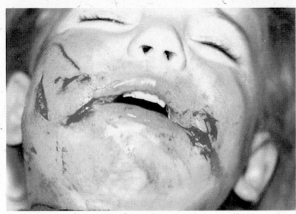

Figure 18-14b Dog bite.

SECTION 2: DRESSING AND BANDAGING WOUNDS

The basic purposes of dressing and bandaging are to control bleeding, prevent further contamination and damage to the wound, keep the wound dry, and immobilize the wound site. Proper wound care also enhances healing. It adds to the comfort of the patient, and it promotes more rapid recovery. Improper wound care can cause infection, severe discomfort and, in rare cases, result in the loss of a limb.

DRESSINGS

A **dressing** is a covering for a wound (Figure 18–15). It should be **sterile** (free of all microorganisms and spores). Ideally, a dressing is layered and consists of coarse mesh gauze. It also should be absorbent and large enough to protect the entire wound from contamination. In an emergency, you can use clean handkerchiefs, towels, sheets, cloth, or sanitary napkins as dressings. Never use elastic bandages, which have a tourniquet effect. Never use toilet tissues, paper towels, or other materials that can shred and cling to a wound.

Types of dressings include:

- *Gauze pads*—These are usually individually wrapped and sealed to prevent contamination. Take care not to touch the portion of gauze that is to make contact with the wound. Unless otherwise specified, all gauze dressings should be covered with open triangular, cravat, or roller bandages.
- *Trauma dressing*—Large and absorbent, this type of dressing is used on larger injuries and when maximum absorbency is needed.
- *Bandage compress*—This is a gauze pad that is attached to the middle of a strip of bandaging material. The pad can be applied directly to an open wound with virtually no exposure to the air or your fingers. The strips of bandage can be folded back and used to tie it in place. When necessary, the sterile pad may be extended to twice its normal size by continued unfolding.

- *Occlusive dressing*—Made of plastic wrap, aluminum foil, petroleum gauze, or other dressing, this dressing is used to form an air-tight, moisture-proof seal over a wound.
- *Petroleum gauze*—This is a sterile gauze saturated with petroleum jelly to prevent it from sticking to a wound.

Large, thick, layered, bulky pads (some with water-proof surfaces) are also available. They come in several sizes for quick application to an extremity or to a large area of the trunk. They are used to help control bleeding and to stabilize impaled objects. These pads are also referred to as bulky dressings, multi-trauma dressings, trauma packs, general purpose dressings, burn pads, or ABD dressings.

If a commercial bulky dressing is not available, you can improvise one with a sanitary napkin. If purchased in individual wrappers, sanitary napkins have the added advantage of cleanliness.

BANDAGES

A bandage does not make contact with a wound. It is used to hold a dressing in place, create pressure to help control bleeding, or provide support for an injured body part. Properly applied, a bandage promotes healing. It also helps the patient to remain comfortable during transport.

Bandages should be applied firmly and fastened securely. They should not be so tight as to stop circulation. They should not be so loose as to let dressings slip. If a bandage becomes unfastened, the wound could bleed or become infected.

Before bandaging, remove the patient's jewelry and other potentially restricting materials such as tape. In case of swelling, these items can restrict circulation. Loosen bandages if the skin around them becomes pale or cyanotic, if pain develops, or if the skin distally is cold, tingly, or numb.

If the pain or discomfort caused by a bandage disappears after several hours, severe damage may have already occurred. Permanent muscle paralysis may result. Please note that improper bandaging can be defined in a court of law as negligence.

TYPES OF DRESSINGS

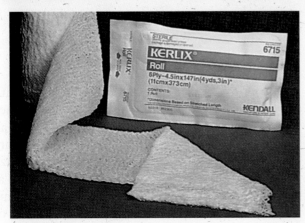

Figure 18-15a Nonelastic, self-adhering dressing and roller bandage.

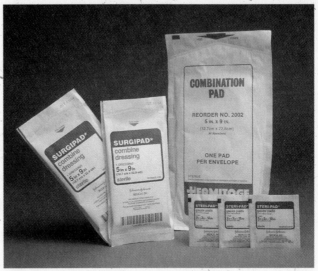

Figure 18-15b Sterile gauze pads.

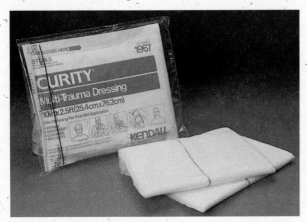

Figure 18-15c Multi-trauma dressing.

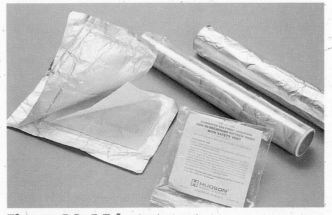

Figure 18-15d Occlusive dressings.

Types of bandages include:

- *Triangular bandage*—This is used to support injured limbs, to secure splints, to form slings, and to make improvised tourniquets. It also can be used to bandage the forehead or scalp (Figure 18–16). The standard triangular bandage is made from a piece of unbleached cotton about 40 inches square, which is folded diagonally and cut along the fold. It can be

handled and applied easily. If applied correctly, it usually remains secure. In an emergency, one can be improvised from a clean handkerchief or clean piece of shirt.

- *Cravat*—This is a triangular bandage that has been folded (Figure 18–17). For a wide cravat, make a one-inch fold along the base of the triangle. Bring the point to the center of folded base, placing the point under the fold. For a medium cravat, fold lengthwise along a line

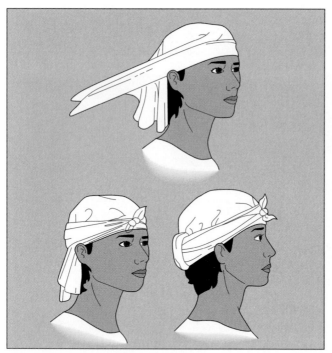

Figure 18-16 Triangular bandage for the forehead or scalp.

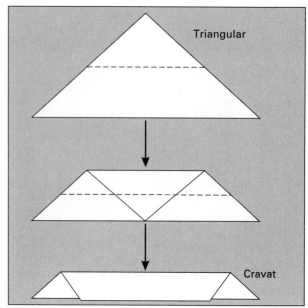

Figure 18-17 Triangular and cravat bandages.

midway between the base and the new top of the bandage. For a narrow cravat, folding is repeated. To complete the procedure, the ends of the bandage are tied securely.

- *Roller bandage*—The self-adhering, form-fitting, nonelastic roller bandage is the most popular and easy to use. Overlapping wraps cling together and can be cut and tied or taped in place. (See Figure 18–18 for how to apply a roller bandage.) Elastic roller bandages should not be used because a tourniquet effect may result.

To apply a pressure dressing to a bleeding wound, follow these steps:

1. Cover the wound with a sterile bulky dressing.
2. Apply hand pressure over the wound until bleeding stops.
3. Apply a firm roller bandage, preferably the self-adhering type. The pressure dressing also may be used to hold some manual pressure while you use a pressure point to stop bleeding.

PRINCIPLES OF APPLICATION

There are no hard-and-fast rules for dressing and bandaging wounds. Often, adaptability and creativity are far more important. In dressing and bandaging, use materials you have on hand and meet the general conditions listed below (Figure 18–19):

- Material used for dressings should be sterile. If sterile items are not available, use a cloth that is as clean as possible.
- Make sure that the dressing is opened carefully. Avoid contaminating it before it reaches the wound surface.
- The dressing should adequately cover the entire wound.
- Do not bandage a dressing in place until bleeding has stopped. The exception is a pressure dressing, which is meant to stop bleeding.
- All edges of a dressing should be covered by the bandage. There also should be no loose ends of cloth or tape.
- Do not bandage a wound too loosely. Bandages should not slip or shift or allow the dressings beneath to slip or shift.
- Bandage wounds snugly, but not too tightly. Be sure to ask the patient how the bandage

APPLYING A ROLLER BANDAGE

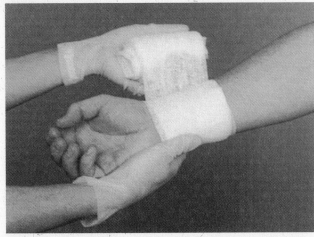

Figure 18-18a Secure the bandage with several overlapping wraps.

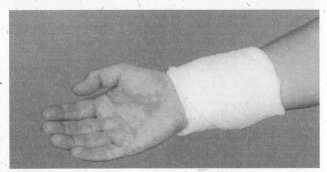

Figure 18-18b When the bandage covers an area larger than the wound, secure it with tape or tie it in place.

BANDAGING

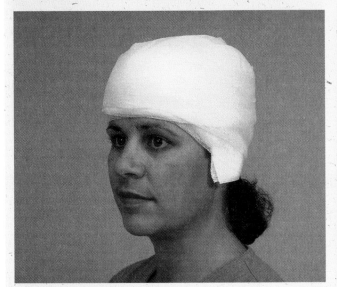

Figure 18-19a Head or ear bandage.

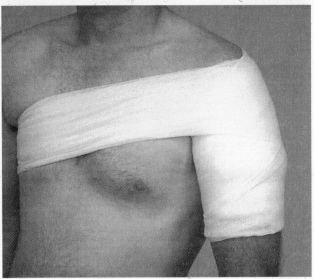

Figure 18-19b Shoulder bandage.

BANDAGING *(Continued)*

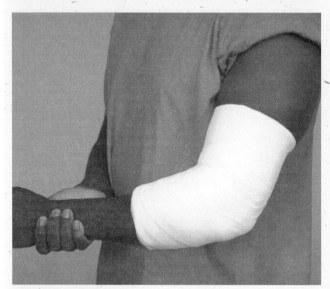

Figure 18-19c Elbow bandage.

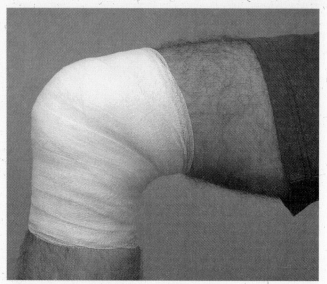

Figure 18-19d Knee bandage.

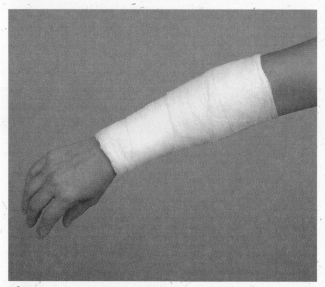

Figure 18-19e Lower arm bandage.

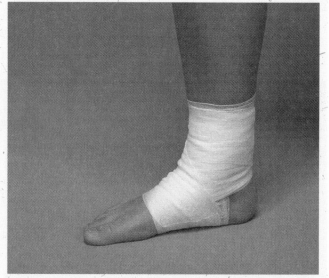

Figure 18-19f Foot or ankle bandage.

feels. Be careful not to interfere with circulation.

• If you are bandaging a small wound on an extremity, cover a larger area with the bandage. This will help avoid creating a pressure point, and it will distribute pressure more evenly.

• Always place the body part to be bandaged in the position in which it is to remain. You can bandage across a joint, but do not try bending a joint after the bandage has been applied to it.

• Tape bandages in place or tie them by using a square knot (Figure 18-20).

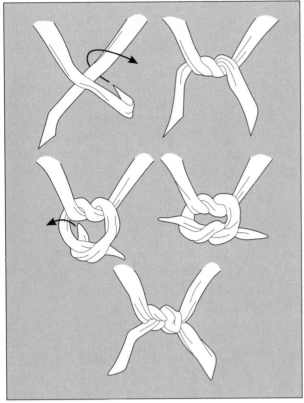

Figure 18-20   Tying a square knot.

- Leave fingers and toes exposed when arms and legs are bandaged, so that you can check for problems with circulation.
- Keep the bandage neat in appearance. You will be perceived as more professional, which can result in easier patient management.

FIRST RESPONDER FOCUS

In your experience as a First Responder, you will come across many patients with soft-tissue injuries. Some injuries will be minor. Others will be large and gaping. Keep your evaluation of these wounds in perspective with the patient's overall condition. If the patient has a laceration that is not bleeding profusely, then it is not your first priority. You must not neglect life-saving care for an obvious but non-life-threatening wound.

This does not mean that care for soft-tissue injuries is unimportant. It is. You must control bleeding as necessary and bandage a wound to keep it clean. Your patient will be very aware of these injuries. Offer reassurance as you provide care. ■

CASE STUDY FOLLOW-UP

At the beginning of this chapter, you read that First Responders were on scene with a female patient with an impaled object in one hand. To see how chapter skills apply to this emergency, read the following. It describes how the call was completed.

PHYSICAL EXAMINATION
A sliver of wood about five inches long had penetrated the palm of the patient's hand. About two inches of wood protruded from each side. The patient's name was Victoria Mashot. Vicky hadn't passed out or fallen after the injury. She had sensation in her fingers distal to the injury. There was no numbness or tingling. I didn't ask her to move

her fingers, because I didn't want to take the chance of causing further problems. Vicky's pulse was 88, strong, and regular. Her respirations were 18 and adequate. Her skin was cool and dry.

My partner stabilized the impaled object while I obtained a patient history.

PATIENT HISTORY
Vicky was still upset that she was so careless as to let this happen. We were able to find out that she had no allergies to medications or the environment. She was in good health and took no medications. Vicky told us she never missed a day of work. She had a doughnut and coffee from the "roach coach" that came onto the mill grounds

CASE STUDY FOLLOW-UP *(Continued)*

about an hour before the injury. She confirmed that she had placed her hand where she wasn't supposed to. She denied any loss of consciousness before or after the object entered her hand.

My partner had done a good job of securing the piece of wood with gauze pads. I continued to stabilize the patient's arm and hand while she secured the object in place.

ONGOING ASSESSMENT

We kept Vicky calm and performed our reassessments. She had calmed down some by then. She was still alert. Her airway and breathing were adequate. There was no bleeding from her wound through the bandage. We made sure the bandage wasn't too tight and that the object was being held securely. Her pulse and respirations were unchanged.

PATIENT HAND-OFF

When the EMTs arrived, we told them what we had:

"This is Victoria Mashot. She is 34 years old and has a five-inch sliver of wood impaled in her left

hand. She never lost consciousness and hasn't fallen or suffered any other injury. We applied some bulky dressings and then bandaged around the object so it wouldn't move. Vicky has no allergies or medications. She tells us that she has no medical problems. She ate a doughnut and coffee an hour ago. Her pulse is 88, strong, and regular. Her respirations are 18 and adequate."

The EMTs took Vicky to the hospital. A plastic surgeon removed the wood from her hand. Fortunately, there was no permanent damage. I heard that Vicky now keeps that sliver of wood over her workbench as a reminder to be more careful.

> Whatever your patient's soft-tissue injuries may be, remember your priorities will always be control of bleeding, preventing further injury, and reducing the risk of infection.

REVIEW QUESTIONS

Page references where answers may be found or supported are provided at the end of each question.

Section 1

1. How are soft-tissue injuries classified? Name the different types. (pp. 300–301, 303–305)
2. What is the recommended emergency care of closed wounds? (pp. 302–303)
3. In general, how would you care for a patient's open wounds? (pp. 305–306)
4. What special considerations are made in caring for open chest injuries? Impaled objects?

Eviscerations? Amputated body parts? (pp. 306–310)

Section 2

5. What are the functions of dressing and bandaging? (p. 312)
6. What are five basic types of dressings? What are the special characteristics of each? (p. 312)
7. What are five or more general principles of dressing and bandaging? (pp. 314, 316–317)

CHAPTER 19

INJURIES TO CHEST, ABDOMEN, AND GENITALIA

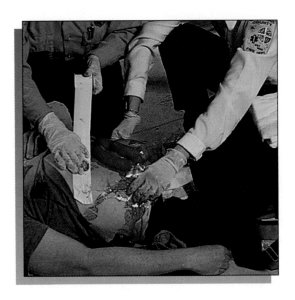

INTRODUCTION

Chest injury is the second leading cause of death from trauma. One third of all deaths caused by car crashes alone involve injuries to the chest. Because the chest contains organs vital to life, all injuries to the chest should be considered life-threatening until proven otherwise.

The abdominal cavity also contains vital organs. Injuries to them can be life-threatening. Remember that both chest and abdominal injuries are serious emergencies that require immediate emergency care, including rapid transport to a trauma center.

Injuries to the external genitalia are rarely life-threatening, but they can cause considerable pain and embarrassment. In addition to caring for injuries to the genitalia, remember to provide emotional support to the patient.

Cognitive, affective, and psychomotor objectives are from the U.S. DOT's 1995 "First Responder: National Standard Curriculum." Enrichment objectives, if any, identify material that is supplemental to the DOT curriculum.

Cognitive

5-2.9 Discuss the emergency medical care considerations for a patient with a penetrating chest injury. (pp. 320–329)

5-2.10 State the emergency medical care considerations for a patient with an open wound to the abdomen. (pp. 329–330)

Affective

5-2.16 Attend to the feelings of the patient with a soft tissue injury or bleeding. (pp. 321–322, 330)

5-2.17 Demonstrate a caring attitude towards patients with a soft tissue injury or bleeding who request emergency medical services. (pp. 321–322, 330)

5-2.18 Place the interests of the patient with a soft tissue injury or bleeding as the foremost consideration when making any and all patient care decisions. (p. 330)

5-2.19 Communicate with empathy to patients with a soft tissue injury or bleeding, as well as with family members and friends of the patient. (pp. 321–322, 330)

Psychomotor

5-2.25 Demonstrate the steps in the emergency medical care of a patient with an open chest wound. (pp. 325–329)

5-2.26 Demonstrate the steps in the emergency medical care of a patient with open abdominal wounds. (p. 330)

Enrichment

* Recognize the signs and symptoms of an injured chest. (pp. 320–322)
* Discuss common chest injuries, such as flail chest, blunt injuries, compression injuries, and broken ribs. (pp. 323–325)
* Describe some complications of chest injuries, such as pneumothorax, hemothorax, and tension pneumothorax. (pp. 327–328)
* Recognize the signs and symptoms of an injured abdomen. (pp. 329–330)
* Describe emergency care of a male patient with injuries to the genitalia, including blunt trauma, avulsion, and amputation. (pp. 330–332)
* Describe emergency care of a female patient with injuries to the genitalia, including special considerations involving sexual assault and the preservation of evidence. (p. 322)

SECTION 1: INJURIES TO THE CHEST

For a quick review of the anatomy of the chest, see Figure 19–1. In addition, now is a good time to review the respiratory and circulatory systems as described in Chapter 4.

PATIENT ASSESSMENT

There are two categories of chest injuries—open and closed. As you would expect, an open chest wound occurs when an object passes through the chest wall. A closed injury is one in which the skin of the chest is not broken. The main types of chest injury include blunt trauma, penetrating injury, and compression injury.

Whether the injury is open or closed, certain signs and symptoms will occur in chest trauma. Many of them may occur simultaneously. The major signs and symptoms include (Figure 19–2):

* Shortness of breath or difficulty breathing.
* Pain during breathing.
* Failure of the chest to expand normally during inhalation.
* Cyanosis.
* Coughing up blood.
* Distended neck veins.
* Rapid, weak pulse.
* Dropping blood pressure.
* Bruising to the chest.

CASE STUDY

DISPATCH
My first response unit was called to a "woman down" at the corner of Hamilton and Lake Shore Drive.

SCENE SIZE-UP
We turned off the lights and sirens before we approached to prevent a crowd from being drawn to the scene. The police on scene waved us in. We still were cautious as we pulled up and put on our gloves and eye wear. There was a woman lying on the ground. An officer was leaning over her.

INITIAL ASSESSMENT
The police officer reported that the woman had been stabbed, probably during a robbery. I saw a hole in the patient's shirt just below the nipple level on the right side of her chest. The woman was moaning and moving around.

> Consider this patient as you read Chapter 19. What else may be done to assess and treat her condition?

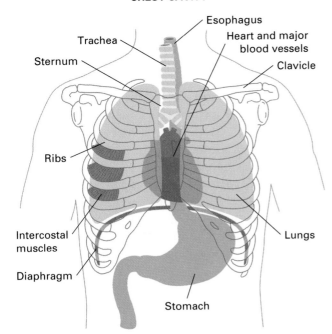

CHEST CAVITY

Esophagus
Trachea
Heart and major blood vessels
Sternum
Clavicle
Ribs
Lungs
Intercostal muscles
Diaphragm
Stomach

Figure 19-1 Chest cavity.

- Chest wall deformity.
- Pain at injury site.
- Shock.

Two of the most important signs are the patient's respiratory rate and the change in normal breathing pattern. In general, a normal breathing rate is from 12 to 20 breaths per minute. Breathing also is done without strain, pain, or difficulty. If a patient breathes more than 20 times per minute and experiences pain with breathing or finds it difficult to take a deep breath, the patient probably has a chest injury.

If the chest is injured, suspect serious underlying damage, even if the skin is not broken. Always assume cardiac damage until it is ruled out. Assume spinal injury if there is any significant mechanism of injury to the chest, including a gunshot wound.

Remember that there is nothing quite so frightening to a patient as a breathing problem.

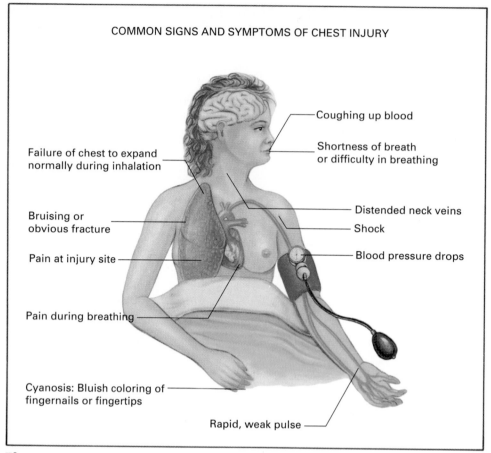

Figure 19-2 Signs and symptoms of chest injury.

Be sure to stay calm. Your demeanor will encourage the patient to stay calm, too. Demonstrate a caring, professional attitude to both the patient and the patient's family.

CLOSED CHEST INJURIES

Guidelines for Emergency Care

In case of any chest injury, update or activate EMS immediately. The patient must be stabilized and transported as quickly as possible to a trauma center or other appropriate medical facility. To provide emergency care for a patient with a closed chest injury, follow the guidelines outlined below:

1. *Maintain an open airway.* Watch for airway obstruction from foreign objects, blood, mucus, and swelling. Suction when needed.

2. *Assure adequate ventilations.* Administer high concentration oxygen, if possible. Be prepared to provide artificial ventilation or CPR if needed. Follow local protocol.

3. *Control any external bleeding.* It is likely for a patient who has a chest injury to have multiple injuries. So perform a quick assessment to detect any source of external bleeding. Treat for shock, if appropriate.

4. *Allow the patient to get in a position of comfort,* if there is no suspected spine injury. Generally, the patient will favor the position that allows for the greatest chest expansion.

5. *Monitor vital signs regularly.*

More information on specific types of closed chest injuries follows. Emergency medical care is basically the same for any closed injury to the chest. Any exceptions are noted below.

NOTE: Always take BSI precautions when there is any possibility that you will come in contact with a patient's blood or other body fluids. Wear protective latex gloves at a minimum.

Blunt Injuries, Compression Injuries, and Traumatic Asphyxia

Severe blunt injuries to the chest are life-threatening emergencies. That includes sudden compression of the chest due to being thrown against a steering wheel in a car crash. These closed injuries cause an increase in pressure inside the chest, which can result in *pulmonary contusions, myocardial contusions*, or *traumatic asphyxia.*

Signs and symptoms of pulmonary (lung) contusions are as follows:

- Severe shortness of breath.
- Rapid pulse.
- Extensive, obvious bruising of the chest wall.

Signs and symptoms of myocardial (heart) contusions are as follows:

- Generalized chest pain.
- Obvious bruising of the chest wall.
- Rapid, sometimes irregular pulse.

When traumatic asphyxia occurs, blood is forced the wrong way out of the heart—from the right side instead of the left. It is then forced back into the veins, particularly the veins of the head and shoulders. Signs and symptoms include:

- Shock.
- Distended neck veins.
- Bloodshot, protruding eyes.
- Cyanotic tongue and lips.
- Coughing up or vomiting blood.
- Swollen, cyanotic appearance of the head, neck, and shoulders.

Guidelines for emergency care are the same as described earlier in the chapter. Note that these conditions are dire emergencies. Time is critical. Be sure EMS has been notified and updated.

Broken Ribs

Rib fractures are not common in children. In adults, direct blows or blunt trauma to the chest often result in broken ribs. The ribs most often broken are those in the middle of the rib cage. Upper ribs are difficult to break because they are protected by the bony shoulder girdle. When they are broken, suspect severe internal injuries. The lower ribs are "floating." They are not attached to the sternum. So they have more ability to move and a greater ability to withstand impact.

Common complications of rib fracture include:

- *Pneumothorax*—an accumulation of air in the pleural cavity. (The pleural cavity is the space between the *visceral pleura*, a membrane that covers the outer surface of the lungs, and the *parietal pleura*, a membrane that covers the internal chest wall.)
- *Hemothorax*—an accumulation of blood in the pleural cavity.
- *Subcutaneous emphysema*—a condition in which air escapes into body tissues, especially in the chest wall, neck, and face.
- *Lacerated intercostal vessels*—blood vessels that surround the ribs are torn and cut.
- *Lung contusions.*
- *Injuries to the liver or spleen.*

The most common symptom of a broken rib is pain at the fracture site. It usually hurts the patient to move, cough, or breathe deeply. The patient will likely want to hold a hand over the area, since stabilization often offers some pain relief (Figure 19–3). Other signs and symptoms may include (Figure 19–4):

- Grating sound upon palpation.
- Chest deformity.
- Shallow, irregular breathing.
- Crackling sensation near the suspected fracture site (subcutaneous emphysema).
- Bruising or lacerations at the suspected fracture site.
- Frothy blood at the nose or mouth, indicating that a rib may have punctured a lung.

The greatest priority of emergency care is to make sure the patient can breathe adequately. Give the patient a pillow or blanket to hold against the broken ribs for support. Apply a sling and swathe to hold the patient's arm against the injured side of the chest.

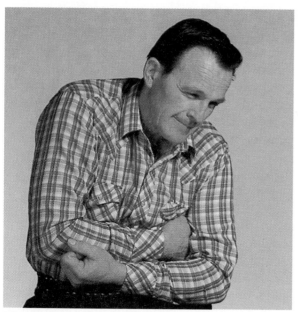

Figure 19-3 Typical "guarding" position.

If the patient is alert, allow him or her to assume a position of comfort. Some EMS systems recommend placing the patient on the injured side. Do not bind, tape, or use other methods that encircle the chest, as they may impair breathing.

Flail Chest

Flail chest, a closed chest injury, results when the chest wall becomes unstable due to fractures of the sternum, fractures of the cartilage connecting the ribs to the sternum, or fractured ribs. Flail chest can affect the front, back, or sides of the rib cage. It most often occurs when two or more adjacent ribs are broken, each in two or more places (Figure 19–5).

In flail chest, an area of chest wall between the broken ribs becomes free-floating. This area is referred to as the **flail segment.** Its motion is opposite the motion of the rest of the chest (Figure 19–6). When the patient inhales, the flail segment collapses or does not expand. When the patient exhales, the flail segment protrudes while the rest of the chest wall contracts. This condition is called **paradoxical breathing.** (You may not notice paradoxical breathing, since the chest muscles may spasm and "splint" the chest.)

Flail chest can be a life-threatening injury. It usually involves bruising of the lung tissues beneath the flail segment. It can lead to inadequate oxygenation of the heart. Fractured ribs also can puncture a lung. Flail chest may involve serious bleeding within the thorax from the arteries and veins between the ribs. This can lead to shock.

Signs and symptoms of flail chest include the following:

BROKEN RIBS

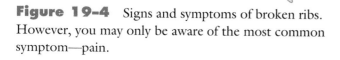

Pain at fracture site.
Pain on moving, coughing, or breathing deeply.
Shallow, uncoordinated breathing.
Chest deformity.
Bruising or lacerations.
Grating sound upon palpation.
Crackling sensation near site.
Frothy blood at nose or mouth (lung puncture).

Figure 19-4 Signs and symptoms of broken ribs. However, you may only be aware of the most common symptom—pain.

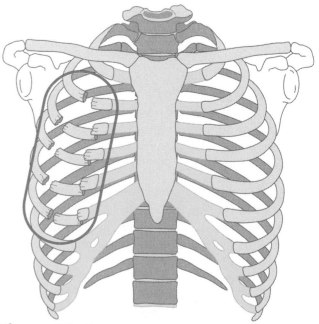

Figure 19-5 In flail chest, two or more ribs are fractured, each in two or more places.

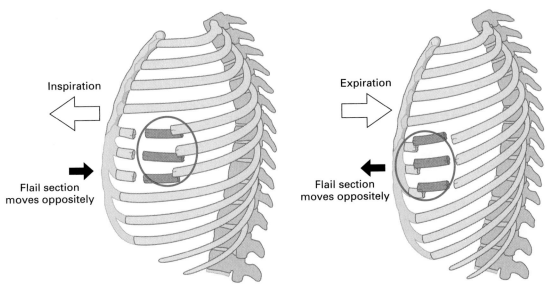

Figure 19-6   In flail chest a free-floating segment of chest wall moves in the opposite direction.

- Shortness of breath.
- Paradoxical breathing, which is almost always accompanied by severe pain.
- Swelling over the injured area.
- Signs of shock.
- Increasing airway resistance.
- Patient's attempt to splint the chest wall with hands and arms.
- Possible grating sounds from bone ends rubbing together.

To check for flail chest, have the patient lie on his or her back. Bare the chest. Watch for a see-saw motion of the chest while the patient breathes. Gently place your hands on the patient's chest. Check for symmetry of the sides as the patient breathes. Note that it can be very difficult to detect flail chest in an obese or muscular patient. In addition, because flail chest can be so painful, the patient may not want to relinquish "guarding" the chest.

In addition to the guidelines for emergency care of chest injuries described above, you must also try to splint the chest. It will help to improve respirations. First, remove clothing from the chest area. Then tape a small pillow or thick, heavy dressing over the injury site. The dressing should weigh less than five pounds. (See Figure 19-7.)

If you suspect internal bleeding or if there is increased pain and discomfort, have the patient lie on the injured side. However, do so only if there is no possibility of spine injury.

OPEN CHEST INJURIES

All chest injuries are serious. However, open chest injuries pose an additional problem because they upset the delicate balance of pressure between the inside and outside of the chest. It is vital for you

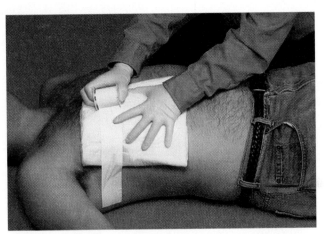

Figure 19-7   Stabilize flail chest by applying a pillow or bulky dressing.

to identify and treat open chest injuries immediately. Remember that the chest cavity has a front, side, and a back. Injuries to the back also may penetrate the chest cavity.

Sometimes an open wound to the chest or back bubbles or makes a sucking noise. Such a wound is typically called a **sucking chest wound.** However, even if a chest wound does not bubble or make a sucking noise, treat it as if it has penetrated the chest cavity.

Guidelines for Emergency Care

Treatment for both an open chest injury and a closed one are basically the same. However, there is one very important difference. You must apply an occlusive dressing to a sucking chest wound (Figure 19–8). The dressing should be at least two inches larger than the wound on all sides, which should be large enough not to be sucked into the wound. Seal the dressing on three sides,

SUCKING CHEST WOUND

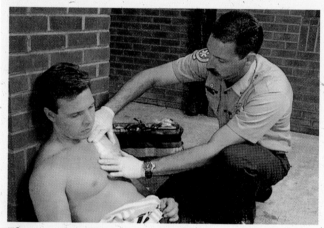

Figure 19-8a Position an occlusive dressing in direct contact with chest wall.

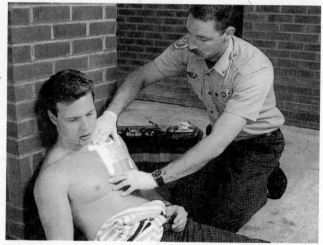

Figure 19-8b Tape the occlusive dressing on three sides.

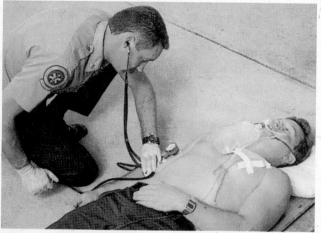

Figure 19-8c Position the patient to help ease breathing.

leaving the fourth side unsealed. The open side of the dressing acts as a "relief valve," which allows air to escape but prevents air from entering the chest cavity. (See Figure 19–9.)

If you have to improvise an occlusive dressing, do not use household plastic wrap. It is not strong enough. If necessary, use material such as a plastic bag. If you have no other choice, use aluminum foil or Vaseline® gauze held in place with a pressure dressing.

If the patient develops increased respiratory distress after application of an occlusive dressing, release the seal immediately. The increased distress usually means pressure is building up within the chest cavity.

There are three conditions that occur inside the chest cavity as a result of an open or closed chest injury. It is not necessary to diagnose them. First Responder emergency care is the same. The three conditions—pneumothorax, hemothorax, and tension pneumothorax—are being presented below to improve your understanding of chest injuries. (See Figure 19–10.)

Pneumothorax

Pneumothorax occurs when air from a wound site enters the chest cavity but not the lungs. The pressure of the air in the chest presses against a lung, separating it from the chest wall and causing it to collapse. The volume of the lung is reduced, resulting in respiratory distress.

Air can enter the chest cavity in one of two ways. It can enter either from a sucking chest wound that allows air to enter from the outside, or air can leak out of a lung laceration. Once the lung is ruptured, it does not expand properly.

In some cases, called *spontaneous pneumothorax*, the lung does not collapse because of injury. It collapses because the patient has a weak area on the surface of the lung that ruptures. The weakened lung loses its ability to expand. The patient then experiences sharp chest pain and mild to severe respiratory distress. Spontaneous pneumothorax is common among smokers or emphysema patients.

Hemothorax

Hemothorax occurs when the pleural space fills with blood, creating pressure on the heart and lungs. The lungs cannot expand, and the same process occurs as with pneumothorax. In addition, severe bleeding can cause shock.

Hemothorax is the result of blunt or penetrating trauma to the chest. It can occur with closed chest wounds, as well as with open ones. It often accompanies pneumothorax. The blood usually originates from lacerated blood vessels in the chest wall or cavity. In rare cases, it results from a lacerated lung. The severity of the hemothorax depends on the amount of blood lost into the pleural space.

On inspiration, dressing seals wound, preventing air entry

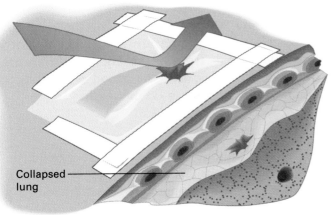

Collapsed lung

Expiration allows trapped air to escape through untaped section of dressing

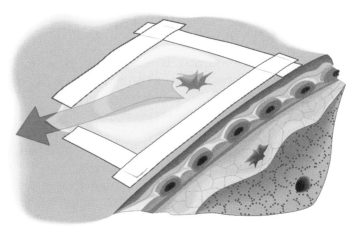

Figure 19-9   A "relief valve" for a sucking chest wound.

COMPLICATIONS OF CHEST INJURIES

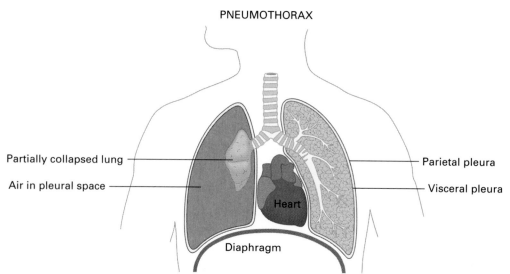

HEMOTHORAX

Partially collapsed lung

Visceral pleura
Parietal pleura

Heart

Blood in pleural space

TENSION PNEUMOTHORAX

Collapsed lung

Compressed lung

Air

Compressed heart

PNEUMOTHORAX

Partially collapsed lung

Air in pleural space

Heart

Parietal pleura

Visceral pleura

Diaphragm

Figure 19-10 Complications of chest injuries.

Tension Pneumothorax

Tension pneumothorax is one of the most life-threatening chest injuries. Air continuously leaks out of a lung and becomes trapped in the pleural space. A process of compression starts and worsens with each breath until the lung on the affected side is reduced to the size of a small ball, sometimes only a few inches in diameter.

Even after the lung is as compressed as it can be, air continues to leak into the pleural space. Pressure continues to rise and may then compress major blood vessels, the heart, or the opposite lung. The extreme pressure in the chest cavity prevents blood from returning to the heart through the veins, and the blood is no longer pumped out. Death can occur rapidly.

Penetrating Injury

Penetrating injuries are open chest wounds in which the chest wall is torn, typically by a foreign object. The most common are caused by stabbing or gunshot. In addition to the possibility of lacerating the great vessels in the chest, penetrating injuries can result in massive bleeding, sucking chest wounds, pneumothorax, hemothorax, or laceration of the heart and lungs. A penetrating injury can be a fatal. Surgery is generally required.

To provide emergency care, follow the guidelines already provided for open chest wounds.

SECTION 2: INJURIES TO THE ABDOMEN

Now is a good time to review the four quadrants of the abdomen as described in Chapter 4.

PATIENT ASSESSMENT

Suspect abdominal injury in patients involved in fights, falls, and car crashes. Injuries could range from severe bleeding and shock to an evisceration. Look for the most common symptom of abdominal injury—pain.

A wound that penetrates the skin and abdominal cavity is dangerous. Internal bleeding may occur. Bacteria may be introduced into the abdomen from the outside and from a penetrated intestine. In the presence of open wounds of the abdomen, assume that organs have been damaged.

In closed abdominal injuries, a severe blow or crushing injury does not break the skin. Such wounds may be extremely dangerous. Serious injury to the internal organs, internal bleeding, and shock may occur.

To assess for a closed abdominal injury, have the patient lie down on his or her back. The knees should be flexed and supported. Remove or loosen clothing over the abdomen. Then look and feel for signs of injury. Look for bruising, lacerations and other open wounds, impaled objects, and protruding organs. Watch how the abdomen moves as the patient breathes. Gently feel all four quadrants. Note rigidity, pain, and tenderness. Also note any guarding, a common reaction to a painful abdomen. If the patient complains of pain in a particular area, palpate that area last. If the

area is palpated first, it may prevent accurate palpation of the remaining quadrants.

General signs and symptoms of an injured abdomen include (Figure 19–11):

• Distended or irregularly shaped abdomen.
• Bruising of the abdomen, back, or flanks.
• Rigid and tender abdomen.
• Mild discomfort progressing to intolerable pain.
• Pain radiating to a shoulder, both shoulders, or the back.
• Abdominal cramping.
• Lying still with legs drawn up in a fetal position (Figure 19–12).
• Rapid, shallow breathing.

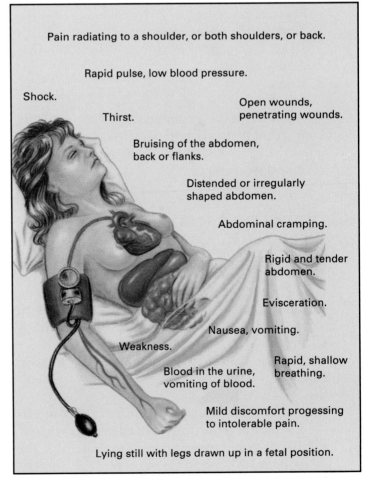

Pain radiating to a shoulder, or both shoulders, or back.

Rapid pulse, low blood pressure.

Shock.

Thirst.

Open wounds, penetrating wounds.

Bruising of the abdomen, back or flanks.

Distended or irregularly shaped abdomen.

Abdominal cramping.

Rigid and tender abdomen.

Evisceration.

Nausea, vomiting.

Weakness.

Blood in the urine, vomiting of blood.

Rapid, shallow breathing.

Mild discomfort progessing to intolerable pain.

Lying still with legs drawn up in a fetal position.

Figure 19-11 Signs and symptoms of abdominal injury.

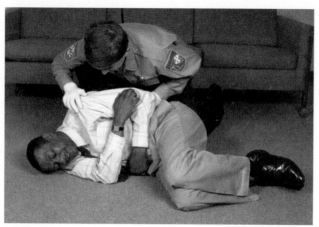

Figure 19-12 Typical "guarding" position.

- Rapid pulse, low blood pressure.
- Open wounds, penetrating wounds.
- Nausea, vomiting.
- Evisceration.
- Blood in the urine, vomiting of blood.
- Shock.
- Weakness.
- Thirst.

Remember to communicate with empathy. Your attitude towards the patient will have an impact, so put his or her needs first. Stay calm, cool, and sympathetic.

GUIDELINES FOR EMERGENCY CARE

As with any patient, your top priorities for a patient with abdominal injuries are airway, breathing, and circulation. Once the ABCs are assessed and treated, update or activate EMS immediately to arrange for transport.

Provide the following emergency medical care:

1. *Maintain an open airway.* Be alert for vomiting. Position the patient for adequate drainage. Be prepared to suction. Do not give the patient anything to eat or drink.
2. *Expose the abdomen.* Remove clothing from the abdominal area to allow proper assessment.

ABDOMINAL EVISCERATION

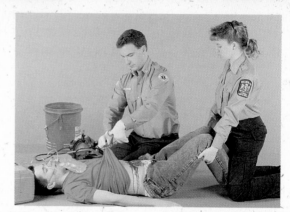

Figure 19-13a Cut away clothing.

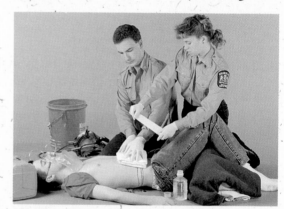

Figure 19-13b Cover the exposed organs with a moist bulky dressing.

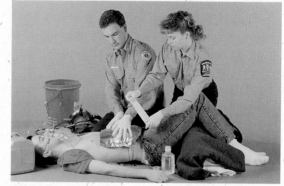

Figure 19-13c Secure an occlusive dressing over the bulky one.

3. *Suspect and treat for shock.* Work diligently to prevent it. Keep the patient warm, but do not overheat. Administer high concentration oxygen, if you are allowed.
4. *Control external bleeding.* Dress open wounds with dry, sterile dressings or follow local protocol.
5. *Position the patient.* The patient usually is most comfortable lying on his or her back with knees flexed. Elevate the feet, if possible. If you suspect a pelvic fracture, also prevent movement. Immobilize the patient on a long backboard if possible.

If there is an abdominal evisceration, you must cover the exposed organs (Figure 19–13). Never touch exposed organs. Never try to replace them. Instead, use a thick, moist, sterile dressing to cover them completely. You can moisten the dressing with sterile saline. Never use absorbent materials as dressings, such as toilet tissue or paper towels, which can shred and cling to the organs. Note that in some parts of the country, dry dressings are recommended. Follow local protocol.

Gently and loosely tape the moist dressing in place. Then loosely cover it with an occlusive dressing such as plastic wrap or aluminum foil. If you use foil, make sure the edges do not cut exposed organs. Tape down the edges to help keep the first dressing moist and warm.

Maintain the temperature of the wound area by covering the dressing with layers of dressings such as a particle-free bath blanket or towel. They may be held loosely in place with a bandage or clean sheet.

SECTION 3: INJURIES TO THE GENITALIA

While assessing injuries to the male or female genitalia, act in a calm professional way. Protect the patient from onlookers. Use sheets, towels or other material as a drape over the area. Provide the same emergency care you would provide for any soft-tissue injury, with the following exceptions.

(Now is a good time to review the reproductive systems as described in Chapter 4.)

MALE GENITALIA

Injuries to the external genitalia of a male can cause severe pain, though they are not usually life-threatening.

Penis

The skin of the penis can be torn or avulsed. Such injuries occur most commonly in accidents and assaults. To give emergency care:

1. Wrap the injured penis in a soft, sterile dressing that is moistened with sterile saline solution.
2. Apply a cold pack to relieve pain and reduce swelling.
3. Never remove impaled objects. Instead, stabilize them and bandage them in place.
4. If you can find avulsed skin, wrap it in sterile gauze that has been moistened with sterile saline. Send it with the patient to the hospital.

In some cases, the penis may be partially or completely amputated. Blood loss may be significant. If so, apply a sterile pressure dressing to the remaining stump to control bleeding. Aggressive direct pressure may be needed also. If you can find the amputated penis, follow the usual procedure for preserving and transporting parts with the patient.

Scrotum and Testicles

A direct blow to the scrotum can cause the testes to rupture. It also can result in a pooling of blood, causing tremendous pain and a feeling of pressure. If a testicle ruptures, it requires surgery.

To care for this emergency, apply an ice pack to the entire area to reduce swelling and pain. If the scrotal skin becomes avulsed, try to find it. Then wrap it in moist, sterile gauze. Send it with the patient to the hospital. Dress the scrotum itself in a sterile dressing moistened with sterile saline. Control bleeding with pressure.

FEMALE GENITALIA

Injuries to the internal female organs are rare. That is because they are small and well protected, except during pregnancy when the uterus is enlarged. Such an injury can result in serious blood loss and shock.

Injuries to the external female genitalia can follow straddle injuries or sexual assault. Because the area is richly supplied with blood vessels and nerves, injuries can cause severe pain and bleeding. However, they are not usually life-threatening.

1. Control bleeding with local pressure, using compresses moistened with sterile saline.
2. Dress wounds. Bandage them in place with a diaper-like bandage. Stabilize any impaled objects and bandage them in place.
3. Use cold packs over the dressing to relieve pain and reduce swelling. Never place anything inside the vagina.

4. Treat the patient for shock.

If you suspect a sexual assault, protect the patient's privacy. Clear the area of bystanders. Provide a cover, such as a blanket or sheet. Discretely question the patient about other potential injuries, such as head trauma. Do not touch or examine the genitals unless there is life-threatening bleeding.

To help preserve evidence in case of sexual assault, do not allow the patient to bathe or douche. Discourage the patient from washing her hair or cleaning under her fingernails. If possible, do not clean any wounds. Handle the patient's clothing as little as possible. Bag all items of clothing and other items separately. If there is blood on any item, do not use plastic bags. Follow local protocol.

FIRST RESPONDER FOCUS

Injuries to the chest and abdomen are potentially very serious. The emergency care you give to the patient—such as applying an occlusive dressing—is vital. Another component of quality care is immediate transport to a hospital, preferably a trauma center if one is available.

It is your responsibility to activate and update EMS when you have a patient with either of these serious conditions. The responding crew will begin to prepare even before they reach the scene, so your call will help expedite care. You also may be asked to help with spinal immobilization and other tasks that will help the EMTs get en route to the hospital faster.

Do not transport the patient in your first response vehicle. The patient will benefit from the additional care he or she will receive from the EMTs and paramedics.

Remember that the care you give is important. But prolonged scene times will hurt rather than help. The care that will ultimately save the patient occurs in the hospital. ■

CASE STUDY FOLLOW-UP

At the beginning of this chapter, you read that First Responders were on scene with a female patient with an open chest wound. To see how chapter skills apply to this emergency, read the following. It describes how the call was completed.

INITIAL ASSESSMENT (*Continued*)
Our immediate priorities were to evaluate the patient's ABCs and seal the chest wound. Fortunately, there were two of us. My partner, Meg, talked to the patient explaining who we were and what we were doing. The patient was alert but in a lot of pain. Meg applied oxygen by nonrebreather mask. I applied an occlusive dressing.

Our general impression was that of a responsive female patient who was in a potentially serious condition. We updated the EMTs from our portable radio.

PHYSICAL EXAMINATION
The patient reported that she had been struck over the head, stabbed, and kicked by a gang of teens. We realized that this was a significant mechanism of injury, so Meg stabilized the patient's head while I began a head-to-toe exam. I got as far as the abdomen when the EMTs arrived.

PATIENT HISTORY
We didn't have time to get much of a history.

ONGOING ASSESSMENT
The EMTs arrived before we could reassess the patient.

PATIENT HAND-OFF
Our hand-off report was as follows:

"This is Andrea MacPurne. She is 34 years old and was assaulted during a robbery. Multiple teens struck, kicked, and stabbed her. She is alert with a strong pulse and adequate respirations. She has a good bump on the left side of her skull. She has a stab wound to the chest to which we have applied an occlusive dressing. We just got to her abdomen and found it reddened. It looks like she took some punches or kicks there, too. We applied oxygen. We didn't get to the history or vitals."

The EMTs understood. There were important things to do. They, too, realized the urgency and quickly immobilized the patient and prepared for transport. Meg and I later found out that the woman's wounds were mostly superficial and that she recovered well.

> Always rely on the mechanism of injury, a high index of suspicion, and a careful physical examination to assess any trauma patient. Early recognition and prompt emergency treatment of injuries to the chest and abdomen especially can save a life.

REVIEW QUESTIONS

Page references where answers may be found or supported are provided at the end of each question.

Section 1

1. What are the major signs and symptoms of an injury to the chest? (pp. 320–321)
2. If a patient's chest is injured—even if the skin is not broken, what serious underlying damage should you suspect? (p. 321)
3. What are the general guidelines for emergency care of a patient with a closed chest injury? (pp. 322–323)
4. How can you recognize flail chest? In addition to the following the general guidelines for emergency care of chest injuries, what else must you do to help this patient? (pp. 324–325)
5. What is the First Responder emergency medical care of a patient with blunt injuries to the

chest, compression injuries to the chest, or traumatic asphyxia? (pp. 322, 323)

6. What are some of the possible complications of a rib fracture? (p. 323)

7. What are the signs and symptoms of a rib fracture? (p. 323)

8. How should you dress a sucking chest wound? What can you do if the patient develops increased respiratory distress after dressing? Explain your answers. (pp. 326–327)

Section 2

9. What are the general signs and symptoms of an injured abdomen? (pp. 329–330)

10. What are the general guidelines for emergency care of a patient with abdominal injuries? (p. 330)

Section 3

11. How should you provide emergency care to a patient with an injury to his penis? (pp. 331–332)

12. What are the emergency care guidelines for injuries to the female genitalia? (p. 332)

CHAPTER 20

BURN EMERGENCIES

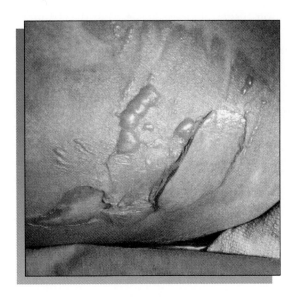

INTRODUCTION

Burns are a leading cause of accidental death in the U.S. More than two million burn accidents occur each year. Of those people who are burned, many die and many more need long-term rehabilitation. In this chapter, you will learn how to assess burns and provide emergency medical care. You also will learn about common causes of burns.

Cognitive, affective, and psychomotor objectives are from the U.S. DOT's 1995 "First Responder: National Standard Curriculum." Enrichment objectives, if any, identify material that is supplemental to the DOT curriculum.

Cognitive

5-2.6 Establish the relationship between body substance isolation (BSI) and soft tissue injuries. (p. 341)
5-2.13 Describe the emergency medical care for burns. (pp. 341–343)

Affective

5-2.17 Demonstrate a caring attitude towards patients with a soft tissue injury or bleeding who request emergency medical services. (p. 343)
5-2.19 Communicate with empathy to patients with a soft tissue injury or bleeding, as well as with family members and friends of the patient. (p. 343)

Psychomotor

No objectives are identified.

Enrichment

* List the classifications of burns. (pp. 337–340)
* Define the characteristics of superficial burns, partial thickness burns, and full thickness burns. (pp. 337–340)
* Establish the relationship between airway management and patients with burns. (p. 343)
* Describe the emergency medical care for a patient with inhalation injuries. (p. 343)
* Describe the emergency medical care for a patient with chemical burns. (p. 344)
* Describe the emergency medical care for a patient with electrical burns. (pp. 344–346)

SECTION 1: GENERAL BURN MANAGEMENT

The skin is the largest organ of the body. Its outermost layer is the epidermis, which contains cells that give the skin its color. The dermis, or second layer, contains a vast network of blood vessels. The deepest layers of the skin contain hair follicles, sweat and oil glands, and sensory nerves. Just below the skin is a layer of fat called **subcutaneous tissue.** (See Chapter 4 for an illustration.)

The function of the skin includes protecting the deep tissues from injury, drying out, and invasion by bacteria and other foreign bodies. It helps to regulate body temperature, and aids in getting rid of water and various salts. It also acts as the receptor organ for touch, pain, heat, and cold. When the skin is damaged by burns, some or all of its functions may be compromised or destroyed.

PATIENT ASSESSMENT

Always make sure the scene of a burn accident is safe before entering. If the emergency involves noxious fumes, chemical spills, or electricity, call for specialized personnel to secure the scene before entering. Never try to rescue people trapped by fire unless you are equipped and trained to do so.

Most burn patients who die in the prehospital setting die from a blocked airway, inhaled toxins, or other trauma, and not from the burn itself. So as with all patients, perform an initial assessment. After you have assessed the ABCs and cared for all life-threats, determine the severity of your patient's burns. (See Table 20–1.)

Severity of a burn depends on many factors, including:

* Depth of the burn.
* Extent of body surface burned.
* Which part of the body was burned.
* Other complicating factors.

CASE STUDY

DISPATCH

It was raining hard that day. As soon as we got back to the station house, my partner and I checked in and readied our truck for the next call. Before long we were dispatched to a "man hit by lightning."

SCENE SIZE-UP

Upon arrival at Costanza's farm, we were met by a woman who told us the patient had been moved into the barn. We drove up to the building, took BSI precautions, and approached the patient.

INITIAL ASSESSMENT

My partner immediately stabilized the patient's head and neck. I found the patient responsive to painful stimuli only. The initial assessment revealed a patent airway, respirations that were adequate and of good quality, and no visible bleeding. We elected to place the patient on oxygen at 15 liters per minute by way of a nonrebreather mask. We also noted a feathery pattern of markings scattered over the patient's left arm.

Our general impression was of a middle-aged male who was responsive only to pain after being hit by lightning.

> What else should be done to assess his condition? What is the proper emergency medical care? Consider this patient as you read Chapter 20.

Depth of Burns

Burns typically are classified by depth (Figure 20–1). A **superficial burn** involves only the first layer of skin. A **partial thickness burn** involves the epidermis and the dermis. In a **full thickness burn,** the burn extends through all layers of skin and may involve subcutaneous tissue, muscles, organs, and bone. Note that burns are seldom only one depth. They usually involve a combination.

You can recognize superficial, partial thickness, and full thickness burns as follows:

- *Superficial burns* (Figure 20–2). A superficial burn is caused by flash, flame, scald, or the sun. It is the most common of all burns and is con-sidered minor. The patient's skin surface will be dry, and there may be some swelling. Though the skin is red and painful, the burn involves only the epidermis. A superficial burn heals in 2 to 5 days with no scarring. Peeling of the burned skin may occur. Some temporary discoloration may result.

- *Partial thickness burns* (Figure 20–3). This type of burn usually results from contact with hot liquids or solids, flash or flame contact with clothing, direct flame from fire, contact with chemicals, or the sun. The skin appears moist and mottled, ranging in color from white to red. The burn area is blistered and intensely painful. It usually requires 5 to 21 days to heal. If infection occurs, healing time can take longer.

TABLE 20-1

DETERMINING SEVERITY OF BURNS

	ADULTS	INFANTS AND CHILDREN
CRITICAL BURNS	Full thickness burns involving the hands, feet, face, or genitalia. Burns associated with respiratory injury. Full thickness burns covering more than 10% of body surface. Partial thickness burns covering more than 30% of body surface area. Burns complicated by painful, swollen, deformed extremity. Burns encompassing any body part, e.g., arm, leg, or chest.	Any full thickness or partial thickness burn greater than 20%, or burns involving hands, feet, face, airway, or genitalia.
MODERATE BURNS	Full thickness burns of 2% to 10% of the body surface area excluding hands, feet, face, genitalia, and upper airway. Partial thickness burns of 15% to 30% of body surface area. Superficial burns of greater than 50% body surface area.	Partial thickness burns of 10% to 20% of body surface area.
MINOR BURNS	Full thickness burns of less than 2% body surface area. Partial thickness burns less than 15% body surface area.	Partial thickness burns less than 10% body surface area.

BURNS: CLASSIFICATION BY DEPTH

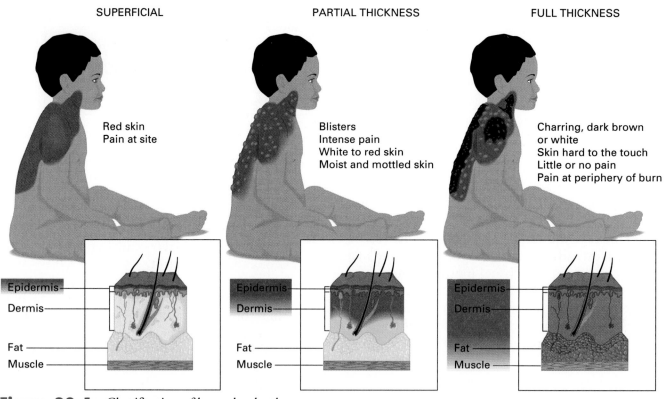

SUPERFICIAL

Red skin
Pain at site

PARTIAL THICKNESS

Blisters
Intense pain
White to red skin
Moist and mottled skin

FULL THICKNESS

Charring, dark brown
or white
Skin hard to the touch
Little or no pain
Pain at periphery of burn

Epidermis
Dermis
Fat
Muscle

Figure 20-1 Classification of burns by depth.

SUPERFICIAL BURNS

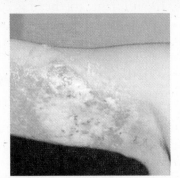

Figure 20-2a

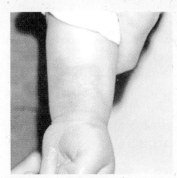

Figure 20-2b

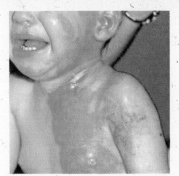

Figure 20-2c

PARTIAL THICKNESS BURNS

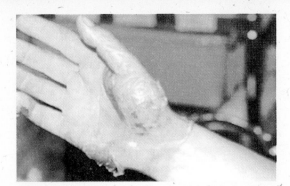

Figure 20-3a

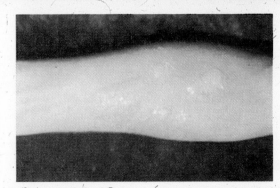

Figure 20-3b

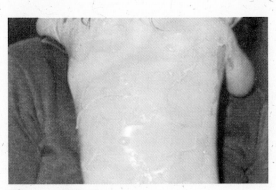

Figure 20-3c

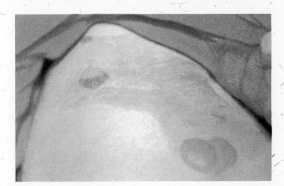

Figure 20-3d

- *Full thickness burns* (Figure 20–4). A full thickness burn results from contact with hot liquids or solids, flame, chemicals, or electricity. The skin is dry and leathery and may be a mix of colors from white to dark brown to charcoal. Often charred blood vessels are visible. While it can be very painful, the patient may feel little if nerve endings have been destroyed. Small full thickness burns require weeks to heal. Large ones, which may need skin grafting and other specialized burn care, can take months or years to heal. These burns often result in scarring.

Extent of Body Surface Burned

The **rule of nines** is a standardized way to estimate the amount of **body surface area** or **BSA** burned. The head and neck region is considered to be 9% of the total body surface area. The posterior trunk is 18%. The anterior trunk is 18%. Each upper extremity is 9%, and each lower extremity is 18%. In an infant, the head is considered to be 18% of BSA and each lower extremity is 14% BSA. External genitalia are estimated as 1% BSA in all patients. (See Figure 20–5.)

An alternative method is called the **palmar surface method.** With this method, use the palm of the patient's hand—approximately 1% of the BSA—to estimate of the size of a burn. For example, if a burn area is equal to "7 palms," the burn would be estimated as 7% BSA.

You will find it useful to use the rule of nines to estimate the BSA of larger burn injuries and the palmar surface method for smaller burns. Follow local protocols. However, do not spend time trying to determine a burn's exact percent of

FULL THICKNESS BURNS

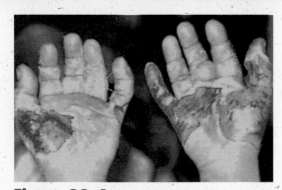

Figure 20–4a

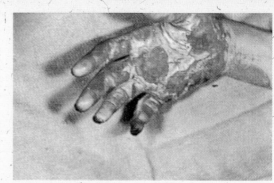

Figure 20–4b

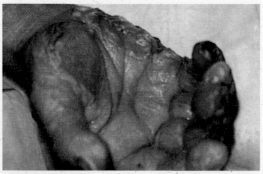

Figure 20–4c

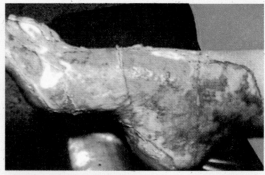

Figure 20–4d

THE RULE OF NINES

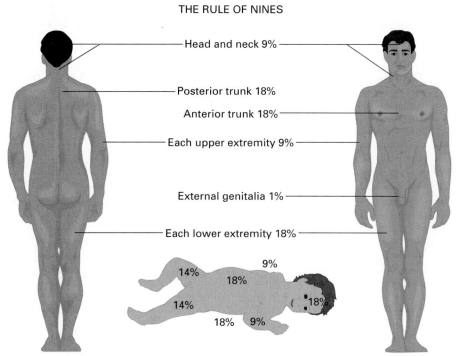

Head and neck 9%

Posterior trunk 18%

Anterior trunk 18%

Each upper extremity 9%

External genitalia 1%

Each lower extremity 18%

9%
14%
18%
14%
18%
18%
9%

Figure 20-5 Rule of nines.

BSA. Slight differences in percentages will not affect proper First Responder care.

Location of Burns

Burns to certain areas of the body are more critical than others. For example, burns to the face can compromise breathing or cause injury to the eyes. Loss of function may be the result of burns to the hands or feet. Burns to the genital area may result in loss or impairment of genitourinary function. Burns that encircle a body part—such as a joint, arm, or leg—are considered critical because of the possibility of blood-vessel and nerve damage. Burns that encircle the chest can limit its ability to expand, which can result in inadequate breathing.

Arrange for patients with burns to any of these areas to be transported to a hospital or burn center immediately.

Complicating Factors

Patients who have chronic diseases such as heart disease or diabetes or who have other injuries will always react more severely to burns, even minor ones. So try to determine the patient's medical history early in the course of care.

The age of a patient also may be a complicating factor. Children under the age of 5 and adults over the age of 55 tolerate burns poorly. In an elderly patient, a burn covering only 20% of body surface can be fatal. Because the elderly and very young generally have thin skin, they can sustain much deeper burns. Fluid loss from a burn also can affect the elderly and young more critically. Even a small fluid loss can result in serious problems. An additional problem concerns the immune system, which is immature in children and usually compromised in the elderly patient.

Please note that burns also may be the result of child abuse. Look for burn patterns that indicate a child might have been dipped in scalding water. Cigarettes also are used to burn children as a form of abuse. Follow local protocols for reporting your observations.

EMERGENCY MEDICAL CARE

Once the patient has been removed from the source of the burn, provide emergency medical care. Take BSI precautions and follow these steps (Figure 20–6):

CARE OF BURN INJURIES

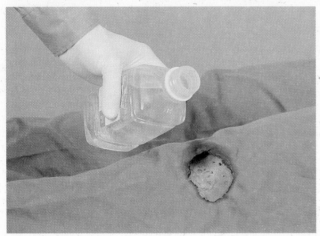

Figure 20-6a Stop the burning process.

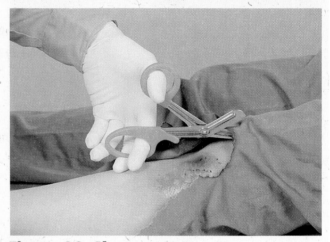

Figure 20-6b Remove all smoldering clothing.

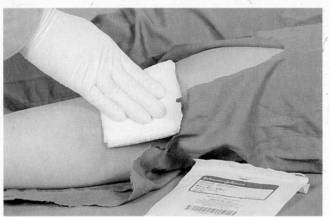

Figure 20-6c After life-threats have been treated and a physical exam completed, cover burns with dry sterile dressings.

1. *Stop the burning process.* Run cold water over scald burns. Flush away chemicals with water for 20 minutes or more. Remove any smoldering clothing and jewelry. If you meet resistance, or if you see bits melted into the skin, cut around the area. Do not try to remove them.

2. *Perform an initial assessment.* Treat all life-threats. Administer oxygen by nonrebreather mask, if allowed. If your patient's breathing is inadequate, provide ventilations with supplemental oxygen.

3. *Determine the severity of the patient's burns* during the physical exam. Take into account the depth of burns, extent of BSA involved, location of burns, and complicating factors. Don't forget to look for other possible injuries.

4. *Cover the burns.* Use dry sterile dressings or a disposable sterile burn sheet. Do not use

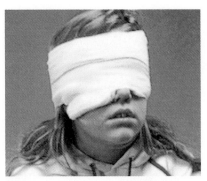

Figure 20-7 Apply dressings to both eyes, even if only one is burned.

grease or fat, ointment, lotion, antiseptic, or ice on the burns. Do not break any blisters. If a burn involves an eye, be sure to apply dressings to both eyes (Figure 20–7).

5. *Keep the patient warm,* and treat other injuries as needed.

Proper care of burns must start as soon as possible after the injury. Loss of body fluids, pain contributing to shock, swelling, and infection may quickly follow a burn injury. Be especially alert to any sign of breathing difficulty. If burns were caused by an electrical source, monitor the patient closely for cardiac arrest. Be prepared to administer CPR and, if you are trained and equipped, to apply an automated external defibrillator (AED). Remember that the patient's status can change suddenly, so monitor vital signs continually.

As always, do your best to calm and reassure the patient. He or she may be in a great deal of pain. The patient and family members also may be afraid of permanent scarring and disfigurement. Tell them that you are doing what is necessary to prevent further injury and contamination. Let them know that additional EMS personnel are on the way.

Also note that patients and family members may have tried to treat the patient's burns before you arrived on scene. Find out what they did. One reason why burns are so often critically damaging or even fatal is that some individuals are poorly informed about methods of care. Include this information in your patient hand-off report.

SECTION 2: SPECIAL TYPES OF BURN INJURIES

INHALATION INJURIES

Greater than half of all fire-related deaths are caused by smoke inhalation. About 80% of those who die in residential fires do so only because they have inhaled heated air or smoke and other toxic gases. Suspect inhalation injury in any patient who was burned in a fire, especially if the patient was confined in an enclosed space.

The severity of an inhalation injury is determined by the following factors:

- Products of combustion (what was burned).
- Degree of combustion (how completely it was burned).
- Duration of exposure (how long the patient was exposed to the smoke or gas).
- Whether or not the patient was in a confined space.

Most upper airway damage from heat inhalation consists of scorched mucous membranes and swelling, which can block the airway. Specific signs and symptoms include (Figure 20–8):

- Singed nasal hairs.
- Burns to the face (Figure 20–9).
- Burned specks of carbon in the sputum.
- Sooty or smoky smell on the breath.
- Respiratory distress.
- Noisy breathing.
- Hoarseness, cough, difficulty speaking.
- Restricted chest movement.
- Cyanosis.

If any of these signs and symptoms are present, administer humidified oxygen if available. Note that this type of injury may appear to be mild at first and then become more severe. Monitor the patient's airway and breathing closely. Be prepared to assist ventilations if necessary.

SIGNS AND SYMPTOMS OF INHALATION BURNS

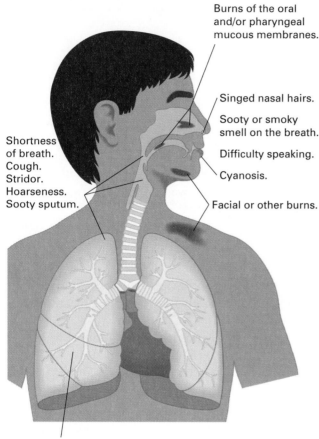

Burns of the oral and/or pharyngeal mucous membranes.

Singed nasal hairs.

Sooty or smoky smell on the breath.

Difficulty speaking.

Cyanosis.

Facial or other burns.

Shortness of breath.
Cough.
Stridor.
Hoarseness.
Sooty sputum.

Respiratory distress.
Noisy breathing.
Restricted chest movement.

Figure 20-8 Signs and symptoms of inhalation burns.

CHEMICAL BURNS

It is very difficult to assess the severity of chemical burns in the field. The general guideline is to treat all chemical burns as critical. Speed is essential. The faster you stop the burning process and initiate care, the less severe the burn will be. Follow these guidelines:

- Remember scene safety. Make sure that it is safe to approach the patient. If not, wait for trained rescue personnel to arrive. When you can approach your patient, wear protective gear to avoid contamination.
- Immediately begin to flush the patient's burns vigorously with water. Do not waste time trying to find an antidote. If the patient is at

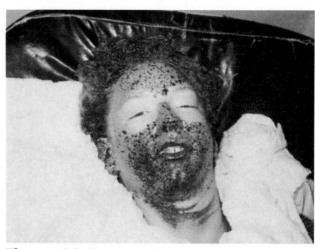

Figure 20-9 Burns to the face.

home, use the shower or a garden hose. Irrigate the area continuously under a steady stream for at least 20 minutes.
- If chemical burns affect the eyes, flush them with water (Figure 20–10). Use a faucet or a hose running at low pressure. If necessary, use a pan, bucket, cup, or bottle. Have the patient remove any contact lenses.
- Minimize further contamination by making sure the water runs away from the injury and not toward any uninjured areas.

Note that you should brush off dry chemicals, such as lime powder, before flushing with water (Figure 20–11). Also wash off phenol or carbolic acid with alcohol first, and then flush the burn with water.

ELECTRICAL BURNS

In any incident involving a car crash into a power pole, look for downed power lines. Sometimes they are hidden from sight by grass or a bush. So look at the next pole down the line. Count the number of power lines at the top crossarm. There should be the same number of lines at the top of the damaged pole. If the number is not the same, then proceed as follows:

- If you suspect that lines are down or the power pole has been weakened, notify all rescue personnel of the possible danger. Then notify the power company and request an emergency crew.

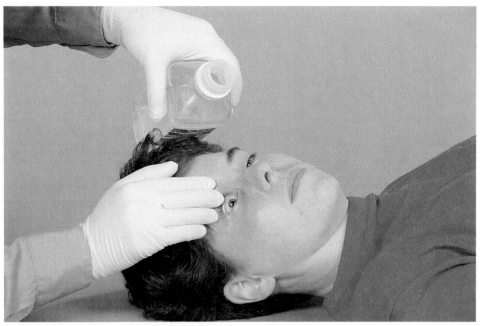

Figure 20-10 Flushing chemical burns to the eye.

- If the soles of your feet tingle when you enter the area, go no further. You are entering an energized zone.
- Assume that a downed power line is live until the power company crew tells you otherwise. Remember that vehicles, guard rails, metal fences, and so on conduct electricity.
- If the patient's vehicle is in contact with a downed power line, tell the patient to stay inside the car. Maintain a safe distance. Never have a patient try to jump clear unless there is immediate danger of fire or explosion. Do not

touch the vehicle and the ground at the same time. If you do, the current can kill you.
- Never try to remove a power line. Personnel from the electrical company must do it. They have the training and the proper equipment to handle the line safely.

If you approach an emergency scene involving other electrical hazards, make a visual sweep for power cords. Pull the plug before you approach or touch the patient. Remember that a power tool does not have to be "on" to present a shock hazard. In general, you should never try to remove a patient from an electrical source unless you are trained and equipped to do so. And never touch a patient still in contact with a electrical source.

Signs and symptoms of electric shock may include:

- Altered mental status.
- Obvious severe burns.
- Weak, irregular, or absent pulse.
- Shallow, irregular, or absent breathing.
- Multiple fractures due to intense muscle contractions.

Care for a patient with electrical burns the same way you would care for any other patient with burns. However, note that an electric shock

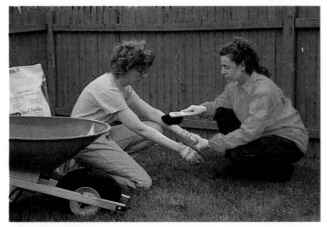

Figure 20-11 Lime powder should be brushed off the skin before flushing.

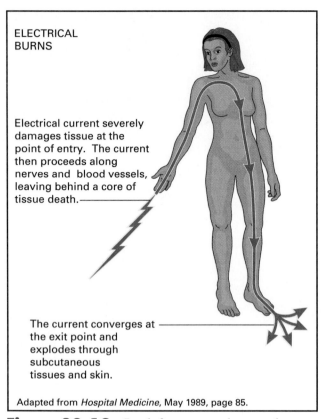

ELECTRICAL
BURNS

Electrical current severely
damages tissue at the
point of entry. The current
then proceeds along
nerves and blood vessels,
leaving behind a core of
tissue death.

The current converges at
the exit point and
explodes through
subcutaneous
tissues and skin.

Adapted from *Hospital Medicine*, May 1989, page 85.

Figure 20-12 Look for an entry burn and an exit burn.

can throw a patient a significant distance. So stabilize the patient's head and neck during assessment and treatment. Also look for both entry and exit burns (Figure 20–12). (See examples of electrical burns, Figure 20–13.)

LIGHTNING INJURIES

Thousands of electrical injuries occur each year in the U.S. About 25% of them are lightning injuries. A lightning bolt can pack more than a trillion watts of electricity and up to 100 million volts. Much of the electrical energy from lightning flows around, not through, a strike victim. A patient who has been struck by lightning does not hold a charge, so it is safe to approach him or her.

People are struck by lightning most often in open fields, under trees, on or near water, near tractors and heavy equipment, on golf courses, and at telephones. A person may be struck

directly by lightning or lightning may "splash" off a nearby object. Whole groups of people can be affected by a ground strike in which lightning hits the ground and electricity ripples outward.

Most victims of lightning are knocked down or thrown, so also assume possible spinal injury. Also assume that a victim of lightning has sustained multiple injuries. Patients generally sustain the following types of injury:

- *The nervous system*—In many instances of lightning strike, the patient becomes unresponsive. Few actually remember being struck. Some patients suffer partial paralysis. Occasionally paralysis of the respiratory system causes death.
- *The senses*—Some patients experience a loss of sight, hearing, and ability to speak. Rupture of one or both eardrums (tympanic membranes) occurs in 50% of patients who have been struck by lightning.
- *The skin*—In a lightning burn the skin may appear to be feathery, patchy, or in a scattered pattern resembling flowers. This is called "ferning." The burn may be red, mottled, blue, white, swollen, or blistered. The ferning fades and disappears within days.
- *The heart*—The lightning strike itself can disrupt the heart's rhythm, but the complications that follow are what generally lead to full cardiac arrest.
- *The vascular system*—Within seconds following the lightning strike, the patient may become unresponsive, appear pale and mottled, have cool arms and legs, and lose pulses. If the injury is moderate, the conditions may correct themselves quickly. In case of severe injury, blood may coagulate and tissues in the arms and legs may die, leading to amputation. Kidney failure may result.

Care for lightning burns as you would any other type of burn. You also should provide manual stabilization of the patient's head and neck during emergency care, and be prepared to provide basic life support. Such measures should continue even if the patient appears to be lifeless. Victims of lightning have been resuscitated as long as 30 minutes after a strike without any lasting damage.

ELECTRICAL BURNS

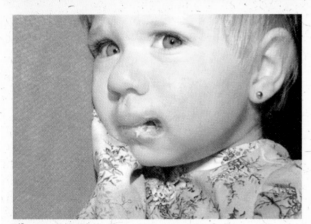

Figure 20-13a Electrical burn caused by chewing on an electrical cord.

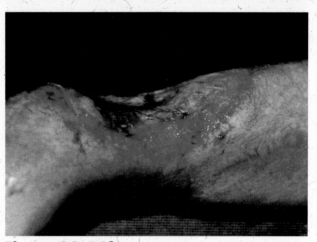

Figure 20-13b Full thickness electrical burn.

FIRST RESPONDER FOCUS

Burns can be painful, disfiguring injuries. The care you provide as a First Responder will be vital for the patient's survival. The most critical complication of burns is the most difficult to observe. Burns to the airway can cause swelling and obstruction, which lead to inadequate breathing or respiratory arrest. Monitor the patient very carefully for these conditions.

Safety also is a primary concern. The source of the burn (such as flames or chemicals) and a smoke- or vapor-filled environment can be a danger to First Responders. Have people who are properly trained and equipped remove the patient from a hazardous scene. Then begin emergency medical care. ∎

CASE STUDY FOLLOW-UP

At the beginning of this chapter, you read that First Responders were on scene with a male patient who had been hit by lightning. To see how chapter skills apply to this emergency, read the following. It describes how the call was completed.

PHYSICAL EXAMINATION
While my partner maintained manual stabilization and monitored breathing, I conducted a head-to-toe exam. I found an entrance burn on the patient's left arm and a larger exit burn on his left foot. There appeared to be no other injuries. I covered the burns with sterile gauze. After I took a set of vital signs, which were within normal ranges, the patient moaned and tried to sit up. We encouraged him to lie still and explained what had happened.

PATIENT HISTORY
The patient was still somewhat confused, so we interviewed witnesses to the incident. They related that the man had been walking to his barn when

CASE STUDY FOLLOW-UP *(Continued)*

he was struck by a lightning bolt. They knew of no medical problems or allergies. We found no medical identification tags or cards.

ONGOING ASSESSMENT
We took the patient's vital signs every 5 minutes or so until the EMTs arrived. There were no changes noted. His oxygen was continued without resistance. When the patient became more alert, he told us his name was Sam Costanza and gave us a brief medical history.

PATIENT HAND-OFF
My hand-off report to the EMTs was as follows:

"This is Sam Costanza. He is 42. He was struck by lightning as he approached his barn some 20 minutes ago. Initially, he responded only to painful stimuli. He presented with good respirations and heart rate. During the physical exam, he slowly became responsive. He remembered nothing about what happened to him. The physical exam revealed full thickness burns on the left arm and left foot. We covered them with sterile dressings. He says he has no significant medical history. His respirations are 20 and of good quality, pulse 90 and strong, BP 140/82. His pupils are equal and reactive. His skin is warm and dry."

After the EMTs took over, we returned to our duty station and prepared our truck for the next call.

Treat all burn injuries in basically the same way: Stop the burning process, remove smoldering clothing, and dress the wounds. However, your job may not be finished there. After the initial assessment and treatment of life-threats, be sure to perform a thorough physical exam to find and treat other injuries the patient may have. Gather a good patient history. And continue with an ongoing assessment until the EMTs arrive to take over patient care.

REVIEW QUESTIONS

Page references where answers may be found or supported are provided at the end of each question.

Section 1

1. When you estimate how severe a patient's burn may be, what four factors should you consider? (p. 336)
2. What is a superficial burn? Briefly describe its characteristics. (p. 337)
3. What is a partial thickness burn? Briefly describe its characteristics. (p. 337)
4. What is a full thickness burn? Briefly describe its characteristics. (p. 340)
5. What is "the rule of nines"? Describe how it is used. (pp. 340–341)
6. What is the "palmar surface method"? (pp. 340–341)

7. Are burns to certain areas of the body more critical than others? Explain. (p. 341)
8. Do age and chronic illness have anything to do with how severe a burn may be? Explain. (p. 341)

Section 2

9. What are the general guidelines for emergency medical care of burns? (pp. 341–343)
10. What special care would you provide if your patient had inhalation burns? (p. 343)
11. How would you stop the burning process if a dry chemical such as lime powder is involved? (p. 344)
12. What special precautions related to scene safety should you take if you are called to the scene of an electrical hazard? (pp. 344–346)

CHAPTER 21

AGRICULTURAL AND INDUSTRIAL EMERGENCIES

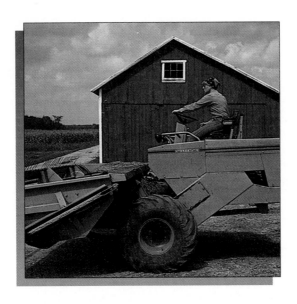

INTRODUCTION

Though more people in the U.S. live in cities, the death rate from accidental trauma is highest in rural areas. Agriculture involves about 3.1 million people, including those in fishing and forestry. According to the National Safety Council, farming is now considered the nation's most hazardous occupation. The number of accidents per work hour is five times higher in agriculture than the national average for major industry. Sadly, there is little on the topic in most First Responder training, even though some form of agricultural activity exists in every state.

Farm-type injuries also occur in urban areas. The pizza dough roller works on the same principles as the printing press or the agricultural combine, for example. Workers who do snow removal, construction work, and factory work also use similar machinery—and are prone to similar accidents.

Cognitive, affective, and psychomotor objectives are from the U.S. DOT's 1995 "First Responder: National Standard Curriculum." Enrichment objectives, if any, identify material that is supplemental to the DOT curriculum.

Cognitive

5-2.8 Describe the emergency medical care of the patient with a soft tissue injury. (pp. 351–352)

Affective

5-2.16 Attend to the feelings of the patient with a soft tissue injury or bleeding. (pp. 351–352)

5-2.17 Demonstrate a caring attitude toward patients with a soft tissue injury or bleeding who request emergency medical services. (pp. 351–352)

5-2.18 Place the interests of the patient with a soft tissue injury or bleeding as the foremost consideration when making any and all patient care decisions. (pp. 351–352, 354, 356, 358, 360)

5-2.19 Communicate with empathy to patients with a soft tissue injury or bleeding, as well as with family members and friends of the patient. (pp. 351–352)

Psychomotor

5-2.24 Demonstrate the steps in the emergency medical care of open soft tissue injuries. (pp. 351–352)

Enrichment

* Identify factors involved in the high rate of injury and fatality among farmers. (p. 350)
* Discuss common mechanisms of injury among agricultural workers. (p. 352)
* Identify common operational controls used on farm machinery. (p. 352)
* Discuss the principles of disentanglement from farm equipment. (pp. 355–360)
* Describe how to safely approach an industrial emegency. (pp. 360–361)

SECTION 1: AGRICULTURAL EMERGENCIES

In recent years 44 of every 100,000 farm workers died in work-related accidents. This is more than workers who die in the mining industry, construction trades, or transportation and public utilities. Why are farm accidents so serious? Consider the following:

* Most farm equipment is very complicated. As machinery becomes more sophisticated, the chances of injury increase.
* Most farmers do not use personal protective equipment.
* Farmers often use old, unsafe equipment because of the tremendous cost of replacement.
* Lengthy extrication is often needed when farmers become entangled in equipment. This can increase the severity of injuries.
* Since many farmers work alone in remote areas, they may not be missed for hours. Many farmers die from injuries that would not have been fatal if they had been discovered in time.
* There often is no phone at the scene. Many rural areas have no 9-1-1 service and no central dispatch.
* Long transport times contribute to the severity of injuries. Farms in rural areas can be long distances from hospitals.

Farmers also are under a great deal of stress. In fact, farming is rated among the top 10% of the most stressful occupations. Farmers work long hours, often seven days a week. They rarely take breaks or vacations. They are exposed to heat, cold, and excessive noise and vibration. They also have the psychological stress of unstable weather conditions and financial difficulties including unfavorable prices at harvest time.

CASE STUDY

DISPATCH

When the Klaxon alarm goes off, it means that an employee is caught in a baling machine. As soon as I heard it, I made sure that someone called 9-1-1. Then I went to the scene of the accident. I knew that a co-worker, Ellen, would meet me with our first-aid kit as planned.

SCENE SIZE-UP

It was quiet when I got to the scene. All equipment around the patient was shut down. Several employees were working to set the man free. They were experts. They told me it would be a few minutes more. When I got a look at the patient, I saw he was an apprentice. He had been pulled by his sleeve into a baler. The workers who were disentangling him said it looked as if he had one or two amputated fingers.

> Consider this patient as you read Chapter 21. What may be done to assess and treat his condition?

GENERAL GUIDELINES FOR EMERGENCY CARE

Emergency care of patients with farm injuries is basically the same as for any other patient. In the case of a patient entangled in equipment and in need of rescue:

- Remember the priorities of airway, breathing, and circulation. Disentanglement can take up to an hour. Do not neglect the airway while the patient is being freed. If you are allowed, administer high-flow oxygen throughout the rescue.
- If you cannot apply direct pressure to a bleeding wound, use the nearest pulse point. Sometimes the farm equipment itself helps to control bleeding by the pressure it exerts on an injury. In these cases, transport the patient while he or she is still entangled in the equipment. Most equipment can be cut to a manageable size.

- Monitor vital signs. Do it constantly so that you will not lose the patient to an undetected injury.
- Preserve amputated parts, despite their appearance. If fingers have been injured, stabilize the wrist joint. It probably is injured, too.

Disentanglement requires appropriate training and assistance at the scene. Rescue should begin only when all of the following have been accomplished:

1. Farm equipment has been stabilized.
2. Engines have been shut down.
3. Other hazards, such as leaking fuel, have been controlled.
4. The patient has been stabilized.

As in any emergency situation, attend to the feelings of the patient as best you can. Explain who you are, what you are doing, and what you plan to do. Keep the patient informed—and his or her family, if they are on scene—as you proceed with emergency care. Be the patient's liaison during extrication, too. As in any emergency, be sure to take all safety precautions continuously. Do not let down your guard.

COMMON OPERATIONAL CONTROLS AND SHUTDOWN

Tractors and other farm equipment have a number of mechanisms that cause injury. (See Figures 21–1 and 21–2.) They include:

- *Pinch points*—two objects meet to cause a pinching or pulling action.
- *Wrap points*—an aggressive component moves in a circular motion.
- *Shear points*—two objects move close enough together to cause a cutting action.
- *Crush points*—two large objects come together to cause a crushing action.
- *Stored energy*—hazards remain after machinery has been shut down.

Become familiar with common operational controls. This knowledge can save you time and frustration during rescue. Some manufacturers use different symbols or colors to help the operator quickly identify controls. Color codes include red, which indicates combine movement controls (throttle, gearshift, ground speed control). Yellow indicates auxiliary power controls (separator control, cylinder speed control, header drive control). Black indicates miscellaneous function controls.

The first step in shutting down farm machinery is to stabilize it. You can use one of several methods: block or chock the wheels, set the parking or operational brakes, or tie the machine to another vehicle. Once the machine is stabilized, shut it down as follows:

1. Enter the cab, if possible. Look at the controls. Locate the ignition switch-on key and throttle lever. *If you have any doubt about how to identify controls, do not touch them. Wait for help.*
2. Slow the engine down with the throttle. Switch off the key. If the machine is fueled with diesel,

the key many not shut off the engine. Locate a fuel or air shutoff lever. Again, if you are in doubt, do not touch the lever.
3. Pull the knob or lever to shut down the engine.
4. If you cannot shut down the engine in the cab, try the fuel tank area.
5. As a last resort, locate the fuel line or filters ahead of the fuel pump or injector pump. Interrupt the flow of fuel. Use extreme caution when cutting a fuel line. Large farm machinery can carry up to 300 gallons of fuel.
6. If the engine is a diesel, loosen the fuel filter. The engine will stall.
7. If all other attempts at shutting down the machine fail, locate the air intake. Discharge a 20-pound CO_2 fire extinguisher into it. Make sure that you hold the trigger of the extinguisher until the engine comes to a complete stop. (Warning: This technique can cause extensive damage to the engine.)

TRACTORS

Tractors are the most common cause of farm-related fatalities. Most involve a tractor turning over backwards or rolling to the side. Of all tractor fatalities, 83% are the result of crushing injuries.

The tractors used today fall into two categories: two-wheel drive and four-wheel drive. Engines may be fueled by gasoline, diesel, or liquid propane. Fuel leaks, fires, and explosions can result from tractor accidents. Fire protection is critical during rescue.

Tractor Stabilization

Before rescue, a tractor engine must be shut down, the fuel controlled, and the tractor stabilized. If you are unfamiliar with the equipment, call for assistance. Local repair shops and area agriculture workers can be good resources. Rescue teams should be capable of handling fire, since there will almost certainly be spilled fuel and hot hydraulic fluid.

To stabilize the tractor, lock up the rear wheels with two one- or two-ton cable hoists and three chains, even if the tractor is upright.

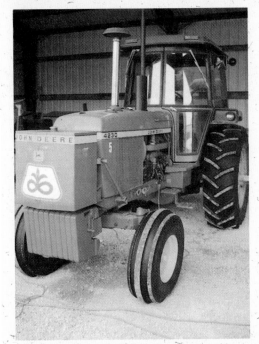

Figure 21-1a Diesel tractor.

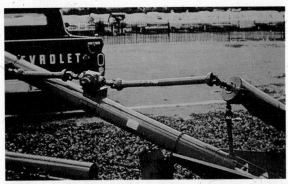

Figure 21-1b Power takeoff (PTO) shaft.

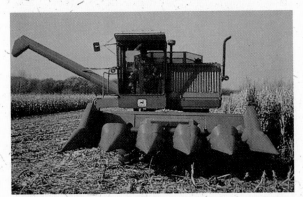

Figure 21-1c Combine with corn head.

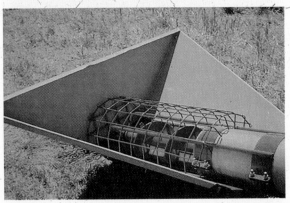

Figure 21-1d Auger and hopper with protective cage.

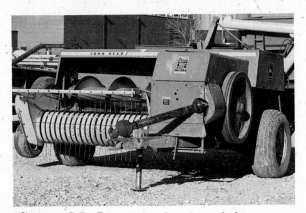

Figure 21-1e Baler for square bales.

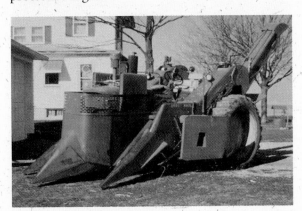

Figure 21-1f Corn picker.

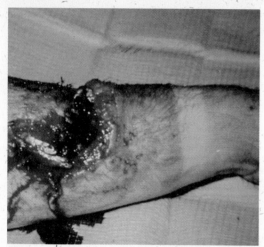

Figure 21-2a Arm injured in a PTO shaft.

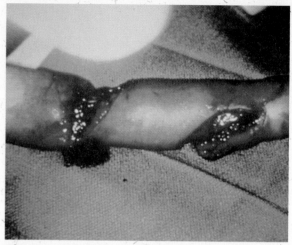

Figure 21-2b Arm injured in an auger.

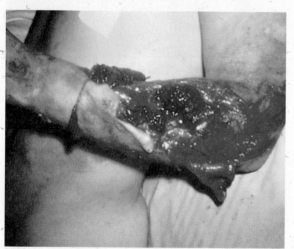

Figure 21-2c Arm injured in an auger.

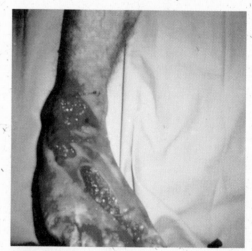

Figure 21-2d Foot injured in an auger.

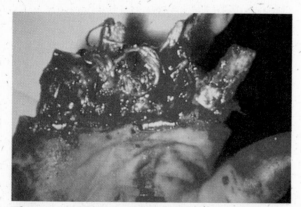

Figure 21-2e Hand injured in snapping rolls.

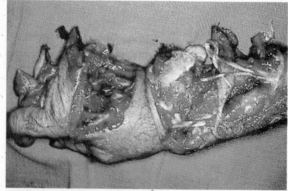

Figure 21-2f Hand and arm injured in hay baler.

1. Wrap one chain around the rear tire and through the high slot in the rim.
2. Wrap the second chain around the same wheel and through the low slot in the rim.
3. Attach the third chain to the front of the tractor and stretch it to a hoist.
4. Attach the other hoist to the two rear chains. If the tractor does not have slots in the rims, stretch the hoist and chains across the rear tire to a strong point on the rear of the tractor. Make sure you do not lift the secure tire off the ground during hoisting.

Patient Assessment and Emergency Care

Scene safety is a priority. Once the equipment is shut down and stabilized, reassess the area before starting patient care. When you are certain the scene is safe, assess the patient. Some points to remember follow:

- As always, determine if there is any immediate threat to life. Give aggressive management to airway, breathing, and circulation.
- Suspect possible chest injuries, including pneumothorax and sucking chest wounds. Since about 85% of all tractor overturns are to the side, expect crushing injuries to the patient's head, chest, and abdomen, as well as multiple lacerations.
- Treat the patient for shock.
- Common tractor rollover injuries include burns from spilled engine coolants, transmission fluid, hydraulic fluid, and battery acid. Pay special attention to the eyes and assess for chemical burns.
- After assessment, stabilize all injuries. When there are open extremity injuries with possible broken bones, immobilize them in splints if you are trained to do so.

When possible, lift or remove the tractor from the patient once he or she is stabilized. Do not stop patient care during lifting operations. Both efforts should continue at the same time. Be sure to call fire crews, extrication crews, and advance care providers as soon as possible.

Lifting Operations

During any lifting operation, a cross-crib capable of supporting the tractor must be built. This is to protect the patient and other rescuers in case lifting devices fail or the tractor has to be let down and repositioned for another lift.

The crib should be as wide as possible. A safe rule of thumb is the crib box should not be taller than it is wide. Also, the cribbing and lifting devices need a solid surface from which to work and function properly. This is sometimes difficult in a soft field or ditch. The rescue squad should carry several quarter-inch tread plates about 24″ × 24″ each. The plates will serve as a firm lifting surface on soft ground or on blacktop.

High-pressure airbags (approximately 90 to 120 psi) are the best tools available to lift a heavy, irregularly shaped machine. The bags must be placed carefully. Keep in mind the tractor's center of gravity. It is 10″ above and 24″ ahead of the rear axle at the platform area where the operator places his or her feet. About 30% of the tractor's weight is in front of this point and 70% behind.

Even though airbags appear to be indestructible, they are not. Airbags are most efficient during the first three to five inches of lift. They may be stacked to get a higher lift, but they become increasingly unstable as they are inflated. Whenever possible, a cross-crib should be built to get the bag within one to two inches of the object. A steel plate should be placed between the bag and the crib to keep the crib from being knocked apart during inflation.

Power spreaders or hydraulic rams also do a good job of lifting. With power hydraulic tools, the steel plate is a must for a good lifting platform. Hydraulic tools move very fast. The operator may have to wait for the crew that is building the cross-crib. The tool operator must continuously take note of the center of gravity. He or she also must watch for unstable conditions, such as changes of angle between the lifting surface of the tool and the tractor, sinking of the tractor on the opposite side of the lift, and so on.

Hand-power hydraulic jacks or manual jacks also can be used to lift a tractor. Use extreme caution if more than one jack has to be used. The cross-crib must be kept as close to the lifting device as possible. If one device becomes overloaded and fails, the other will almost certainly do the same. Cranes, wreckers, and boom trucks also can be used, if readily available, especially if you are dealing with a very large tractor. Regardless, cribs should still be built to protect the patient and rescuers from equipment failure or operator error.

When you lift or remove the overturned tractor from a patient, follow these basic rules:

- All rescuers should know exactly what their roles will be. They should also know who is responsible for hoisting commands before lifting is done. During any extrication, only one rescuer should give lifting instructions. Instructions from more than one will result in injury to rescuers and patients.
- Always try to determine the tractor's center of gravity. Always build a crib to guard against equipment failures or operator error.
- Watch the patient during the lift to ensure that the part to be lifted is moving properly and that another part is not putting more pressure on the patient. If conditions change, the rescuer leading the lifting operation should be advised.
- Anytime more than one lifting device has to be used, use extra care in coordinating the lift to keep loads from shifting.

Lifting a tractor is not like lifting an automobile. A tractor usually is heavier. (A tractor can weigh up to 15 tons.) It also is difficult to stabilize because of its irregular shape and because many accidents occur on soft ground. To be sure, a tractor rollover presents a difficult challenge. However, if safety precautions are taken and if patient care and extrication are provided at the same time, this complex situation can be handled with confidence.

Power Takeoff Shafts

The power takeoff (PTO) shaft is a high-speed drive shaft that connects a tractor to farm implements such as balers, mowers, corn pickers, forage harvesters, and so on. It is the second most common cause of agricultural fatalities.

PTO-related accidents most often occur in fall or winter when the farmer's heavy clothing gets caught in the shaft and pulls the farmer in. Most of these accidents involve the arms, which are usually amputated. The farmer also can get wrapped around the shaft. PTO shaft injuries are not common. They make up only 8% of farm injuries. However, they usually are fatal.

To shut down a PTO shaft, turn off the source of power—the tractor. Some PTO shafts will free-wheel in either direction when the power is shut off. Some lock up immediately. Take care, because energy can be stored in the shaft.

To disentangle the patient, do the following:

- Always assume that the patient has sustained neck and back injuries. Stabilize the patient's spine as soon as possible. Immobilize him or her before transport.
- If the patient is wrapped on the shaft, determine if clothing could be cut to free the patient. The PTO shaft will wrap the patient's clothing into multiple layers, making cutting difficult and time-consuming. Look for the end of the wrap where clothing is only one layer thick. Cut at this point with rescue knives.
- If you must remove the PTO shaft with the patient, place a fire pry bar (42″ or longer) into the implement side of the PTO shaft to hold the stored energy. If pressure is on the coupling, the shaft will not slide apart. By reversing the shaft one-sixteenth of an inch, the coupling will move. Uncouple the shaft. Slide it apart. Have the patient sent to the hospital with the section.
- If you cannot uncouple the shaft, cut it with a power saw, gasoline-powered circular saw, or hack saw. Cutting should be done if nothing else will extricate the patient. This procedure will release the stored energy in the shaft very quickly. So, when cutting the shaft, take extreme care to prevent it from spinning. Lock the PTO shaft in place with a fire pry bar through the universal joint on both ends.
- As you remove the patient, make sure that all rescuers and bystanders stand clear to avoid further injury.
- Locate amputated parts if possible, but do not delay transport. Send parts with the patient.

Because of the energy involved, injuries to the patient can be quiet severe. The patient would need rapid treatment and transport. Aggressively control bleeding with trauma dressings at the site of an avulsion or amputation. If advanced care is available (air transport, ground paramedics), call as soon as possible.

OTHER EQUIPMENT

Other types of agricultural equipment include the combine, auger, corn picker, snapping rolls, and hay baler.

Combines, Snapping Rolls, and Gathering Chains

The combine is a machine used to harvest and thresh all kinds of grain. It is assembled with multiple augers, shafts, belt and pulleys, roller chains, and sprockets. Many times a farmer is injured while doing routine maintenance on the combine, such as greasing bearings or tightening belts. Combines commonly cause partial and complete amputations.

The snapping rolls and gathering chains on an older model combine (two- to four-row units) require power rescue tools and airbags along with wooden wedges to spread the rolls. The rolls on the new models cannot be spread with conventional rescue tools. (See "Corn Pickers, Snapping Rolls, and Gathering Chains" later in this chapter.)

Just behind the combine header, and just ahead of the wheels, is a coupling device that attaches the head to the driving mechanism. This device could be a shaft with a pin in it. It could also be a set of flat gears sitting side by side with a common roller chain wrapped around them. Since it has to be released any time the head is changed, the device will be easy to get to and remove.

If you release the coupling device, you will be able to turn the header backward slowly and keep it under control. However, because of stored energy, you may need to use a pipe wrench or a large channel-lock pliers to move the shaft a sixteenth of an inch forward to remove the coupling. Once the coupling has been disconnected, manual pressure on the wrench should be released with care.

Never use the self-reversing features on modern combines to remove a trapped person. The reversing feature moves too fast and for too long for you to remove a patient without causing further injury. By turning the shaft backward, you will only reverse the head.

If the patient has been pulled into the feeder-conveyor, where the head attaches to the combine, you will have to disassemble a portion of the head and the shroud that surrounds the conveyor. This should be done by using an air chisel to cut away the sheet metal in the area.

If a torch is used, consider the fire hazards first. One spark could start a fire quickly. A charged fire line should be available after the surrounding area of the field and the combine itself is washed down with water. Any dust standing around the work area should be removed with water. Flush down the inside of the combine header, feeder house, and up into the main combine.

Augers and Elevators

Combines and corn pickers are equipped with augers and elevators that move the grain through the machine. Many augers and elevators have clean-out doors and inspection covers that, if opened while the machine is in operation, become traps to the unwary operator.

Augers are used to move the threshed, separated, and cleaned grain from the cleaning shoe to the wagon or truck for transport. An auger is generally 4 to 12 inches in diameter with flights 3 to 11 inches apart. The elevator has a series of rubber or steel paddles attached to a drive chain that moves at about 350 feet per minute.

The power for the majority of these devices comes from the belt and pulley system on the combine. If a patient becomes trapped in the auger, the drive should be disconnected. Before cutting the belt or chain, place a large pipe wrench on the shaft that drives the auger. This will hold the stored energy and prevent further injuries. After the belt or chain is cut, slowly release the pressure on the shaft. Monitor the patient to be sure no further injury is being done.

Augers can pull in victims with extreme force. They often cause complete amputation, usually of the hands and arms and sometimes of the feet and legs. Auger accidents often involve children who are not experienced enough to avoid an accident. Entanglement in augers is so severe that it often cannot be handled in the field. You may need to cut the auger free and have it transported with the patient.

If amputation is complete, you may be able to slowly rotate the auger in its natural direction until the amputated part emerges at the end. (Never reverse an auger. It can cause increased tissue damage.) If that is not possible, you may have to dissemble the auger.

If the auger tube is held by bolts, remove them first. If not, then the tube will have to be split or cut with an air chisel or a reciprocating saw. Do not use a torch. The danger of heat transfer to the patient and the threat of fire is too great. Cut a few feet from the patient. Look for spot welds on the flighting. Cut so the end of the flighting nearest the patient will not spring back to cause further injury. Take care to avoid excessive vibration or movement.

Corn Pickers, Snapping Rolls, and Gathering Chains

Corn pickers can be mounted on a tractor, pulled by a tractor, or they may be self-propelled. Each uses a system of rollers, chains, belts, and blades to remove corn from the stalk and then shear the corn away from the cob. Power for corn pickers is usually taken from the tractor PTO and hydraulic systems.

Corn picker accidents usually involve a hand that is crushed when a farmer tries to free trapped material in the picker. Amputation is rare, but the hand is often lost as a result of damage or infection. Extrication is extremely difficult, since the machinery is in heavy metal housings and cannot be reversed.

Snapping rolls move at a normal speed of 12 feet per second. Generally, they can cause severe crushing injuries to the hand. Often a weed or stalk catches between the rolls and stops them. A farmer who tries to remove the trapped material can cause the snapping rolls to start up with the slightest movement—and the rolls move more quickly than the farmer can pull back.

The majority of snapping rolls on corn pickers can be spread with the use of two wooden wedges plus a small hydraulic wedge. Use the wooden wedges for cribbing the rolls as they are separated by the hydraulic wedge. Insert one wooden wedge from the top of the rolls, while the other wooden wedge is pushed in from below. Equip the bottom wedge with a rope that allows the operator to pull it through from above.

The two wedges are a must. If only one is used and the hydraulic wedge slips or is released, the one wooden wedge will be shot from the machine. If this is allowed to happen, your patient may be further injured and rescuers jeopardized.

Snapping rolls also may be spread with the use of high-pressure airbags and two wooden wedges. The majority of power hydraulic tools may be used with the two wooden wedges. Whatever tool you use, remember these basic rules: Always use the wooden wedges for cribbing. Only open the roll as wide as necessary to remove your patient. Make sure that rescue efforts are coordinated with medical personnel.

Husking Beds

After the ears of corn pass through the snapping rollers, they enter the husking beds, one on each side of a mounted picker. The husking beds pull the leaves from the ear, exposing the kernels of corn still attached to the cob. The ear is then moved to the elevator and dropped in a wagon.

Husking beds present the greatest challenge. They are mounted to the picker with heavy duty bearing housings (normally cast iron) and are held together with strong springs. They are also enclosed by sheet metal, which can be removed by cutting off the bolt heads with an air chisel or just by taking the machine apart with wrenches.

Once the rolls have been reached, take care to avoid uncontrolled release of the springs that hold them together. At this point, you should release the tension-adjusting nuts or bolts. Then remove the bolts that fasten the bearing housings to the husking bed housing, again avoiding explosive release of stored energy in the springs. If you can reach the bearing housings with a power rescue tool, try to break them. However, removing the bolts by hand is the recommended and more controlled method.

Hay Baler

The hay baler compacts straw and hay into bundles. Some are small rectangular bundles. Others are massive rounded ones. The hay baler exerts force of up to 1300 pounds between spring-loaded rollers. Amputations are often the result. Hay balers also commonly cause compression, avulsion, and wringer injuries. Because the springs can be released and the bolts cut, it is not as difficult to free a patient from a hay baler as it is from other farm equipment.

AGRICULTURAL STORAGE DEVICES

Grain Tank

Farmers who fall into the grain tanks risk death from suffocation. Always assume that a patient in a grain tank is alive, even if he or she has been trapped there for hours. Turn off electric power to the structure as soon as possible. Call the fire department and extrication teams to the scene. If advanced care providers are available, have them dispatched to the scene as soon as possible. Do not enter the structure without other rescuers to help. Any rescuer entering should be tied to a safety lifeline and wearing a disposable mechanical filter respirator rated for dust particles.

Do not use the gravity gate or auger to release the grain. The grain flows from top to bottom, and the patient can be pulled further into the tank. Instead, cut uniform 18" triangular holes as high as possible but still below the level of the grain. Cut in the middle of the bin sheets, avoiding bolts, seams, and stiffeners. Open the holes simultaneously so that the grain flows out evenly. This will prevent the walls of the tank from collapsing. Once the tank begins to empty, rescuers with shovels, tractors and loads, or skid loaders may be needed to remove grain.

Once the patient is exposed, secure him or her with a lifeline. Then aggressively clear the patient's airway of grain by suctioning. After the airway has been assured, assess for other injuries. Then a trained rescuer must fully immobilize the patient. Move the patient onto a long backboard and position a basket stretcher for extrication. A 24" × 24" hole can be cut at the surface of the grain to allow the stretcher to be lowered to the ground. If the grain feels cool or cold, treat the patient for hypothermia.

If the patient is only partially submerged, lower a rescuer on a harness secured with lifelines. Clear the area around the patient's head to make breathing possible and to establish an airway. Use plywood, sheets of metal, or a 55-gallon drum with both ends removed to keep grain away from the patient's face during extrication.

Silo

When crops are stored in silos, gas is formed by natural chemical fermentation. Fermenting crops can release high levels of carbon monoxide, methane, and nitrogen dioxide. These gases can cause serious injury or death. The presence of silo gas may be recognized by any of the following signs:

- Bleach-like odor.
- Yellowish or reddish vapor hovering over the product.
- Stains of red, yellow, or brown on the product or other surfaces touched by the gas.
- Dead birds or insects near the silo.
- Nearby livestock with signs of illness.

The greatest danger of silo gas is just after harvest. However, fumes can persist and occur when a silo is opened months later. Most silo injuries occur when a victim falls into the silo and either becomes trapped in the unloading device or is overcome by gas. Some suffer cardiac arrest in the silo.

Unfortunately, silo gas causes little immediate pain. A victim may not be aware of an injury and die hours later because the injured lungs fill with fluid during sleep. Common reactions to silo gas include:

- Eye irritation.
- Cough, possibly with labored breathing.
- Fatigue.
- Nausea, vomiting.
- Cyanosis.
- Dizziness or sleepiness.

Two teams are usually needed to rescue a patient from a silo. Rescuers should be lowered in, and the patient lifted out through the top on a litter. Always use a self-contained breathing apparatus (SCBA) when doing rescue work at a silo. Place a SCBA with supplementary oxygen on the patient as soon as possible. If the extrication team is delayed or if no SCBA is available, the silo blower may be turned on to purge the air.

Be sure all patients exposed to silo gas are transported to a hospital for monitoring. Complications can develop up to 12 hours after exposure.

Manure Storage Areas

Large livestock facilities handle manure by flushing down the confinement buildings with water. The liquid is then sent to an open pond for storage. In some cases, liquid manure is stored in a structure similar to a silo.

There are two potential injuries from liquid manure: drowning and inhaling toxic fumes. (The liquid manure releases ammonia, carbon monoxide, carbon dioxide, methane, and hydrogen sulfide.) Agitation of a manure pit can cause the sudden release of hydrogen sulfide. Signs and symptoms of hydrogen sulfide poisoning may include:

- Cough.
- Irritation of mucous membranes.
- Nausea.
- Sudden collapse and respiratory paralysis (with high concentrations).

The primary goal of rescue is to provide ventilation to the patient. Always use back-up rescuers. Always wear a self-contained breathing apparatus (SCBA) and lifelines. Provide aggressive airway management to the patient and, if needed, basic life support. Monitor the patient's vital signs. Treat for shock. Place the patient on high-flow oxygen. If advanced care is available (air transport, ground paramedics), call as soon as possible.

After the patient has been pulled from the storage area, remove all clothing from the patient and rescuers. Flush thoroughly with water and wash with green soap. All contaminated clothing must be removed before transport. If not, the clothing will give off fumes that can overcome the ambulance crew.

SECTION 2: INDUSTRIAL RESCUE

Like rural emergencies, industrial emergencies are anything but routine. Often hazardous materials are at the scene. Heavy machinery may be involved. More than one person is usually injured, and patients may be in unusual positions, crushed beneath fallen debris or trapped at high angles.

In any industrial rescue, follow these safety guidelines:

- If you are not familiar with the company's operations, check with staff to determine potential hazards at the scene. Make sure all hazards are controlled before you approach the patient.
- Never assume that any machine is locked and secured. Verify with company officials that all valves, switches, and levers that allow a machine to operate have been secured to the "off" position.
- If the patient is in a confined space, or if he or she has been injured by an airborne or spilled agent, wait for specialized personnel or hazardous materials teams to arrive and decontaminate the scene and the patient.

Your first priority in responding to the scene of an industrial accident is to protect your own safety. If there are hazardous materials or chemical spills at the scene, all rescuers must be protected. Call multiple response teams, including teams who can fight fire and handle hazardous materials if needed. If the site is large, designate an area where responding units should report. Assign a rescuer to stand at the gate or site to meet incoming units and to direct them to the patients. If patients are buried by heavy debris (such as concrete, steel reinforcements, heavy machinery, or roofing materials), call specialty teams who can hoist it away. A member of an EMS team should supervise removal of heavy objects. Removal must be closely monitored to prevent further injury to the patient.

If a patient has been contaminated by hazardous materials, decontamination is necessary.

Rescuers should not assess or treat a contaminated patient, or they may become contaminated themselves. In cases of gross contamination, specially equipped rescuers may need to scrape or dissolve chemicals from the patient before assessment and treatment can take place.

If the patient is trapped at a high angle, get enough rescuers who are properly equipped for the rescue. Secondary safety belts, full-body harnesses, and rappelling harnesses can be used in high-angle rescues. Patients who are not severely injured can be lowered with full-body and rappelling harnesses. Those who are more severely injured or who require immobilization prior to being moved can be lowered in a basket stretcher. Regardless of which method is used, a rescuer must be lowered alongside the patient to monitor his or her condition and provide reassurance during descent.

(Specific information on how to handle hazardous materials and multiple-casualty incidents is offered in Chapters 28 and 29. Also see Chapter 32 for other special rescue situations.)

FIRST RESPONDER FOCUS

Agricultural and industrial emergencies may be catastrophic. The machinery used in these settings are capable of causing serious injury or death by way of their moving parts, sharp edges, and even extreme weights. These same mechanisms of injury also work against the First Responder. So unless you are trained to do so, do not attempt a rescue. You too may fall victim to the weight of the overturned tractor, the hazardous atmospheres and shifting materials in a silo, or the grasp of a baler. ■

CASE STUDY FOLLOW-UP

At the beginning of this chapter, you read that First Responders were on scene with a male patient who was pulled into a baler. To see how chapter skills apply to this emergency, read the following. It describes how the call was completed.

INITIAL ASSESSMENT

Ellen and I quickly sorted out our priorities, remembering that the ABCs are always first. When the patient was free and a safe distance away from the machine, we saw that the others had been correct. There were two fingers missing, the hand was badly mangled, and the patient was going into shock. Ellen had him lie down and positioned him. I assessed his airway and breathing. Ellen applied oxygen as I worked on controlling the bleeding.

Because the plant was so large, I knew that the ambulance crew would need help to find us. Another employee volunteered to go to the main gate to meet them when they arrived.

PHYSICAL EXAMINATION

After bleeding was under control, I performed a quick head-to-toe. I bandaged and splinted the patient's injured hand and wrist. A worker yelled out that he found one of the patient's amputated fingers. I wrapped it in sterile gauze, and instructed him to go to the cafeteria to get some cold packs, a container with a tightly fitting lid, and at least two plastic bags. I wanted to make sure it was stored safely in case it could be reattached.

PATIENT HISTORY

The patient reported that he was allergic to penicillin but had no other problems. He answered the rest of our questions, but he was in a lot of pain.

ONGOING ASSESSMENT

Each time I took vital signs, I wrote them down. I did that a few times. We monitored the patient closely, kept him warm, and kept checking the oxygen until the ambulance crew arrived.

CASE STUDY FOLLOW-UP *(Continued)*

PATIENT HAND-OFF

When the EMTs arrived, I gave them the hand-off report:

> "This is Tom Robinson. He is 22. About 15 minutes ago his right arm got pulled into the baler, which amputated two fingers. Tom is responsive. We had him lie down, and applied oxygen. The physical exam did not turn up anything except the injured hand, so we bandaged and splinted it. We wrapped and bagged one of the amputated fingers. The patient had some coffee about two hours ago, nothing else today. He is allergic to penicillin. His vitals are pulse 110, respirations 18. Skin is cool and moist."

We found out later that the doctors were able to reattach the one finger. The apprentice thanked Ellen and me for saving his life when we saw him. I don't think we saved his life. He wouldn't have died from his injuries, but I'm real glad we had the training to help him.

> No matter where or how your patient is found, follow the First Responder's patient assessment plan—scene size-up through patient hand-off. If special rescue teams are needed to extricate the patient, assure continued emergency medical care throughout the procedure.

REVIEW QUESTIONS

Page references where answers may be found or supported are provided at the end of each question.

Section 1

1. What are the general procedures of emergency care for farm-related injuries? (pp. 351–352)
2. If a patient is caught in machinery, what four steps must be accomplished before disentanglement should begin? (p. 351)
3. What are some mechanisms of injury associated with farm machinery? (p. 352)
4. When a patient has debris or machinery on top of him or her, why should medical personnel monitor lifting during rescue? (p. 356)

Section 2

5. What are three safety guidelines that you should follow at the scene of any industrial accident? (p. 360)

INJURIES TO THE HEAD, FACE, AND NECK

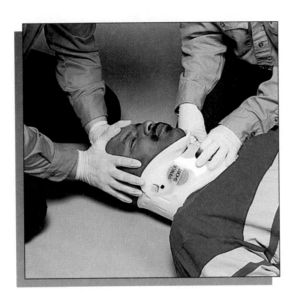

INTRODUCTION

Injuries to the head are among the most serious emergencies. They run a high risk of causing life-long complications and death. Your role as the first medically trained rescuer on scene can be critical.

While some injuries to the face and throat are minor, many can be life-threatening. They can compromise the upper airway and impair the patient's ability to breathe. In addition, many injuries to the face and neck stem from impacts strong enough to cause hidden facial fractures, cervical-spine damage, and skull fractures.

OBJECTIVES

Cognitive, affective, and psychomotor objectives are from the U.S. DOT's 1995 "First Responder: National Standard Curriculum." Enrichment objectives, if any, identify material that is supplemental to the DOT curriculum.

Cognitive

5-3.7 List the signs and symptoms of injury to the head. (pp. 364–366)
5-3.8 Describe the emergency medical care for injuries to the head. (pp. 366–368)

Affective

No objectives are identified.

Psychomotor

No objectives are identified.

Enrichment

* Describe the emergency care of injuries to the face, including injuries to the jaw, cheek, nose, and ear. (pp. 368–371)
* Establish the relationship between airway management and injuries to the face. (p. 368)
* Describe the emergency care of injuries to the neck. (pp. 371–372)
* Describe the emergency care of injuries to the eyes. (pp. 372–379)

SECTION 1:
INJURIES TO THE HEAD

A head injury may be open or closed. An open head injury is accompanied by a break in the skull, such as that caused by a fracture or an impaled object. It involves direct local damage to tissue. It also can result in brain damage.

A closed head injury does not involve a break in the skull. Even so, the brain can be seriously injured. The skull holds brain tissue, blood, and cerebrospinal fluid. The volume of each can vary, but the total volume cannot. Because the skull is rigid, its capacity is limited. If brain tissue swells or if bleeding occurs, pressure can build up inside the skull causing damage to the brain.

PATIENT ASSESSMENT

The general signs and symptoms of a head injury include the following:

- Altered mental status, from confusion to unresponsiveness.
- Irregular breathing.
- Open wounds to the scalp.
- Penetrating wounds to the head.
- Softness or depression of the skull.
- Blood or cerebrospinal fluid leaking from the ears or nose (Figure 22–1).
- Facial bruises.
- Bruising around the eyes ("raccoon eyes").
- Bruising behind the ears ("Battle's sign").
- Abnormal findings in an assessment of pulses, movement, and sensation.
- Headache severe enough to be disabling or which appears suddenly.
- Nausea, vomiting.

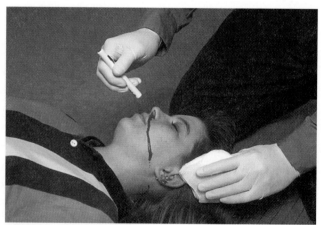

Figure 22-1 Blood or cerebrospinal fluid may come from the ears and nose of a patient with head injury.

was 0750

700 Mill

of the fac-

SIZE-UP

Although dispatch did not give us reason to anticipate an unsafe scene, we approached with caution. The foreman met us at the gate and immediately directed us to the patient's location. The crowd gathered around the patient was being controlled by the company security guards. We identified ourselves and approached the patient.

INITIAL ASSESSMENT

My partner held the patient's head and neck, while I began the assessment. The patient was not responsive to voice or painful stimuli. I opened and assessed his airway and heard gurgling sounds from his throat. Without delay, I suctioned the mouth, and the gurgling sounds ceased.

The patient's respirations appeared to be adequate. We elected to place him on oxygen at 15 liters per minute with a nonrebreather mask. There was no visible bleeding present. Our general impression was of a male in his 30s who was unresponsive after a fall.

> Consider this patient as you read Chapter 22. What would you do to assess and treat his condition?

- Unequal pupil size with altered mental status.
- Seizure activity.

Suspect spine injury in any patient with a head injury (Figure 22–2). If there is an obvious head injury, if the mechanism of injury suggests a head or spine injury, or if a trauma patient is unresponsive, immediately stabilize the patient's head and neck. Maintain manual stabilization until the patient is completely immobilized (Figure 22–3). If you are alone with an injured patient, you may be allowed to place a rigid item on each side of the patient's head to prevent movement. Follow local protocols.

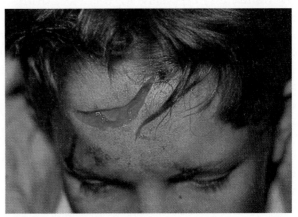

Figure 22-2 Always suspect spine injury in a patient with a head injury.

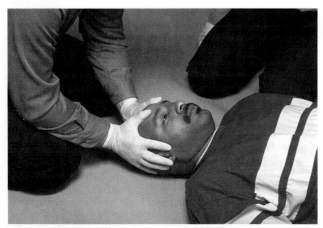

Figure 22-3 Maintain manual stabilization until the patient is properly immobilized.

During your initial assessment, use a jaw-thrust maneuver to open, assess, and maintain the airway. Also note that bleeding from the scalp may be profuse because of the large number of blood vessels there.

During your physical exam of the patient, look for open injuries to the head. Closed injuries may present with swelling or depression of the bones of the skull. Check for cerebrospinal fluid, which appears as a clear liquid, possibly tinged pink with blood, leaking from an open head wound or from the ears or nose.

For the head-injured patient, it is especially important for you to assess pulses, movement, and sensation in the extremities. Also pay attention to the function of the patient's eyes and note any numbness, especially of the face, arms, or legs.

When you take the patient's history, be sure to try to find out when the injury occurred, if the patient lost consciousness, and if the patient was moved after the injury occurred. Details about what happened are crucial to his or her medical care.

During your ongoing assessment, monitor the patient for any change in his or her level of responsiveness. Keep in mind that change in a patient—not the patient's status at any one time—may be the most important sign of how a patient is doing.

GENERAL GUIDELINES FOR EMERGENCY CARE

If you suspect injury to the head, be sure EMS has been activated. After taking BSI precautions and establishing manual stabilization of the patient's head and neck, proceed with emergency care as follows:

1. *Make the airway a top priority.* Note that oxygen deficiency in the brain is the most frequent cause of death following a head injury. So monitor the airway and breathing closely, and suction as needed. Administer oxygen in high concentrations. If ventilation is needed, use 100% oxygen at a rate of 22 to 25 times per minute. Follow local protocol.

2. *Control bleeding and dress open wounds.* Scalp wounds may bleed profusely, but they usually are easy to control with direct pressure. Note: never apply direct pressure to a head wound that is accompanied by an obvious or depressed skull fracture. It could drive fragments of bone into brain tissue and cause further injury.

   Do not try to stop a flow of cerebrospinal fluid. If the fluid is leaking from the ears or a head wound, cover the opening loosely with sterile gauze dressings.

   If there is a penetrating object, do not try to remove it. Instead, stabilize it with bulky dressings.

3. *Apply a rigid cervical immobilization device,* if you are trained and allowed to do so. (See Chapter 23 for instructions.) Maintain manual stabilization of the head and neck before, during, and after application and until the patient is immobilized on a long backboard.

4. *Monitor vital signs closely.* Watch for any sign of deterioration or change in the patient's status. If the patient has convulsions, protect him or her from injury.

5. *Calm and reassure the patient.* Continue to talk with him or her. If you can stimulate the patient, you may be able to prevent loss of consciousness.

SPECIFIC HEAD INJURIES

Injuries to the head include skull fracture, injuries to the brain, concussion, and penetrating wounds.

Skull Fracture

The primary function of the skull is to protect the brain from injury. Because of its shape and thickness, the skull usually is broken only by extreme trauma. Suspect skull fracture with any significant trauma to the head, even if the injury is a closed one.

A skull fracture accompanied by brain injury is a serious condition that needs immediate management. Signs and symptoms include (Figure 22–4):

- Damage to the skull, visible through lacerations in the scalp.
- Deformity of the skull or face.
- Pain or swelling at the injury site.

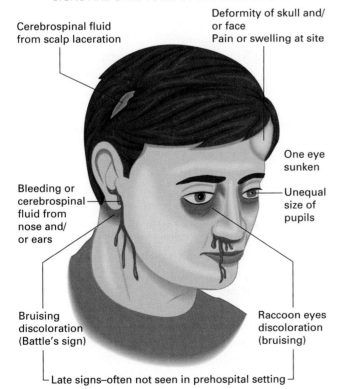

SIGNS AND SYMPTOMS OF SKULL FRACTURE

Cerebrospinal fluid from scalp laceration

Deformity of skull and/or face
Pain or swelling at site

Bleeding or cerebrospinal fluid from nose and/or ears

One eye sunken

Unequal size of pupils

Bruising discoloration (Battle's sign)

Raccoon eyes discoloration (bruising)

Late signs–often not seen in prehospital setting

Figure 22-4 Signs and symptoms of skull fracture.

- Clear or pinkish fluid dripping from nose, ears, mouth, or head wound.
- Unusual size of pupils, one eye sunken.
- Purplish bruising under or around the eyes ("raccoon eyes").
- Purplish bruising behind the ear ("Battle's sign").

Injuries to the Brain

Whether a head wound is open or closed, brain damage can be extensive. In fact, it is often more severe in closed injuries than in open ones. Severity depends mainly on the mechanism of injury and the force involved. However, consider all suspected head injuries to be serious. Signs and symptoms include:

- Changes in mental status, ranging from confusion to unresponsiveness.
- Paralysis or flaccidity, usually only on one side of the body.
- Unequal facial movements, squinting, drooping, unequal or unresponsive pupils, disturbances of vision in one or both eyes.
- Ringing in the ears, loss of hearing in one or both ears.
- Rigidity of all limbs (present with severe injury).
- Loss of balance, staggering or stumbling gait.
- Slow, strong heartbeat that gradually becomes rapid and weak (late sign).
- High blood pressure with a slow pulse.
- Rapid, labored breathing or disturbances in the pattern of breathing.
- Vomiting after head injury.
- Incontinence.

Concussion

A concussion is a temporary loss of the brain's ability to function. There is no detectable damage to the brain. A concussion is classified as mild, moderate, or severe, based on the time interval before return to responsiveness. The key distinguishing factor of concussion is that its effects appear immediately or soon after impact. Then they disappear, usually within 48 hours. If symptoms develop several minutes after impact or do not subside over time, the injury is probably more serious than a concussion.

- Restlessness.
- Seizures.
- Brief loss of consciousness.

Penetrating Wounds

A penetrating wound occurs when an object passes through the skull and lodges in the brain. It often involves bullets, knives, or ice picks. An extreme emergency, a penetrating wound almost always results in long-term damage.

If the object is impaled in the skull, do not try to remove it. Stabilize it with soft bulky dressings instead. Then dress the area around it with sterile gauze. If an object has penetrated the skull but you cannot see it, cover the wound lightly with sterile dressings. In both cases, permit blood to drain. Never apply firm pressure to a head injury that might involve a skull fracture.

SECTION 2: INJURIES TO THE FACE AND NECK

General Principles of Care

While some injuries to the face and neck are minor, many can be life-threatening (Figures 22–5 and 22–6). They can result from impacts strong enough to cause hidden facial fractures, cervical-spine damage, and skull fractures.

For injuries of the face and neck, follow the patient assessment and general guidelines for emergency care described at the beginning of this

FACIAL INJURIES

Face

Whenever there are significant soft-tissue injuries to the face, there also may be underlying fractures. Signs and symptoms include:

- Distortion of facial features.
- Numbness or pain.
- Bruising and swelling.
- Bleeding from the nose or mouth.
- Limited jaw motion.
- Teeth that do not meet normally, teeth that are missing.
- Double vision (with fracture of bones around the eyes).
- Asymmetry of bones in face (before swelling).

Jaw

Patients with injuries to the face also may have a broken jaw (Figure 22–7 p. 371). Such an injury can cause problems with the airway and breathing. Monitor both closely. Signs and symptoms of injuries to the jaw include:

- Mouth will not open or close.
- Drooling of saliva mixed with blood.
- Difficulty swallowing.
- Pain with talking, or difficulty talking.
- Missing, loosened, or uneven teeth.
- Teeth that do not meet normally.
- Pain in areas around the ears.

INJURIES TO THE FACE

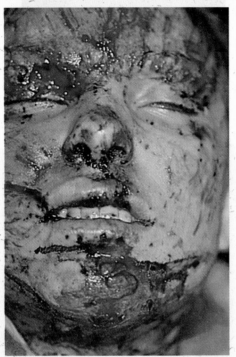

Figure 22-5a Injury to the face.

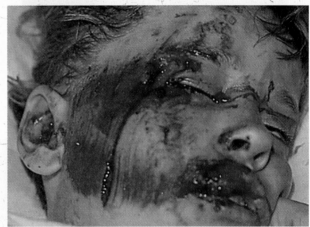

Figure 22-5b Injury to the face.

If a tooth has been lost, try to find it. Control bleeding from the socket with a gauze pad. If you find the missing tooth, be sure to handle it by the crown, not by the roots. Then, rinse it with tap water and be careful to protect any remaining tissue. Gently pick off debris. Then put the tooth in a glass of milk. If milk is not available, wrap the tooth in moistened gauze. Do not allow the tooth to dry. Send it with the patient to the hospital. (These steps will help to maximize the chances for a successful reimplantation.)

If dentures are in place and unbroken, let them stay in place. They can help support the structures of the mouth. If dentures are broken, remove them. Send them with the patient to the hospital so that the surgeon can use them to establish proper alignment.

Cheek

If there is an impaled object in the cheek, stabilize it with bulky dressings unless it has penetrated all the way through. If it has penetrated all the way through, it may cause enough bleeding to block the airway. So remove it carefully. Be prepared to suction the airway.

Nose

Care for soft-tissue injuries to the nose (Figure 22–8) in the same way you would care for other such injuries. Take special care to maintain an open airway. Position the patient to prevent blood from draining into the throat.

The nose is the most commonly broken bone in the face. When it is broken, it will swell and appear to be deformed. To treat, apply cold

Figure 22-6a Injury to the throat, mouth, and jaw.

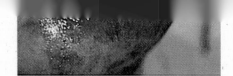

Figure 22-6b Injury to the cheek, mouth, and jaw.

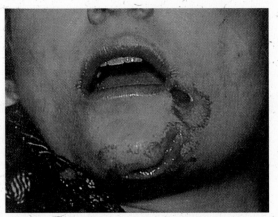

Figure 22-6c Injury to the mouth and jaw.

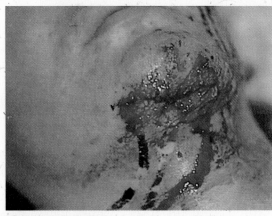

Figure 22-6d Injury to the jaw.

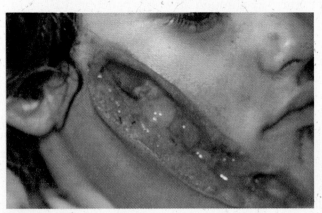

Figure 22-6e Injury to the cheek and jaw.

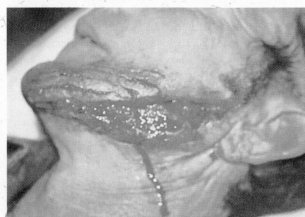

Figure 22-6f Injury to the jaw.

COMMON FRACTURES OF THE FACE AND JAW

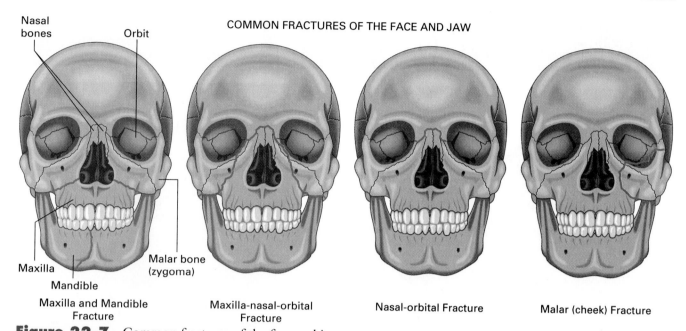

Figure 22-7 Common fractures of the face and jaw.

packs to reduce swelling. Arrange for patient transport.

Foreign objects in the nose usually are a problem among small children. Reassure the child and parent, and arrange for transport to a hospital. Do not probe or try to remove the object, because special lighting and instruments are required.

Ear

Soft-tissue injuries to the ear, including avulsions, are common (Figure 22–9). Treat them as you would treat any such injury. Keep in mind that when dressing an injured ear, place part of the dressing between it and the side of the head.

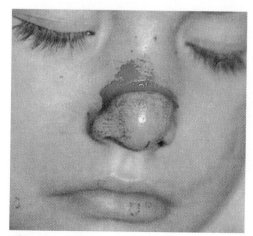

Figure 22-8 Injury to the nose.

Never probe the ear. Never pack it to stop bleeding from the ear canal. Blood, clear fluid, or blood-tinged fluid draining from the ear may indicate skull fracture. Place a loose, clean dressing across the opening to absorb the fluids. Do not apply pressure.

Foreign objects in the ear, such as beans or peanuts, are common among children. The patient should be transported to the hospital where good lighting and appropriate equipment are available.

NECK INJURIES

Common causes of neck injury include hanging (attempted suicide), impact with a steering wheel, or running into a stretched wire or clothesline. (See Figure 22–10.) Large wounds may involve injuries to the major vessels in the neck, which can produce massive, even fatal bleeding. If a wound to the neck is left uncovered, air may be sucked into the vessels causing an obstruction (air embolism).

Signs and symptoms include the following:

- Obvious lacerations or other wounds.
- Deformities or depressions.
- Obvious swelling, which sometimes occurs in the face and chest.
- Difficulty speaking, loss of the voice.
- Airway obstruction.

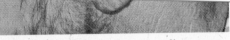

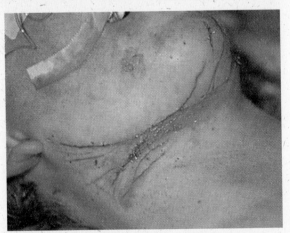

Figure 22-9a Injury to the ear.

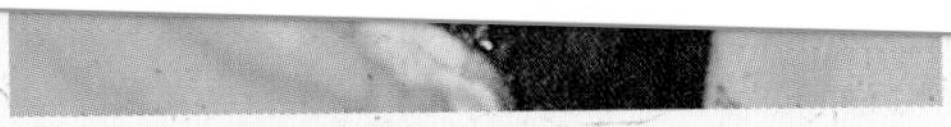

Figure 22-9b Injury to the ear.

- Crackling sensations under the skin due to air leaking into the soft tissues (subcutaneous emphysema).

If there is bleeding from a neck wound, apply slight to moderate pressure with an occlusive dressing. Tape down the edges of the dressing to form an airtight seal. Add a bulky dressing over the occlusive one (Figure 22–11). Never apply pressure to both sides of the neck at the same time. Never apply a pressure dressing around the neck.

INJURIES TO THE NECK

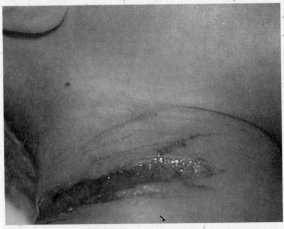

Figure 22-10a Injury to the neck.

Figure 22-10b Injury to the neck.

SEVERED NECK VEINS

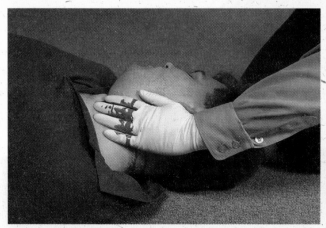

Figure 22-11a Do not delay! Place your gloved palm over the wound.

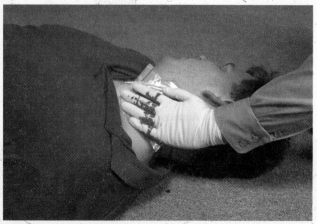

Figure 22-11b Apply moderate pressure with an occlusive dressing.

CAUTION: Do not compress blood vessels on both sides of the neck at once.

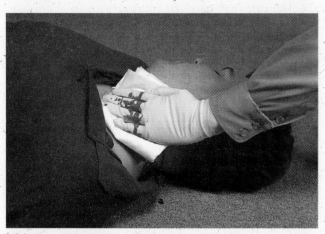

Figure 22-11c Add a bulky dressing.

If there is an impaled object in the neck, stabilize it in place with bulky dressings. Do not remove it.

EYE INJURIES

For the anatomy of the eye, see Figure 22–12. When you assess a patient with eye injuries, find out when the injury occurred, whether or not both eyes were affected, and what symptoms the patient first noticed. Then carefully examine the eyes separately and together with a small penlight. Proceed as follows:

- *Orbits* (the bones in the skull that hold the eyeballs). Check for bruising, swelling, lacerations, tenderness, depression, and deformity.
- *Eyelids.* Check for bruising, swelling, and lacerations.
- *Mucous membranes.* Check for redness, pus, and foreign objects.

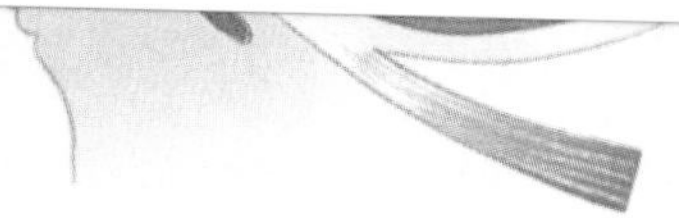

Figure 22-12 Anatomy of the eye.

- *Globes* (eyeballs). Check for abnormal coloring, laceration, and foreign objects.
- *Pupils*. Check for size, shape, equality (Figure 22–13). Also check for reaction to light. The pupils should be black, round, and equal in size. They should react to light by constricting.
- *Eye movement*. Check to see that the eyes can move in all directions. Check for abnormal gaze or pain upon movement.

Basic rules for emergency care of an injured eye include the following:

- Many EMS systems do not allow flushing of an injured eye unless it has a chemical injury. If the eye has been perforated, damage done during flushing will be irreversible. Follow local protocol.

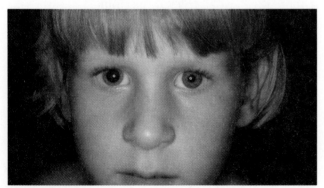

Figure 22-13 Unequal pupils.

- Do not put salves or medications in the injured eye. This is a physician's responsibility.
- Do not remove blood or blood clots from the eye. But you can sponge blood from the face to help keep the patient comfortable.
- Do not try to force the eyelid open unless you have to flush out chemicals.
- Do not let a patient with an eye injury walk without help, especially up or down stairs.
- Patch both eyes, even if only one is injured. Eyes move together, patching both eyes will help keep the injured eye from moving excessively.
- Do not allow the patient to eat or drink.
- Never panic. It will upset the patient, and you may lose his or her trust.
- An eye injury should always be examined by a physician.

Foreign Objects

Foreign objects frequently are blown or driven into the eye (Figure 22–14). They include particles of dirt, sand, cinders, coal dust, or fine pieces of metal. If not removed, they can cause inflammation, scarring, or infection. They also may scratch the cornea. Signs and symptoms of foreign objects in the eye include pain, excessive tearing, and abnormal sensitivity to light.

Do not allow the patient to rub his or her eyes. Rubbing can force a particle with sharp edges into the tissues, making removal difficult.

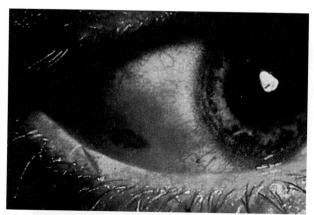

Figure 22-14 Foreign object lodged in the eye.

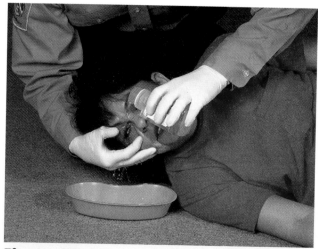

Figure 22-15 Flushing a foreign object from the eye.

It is always safer for a First Responder to allow EMS personnel with more training to remove a foreign object. However, if removal is necessary and local protocols allow it, there are several ways in which you might proceed. They are as follows:

- Hold the lids apart, and flush the eye with clean water (Figure 22–15). Note that some EMS systems do not allow flushing except for chemical burns. Follow local protocol.
- If the object is under the upper eyelid, draw the upper lid down over the lower lid. When you let it return to its normal position, its undersurface will be drawn over the lashes of the lower lid. The lashes will "sweep" away the foreign object.
- Grasp the eyelashes of the upper lid. Turn up the lid over a cotton swab. The foreign object then may be carefully removed with the corner of a piece of sterile gauze.

If the object is under the lower eyelid, pull down the lower lid to expose the inner surface. Then use the corner of a piece of sterile gauze to remove the object. (See Figure 22–16.)

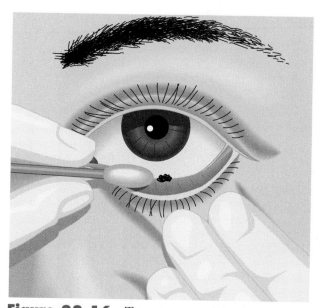

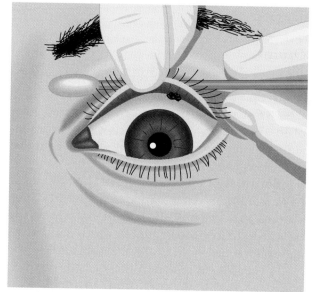

Figure 22-16 To remove particles from the white of the eye, pull down the lower lid while the patient looks up or pull up the upper lid while the patient looks down.

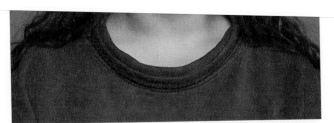

Figure 22-17 Place a rigid shield over the eye with the imbedded foreign object. Cover the opposite eye with gauze.

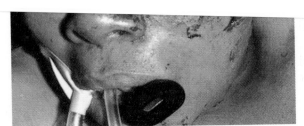

Figure 22-18 Eye orbit injury.

Should a foreign object become lodged in the eyeball, do not try to remove it. If you do, it could be forced deeper into the eye, causing further damage. In this case, place a rigid eye shield over the injured eye (Figure 22–17). Cover the opposite eye with gauze. Arrange for immediate transport to a hospital.

Orbits

Trauma to the face may result in fracture of the bones that form the orbits, or eye sockets (Figure 22–18). A patient with an orbit injury may complain of double or decreased vision, numbness above the eyebrow or over the cheek, or massive discharge from the nose.

Fractures of the lower part of the orbit are the most common. They can cause paralysis of the upward gaze. That is, the patient's eyes would not be able to follow your finger upward. Patients with an orbit fracture need hospitalization and surgery.

If there is no injury to the eyeball, place cold packs over the injured orbit to help reduce swelling. However, if the eyeball is injured or if you are in doubt, do not apply cold packs.

Eyelids

Lid injuries include discoloration, burns, swelling or drooping, and laceration (Figure 22–19). Anything that damages the lid also may damage the eyeball. In general, little can be done for these injuries in the field beyond gentle patching.

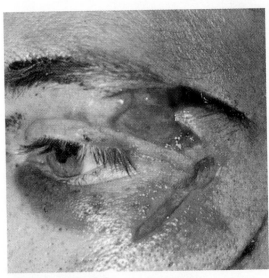

Figure 22-19 Eyelid injury.

To control bleeding from the eyelid, apply light pressure. No pressure should be used if the eyeball itself is injured.

Never attempt to remove embedded material, such as gravel. Use sterile gauze soaked in saline to keep the wound from drying. If the lid is avulsed, preserve and send it with the patient for later grafting.

Globes

Injuries to the globe include bruises, lacerations, foreign objects, and abrasions. These generally are best treated in the hospital where specialized equipment is available. In the field, keep the patient supine. Lightly apply patches to both eyes since eyes move together. Keep in mind that patients who have both eyes covered need a bit more patience and understanding. This is a very frightening experience for them.

Chemical Burns to the Eye

Chemical burns to the eye are quite common (Figure 22–20). They are the most urgent emergency related to the eyes. Permanent damage can occur within seconds of the injury. The first 10 minutes are crucial to the final outcome. Remember, burning and tissue damage will continue as long as the chemical remains in the eye, even if it is diluted.

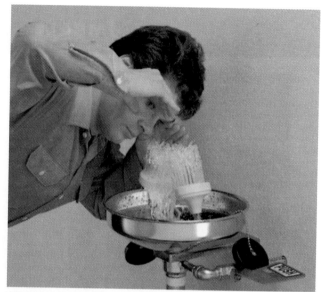

Figure 22-21 If possible, irrigate chemical burns to the eye in an eye-wash system. (Courtesy of Lab Safety Supply, Inc., Jamesville, WI)

To provide emergency care, begin immediate, continuous irrigation with water (Figure 22–21). Do not use anything other than water. The water does not need to be sterile, but it must be clean. Be sure to wear protective glasses. Gently hold the patient's eyelid open so that all of the chemical can be flushed away. You may have to force the eyelid open because of the patient's pain.

Pour water from the inside corner across the eyeball to the outside edge. This will help to avoid contaminating the uninjured eye. Irrigate continuously for 30 to 60 minutes.

Remove any solid particles from the surface of the eye with a moistened cotton swab. Contact lenses must be removed or flushed out. If not, they can trap chemicals between the lens and the cornea. Follow local protocol.

Following irrigation, wash your hands thoroughly. Avoid contaminating your own eyes.

Impaled Objects

Objects impaled in the eye should be removed only by a physician. You must protect the patient from further injury until he or she can reach a doctor. So stabilize the object in place (Figure 22–22).

Begin by stabilizing the patient's head with sandbags or large pads. Keep the patient supine.

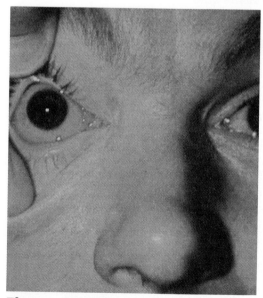

Figure 22-20 Chemical burn of the eye.

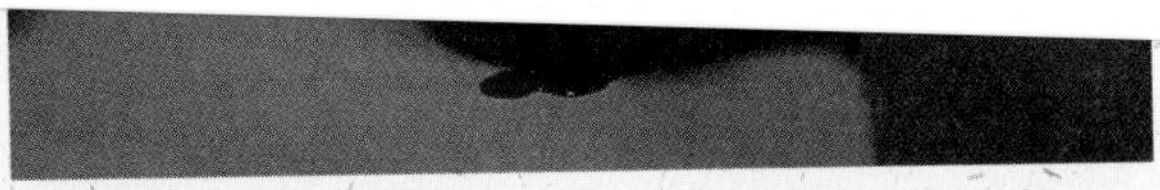

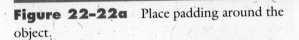

Figure 22-22a Place padding around the object.

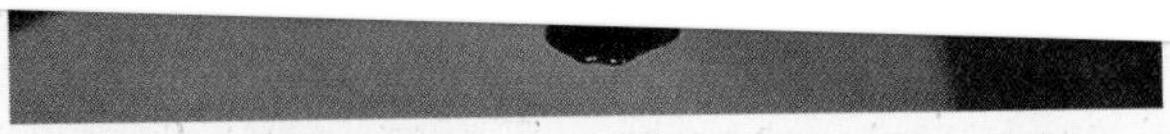

Figure 22-22b Stabilize the object with a cup.

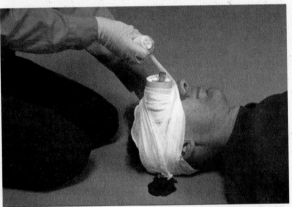

Figure 22-22c Secure the cup in place.

Then encircle the eye with a gauze dressing or soft sterile cloth. Do not apply pressure. You can then cut a hole in a single bulky dressing and slip it over the impaled object. Then place a metal shield, a crushed cup, or a cone over the object and the eye. The sides of the shield or cup should not touch the object at all. Hold the cup and the dressing in place with a self-adhering bandage and a roller bandage that covers both eyes.

After covering the patient's eyes, do not leave him alone. He could panic. Keep him in hand contact so that he knows someone is there.

Extruded Eyeball

During a serious injury, the eyeball may be knocked out of the socket, or extruded (Figure 22–23). Do not try to replace it. Instead, cover it with a moist dressing and protective cup. Do not apply any pressure. Then apply a bandage that covers both eyes.

Other Eye Injuries

In all other emergencies involving the eye, patch both eyes and arrange for transport. Such emergencies include eye infections, "black eye," cornea

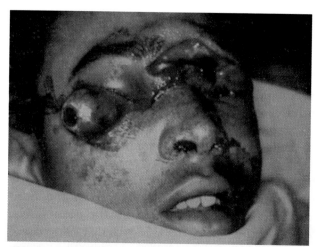

Figure 22-23 Extruded eyeball.

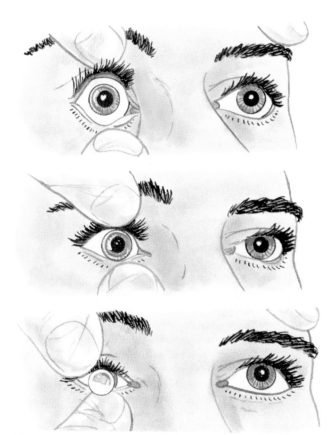

Figure 22-24 Removing hard contact lenses.

abrasions, light burns, and heat burns. Follow local protocols.

Removing Contact Lenses

An estimated 18 million people in the U.S. wear contact lenses. Some may only wear a lens in one eye, so be sure to examine both eyes carefully. Other patients, especially the elderly, wear both contact lenses and eyeglasses. To detect lenses, shine a penlight into each eye. A soft lens will show up as a shadow on the outer portion of the eye. A hard lens will show up as a shadow over the iris. In general, remove contacts only when there has been a chemical burn to the eye or when it is medically necessary. Always follow local protocols.

To remove hard contact lenses, first separate the eyelids (Figures 22–24 and 22–25). Position the lens over the cornea by manipulating the eyelids. Place your thumbs gently on the top and bottom eyelids, and open the lids wide. Gently press them down and forward to the edges of the lens. Press the lower lid slightly harder, and move it under the bottom edge of the lens. Move the eyelids toward each other, allowing the lens to slide out between them. Finally, remove the lens and put it in a safe place.

To remove soft contact lenses, place several drops of saline onto the lens. Then gently lift it off by pinching it between your thumb and index finger (Figure 22–26).

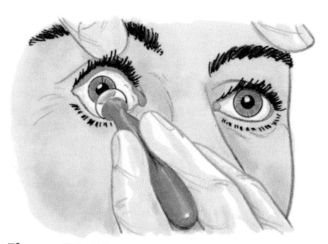

Figure 22-25 Using a moistened suction cup to remove hard contact lenses.

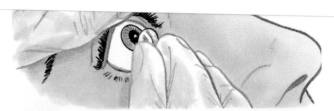

Figure 22-26 Removing soft contact lenses.

cause injuries to the spine. Take spinal precautions whenever a patient's chief complaint or mechanism of injury suggests the possibility of a spine injury. ■

CASE STUDY FOLLOW-UP

At the beginning of this chapter, you read that First Responders were on scene with an unresponsive male patient. To see how the skills in this chapter apply to this emergency, read the following. It describes how the call was completed.

PHYSICAL EXAMINATION

My partner continued to monitor the airway and breathing, while I conducted a head-to-toe exam. I found only a large bruise on the left side of the patient's head. His vital signs were within normal ranges.

During the exam, the patient opened his eyes and responded to my voice. I cautioned him to be very still, told why my partner was holding his head, and explained what I knew of what happened. Although he was somewhat drowsy, he indicated he understood by whispering, "Okay."

PATIENT HISTORY

A company personnel officer provided the medical history that was kept on record. The patient was also able to answer some of our questions.

His chief complaint was that he "hurt all over." He had no known allergies and took no medications recently. He had eaten breakfast at 0500. The patient did not remember what happened, but coworkers said he was performing his job when he tripped and flipped over the roof ledge. There were no eyewitnesses to the fall to the ground.

ONGOING ASSESSMENT

The patient required careful monitoring due to changes in his level of responsiveness. He did not resist the oxygen mask, so we elected to continue administration. The patient was able to wiggle his toes and fingers, and he continued to respond to questions appropriately.

PATIENT HAND-OFF

When the EMTs arrived, I gave them the hand-off report:

"This is Ray Gonzalez. He is 38 years old. About 15 minutes ago he fell approximately 25 feet from the roof of this building onto the grass. No one

CASE STUDY FOLLOW-UP *(Continued)*

moved him before or after we arrived on scene. Initially he did not respond to voice or painful stimuli. He presented with adequate respirations but needed suctioning of the airway early in the initial assessment. During the physical exam, he began to respond to our voices. The exam revealed a large bruise to the left side of his head. There was no bleeding at the wound site. There is no record of previous medical problems. His vital signs are pulse 88, respirations 18, blood pressure 130/82, skin warm and dry, and pupils equal and reactive."

The EMTs took over care of the patient and told us that we had done a good job. We learned

when we started our next shift that Mr. Gonzalez was diagnosed with a concussion and would be released from the hospital the next day.

By being the first medically trained rescuer on scene, you have the opportunity to really make a difference in the head-injured patient's life. Proper assessment and treatment could save him or her from further injury, permanent disfigurement, and even death.

REVIEW QUESTIONS

Page references where answers may be found or supported are provided at the end of each question.

Section 1

1. What are the signs and symptoms associated with a head injury? (pp. 364–365)
2. What are the general guidelines for emergency care of a patient with a head injury? (p. 366)
3. Under what conditions should you immediately take spinal precautions with a patient who has a head injury? (p. 365)

Section 2

4. Should you remove an object impaled in the skull of a patient? Describe what you should do. (p. 368)

5. What are the general principles of emergency care of a face or neck wound? (p. 368)
6. Why would you want to remove a penetrating object from a patient's cheek? (p. 369)
7. How would you provide emergency care to a patient with an open and bleeding neck wound? (pp. 371–372)
8. How would you care for a patient with a chemical burn to the eye? (p. 377)
9. How would you care for a patient with an object impaled in the eye? (pp. 377–378)

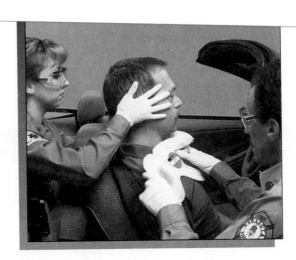

INTRODUCTION

A major goal of EMS has always been the prevention of problems related to spine injury. So, from the moment you arrive on scene, consider the possibility of spine injury and act accordingly. To appreciate the importance of this task, remember that failing to accomplish it can condemn a patient to a life in a wheelchair or even to death.

Cognitive, affective, and psychomotor objectives are from the U.S. DOT's 1995 "First Responder: National Standard Curriculum." Enrichment objectives, if any, identify material that is supplemental to the DOT curriculum.

Cognitive

5-3.4 Relate mechanism of injury to potential injuries of the head and spine. (pp. 384–385)
5-3.5 State the signs and symptoms of a potential spine injury. (pp. 385, 387)
5-3.6 Describe the method of determining if a responsive patient may have a spine injury. (pp. 385, 387)

Affective

5-3.10 Demonstrate a caring attitude towards patients with a musculoskeletal injury who request emergency medical services. (p. 387)
5-3.11 Place the interests of the patient with a musculoskeletal injury as the foremost consideration when making any and all patient care decisions. (pp. 387, 398)
5-3.12 Communicate with empathy to patients with a musculoskeletal injury, as well as with family members and friends of the patient. (p. 387)

Psychomotor

5-3.14 Demonstrate opening the airway in a patient with suspected spinal cord injury. (pp. 385, 387)
5-3.15 Demonstrate evaluating a responsive patient with a suspected spinal cord injury. (pp. 385, 387)
5-3.16 Demonstrate stabilizing the cervical spine. (p. 387)

Enrichment

* Describe the implications of not properly caring for potential spine injuries. (pp. 383, 398)
* Relate emergency airway techniques to the patient with a suspected spine injury. (pp. 385, 387)
* Discuss sizing and using a cervical spine immobilization device. (p. 389)
* Describe how to log roll a patient with a suspected spine injury. (pp. 389, 391–392)
* Describe how to secure a patient to a long backboard. (pp. 389, 391–392)
* Describe when and how to perform a rapid extrication. (pp. 393, 396)
* Discuss the circumstances in which a helmet should remain on a patient and when it should be removed. (p. 396)
* Explain the preferred methods of removing a helmet. (pp. 396–397)

SECTION 1: ANATOMY OF THE SPINE

The spinal cord lies within the spinal column. It is responsible for sending signals from the brain to the body and for receiving signals from the body and relaying them to the brain. If these signals are interrupted by injury or illness, we could lose the ability to move, feel, or even breathe. (Review Chapter 4 for more on the musculoskeletal and nervous systems of the body.)

The spinal column is made up of 33 bones, one stacked on top of another. The vertebrae *articulate,* or fit and move together, so we can bend, turn, and flex.

The spine is divided into five regions—the cervical, thoracic, lumbar, sacral, and coccygeal (Figures 23–1 and 23–2). The cervical spine starts at the base of the skull where the spinal cord begins. Its seven vertebrae not only house delicate nerve tissue, they also support the weight of the head. This makes them especially vulnerable to injury.

The thoracic spine is supported by the rib cage. There are 12 thoracic vertebrae, one for each rib. Because the ribs help protect this part of the spine, it is less frequently injured.

The next group of five vertebrae make up the lumbar spine. They carry the weight of most of the body. For this reason they are heavier and larger. The discs between the lumbar vertebrae

head and neck. He quickly told us that the player appeared to be unc...
noticed the helmet was cracked along the top. We called for EMS support immediately.

INITIAL ASSESSMENT

My partner and I assisted the trainer who was experienced in helmet removal. Then we used a jaw-thrust to open his airway. It was clear of blood and secretions. Breathing was adequate but irregular. We applied 100% oxygen by nonrebreather mask, using a small portable oxygen tank. The patient's pulse was strong and bounding, and his skin was warm and dry. No bleeding was noted. We carefully applied a rigid cervical immobilization device.

> Consider this patient as you read Chapter 23. What else might be done to assess and treat his condition?

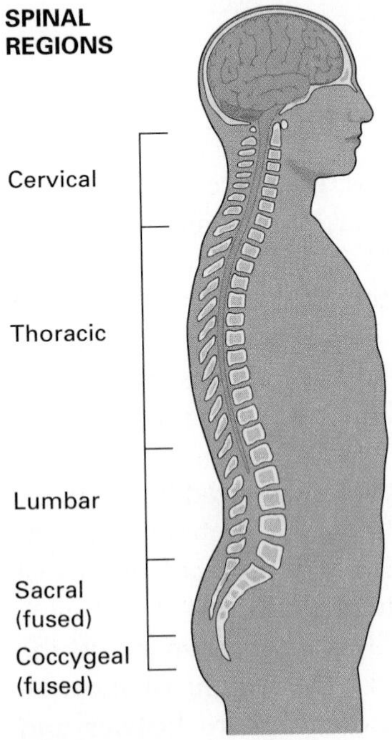

SPINAL REGIONS

Cervical

Thoracic

Lumbar

Sacral (fused)

Coccygeal (fused)

Figure 23-1 Regions of the spine.

are thicker than in other parts of the spine. Sometimes, a disc can shift, slip, or rupture. Injuries to the lumbar spine cost millions of dollars in medical expenses and lost wages every year.

The last two regions of vertebrae are the sacral and coccygeal spines. The sacrum has five fused vertebrae. The coccyx has four. Together they form the posterior portion of the pelvis. Because they are fused, these parts of the spine do not bend easily.

SECTION 2: SPINE INJURIES

During scene size-up, you as a First Responder must identify the mechanism that injured your patient. In doing so, you consider what occurred and what injuries may have resulted. Your index of suspicion for a spine injury should be very high in any of the emergencies described below:

- Motor vehicle crashes.
- Motorcycle crashes.
- Pedestrian-car crashes.
- Falls.
- Diving accidents.
- Hangings.
- Blunt trauma.
- Penetrating trauma to the head, neck, or torso.
- Gunshot wounds.
- Any speed sport accident, such as roller blading, bicycling, skiing, surfing, or sledding.
- Any unresponsive trauma patient.

See also Figure 23–3. Note that if the mechanism of injury suggests it, proceed as if the patient has a spine injury—even if he says he is not injured at all. The lack of back pain or the ability to walk, move arms and legs, or feel sensation does not rule out spine injury.

PATIENT ASSESSMENT

If you suspect spine injury in your patient, you must protect the spine from further injury. Immediately upon completing your scene size-up, stabilize the patient's head and neck. Then assess the ABCs. Be sure to use the jaw-thrust maneuver to open and maintain the airway. Remember that a cervical-spine injury can result in severe breathing problems, even respiratory arrest. So be sure to monitor the patient's airway and breathing continuously.

There may be no signs at all of spine injury. However, when they do appear, they typically include one or more of the following:

- Respiratory distress.
- Tenderness at the site of injury on the spinal column.
- Pain along the spinal column with movement. (Do not move the patient or ask the patient to move to test for this pain.)
- Constant or intermittent pain without movement along the spinal column or in the lower legs.
- Obvious deformity of the spine. (This is rare.)

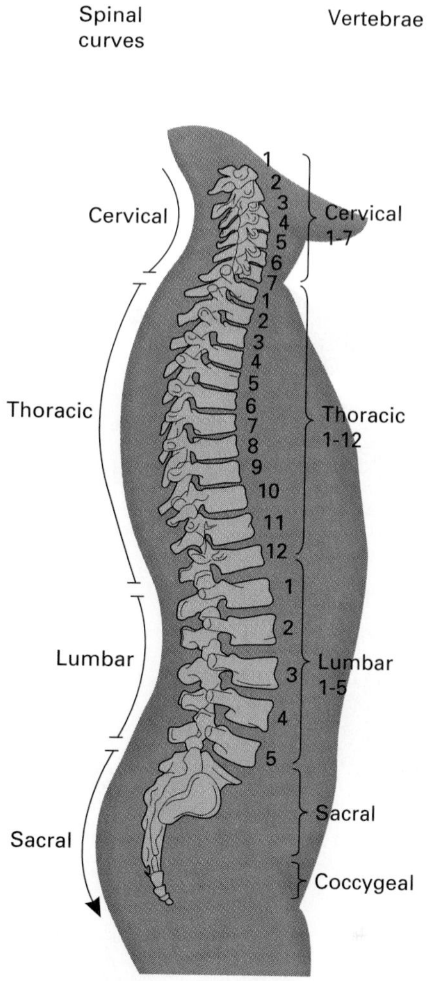

Figure 23-2 Regions of the spine.

- Soft-tissue injuries to the head, neck, shoulders, back, abdomen, or legs.
- Numbness, weakness, or tingling in the arms or legs.
- Loss of sensation or paralysis in the upper or lower extremities or below the injury site.
- Incontinence, or loss of bowel or bladder control.
- Priapism, or a constant erection of the penis (a classic sign of cervical-spine injury).

During the physical exam, do not risk moving the spine by taking off the patient's shirt or coat. Cut off the patient's clothes if necessary. Be sure to ask the patient if and where the spine hurts. If the patient complains of pain upon palpation of the spine, stop. Continue the assessment in other areas of the body.

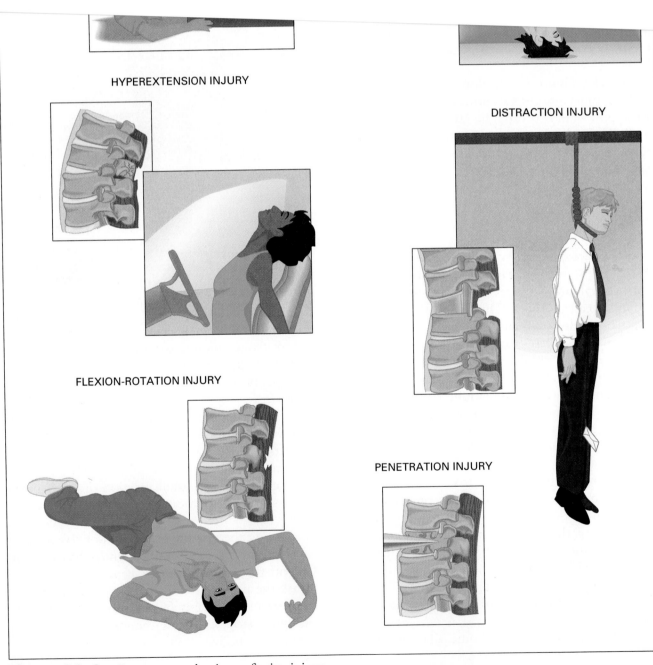

Figure 23-3 Common mechanisms of spine injury.

If the patient is unresponsive or unable to follow your instructions, apply a painful stimulus to check response. Either pinch the webbing between the toes and fingers or apply pressure with a pen across the back of a fingernail. The patient should withdraw from the pain. Note the response to pain in all four extremities.

After the assessment of the front of the patient, perform a log roll so you can assess the back. However, do so only if you are trained in its use and have enough help to do so safely. Details on how to perform a log roll are provided later in this chapter.

Remember that a patient may be uncomfortable, confused, and possibly afraid of paralysis or death. It is important for you to show a caring attitude. As you proceed with the physical exam, for example, be careful how you communicate your findings to your partner. An off-hand remark could terrify the patient. When you speak to his or her family, be honest but do not alarm them unnecessarily.

GENERAL GUIDELINES FOR EMERGENCY CARE

If the mechanism of injury suggests a possible spine injury, immediately stabilize the patient's cervical spine. That is, place your gloved hands just behind the patient's ears. Then hold the patient's head firmly and steadily in a neutral, in-line position. *Neutral* means the head is not flexed forward or extended back. *In-line* means the patient's nose is in line with the navel.

1. Take BSI precautions. Observe the mechanism of injury.
2. Stabilize the patient's head and neck immediately (Figure 23-5). Keep the patient from moving.
3. Then perform an initial assessment and provide treatment. Be sure to open and maintain the airway with a jaw-thrust maneuver. Insert an oropharyngeal or nasopharyngeal airway if needed. Suction without turning the patient's head.
4. Provide high-concentration oxygen via a nonrebreather mask. If the patient stops breathing or if breathing is inadequate, assist with artificial ventilation. Maintain neutral, in-line stabilization throughout.
5. Perform a physical exam and provide treatment. Be sure to monitor the patient's airway and breathing continuously.
6. Maintain manual stabilization until the patient is completely immobilized.

IMMOBILIZATION TECHNIQUES

Many EMS systems allow First Responders to immobilize a suspected spine-injured patient. Even if your system does not, you may be called to assist EMTs. So become familiar with the techniques. They include cervical immobilization, long backboard immobilization, rapid extrication, and helmet removal.

Remember: Never attempt to treat or move a spine-injured patient unless you have the proper equipment, training, and personnel.

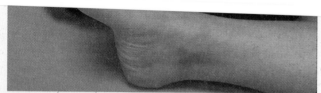

Figure 23-4a Feel for a pulse in all extremities.

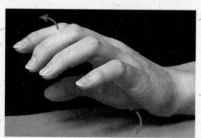

Figure 23-4c See if hands and fingers can move.

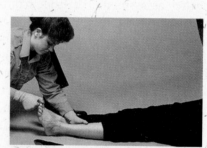

Figure 23-4d Touch the toes to assess for sensation.

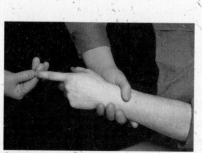

Figure 23-4e Touch the fingers to assess for sensation.

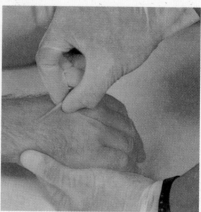

Figure 23-4f If the patient is unresponsive, see if he or she responds to painful stimuli.

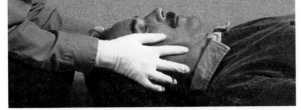

Figure 23-5 Manual stabilization means holding the patient's head firmly and steadily in a neutral, in-line position.

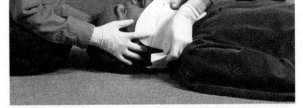

Figure 23-6 If allowed, apply a rigid cervical immobilization device to the patient.

Cervical Immobilization

After an initial assessment, a rigid cervical immobilization device, or extrication collar, should be applied to the patient (Figure 23–6). There are a variety available. However, never use a "soft" collar in the field. They are nothing more than cotton-covered foam rings, which do not prevent movement of the head and neck.

Use rigid or hard collars in the field. They are designed to prevent the patient from turning, flexing, and extending the head. They can restrict movement by up to 70%. The remaining 30% must be accomplished by manual stabilization.

Follow manufacturer's instructions for applying a collar. Though instructions will vary, all collars are supported at the same points: the maxilla (jaw), shoulders, and clavicles. Note that failure to fit a patient properly can aggravate the injury.

Before application, be sure that jewelry and long hair have been moved away from the area. Also, examine and palpate the patient's neck before the collar is applied.

In general, to apply a rigid cervical collar to a supine patient, follow these steps (Figure 23–7):

1. Slide the posterior portion of the collar in the gap under the patient's neck.
2. Then flip the anterior portion over the chin.
3. Secure the collar with the Velcro strap. Be careful not to pull too hard on one end. It can twist the patient's head.

If your patient is sitting, bring the collar up the chest until the chin is trapped. Then slide the posterior portion around the back of the neck and fasten it. Whatever position your patient is in, you must maintain manual stabilization of the head and neck. Release it only when the patient is completely immobilized on a long backboard.

Long Backboard Immobilization

All patients with suspected spine injury must be immobilized onto a long backboard. To immobilize a supine or prone patient, you must first roll the patient onto his side, slip the board under him, and then roll the patient back. This procedure is called a **log roll.**

To perform a log roll safely, you need at least three rescuers, and preferably four, who are

overextend the neck, force the jaw closed, and limit access to the airway. Too short can lead to inadequate immobilization. Too tight can impede blood flow. One way to measure collar size is to use your fingers to compare the neck size to the corresponding area of the collar.

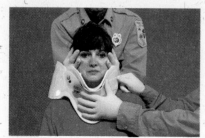

Figure 23-7c

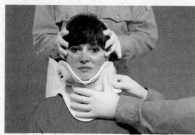

Figure 23-7d

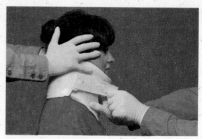

Figure 23-7e

SEATED APPLICATION

The patient's chin must be well supported by the chin piece. To accomplish this, slide the collar up the patient's chest wall. If the collar is pushed directly inward, it may be difficult to position the chin piece and, therefore, to apply the collar tightly enough.

TIGHTENING

Grip the trach hole as you tighten the collar. Then check to see that the collar fits according to the manufacturer's instructions.

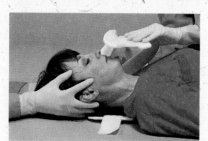

Figure 23-7f

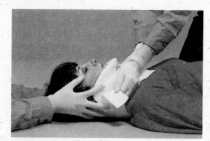

Figure 23-7g

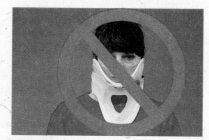

Figure 23-7h

SUPINE APPLICATION

Slip the collar underneath the patient's neck. Then rotate the collar up along the chest until the chin piece is properly positioned.

WARNING

Always check for neutral alignment and proper fit. Improper sizing or application may allow the patient's chin to slip inside the collar. This must be prevented.

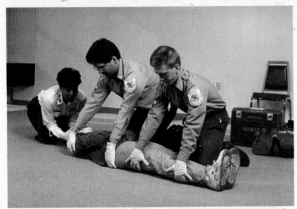

Figure 23-8a Maintain the head and neck in a neutral in-line position.

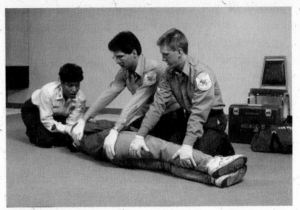

23-8b Roll the patient onto his or her side.

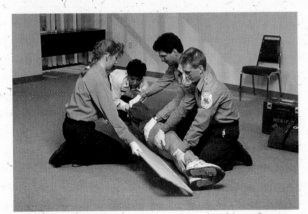

Figure 23-8c A bystander or one of the three rescuers should move the long backboard into place.

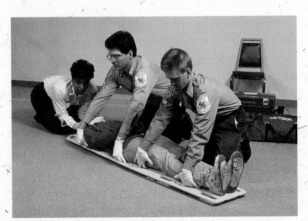

Figure 23-8d Lower the patient onto the long backboard.

of the spine. Never push a patient over to the middle of the backboard.

9. Reassess pulses, movement, and sensation in all four extremities. Report any change to the incoming EMTs.

Once in place, pad the spaces between the patient and the board (Figure 23–9). In an adult, pad anywhere along the length of the body to maintain neutral alignment and provide comfort. In the infant and child, also pad under the shoulders. This is to keep the relatively larger head from flexing forward. Take care to avoid extra movement.

Your next step is to secure the patient to the long backboard. It should always be done in this order (Figure 23–10):

1. Immobilize the torso first.
2. Immobilize the head next. The head must always be immobilized after the torso. Take a

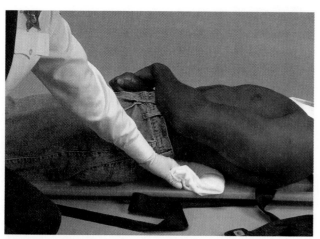

Figure 23-9 Pad the voids between the patient and the board.

a long backboard.

To apply a short backboard to a seated patient, follow the steps outlined below. Remember to maintain manual stabilization throughout and until the patient is completely immobilized. Proceed as follows (Figure 23–11):

1. Maintain manual stabilization of the patient's head and neck. If possible, hold the patient's head and neck from behind.
2. Apply a rigid cervical immobilization device.
3. Assess pulses, movement, and sensation in all four extremities.
4. Slide the short backboard behind the patient. Slip it as far down into the seat as possible, but not below the patient's coccyx. The top of the short backboard should be level with the top of the patient's head. The body flaps should fit snugly under the patient's armpits. Try not to jostle the patient or the rescuer who is holding manual stabilization.
5. Secure the patient to the backboard. Strap up the patient's torso first. If the device has leg straps, tighten those next. Finally, secure the patient's head. To make sure the head and neck remain in neutral alignment with the rest of the spine, you may need to pad behind them.

To move the patient to a long backboard, position it under or next to the patient's buttocks. Rotate the patient until his back is in line with it. Then lower the patient onto the long backboard. Follow the instructions outlined above for securing the patient. Release manual stabilization when the patient is completely immobilized.

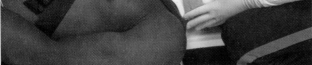

Figure 23-10a Immobilize the patient's torso first.

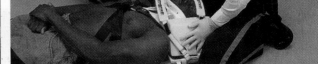

Figure 23-10b Immobilize the head next.

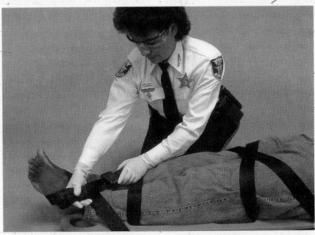

Figure 23-10c Finally, immobilize the patient's legs.

Rapid Extrication

In general, rescuers should move a sitting spine-injured patient only after short backboard immobilization. However, in certain emergencies there is not enough time. A rapid extrication may need to be performed instead when:

- The scene is not safe. For example, there is a threat of fire or explosion, a hostile crowd, or extreme weather conditions.

- Life-saving care cannot be given because of the patient's location or position.
- There is an inability to gain access to other patients who need life-saving care.

In general, a rapid extrication must be performed by a team of three or more rescuers. The objective is to move a sitting patient to a long backboard with only manual stabilization of the spine. To do so, proceed as follows (Figure 23–12):

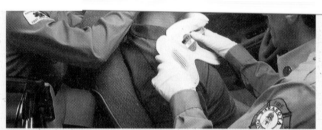

Figure 23-11a Manually stabilize the head and neck. Then apply a rigid cervical collar.

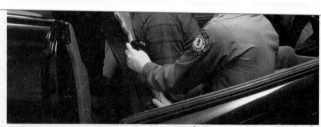

Figure 23-11b Position the short backboard behind the patient.

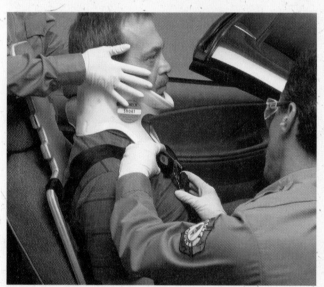

Figure 23-11c Secure the torso to the board.

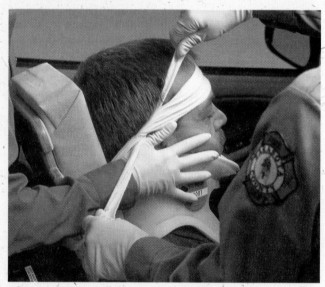

Figure 23-11d Pad behind the head and secure it to the board.

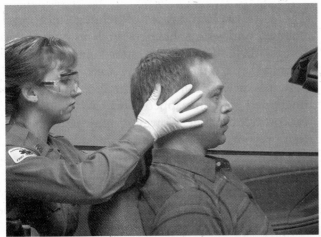

Figure 23-12a Bring the patient's head into a neutral, in-line position.

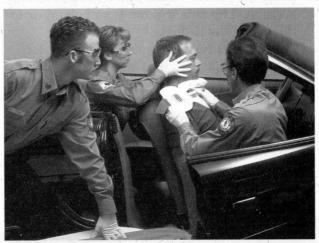

Figure 23-12b Apply a rigid cervical immobilization device.

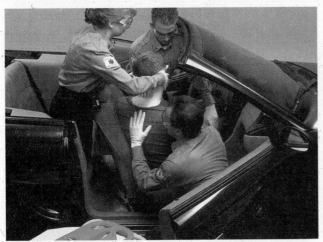

Figure 23-12c Rotate the patient into position.

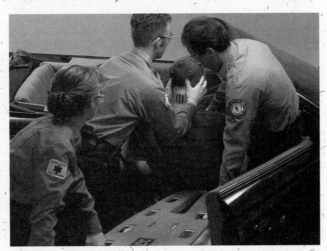

Figure 23-12d Bring the long backboard in line with the patient.

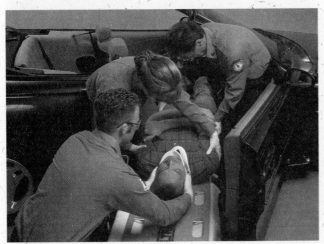

Figure 23-12e Lower the patient onto the long backboard.

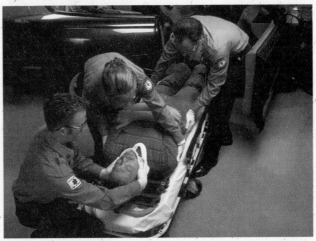

Figure 23-12f Slide the patient into position in small steps, and secure the patient to the backboard.

nated moves.

6. Secure the patient to the backboard. Release manual stabilization only when the patient is completely immobilized on a long backboard.

Note that it may be necessary to hand off manual stabilization during the procedure. Be sure it is maintained continuously until the patient is completely immobilized.

removed, then follow these steps (Figures 23–13 and 23–14):

1. Stabilize the helmet to prevent movement. The rescuer at the head holds each side of the helmet. He then places his fingers on the lower jaw.
2. Loosen the chin strap. The second rescuer does this, while the first maintains manual stabilization.

HELMET REMOVAL

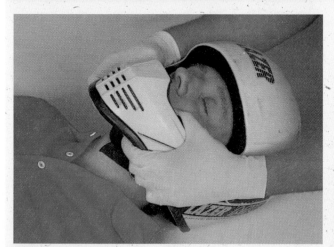

Figure 23-13a Stabilize the helmet, head, and neck to prevent movement.

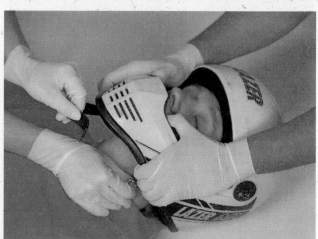

Figure 23-13b Loosen the chin strap, while maintaining manual stabilization.

HELMET REMOVAL *(Continued)*

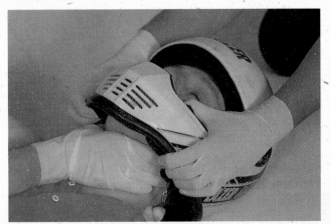

Figure 23-13c Transfer stabilization.

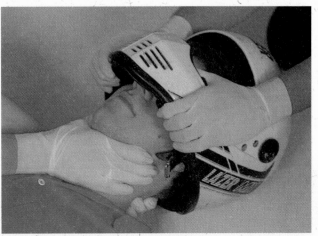

Figure 23-13d Slip off the helmet about half way so your partner can maintain an in-line position of the head.

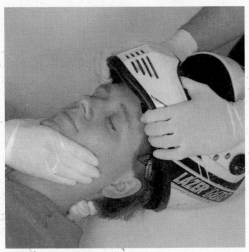

Figure 23-13e When the helmet is completely removed, transfer manual stabilization to the rescuer at the head.

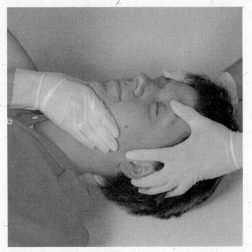

Figure 23-13f Maintain manual stabilization until the patient is completely immobilized.

3. Transfer stabilization next. To do so, the second rescuer places one hand anteriorly on the mandible at the angle of the jaw. He then places the other hand at the back of the head.
4. Slip off the helmet about half way. Be sure to spread it so it can clear the ears. The second rescuer then re-adjusts his hands in order to maintain alignment of the head.
5. Remove the helmet completely. The rescuer at the head then takes over manual stabilization until the patient is completely immobilized.

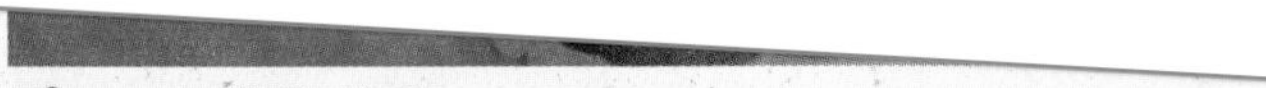

Figure 23-14a Stabilize the helmet, head, and neck to prevent movement.

Figure 23-14b Remove the ... maintaining manual stabilization.

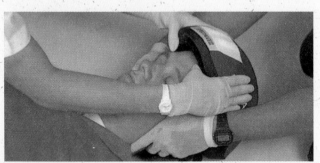

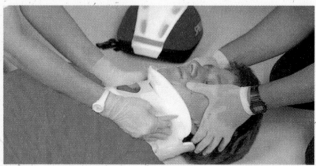

Figure 23-14c Full-face helmets will have to be tilted back to clear the nose.

Figure 23-14d Apply a rigid cervical collar, and maintain manual stabilization until the patient is completely immobilized.

FIRST RESPONDER FOCUS

Even after a collision with heavy damage to the crash vehicles there may be patients with a complaint of only minor pain or no pain at all. Note that it is just as important to take spinal precautions with these patients as with patients who complain of pain. Never assume a patient is uninjured if the mechanism suggests injury. That is for the hospital physicians to decide.

An EMS instructor wrote this simple but powerful message on the chalkboard during a First Responder class: "Quadriplegia is forever." (Quadriplegia is the inability to use any of the extremities because of a spinal-cord injury.) Use caution with every patient who has a possible spine injury. The consequences of not doing so are extremely serious! ∎

CASE STUDY FOLLOW-UP

At the beginning of this chapter, you read that First Responders were caring for a male patient with possible head and spine injuries. To see how chapter skills apply to this emergency, read the following. It describes how the call was completed.

PHYSICAL EXAMINATION

The ETA of the ambulance was about three minutes. I began a physical exam as the team trainer carefully removed the patient's pads. My partner held manual stabilization and asked the coach about the patient's history.

My first obvious finding was a deformity and swelling on the top of the patient's head. Clear fluid and blood seeped out of his ears. His facial bones all appeared to be intact.

PATIENT HISTORY

The coach got the patient's medical history card from his pack at the sideline. It indicated that the player had no known allergies and that he did not take any medications regularly. His last physical by the team doctor was unremarkable. He had no other significant past medical history.

The coach told my partner that the team players ate lunch about an hour before the game.

ONGOING ASSESSMENT

We maintained manual stabilization. Since the patient was unresponsive and his respirations were somewhat irregular, we watched breathing carefully. We also checked his pulse again. We radioed for the ambulance to bring immobilization equipment and to drive right onto the field.

PATIENT HAND-OFF

When the EMTs arrived, I told them:

"This is Henry Jones, 21 years old. He struck a steel goal post, shattering his helmet and sustaining a head injury. He was unresponsive upon our arrival and that hasn't changed. His respirations have been irregular but deep. We'll have to assist his breathing soon. Pulse has dropped from 80 to 56. We removed the helmet and pads with the assistance of the trainer. We manually stabilized his head and neck the whole time. The coach has his history—nothing of note."

We helped to log roll the patient onto a long backboard. The EMTs radioed the trauma center to report a possible neurosurgical emergency.

> Head and spine injuries are among the most devastating injuries a patient can suffer. Always be alert to the possibility that an injury to the spine may have occurred. Then do everything you can to protect it from further harm. Remember, if the mechanism of injury suggests it, treat for it.

REVIEW QUESTIONS

Page references where answers may be found or supported are provided at the end of each question.

Section 1

1. Which of the five regions of the spine is most vulnerable to injury? Why? (pp. 383–384)

Section 2

2. What are five emergencies in which your index of suspicion for spine injury should be high? (p. 385)
3. When should you begin manual stabilization of the cervical spine? When may you release it? (p. 385)
4. What is the basic emergency care for a suspected spine-injured patient? (p. 387)

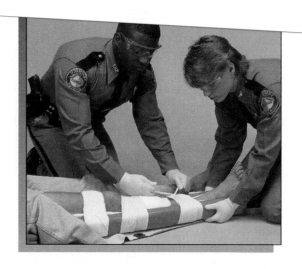

INTRODUCTION

Injuries to muscles, joints, and bones are some of the most common emergencies you will encounter in the field. They can range from a pulled muscle or twisted ankle to life-threatening breaks in a femur. Regardless of whether the injury is mild or severe, your ability to assess your patient and provide the appropriate emergency care can help prevent permanent disability and disfigurement.

Cognitive, affective, and psychomotor objectives are from the U.S. DOT's 1995 "First Responder: National Standard Curriculum." Enrichment objectives, if any, identify material that is supplemental to the DOT curriculum.

Cognitive

5-3.1 Describe the function of the musculoskeletal system. (p. 402)

5-3.2 Differentiate between an open and a closed painful, swollen, deformed extremity. (pp. 402–403)

5-3.3 List the emergency medical care for a patient with a painful, swollen, deformed extremity. (pp. 403, 405–406)

Affective

5-3.9 Explain the rationale for the feeling patients who have need for immobilization of the painful, swollen, deformed extremity. (pp. 403, 407)

5-3.10 Demonstrate a caring attitude towards patients with a musculoskeletal injury who request emergency medical services. (pp. 403, 407)

5-3.11 Place the interests of the patient with a musculoskeletal injury as the foremost consideration when making any and all patient care decisions. (pp. 403, 406, 407, 414)

5-3.12 Communicate with empathy to patients with a musculoskeletal injury, as well as with family members and friends of the patient. (pp. 403, 407)

Psychomotor

5-3.13 Demonstrate the emergency medical care of a patient with a painful, swollen, deformed extremity. (pp. 403, 405–406)

Enrichment

* State the reasons for splinting. (p. 406)
* List the general rules of splinting. (p. 407)
* List the complications of improper splinting. (p. 407)
* Describe several different types of splints. (pp. 406–407)
* Describe splinting of the upper extremities. (pp. 409–411)
* Describe splinting of the lower extremities. (pp. 411–415)

SECTION 1: INJURIES TO BONES AND JOINTS

The musculoskeletal system is made up of more than 200 bones and over 600 muscles. Together they give the body shape, protect internal organs, and provide for movement. Any time bones and muscles are injured, one of those functions is either temporarily or permanently impaired. Turn to Chapter 4 to review system components now.

Bones and muscles may be injured in four basic ways:

* A bone is broken (fracture).
* A muscle or a muscle and tendon are overextended (strain).
* A joint and ligament are injured (sprain).
* A bone is moved out of its normal position in a joint and remains that way (dislocation).

MECHANISMS OF MUSCULOSKELETAL INJURY

As you conduct your scene size-up, consider the mechanism of injury. A mechanism of musculoskeletal injury may involve direct, indirect, or twisting forces (Figure 24–1). They can give you a good idea of how extensive an injury may be.

With a direct force, an injury occurs at the point of impact. For example, imagine that a patient is in a car crash. When he is thrust forward, one of his knees strikes the dashboard. The resulting broken kneecap is caused by that direct force, or direct blow.

With an indirect force, the energy of a blow travels along a path away from the point of impact. For example, think of a patient who falls onto her outstretched hand. The force of the blow can travel from her hand and wrist up through her arm and shoulder. The injuries

off the road and against the guardrails. We were just stepping
cruiser slide into a slow spin and glide past us.

We exited our unit when the road was flared off and the scene was safe. The police
then directed us to vehicle #3. It had been struck by another vehicle and had skidded into
the guardrail.

INITIAL ASSESSMENT

Our patient was a 19-year-old woman who was in the driver's seat. Her left thigh was
bulging so much that we could see the deformity through her jeans. She was holding her
leg tightly and appeared to be in a great deal of pain. My partner stabilized her head
and neck, while I began the initial assessment.

The patient was alert and cooperative. Her speech was clear. Her pulse was strong
and fast, and her skin was cold and dry. There was no gross external bleeding. She had no
trouble breathing, no chest pain, and no apparent injuries to her head. She did not have
her seat belt on when the car crashed into the guardrail.

Consider this patient as you read Chapter 24.
What may be done to assess and treat her
condition?

caused by the indirect force could include broken arm bones and even a broken clavicle. So, look beyond the injury caused by a direct force when you examine a trauma patient. Additional injuries may be involved.

With a twisting force, one part of a limb remains stationary while the rest of it twists. An example would be the case of a jogger who steps into a hole and gets his foot caught. When he falls, the body would pull the leg one way, while the trapped foot would hold it firmly in its origi-nal position. That could twist the limb, causing any of its bones or joints to break. Again, suspect injuries beyond the most obvious one when you examine your patient.

PATIENT ASSESSMENT

A musculoskeletal injury is classified as either closed or open (Figure 24–2). In a closed extremity injury, the skin is not broken at the

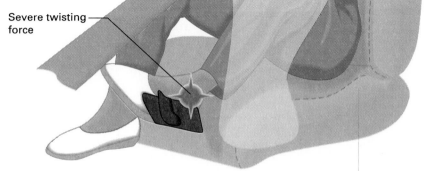

Severe twisting force

Figure 24-1 Different types of force can cause different types of injuries.

injury site. It remains intact. In an open extremity injury, the skin is broken, perhaps by protruding bone ends.

Signs and symptoms of musculoskeletal injury include (Figure 24–3):

- Deformity or angulation. When compared to the uninjured limb, the injured one is a different size or has a different shape.
- Pain and tenderness.
- Grating, or **crepitus.** This is the sound or feeling of broken bones grinding against each other.
- Swelling.
- Bruising, or discoloration.
- Exposed bone ends (Figure 24–4).
- Joint locked in position.

An injury that causes pain, swelling, or deformity in an extremity may be the result of a fracture, sprain, strain, or dislocation. Because these injuries look so much alike in the field, you do not

need to figure out which is which. Instead, always treat a painful, swollen, or deformed extremity as if it involved a broken bone.

When examining a patient with a musculoskeletal injury, remember that he or she may be in a great deal of pain. Be careful not to move the injured limb or jar the body. Be gentle and reassuring to the patient and his or her family.

GENERAL GUIDELINES FOR EMERGENCY CARE

As a First Responder, you must not be distracted by gruesome-looking injuries, especially when treating a patient with multiple trauma. Simply put, your priority is life before limb. Remain focused on treating the life threats you identify in the initial assessment. Once that is done, you can turn to limb-threatening injuries.

Generally, emergency care proceeds in the following manner:

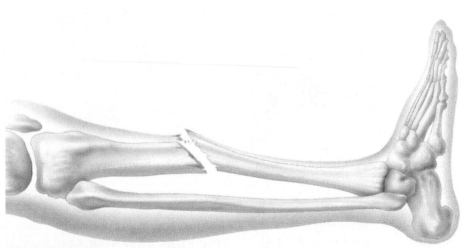

Figure 24-2 A closed injury vs. an open one.

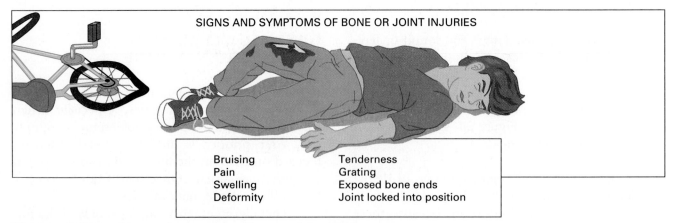

SIGNS AND SYMPTOMS OF BONE OR JOINT INJURIES

Bruising	Tenderness
Pain	Grating
Swelling	Exposed bone ends
Deformity	Joint locked into position

Figure 24-3 Signs and symptoms of bone or joint injuries.

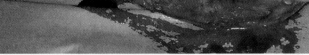

Figure 24-4a Open injury.

Figure 24-4b X-ray of limb in Figure 24-4a, showing broken bones both above and below surface.

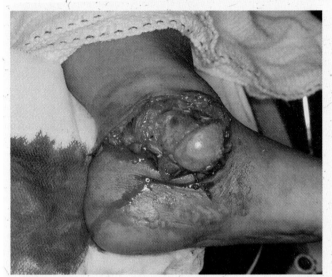

Figure 24-4c Open injury.

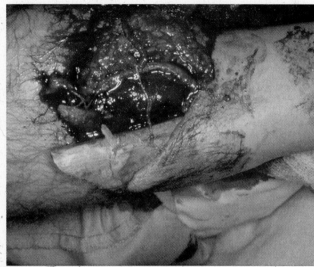

Figure 24-4d Open injury.

1. *Take BSI precautions.*
2. *Identify and treat life threats.* Maintain manual stabilization of the patient's spine, if indicated. Administer oxygen, if it is available.
3. *Stabilize the injured extremity* after you have completed a physical exam. Hold it manually above and below the injury site. Maintain manual stabilization until the limb is completely immobilized in a splint.
4. *Expose the injury site.* To avoid jarring the limb, you may need to cut away clothing. Remove jewelry, too, if possible.

5. *Treat any open wounds.* Control bleeding. If necessary, apply pressure to the appropriate pressure point. Be careful to avoid applying any pressure to broken bone ends. Then dress any open wounds with sterile dressings.
6. *Allow the patient to rest in a position of comfort* while you wait for the arrival of the EMTs. Apply a cold pack to the injured area. If you have one available, it can help reduce pain and swelling. You also may wish to pad under the patient's injured limb to prevent discomfort. Continue to assess for pulse,

except when you are [illegible] trained medical personnel should attempt traction in the field. Be sure to follow all local protocols.

Maintain manual stabilization of an injured extremity until it is completely immobilized with a splint. Even if you find that you have to stay in an uncomfortable position for some time, maintain stabilization. The patient's best interests must be your foremost consideration. If you are trained and allowed to do so, splint the injured extremity after you have performed the steps described above.

SECTION 2: SPLINTING MUSCULOSKELETAL INJURIES

Any device used to immobilize a body part is called a **splint.** A splint may be soft or rigid. It can be commercially manufactured or it can be improvised from virtually any object that can immobilize the limb. (See Figure 24–5.)

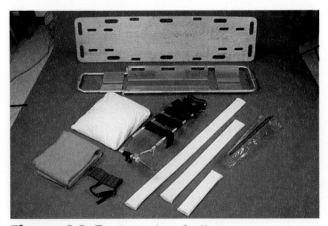

Figure 24-5 Examples of splints.

your EMS system. Make sure you [illegible] protocols.

TYPES OF SPLINTS

Some common types of splints are rigid splints, traction splints, circumferential splints, improvised splints, and the sling and swathe. All are designed to accomplish the same task. They must immobilize an injured extremity.

Rigid Splints

Rigid, padded boards are the most common type of splint. They may be made of wood, aluminum, wire, plastic, cardboard, or compressed fibers. Some are shaped specifically for arms or legs. Others are pliable enough to be molded to fit any appendage. Some come with washable pads. Others must be padded before being applied.

A rigid splint must be applied in line with the bone. Then it must be anchored to the limb with cravats that are secured with square knots (or straps or Velcro closures). Remember, never place a cravat across the injury site. It could cause further injury and pain.

Traction Splints

A traction splint is a mechanical device that provides a counter-pull to alleviate pain, reduce blood loss, and minimize further injury. It does not realign broken bones. Several types of traction splints are available, and application procedures vary according to manufacturer. As a First Responder, you should use a traction splint only if you are specifically trained and allowed to do so. Follow local protocols.

shin guard, or any similar object. It must be long enough to extend past the joints and prevent movement on both sides of the injury. It also should be as wide as the thickest part of the injured part.

A "self-splint" also may be effective. In fact, in some cases, a patient will not permit any other type of splint to be applied. In a "self-splint," the injured limb is secured against the patient's body with a cravat or roller bandage. Voids between the limb and body are then padded with bulky dressings or similar material as appropriate.

Sling and Swathe

An injured limb can be supported by the sling, while a swathe keeps the limb protected and immobile against the body. When applying a sling, be sure to keep the knot off the back of the patient's neck. It can be very uncomfortable there.

GENERAL RULES OF SPLINTING

Keep these general rules of splinting in mind (Figure 24–6):

- Be sure you have taken BSI precautions before splinting.
- Do not release manual stabilization of an injured extremity until it is properly and completely immobilized.
- Never intentionally replace protruding bones or push them back below the skin.

the injury site, align it with gentle manual traction (pulling). If there is pain or grating (crepitus), stop pulling immediately. Perform this procedure *only if you are specifically trained and allowed to do so.* Follow all local protocols.
- Pad a splint before applying it to help keep the patient as comfortable as possible.
- Before and after applying a splint, assess pulse, movement, and sensation below the injury site. Reassess every 15 minutes after applying a splint, and record your findings.

For all the obvious benefits splints provide, they also can cause complications if they are applied incorrectly. *Improper* splinting can:

- Compress nerves, tissues, and blood vessels under the splint, which can aggravate the injury and cause further damage.
- Move displaced or broken bones, causing even further injury to nerves, tissues, and blood vessels.
- Reduce blood flow below the injury site, risking the life of the limb.
- Delay transport of a patient who has a life-threatening problem.

Remember that patients who have a painful, swollen, deformed extremity may be in considerable pain. They also may be concerned about regaining full use of the limb. So, as you provide emergency care, consider their feelings. Be gentle and reassuring.

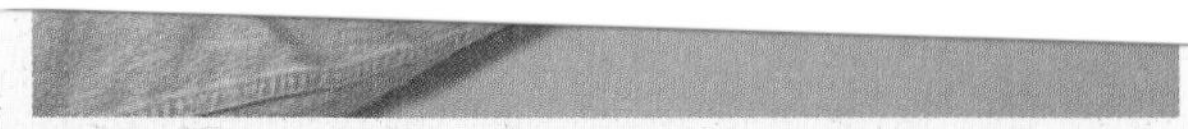

Figure 24-6a Stabilize the limb, and assess pulse, movement, and sensation below the injury site.

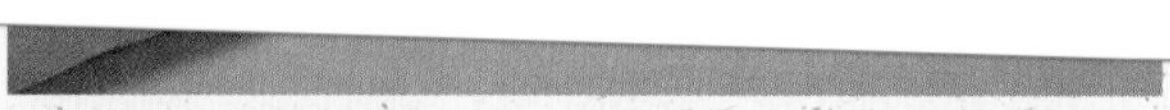

Figure 24-6b Cut away clothing to expose the injury.

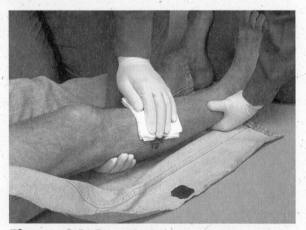

Figure 24-6c After controlling bleeding, place a sterile dressing over open wounds, if any.

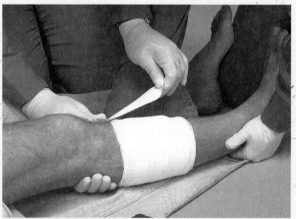

Figure 24-6d If there is severe deformity, absence of pulse, or cyanosis in the extremity, align it with gentle traction. Maintain it until the limb is completely immobilized.

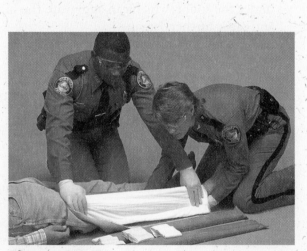

Figure 24-6e Pad the splint.

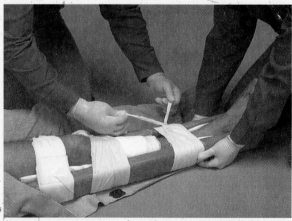

Figure 24-6f Secure the limb to the splint, and reassess pulse, movement, and sensation.

SPLINTING THE UPPER EXTREMITIES

Clavicle

Often an injury to a shoulder will result in a fracture of a clavicle. When a clavicle is broken, the patient's shoulder may appear to have "dropped." The clavicle itself may look crooked and deformed. The best way to splint it is to apply a sling and swathe (Figure 24–7).

Shoulder

A dislocated shoulder is a common injury. Patients with one often have had the same injury many times before. The dislocated shoulder will appear to be deformed. You also may see a "hollow" in the upper arm below the clavicle. The patient frequently complains of severe pain and may refuse to let anyone touch the arm.

Attempt to apply a sling and swathe to the arm. Padding the void between the body and the arm may be helpful. Use a small pillow, towels, or even trauma dressings for padding.

In a shoulder dislocation, there is a danger of injuring nerves and arteries. So a great deal of care must be taken when applying the sling and swathe.

Shoulder and Humerus

The humerus may break at midshaft or at the shoulder. It is thick and fairly strong. So if it is injured, suspect other injuries nearby.

Manually stabilize the arm as soon as possible. Then check for pulse, movement, and sensation below the injury site. Apply a rigid splint to the outside of the arm, and pad the voids. Then apply a sling and swathe (Figure 24–8). Do not forget to reassess pulse, movement, and sensation. (See alternative, Figure 24–9.)

Elbow

The elbow should be splinted in the position in which it was found. Do not attempt to straighten it. If the arm is bent at the elbow, splint the injury with a sling and swathe (Figure 24–10). However, if the deformity is severe, you may elect to use a large, flat pillow or even a blanket wrapped around the limb and secured to the chest with a strap.

If the elbow is straight, then the entire arm should be splinted from the armpit to the fingertips on two sides (Figure 24–11).

Forearm and Wrist

Forearm and wrist injuries are very common. They must be supported from the elbow to the fingertips. First splint the injured area with a

APPLYING A SLING AND SWATHE

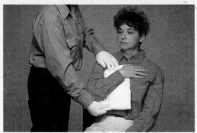

Figure 24-7a Place a pad between the arm and chest.

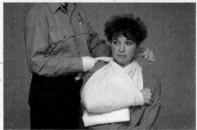

Figure 24-7b Support the injured arm with a sling.

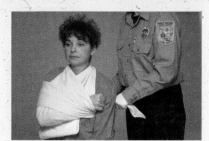

Figure 24-7c Immobilize the arm with a swathe.

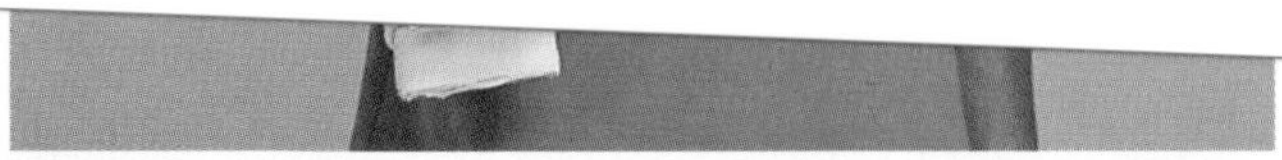

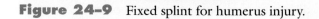

Figure 24-8   Fixation or rigid splint with a sling and swathe.

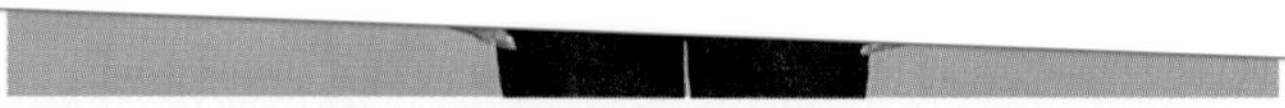

Figure 24-9   Fixed splint for humerus injury.

short arm board. Then a sling and swathe should be applied (Figure 24–12).

If the injury is a closed one, a circumferential splint may be used instead. Be sure the splint extends from the elbow to beyond the hand (Figure 24–13).

Hands and Fingers

If just one finger is injured, then it may be taped to the uninjured finger beside it. This is called "buddy taping." You may also use a tongue depressor as a splint (Figure 24–14).

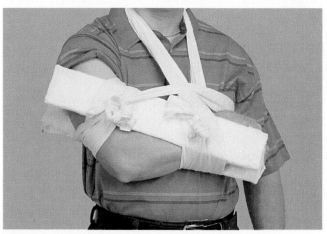

Figure 24-10   Injured elbow immobilized in a bent position.

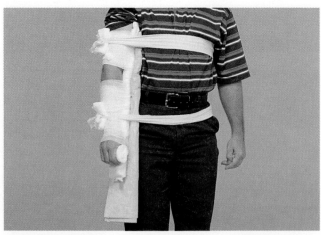

Figure 24-11   Injured elbow immobilized in a straight position.

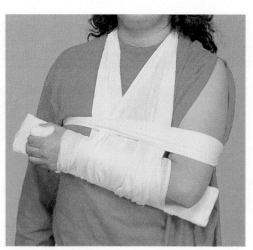

Figure 24-12   Immobilization of an injury to the forearm, wrist, or hand.

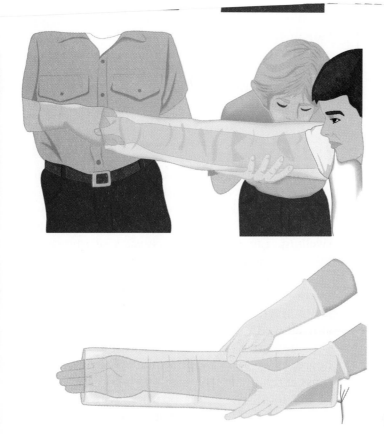

Figure 24-13 Applying an air splint.

If there is more than one finger involved, or if the hand injury is the result of a fight, then the entire hand needs to be immobilized.

A hand must be splinted in the position of function. The easiest way to do it is to place a four-inch roll of bandage, a rolled hand towel, or a small ball inside the palm of the injured hand. Then wrap the entire hand and place it on an arm board to immobilize the wrist (Figure 24–15).

SPLINTING THE LOWER EXTREMITIES

Pelvis

Pelvis injuries can be life-threatening, because a large amount of blood can be lost into the lower abdomen quickly. So suspect shock with any pelvis injury.

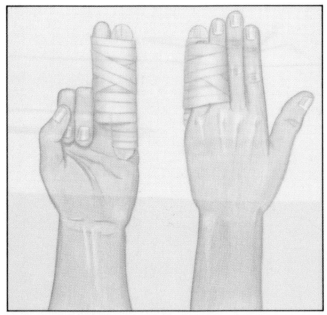

Figure 24-14 A tongue depressor used as a splint.

The patient must be placed on a long backboard. Pad between the legs, and consider putting a blanket on each side of the patient's hips. Then secure the patient's whole body to the backboard. Keep the patient warm. If you suspect shock, the foot end of the backboard may be elevated slightly if it does not compromise the splinting.

Hip

The hip is actually the proximal end of the femur, where the femur fits into the pelvis. Fractures of the hip are common to severe frontal car crashes.

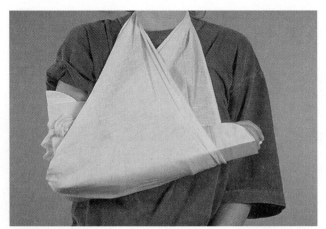

Figure 24-15 Cardboard splint of the forearm, wrist, or hand.

They also are common in the elderly as the result of a fall.

Any femur fracture can be dangerous. The femoral arteries lie next to the femur and can be lacerated by broken bone ends. Bleeding in this location can be very difficult to detect. Sometimes the only outward sign is swelling in the thighs. With a broken hip, the leg on the injured side may be shorter than the other leg and rotated. The patient will complain of pain when the leg is moved or when the hips are gently compressed.

When you perform an initial assessment of a patient with a possible hip injury, be sure to assess and treat for life-threatening problems first, including shock. Then stabilize the patient's hip. The best method is to immobilize the patient's whole body on a long backboard.

Femur

It takes a great deal of force to break a femur, such as in sky diving and skiing accidents. The result of a break is usually a marked deformity of the thigh, as well as a great deal of pain and swelling. Emergency care consists of immobilizing the bone ends to prevent further injury.

The preferred method of immobilization is a traction splint (Figure 24-16). Remember, only use a traction splint if you are specially trained and allowed to do so.

Alternative care involves using two long boards to create a fixation splint. The inner board must extend from the groin to below the bottom of the foot. The outer board must extend from the armpit to below the bottom of the foot (Figure 24-17). Pad the voids, then secure the boards to the patient with cravats at the shoulders, hips, knees, and ankles.

Knee

There are many types of knee injuries. Emergency treatment is basically the same. If you find the injured leg in a straight position, use two padded long boards to splint it in the position found. Place the first on the inner thigh so it extends from the groin to beyond the foot. Place the second on the outer thigh so it extends from the hip

APPLYING A TRACTION SPLINT

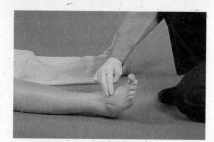

Figure 24-16a Assess pulse, movement, and sensation below the injury site.

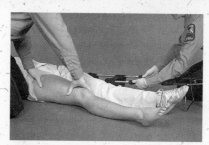

Figure 24-16b Manually stabilize the limb.

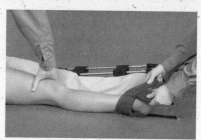

Figure 24-16c Apply the ankle hitch.

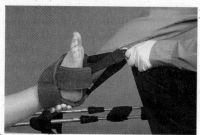

Figure 24-16d Apply and maintain manual traction. Position the splint.

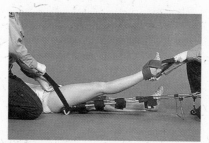

Figure 24-16e Attach the ischial strap.

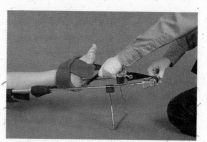

Figure 24-16f Fasten the splint to the ankle hitch. Apply mechanical traction.

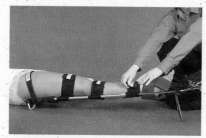

Figure 24-16g Fasten leg support straps in place.

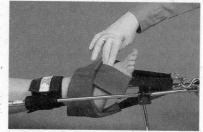

Figure 24-16h Reassess pulse, movement, and sensation below the injury site.

to beyond the foot. Then secure the boards to the patient with cravats.

If you find the knee in a bent position, immobilize it in the position found. The bones above and below it should be splinted with two padded short boards. (See Figure 24–18.)

Tibia and Fibula

Open fractures of the tibia are common because only thin layers of skin protect it. Usually fractures of the fibula are not so readily apparent, since it is not a weight-bearing bone. Whichever

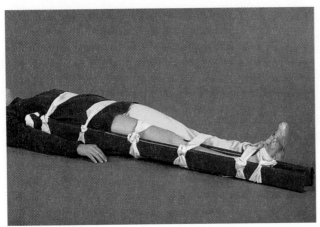

Figure 24-17 A high femur fracture immobilized in a fixation splint.

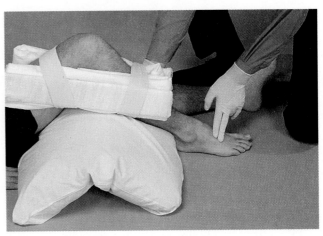

Figure 24-18 A splinted knee.

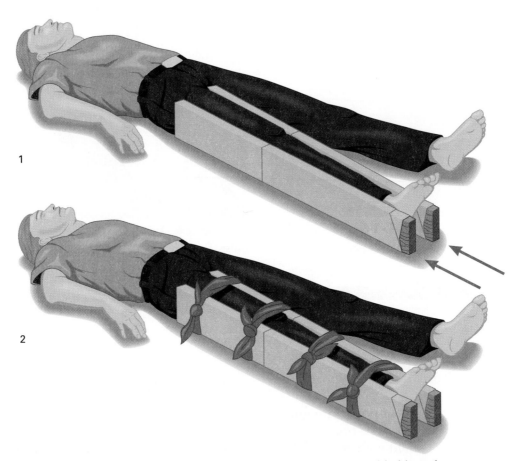

1

2

Figure 24-19 Fixation splint of the tibia/fibula using padded boards.

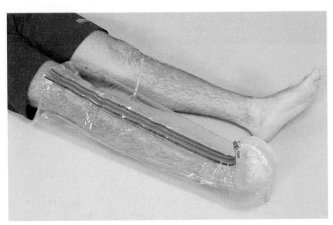

Figure 24-20   Air splint of the lower leg.

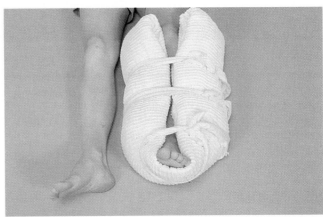

Figure 24-21   Blanket-roll splint of the ankle and foot.

one of the two bones is injured, the procedure for splinting remains the same.

Use two padded long boards (Figure 24–19). Place the first on the inner thigh so it extends from the groin to below the foot. Place the second on the outer thigh so it extends from the hip bone to below the foot. Then secure the boards to the patient with cravats.

An alternative method for a closed injury to the tibia or fibula is to use a circumferential splint. Make sure it extends beyond the knee and covers the entire foot (Figure 24–20).

Ankle and Foot

The foot is commonly injured by heavy objects falling onto it or twisting forces during a fall. The ankle bears so much weight, it does not take much movement in the wrong direction to make it unstable. No matter if the injury is to the ankle or foot, it is splinted in the same way.

Circumferential splints work well in these cases. However, the easiest splint may be a pillow. Simply wrap the pillow, or a blanket, around the foot. Then secure it with cravats at the toes and the shin. The more cravats applied, the better (Figure 24–21).

FIRST RESPONDER FOCUS

Patients may be aware of only one obvious injury, but it is your responsibility to perform a thorough patient assessment. Do not let an injury that is gruesome but relatively minor make you miss life threats such as an open chest wound or shock. So as you assess a patient with musculoskeletal injuries, keep the following tips in mind:

• The mechanism of injury can alert you to hidden injuries.
• Broken bones can be serious. They bleed, and they cause shock. If there is a possibility that your patient has more than one broken bone, the potential for shock and other hidden injuries is very high.
• Examine the extremities last. More important areas—the head, neck, chest, and abdomen—must be examined before them because they contain the vital organs.

In the first 10 minutes, it is important to make accurate decisions based on your assessment findings. Treat injuries and conditions that are a threat to life first. ∎

CASE STUDY FOLLOW-UP

At the beginning of this chapter, you read that First Responders were caring for a patient with a painful, swollen, deformed thigh. To see how chapter skills apply to this emergency, read the following. It describes how the call was completed.

PHYSICAL EXAMINATION

A quick physical exam revealed no other deformities, open injuries, tenderness, or swelling. At this point a police officer took manual stabilization of the femur above and below the injury site. I cut open the patient's jeans and saw that there was no obvious bleeding. The skin was unbroken.

PATIENT HISTORY

During the interview, I asked the patient if she had heard a popping or snapping sound. "Yes," she answered. Then I asked her to describe the pain on a scale of 1 to 10, with 10 being the worst. "10," she told us. She also said that she had consumed some alcohol, "two or three beers," but had not taken any type of medication.

ONGOING ASSESSMENT

We monitored the patient carefully. We were especially concerned about shock because of the possible femur fracture. So we continued to check her pulse and respiration every five minutes. Her airway remained clear. Her respirations remained at 24 and adequate. Her pulse was 106 and strong.

PATIENT HAND-OFF

When Ambulance 40 arrived, I gave a quick hand-off report:

"This is Lynn Solomon. She is 19, and was involved in a low-speed auto collision. Her chief complaint is pain in her left mid-thigh. She is awake, alert, and her airway is patent. Her breathing is rapid. She is not having trouble breathing. We put her on oxygen by nonrebreather mask. She is not bleeding externally. Her vital signs are: respirations 24, pulse 100, blood pressure 120/90, and skin is cold and dry. She said she has had 2 or 3 beers."

The ambulance crew took over manual stabilization of the patient's femur and further medical care. It wasn't long before the patient was extricated, packaged, and on the way to the trauma center. We proceeded to keep our promise to contact her parents and tell them where she and her wrecked car were being taken.

Musculoskeletal injuries usually are painful and obvious. Even so, you should always assess for and treat life-threatening problems first. Remember—life before limb!

REVIEW QUESTIONS

Page references where answers may be found or supported are provided at the end of each question.

Section 1

1. What is the function of the musculoskeletal system? (p. 402)

2. What is the difference between an open and a closed painful, swollen, deformed extremity? (pp. 402–403)

3. Is the emergency care you give to a patient with a fracture any different from the care you give to a patient with a strain, a sprain, or a dislocation? Why or why not? (p. 403)

REVIEW QUESTIONS *(Continued)*

4. What are the general emergency care guidelines for a painful, swollen, deformed extremity? (pp. 403, 405–406)

Section 2

5. What are the reasons for splinting a painful, swollen, deformed extremity? (p. 406)

6. What are five general rules of splinting? (p. 407)

7. What are some of the possible complications of improper splinting? (p. 407)

CHAPTER 25

CHILDBIRTH

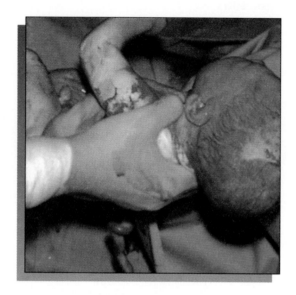

INTRODUCTION

A pregnant woman is too often rushed to a hospital, usually because the First Responder is afraid that the baby will be born before the mother can get there. In most cases there is no need for haste. Childbirth is a normal, natural process. Only in a few situations will you need to see that the mother reaches the hospital quickly.

First Responders are often called to help pregnant patients. So become familiar with the nature of childbirth and the emergency medical care of both the mother and the newborn.

Cognitive, affective, and psychomotor objectives are from the U.S. DOT's 1995 "First Responder: National Standard Curriculum." Enrichment objectives, if any, identify material that is supplemental to the DOT curriculum.

Cognitive

6-1.1 Identify the following structures: birth canal, placenta, umbilical cord, amniotic sac. (p. 420)

6-1.2 Define the following terms: crowning, bloody show, labor, abortion. (pp. 419, 421, 429)

6-1.3 State indications of an imminent delivery. (pp. 422–423)

6-1.4 State the steps in the pre-delivery preparation of the mother. (pp. 423–424)

6-1.5 Establish the relationship between body substance isolation and childbirth. (p. 424)

6-1.6 State the steps to assist in the delivery. (pp. 425–427)

6-1.7 Describe care of the baby as the head appears. (pp. 425–427)

6-1.8 Discuss the steps in delivery of the placenta. (pp. 427–428)

6-1.9 List the steps in the emergency medical care of the mother post-delivery. (pp. 427–428)

6-1.10 Discuss the steps in caring for a newborn. (p. 428)

Affective

6-1.11 Explain the rationale for attending to the feelings of a patient in need of emergency medical care during childbirth. (pp. 423, 429)

6-1.12 Demonstrate a caring attitude towards patients during childbirth who request emergency medical services. (pp. 423, 429)

6-1.13 Place the interests of the patient during childbirth as the foremost consideration when making any and all patient care decisions. (pp. 422–423, 432)

6-1.14 Communicate with empathy to patients during childbirth, as well as with family members and friends of the patient. (pp. 423–429)

Psychomotor

6-1.15 Demonstrate the steps to assist in the normal cephalic delivery. (pp. 425–427)

6-1.16 Demonstrate necessary care procedures of the fetus as the head appears. (pp. 425–427)

6-1.17 Attend to the steps in the delivery of the placenta. (pp. 427–428)

6-1.18 Demonstrate the post-delivery care of the mother. (pp. 427–428)

6-1.19 Demonstrate the care of the newborn. (p. 428)

Enrichment

* Describe emergency medical care of a patient who is suffering from the complications of pregnancy. (pp. 429–430)

* Discuss specific complications of pregnancy, including toxemia, spontaneous abortion, ectopic pregnancy, placenta previa, and abruptio placenta. (pp. 429–430)

* Describe emergency medical care of a patient who is suffering from the complications of childbirth. (pp. 430–432)

* Discuss specific complications of childbirth, including prolapsed umbilical cord, breech birth, limb presentation, multiple births, and premature birth. (pp. 430–432)

SECTION 1: THE PROCESS OF CHILDBIRTH

ANATOMY OF PREGNANCY

The **uterus** is the organ that contains the developing fetus, or unborn infant. (See Figure 25–1.) A special arrangement of smooth muscles and blood vessels in the uterus allows for great expansion during pregnancy and forcible contractions during labor and delivery. It also allows for rapid contractions after delivery, which help to constrict blood vessels and prevent excessive bleeding.

During pregnancy, the wall of the uterus becomes thin. The **cervix** (neck of the uterus) contains a mucous plug that is discharged during labor. The expulsion of this plug is known as the **bloody show** and appears as pink-tinged mucus in the vaginal discharge.

CASE STUDY

DISPATCH

My radio sounded the alert tones for an ambulance to respond to a call for a 28-year-old woman in labor. Before I was able to acknowledge the dispatcher, I heard: "Be advised the winter snow advisory has been posted and all roads are considered hazardous for travel." A snow plow was being asked to respond to the ambulance station. As the deputy sheriff, I had access to a four-wheel drive and knew I could get to the scene.

I informed dispatch that my ETA would be 5 to 10 minutes. She reported back that the ambulance could be 20 to 30 minutes. I found the OB kit, got my jacket on, and went out the door.

SCENE SIZE-UP

I arrived at the residence, a farm house, and did a quick safety check of the area. I then advised the dispatcher of the road conditions and best access for the ambulance. Once inside the house, I was met by the husband who informed me that his wife was due to deliver in a few weeks but her "water broke" and she was in labor. I was led to the bedroom, where the wife was lying on the bed.

INITIAL ASSESSMENT

The patient looked up at me and said, "The baby is coming—now."

Consider this patient as you read Chapter 25. How would you proceed?

The **placenta** is a disk-shaped organ on the inner lining of the uterus. Rich in blood vessels, it provides nourishment and oxygen to the fetus from the mother's blood. It also absorbs waste from the fetus into the mother's bloodstream. The mother's blood and the baby's blood do not mix. The placenta also produces hormones such as estrogen and progesterone that sustain the pregnancy.

After the baby is delivered, the placenta separates from the uterine wall and delivers as the **afterbirth.** It usually weighs about a pound or about one-sixth of the infant's weight.

The **umbilical cord** is the unborn infant's lifeline. It is an extension of the placenta through which the fetus receives nourishment. The umbilical cord contains one vein and two arteries. The vein carries oxygenated blood to the fetus. The arteries carry deoxygenated blood back to the placenta. When the baby is born, the cord resembles a sturdy rope about 22 inches long and one inch in diameter.

The **amniotic sac,** or *bag of waters,* is filled with a fluid in which the fetus floats. The amount of fluid varies. It is usually from 500 to 1000 milliliters. The sac of fluid insulates and protects the fetus during pregnancy. During labor, part of the sac usually is forced ahead of the baby, serving as a resilient wedge to help dilate (expand) the cervix.

The **birth canal** is made up of the cervix and the vagina. The vagina is about 8 to 12 centime-

ANATOMY OF PREGNANCY

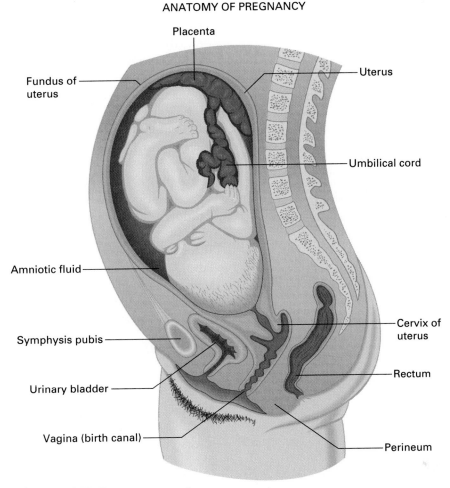

Figure 25-1 Anatomy of pregnancy.

ters in length. It originates at the cervix and extends to the outside of the body. Its smooth muscle layer stretches gently during childbirth to allow the passage of the infant.

A full-term pregnancy lasts approximately 280 days. Towards the end, the baby usually is in a head-down position, which brings the uterus down and forward. Mothers often can feel the difference and say that the baby has "dropped." This position is most favorable for the baby's passage through the birth canal.

STAGES OF LABOR

Labor is the term used to describe the process of childbirth. It consists of contractions of the uterine wall, which force the baby and later the pla-

centa into the outside world. Normal labor is divided into three stages: *dilation*, *expulsion*, and *placental* (Figure 25–2). The length of each stage varies greatly in different women and under different circumstances.

First Stage: Dilation

During this first and longest stage, the cervix becomes fully dilated (expanded). This allows the baby's head to progress from the uterus into the birth canal. Through uterine contractions, the cervix gradually stretches and thins until the opening is large enough to allow the baby to pass through.

The contractions may begin as an aching sensation in the small of the back. Within a short time, the contractions become cramp-like pains in

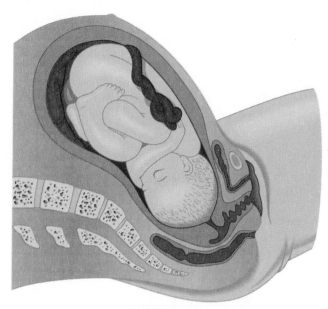

FIRST STAGE:
First uterine contraction to dilation of cervix

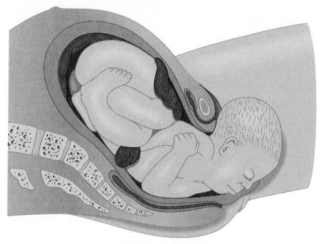

SECOND STAGE:
Birth of baby or expulsion

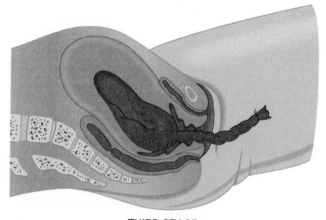

THIRD STAGE:
Delivery of placenta

Figure 25-2 Three stages of labor.

the lower abdomen. These recur at regular intervals, each one lasting about 30 to 60 seconds. At first, the contractions usually occur 10 to 20 minutes apart and are not very severe. They may even stop completely for a while and then start again. Appearance of the mucous plug, or bloody show, may occur before or during this stage of labor. Also before or during this stage, the amniotic sac may rupture, resulting in a gush of fluid from the vagina. The patient may say something like "my water broke" when this occurs.

Stage one may continue for as long as 18 hours or more for a woman having her first baby. Women who have had a child before may only have two or three hours of labor. By the end of the first stage of labor, contractions are at regular three- to four-minute intervals, last at least 60 seconds each, and feel very hard. The patient may indicate that she is having a considerable amount of discomfort.

Second Stage: Expulsion

During this stage, the baby moves through the birth canal and is born. Contractions are closer together and last longer—45 to 90 seconds each. As the baby moves downward, the mother experiences considerable pressure in her rectum, much like the feeling of a bowel movement.

When the mother has this sensation, she should lie down and get ready for the birth of her child. The tightening and bearing-down sensations will become stronger and more frequent. The mother will have an uncontrollable urge to push down, which she may do. There probably will be more bloody discharge from the vagina at this point.

Soon after, the baby's head appears at the opening of the birth canal. This is called **crowning.** The shoulders and the rest of the body follow.

Third Stage: Placental

During this stage, the placenta separates from the uterine wall. Usually, it is then spontaneously expelled from the uterus.

PATIENT ASSESSMENT

Childbirth is a natural, normal process. It is not an illness or disease. It is, however, physically traumatic. Complications can be life-threatening to both the mother and the baby.

If you are called to the scene of a childbirth, perform a scene size-up and initial assessment and treatment as you would for any patient. Give the mother calming reassurance. Then assess her condition to see if there will be time for transport to the nearest medical facility or if she will have the baby in her present location. Update EMS.

Generally, you should expect to assist in the delivery of the baby on scene if:

- You have no suitable transportation.
- The delivery of the baby can be expected within five minutes.
- The hospital or physician cannot be reached due to a natural disaster, bad weather, or some kind of catastrophe.

To determine if you should have the patient transported, time the contractions. Follow these steps:

1. Place your gloved hand on the mother's abdomen, just above her navel. Feel the involuntary tightening and relaxing of the uterine muscles.
2. Time these involuntary movements in seconds. Start from the moment the uterus first tightens until it is completely relaxed.
3. Time the intervals in minutes from the start of one contraction to the start of the next.

If the contractions are more than five minutes apart, the mother usually has time to be transported to a hospital safely, as long as traffic or weather conditions are not a problem. If the contractions are two minutes apart, she probably does not have time. So prepare to help deliver the baby where you are.

If the contractions are between two and five minutes apart, you must make a decision based on a number of factors. Ask the mother a few questions and conduct a simple assessment. The mother is usually nervous and apprehensive, so be gentle and kind. Show confidence and support. Ask these questions:

- Have you had a baby before? (The birth may take longer in a first pregnancy.) Are you having contractions? How far apart are they? Has the amniotic sac ruptured (or did your water break)? If so, when?

- Do you feel the sensation of a bowel movement? (If yes, the baby's head is pressing against the rectum and will soon be born. Do not let the mother sit on the toilet.)
- Do you feel like the baby is ready to be born?

Examine the mother. She should be on her back with knees bent and legs spread. Inspect the vaginal area, but do not touch it except during delivery and when your partner is present.

Determine if there is crowning. If you can see bulging in the vaginal area, and either the head or other part of the baby is visible, prepare to deliver the baby where you are. Report your findings to EMS.

Never ask the mother to cross her legs or ankles. Never tie or hold her legs together to try to delay delivery. Never delay or restrain delivery in any way. The pressure could result in death or permanent injury to the infant.

Also, be alert to the possibility of a condition known as *supine hypotensive syndrome*. This condition may occur when the pregnant patient lies on her back. The combined weight of the uterus and the fetus presses on the great vein that collects blood from the lower body and delivers it to the heart. This vein is called the *inferior vena cava*. That pressure can limit the blood that must return to the heart, causing the amount of blood that circulates through the body to decrease. You may observe signs of shock in your patient, including reduced blood pressure, increased pulse, and pale skin color. Also be alert for fainting.

To avoid supine hypotensive syndrome, the patient should be in a sitting position, if appropriate, or lying on her left side. If you suspect the condition, position the patient on her left side and treat for shock.

PREPARATION FOR DELIVERY

Always act in a professional manner. Be calm. Reassure the mother. Tell her that you are there to help with the delivery. Provide as much quiet and privacy for her as you can. Get rid of distractions. Hold her hand and speak encouragingly to her. Help the mother concentrate on breathing regularly with the contractions. Wipe the mother's face. Give her ice chips only if allowed by local protocol. (The mother should not eat or drink anything once labor starts.) The father or another rescuer can help.

At a minimum, the following materials and equipment should be included in your obstetrical (OB) kit. They are:

- Sheets and towels, sterile if possible.
- One dozen four-inch square gauze pads.
- Two or three sanitary napkins.
- Rubber suction syringe.
- Baby receiving blanket.
- Surgical scissors for cutting the umbilical cord.
- Cord clamps or ties.
- Foil-wrapped germicidal wipes.
- Wide tape or sterile cord.
- Large plastic bags.

All materials used during delivery should be sterile, or at least as clean as possible. This is to protect both the baby and the mother from contamination and infection.

In addition, because delivery results in exposure to a great deal of blood and other body fluids, you must wear personal protective equipment. Put on eye wear, a face mask, protective gloves, a disposable gown, and shoe coverings if possible. Handle soaked dressings, pads, and linens carefully. Place them in separate bags that will not leak. Then seal and label the bags. Scrub your arms, hands, and nails thoroughly *before and after* the delivery, even if you wore gloves.

Other guidelines include:

- Be prepared to provide basic life support to both the mother and the infant, including treatment for shock.
- Help the mother relax with each contraction. Inhaling causes muscles to tighten, so have her exhale with each contraction. Encourage her to keep her breathing slow but comfortable. Tell her not to strain or push during the first stage of labor.
- The amniotic sac may rupture, if it has not already done so. There also may be some blood-tinged mucus. These fluids increase as

labor progresses. If you have a clean towel, place it under the mother's buttocks to absorb the fluids. Always wipe in a down-and-away direction to minimize contamination. Discard soiled towels or sheets used for this purpose. Replace them frequently with clean ones.

- If the patient feels more comfortable sitting, reclining, or in some other position during the first stages of labor, let her do so.
- As contractions become longer and closer together, the patient should lie down on a flat, firm surface that she can push against. It is easiest for you if the mother is on an elevated surface. However, if the floor is the only firm surface available, use it. Pad it with folded sheets, towels, or blankets. Elevate the mother's buttocks about two inches with an additional pad of folded sheets or towels. The pad, which should extend about two feet in front of her, will help to support the slippery baby when it is born.
- When the mother is in position, her feet should be flat on the surface beneath her. Her knees will naturally spread apart because of the size of her abdomen. Do not pull them apart any further. Remove any constricting clothing, or push clothing above the mother's waist.
- Create a sterile field around the opening of the vagina. Place a sterile or clean sheet under the mother's hips. Touching only the corners of the sheet, have the mother lift her hips while you place one fold well under her hips. Unfold it toward her feet. If you have time, place another sheet or towel over the mother's abdomen and legs, leaving the vaginal area uncovered. Direct the best possible light toward the mother's genitals. Do not touch the vagina at any time.
- During the second stage of labor, when the mother bears down, remind her not to arch her back. She should curve it and bring her chin to her chest to avoid excessive straining. Have her hold her breath for 7 to 10 seconds as she bears down. Holding the breath longer will cause too much straining, broken blood vessels, and tearing of the area around the vagina.

DELIVERY OF THE BABY

(See Figure 25–3 for photographs of the delivery of a baby and the placenta.)

1. *Place the palm of your hand on top of the baby's head.* When it crowns, apply very gentle pressure to prevent an explosive delivery.

2. *Break open the amniotic sac if it has not already broken.* Tear it or pinch it open with your fingers and push it away from the infant's head and mouth. Note that the baby can safely inhale clear amniotic fluid. However, if there is **meconium staining** (greenish or brownish fluid), the baby has had a bowel movement, which could cause pneumonia if inhaled.

In the case of meconium staining, clean the area around the mouth and nose once the head is delivered. Suction the mouth first and then the nose with a rubber suction syringe. Expel all air from the suction bulb prior to placing it in the baby's mouth or nose. Release the bulb to create suction. Suctioning may need to be repeated in order to clear the airway. Note that meconium staining can be a life-threatening event. Consider requesting an advanced life support unit to assist.

CHILDBIRTH

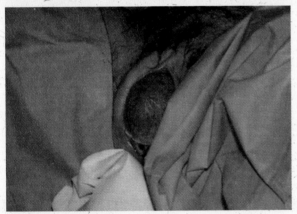

Figure 25-3a Crowning.

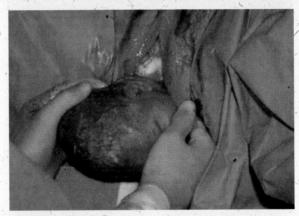

Figure 25-3b Head delivers and turns.

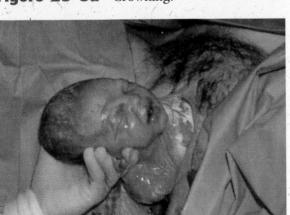

Figure 25-3c Shoulders deliver.

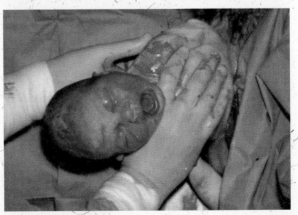

Figure 25-3d Chest delivers.

CHILDBIRTH *(Continued)*

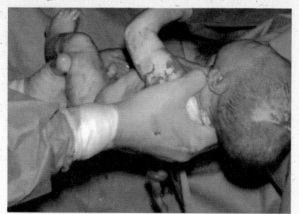

Figure 25-3e Legs and feet deliver.

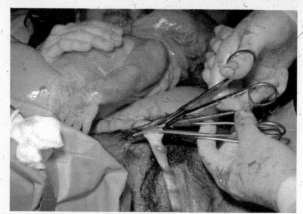

Figure 25-3f Cutting of cord.

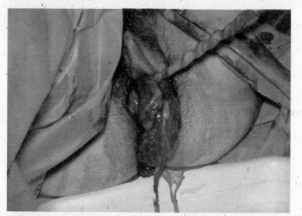

Figure 25-3g Placenta begins delivery.

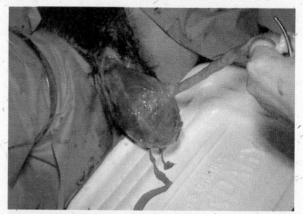

Figure 25-3h Placenta delivers.

3. *Determine the position of the umbilical cord.* When the baby's head delivers, check to see if the umbilical cord is around the baby's neck. If it is, use two gloved fingers to slip the cord over the shoulder. Only if you cannot dislodge it, attach two clamps a few inches apart. Then cut between the clamps.

4. *Support the baby's head.* As soon as the baby's head is born, place one hand below it. Spread the fingers of your other hand gently around it. Avoid touching the fontanel (the soft spots at the top of the head). In most normal presentations, the baby's head faces down. Then it turns so that the nose is toward the mother's thigh.

5. *Remove fluids from the infant's airway.* Use a rubber bulb syringe to suction mucus from the baby's mouth first and then the nose. Make sure you fully compress the syringe before you bring it to the baby's face. Avoid contact with the back of the mouth. Insert the tip no more than an inch into the mouth. Slowly release the bulb to allow fluid to be drawn into the syringe. If a syringe is not available, wipe the baby's mouth and then the nose with gauze.

6. *Support the baby with both hands as the rest of the body is born.* Once the shoulders are delivered, the rest of the body will appear rapidly. Note that you should never pull the baby from the vagina. Never touch the mother's vagina or anus. Handle the baby's slippery body carefully. Do not put your fingers in the baby's armpits. Pressure on the nerve centers there can cause paralysis.

7. *Grasp the feet as they are delivered.* Do not pull on the umbilical cord. Position the baby level with the mother's vagina until the umbilical cord is cut. The neck should be in a neutral position. Note the time of birth.

8. *Dry, wrap, and position the newborn.* Gently dry the infant with towels. Then wrap him or her in a clean, warm blanket. Place the baby on his or her side, head slightly lower than the trunk. Turn the baby's head slightly to one side to allow mucus and fluid to drain from the nose and mouth. Only the face should be exposed.

9. *Clean the newborn's mouth and nose.* Wipe blood and mucus from the baby's mouth and nose with sterile gauze. Suction the mouth first and then the nose again. The infant should cry almost immediately.

10. *Provide tactile stimulation, if the baby is not breathing.* Rub the back gently or slap the soles of the feet (Figure 25–4). Administer oxygen as soon as possible. Usually, placing an oxygen mask near the baby's face and allowing the oxygen to blow by is effective.

Do not use oxygen tubing without a mask. The force of the oxygen coming out of the tube can be harmful. If you still get no response, start artificial ventilation. (See "Newborn Care" below for details.)

11. *Clamp, tie, and cut the umbilical cord when it stops pulsating,* if your EMS system allows you to do so (Figure 25–5). Place two clamps or ties on it about three inches apart. Position the first clamp about four finger-widths (six inches) from the infant. Use sterile surgical scissors to cut the cord between the two clamps or ties. Periodically check the end of the cord for bleeding, and control any that occurs.

12. *Record the time of delivery.*

DELIVERY OF THE PLACENTA

1. *Observe for the delivery of the placenta.* When it starts to separate from the uterus, the cord will appear to be longer.

2. *Feel for contractions.* The contracting uterus should feel like a hard, grapefruit-size ball.

3. *Encourage the mother to bear down as the uterus contracts.* It usually delivers within 10 minutes of the infant, and almost always within 30 minutes. Normally, there will be some bleeding as the placenta separates.

4. *Wrap the placenta when it delivers.* When the placenta appears, slowly and gently guide it from the vagina. Never pull. If you have not cut the cord, wrap the placenta in a sterile

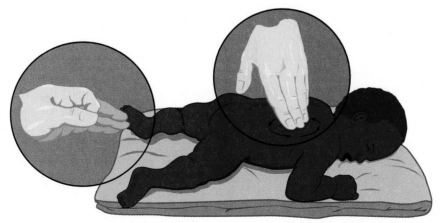

Figure 25-4 Stimulate breathing by rubbing back or flicking feet.

CUTTING THE UMBILICAL CORD

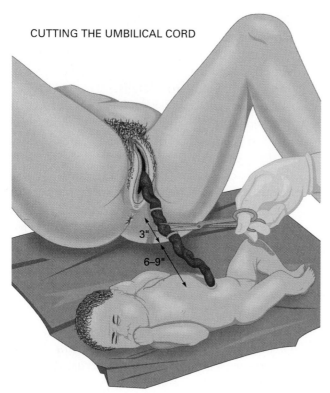

3"

6–9"

Figure 25-5 Cutting the umbilical cord.

towel and place it next to the baby. Wrap the baby and the placenta in a third sheet or blanket. If the cord is cut, place the placenta in a plastic bag to be taken to the hospital where a physician can confirm the delivery is complete.

After the placenta delivers, check the mother's vaginal bleeding. Up to 500 cc of blood loss is normal and usually well tolerated by the mother. Place two sanitary napkins over the opening of the vagina. Touch only the outer surfaces of the pads. Do not touch the mother's vagina. Note that at this time, ask the mother if she plans to breastfeed the infant. If so, now is a good time to encourage the mother to start. Breastfeeding helps the uterus to contract, which decreases the size of the uterus and helps to stop bleeding.

Make sure that the mother and the baby are covered and warm. The mother as well as the infant can chill easily following birth. Activate the EMS system if you have not already done so. The mother and the baby should be taken together to the hospital for evaluation by a physician.

If after the delivery of the placenta, bleeding appears to be excessive, treat the mother for shock and arrange for immediate transport. Then massage the uterus as described below to stimulate uterine contractions:

1. Place the medial edge of one hand horizontally across the abdomen, just superior to the symphysis pubis. Extend your fingers.
2. Cup your other hand around the uterus. Use a kneading or circular motion to massage the area. It should feel like a hard ball.
3. If bleeding continues to appear to be excessive, check your massage technique.

Replace any blood-soaked sheets and blankets while waiting for transport. Place all soiled items in a marked infection control bag and seal.

NEWBORN CARE

Perform artificial ventilation on the newborn if any of the following three conditions exist:

- The newborn is not breathing after drying, warming, and tactile stimulation or there are gasping respirations.
- The newborn's pulse rate is less than 100 beats per minute.
- There is persistent central cyanosis, or bluish discoloration around the chest and abdomen after 100% oxygen as been administered.

The recommended rate for assisting a newborn's ventilations is between 40–60 breaths per minute. Keep in mind that a baby's lungs are very small and require very small puffs of air. Never use mechanical ventilation on a newborn. A bag-valve-mask device may be used but it must be the appropriate size for a newborn. Remember to observe for chest rise. Reassess after 30 seconds. For proper positioning of the head, a towel may be placed under the baby's shoulders.

If breathing and pulse are absent or if pulse rate is less than 60 beats per minute, or 60–80 beats per minute and not rising when oxygen is administered, then start CPR. The rate of compressions is 120 per minute. The ratio of compressions to breaths for the newborn is 3:1.

SECTION 2: COMPLICATIONS OF CHILDBIRTH

COMPLICATIONS OF PREGNANCY

Toxemia of Pregnancy

About 5% of women develop toxemia (or "poisoning" of the blood) during pregnancy. It occurs most frequently in the last trimester (last three months). It most often affects women in their twenties who are pregnant for the first time. Women with a history of diabetes, heart disease, kidney problems, or high blood pressure are at greatest risk.

Signs and symptoms of toxemia may include:

- High-blood pressure (most common).
- Swelling in the extremities (most common).
- Sudden weight gain (two pounds or more per week).
- Blurred vision or spots before the eyes.
- Pronounced swelling to the face.
- Decreased urinary output.
- Severe and persistent headache.
- Persistent vomiting.
- Pain in the upper abdomen.
- Sudden seizures.

To provide emergency medical care for toxemia of pregnancy, arrange for immediate transport. Position the patient on her left side to avoid compressing the inferior vena cava. Keep the patient calm. Administer oxygen, if you are allowed to do so.

If the mother suffers a seizure, monitor her breathing closely. When the seizure stops, elevate her head and shoulders and administer high-flow oxygen.

Spontaneous Abortion

Sometimes called a "miscarriage," a **spontaneous abortion** is the loss of pregnancy before the twentieth week. It occurs naturally, unlike abortions that are deliberately performed under legal or criminal settings. Signs and symptoms include:

- Vaginal bleeding, often heavy.
- Pain in the lower abdomen that is similar to menstrual cramps or labor contractions.
- Passage of tissue from the vagina.

To provide emergency care, arrange for immediately transport. Treat the patient for shock. Save any passed tissue by packaging it in a sealed bag. The bag should then be transported with the patient for evaluation by a physician.

Ectopic Pregnancy

A woman has two fallopian tubes. Each one extends up from the uterus to a position near an ovary. Each month an egg drops from an ovary into a fallopian tube. The fallopian tube then conveys the egg to the uterus and sperm from the uterus toward the ovary.

In a normal pregnancy, a fertilized ovum (egg) is implanted in the uterus. In an ectopic pregnancy a fertilized ovum is implanted outside the uterus. It could be in the abdominal cavity, on the outside wall of the uterus, on the ovary, or on the outside of the cervix. In 95% of cases, the ovum is implanted in a fallopian tube.

An ectopic pregnancy is a severe medical emergency. The expanding fertilized ovum eventually causes rupture of a blood vessel and severe abdominal bleeding. It is the leading cause of death in pregnant women in their first trimester (first three months).

Signs and symptoms include:

- Sudden, sharp abdominal pain on one side. If bleeding is extensive, pain will become more diffuse.
- Pain under the diaphragm, or pain radiating to one or both shoulders.
- Tender bloated abdomen.
- Vaginal spotting or bleeding.
- Missed menstrual periods.
- Weakness when sitting.
- Signs of shock.

Suspect ectopic pregnancy in any woman of childbearing age when the above signs and symptoms are present. To provide emergency care, arrange for immediate transport. Place the patient on her back with knees elevated. Keep the patient warm. Administer oxygen, if you are allowed.

Placenta Previa

Placenta previa occurs when the placenta is positioned in the uterus in an abnormally low position. So when the cervix dilates (expands), the fetus moves, or labor begins, the placenta separates from the uterus. This puts both the mother and the baby in danger.

Signs and symptoms include:

- Severe, usually painless bleeding from the vagina.
- Signs of shock.

To provide emergency care, arrange for immediate transport. Elevate the patient's legs. Maintain body temperature. If possible, administer 100% oxygen by mask.

Abruptio Placenta

Another major cause of bleeding during pregnancy is abruptio placenta. It is the leading cause of fetal death after blunt trauma. Life-threatening for both the mother and the baby, it needs to be recognized and treated rapidly.

There are several causes, including toxemia and trauma. Whatever the cause, the normally implanted placenta begins separating from the uterus sometime during the last three months of pregnancy. Bleeding begins, but it is often behind the placenta and the mother is unaware of it. Shock then develops in the mother, and the baby does not get enough oxygen.

Signs and symptoms include:

- Bleeding from the vagina, not usually in great quantities.
- Severe abdominal pain.
- Rigid abdomen.
- Signs of shock.

To provide emergency care, arrange for immediate transport. Monitor vital signs carefully, and treat for shock. Administer 100% oxygen by mask, if you are allowed.

COMPLICATIONS OF DELIVERY

Prolapsed Umbilical Cord

In some situations, the umbilical cord comes out of the birth canal before the infant. When this happens, the baby is in great danger of suffocating. The cord is compressed against the birth canal by the baby's head, which cuts off the baby's supply of oxygenated blood from the placenta. Emergency care is extremely urgent. Arrange for immediate transport. Follow these steps:

1. Have the mother lie down on her left side, if possible. Knees should be drawn to her chest, or her hips and legs should be elevated on a pillow.
2. Administer high-flow oxygen, if possible.
3. With your gloved hand, gently push the baby up the vagina far enough so that the baby's head is off the umbilical cord. Maintain pressure on the baby's head and keep the cord free until medical help arrives. This is controversial in some areas. Follow local protocol.
4. Do not try to push the cord back into the vagina. Cover the cord with a sterile towel moistened with clean, preferably sterile, water.

Breech Birth

In a breech birth, the baby's feet or buttocks are delivered first (Figure 25–6). Whenever possible, the mother should be taken to the hospital for the birth. If that is not possible, then follow these guidelines:

1. Position and prepare the mother for a normal delivery.
2. Let the buttocks and trunk deliver on their own. Note, never try to pull the baby from the vagina by the legs or trunk.
3. Place your arm between the baby's legs. Let the legs dangle astride your arm. Support the baby's back with the palm of your other hand.
4. The head should follow on its own within three minutes. If not, you need to prevent the baby from suffocating. If you do not, the baby's head will compress the umbilical cord, preventing the flow of oxygenated blood from the placenta.

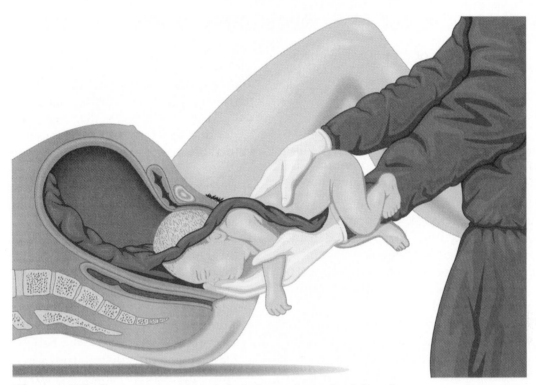

Figure 25-6 In breech birth, baby's feet or buttocks deliver first.

5. Place the middle and index fingers of your gloved hand alongside the infant's face. Your palm should be turned toward the face. Form an airway by pushing the vagina away from the baby's face until the head is delivered. Hold the baby's mouth open a little with your finger so that the baby can breathe.

Umbilical Cord Around the Neck

If the umbilical cord is wrapped around the baby's neck in the birth canal:

1. Try to slip the cord gently over the baby's shoulders or head.
2. If you cannot, and the cord is wrapped tightly around the neck, place clamps or ties three inches apart on the cord. Quickly but carefully cut between them. Unwrap the cord from around the neck.
3. Deliver the shoulders and body, supporting the head at all times.

Limb Presentation

If the baby's arm or leg comes out of the birth canal first, it means that the baby has shifted so much in the uterus that a normal delivery is not possible. The baby will have to be delivered by a physician. Delay can be fatal. Never pull on the baby by the arm or leg. The mother must be taken immediately to a hospital. Transport without delay.

Multiple Births

Twins are delivered the same way as single babies, one after the other. In fact, since twins are smaller, delivery is often easier. Identical twins have two umbilical cords coming out of a single placenta. If the twins are fraternal (not identical), there will be two placentas.

The mother may not be aware that she is carrying twins. You should suspect them if one or more of the following conditions exists:

- The abdomen is still very large after one baby is delivered.
- If the baby's size is out of proportion with the size of the mother's abdomen.
- If strong contractions begin again about 10 minutes after one baby is born.

The second baby is usually born within minutes and almost always within 45 minutes. To manage a multiple birth, follow these guidelines:

- After the first baby is born, clamp and cut the cord to prevent bleeding to the second baby. About one-third of second twins are breech.
- If the second baby has not delivered within 10 minutes, the mother should be transported to the hospital for the birth.
- After the babies are born, the placenta or placentas will be delivered normally. You can expect bleeding after the second birth.
- Keep the babies warm. Twins are often born early and may be small enough to be considered premature. Guard against heat loss until they can be taken to a hospital.

Premature Birth

If a woman gives birth before the thirty-sixth week of pregnancy, or if the baby weighs less than five and one-half pounds, the baby is considered to be premature. Premature babies are smaller and redder. They have heads that are proportionately larger than full-term babies. Because they are very vulnerable to infection, special care must be taken.

- Keep the baby warm with a blanket or swaddle. If you lack other supplies, use aluminum foil as an outer wrap.
- Keep the baby's mouth and nose clear of fluid by gentle suction with a bulb syringe.
- Prevent bleeding from the umbilical cord. A premature infant cannot tolerate losing even a little blood without being at risk for shock.
- Administer oxygen, if you are permitted, by blowing it gently across the baby's face. Never blast oxygen directly into the face.
- Since premature babies are so vulnerable to infection, do not let anyone breathe into the baby's face. Do everything you can to prevent contamination.

FIRST RESPONDER FOCUS

Calls for emergency childbirth are rare when compared to other types of calls. Unlike other calls, childbirth is not an injury or illness. Families have delivered babies outside of hospitals for eons. In modern times, hospital deliveries usually are preferred.

If you are called to the scene where the delivery of a baby is imminent, remain calm. Remember what you have learned, and keep in mind that you are assisting a natural process.

Become familiar with procedures and protocols in your area. In the event of complications, you will need to care for the infant and the mother until they are turned over to EMTs for transport to a hospital.

Boiling water is not performed by First Responders. ■

CASE STUDY FOLLOW-UP

At the beginning of this chapter, you read that a First Responder was on scene with a patient who was preparing to give birth in her home. To see how chapter skills apply to this emergency, read the following. It describes how the call was completed.

INITIAL ASSESSMENT (*Continued*)

I introduced myself to the patient and assured her that I had been trained to handle this type of situation. As we talked, I determined that she was alert and oriented with a good airway and adequate respiration. Her pulse was strong and regular, and her skin warm and slightly sweaty. There was no evidence of bleeding.

I moved next to the patient and explained that the ambulance was on the way. At this point I told both parents what needed to be done until the paramedics arrived and how they could help. I then updated dispatch.

PATIENT HISTORY

The patient, Mrs. Frieda Whitney, told me that this was her second pregnancy and that there had been no problems with the first baby. The doctor had told her that this pregnancy was normal. She reported that her water broke 45 minutes before and contractions were two minutes apart with a 50-second duration. She said she felt pressure on her rectum, as if she had to move her bowels.

I asked where her other child was, and she said her daughter was at a neighbor's.

PHYSICAL EXAMINATION

I asked Mrs. Whitney's permission to examine her for crowning and to prepare her for delivery. She agreed. Acting quickly, I made sure I had on all appropriate personal protective equipment. The husband was next to his wife holding her hand and trying to reassure her.

The baby's head had crowned. I placed my hands gently on the head. The shoulders and the rest of the baby followed rapidly. Using the bulb syringe from the OB kit, I suctioned the mouth first and then the nose. The baby cried loudly. It was a girl. I wrapped her in a warm towel and placed her on her mother's belly. I then clamped the umbilical cord.

ONGOING ASSESSMENT

Not long after the birth, Mrs. Whitney delivered the placenta. I placed it in a container for the paramedics to transport with the patients. Although the mother was tired, she was in good spirits and had no unusual complaints or distress. Her mental status was normal and vitals were stable.

After being cleaned up a bit, the baby's color also appeared to be normal. Her respirations were 48. Pulse was 146 and regular. She was actively moving around and had a good strong cry.

PATIENT HAND-OFF

When the EMTs arrived, I gave them the hand-off report. They quickly packaged the two patients and moved them to the ambulance. They had gotten to the residence quickly, considering the weather. The snow plow driver was my new hero. Even though there were no complications, and you could say it had been a "textbook" delivery, my heart was still racing as I watched them drive away.

> Childbirth is a rare and exciting event for a First Responder. Remember that birth is a natural process. You are there to assist the mother and then care for her and the baby after delivery. Your top priorities are the same as for any call. They are scene safety and the ABCs of your patients—both mother and child.

REVIEW QUESTIONS

Page references where answers may be found or supported are provided at the end of each question.

Section 1

1. What is the function of each of the following: placenta, umbilical cord, amniotic sac? (p. 420)
2. What happens during the first stage of labor? The second stage? The third stage? (pp. 421–422)
3. What information must you have in order to decide if a birth is imminent? (p. 423)
4. How can you determine how fast and how close together contractions may be? (p. 423)
5. What is supine hypotensive syndrome? How can you avoid it? (p. 423)

6. What part of the baby usually presents first in a normal delivery? (p. 422)
7. What can you do to assist a mother in the delivery of the baby? Describe the process briefly. (pp. 425–427)
8. When does the placenta usually deliver? What should you do with it when it does? (pp. 427–428)

Section 2

9. What would you observe in a breech birth? A prolapsed cord? A limb presentation? (pp. 430–431)
10. How does a multiple birth differ from a single birth? (pp. 431–432)

CHAPTER 26

INFANTS AND CHILDREN

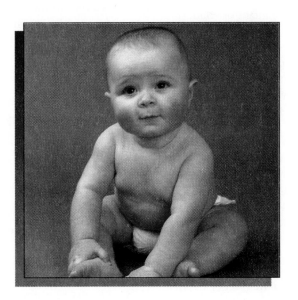

INTRODUCTION

Nearly 45,000 children die in the U.S. each year. Approximately one in four children will sustain an injury that will require medical care. Most children are injured as a result of motor vehicle crashes. Burns and drowning are the next most frequent type of injuries. Respiratory problems are the most serious of medical emergencies.

While your assessment approach to the ill or injured child is somewhat different from your approach to an adult, your patient care plan is the same. This chapter focuses only on the particular needs of children and how you can address those needs in emergency situations. It is meant to supplement the emergency care information found in the rest of the book.

Cognitive, affective, and psychomotor objectives are from the U.S. DOT's 1995 "First Responder: National Standard Curriculum." Enrichment objectives, if any, identify material that is supplemental to the DOT curriculum.

Cognitive

6-2.1 Describe differences in anatomy and physiology of the infant, child, and adult patient. (pp. 440–441, 444, 448–449)

6-2.2 Describe assessment of the infant or child. (pp. 440–446)

6-2.3 Indicate various causes of respiratory emergencies in infants and children. (pp. 441–442)

6-2.4 Summarize emergency medical care strategies for respiratory distress and respiratory failure/arrest in infants and children. (pp. 441, 448–450)

6-2.5 List common causes of seizures in the infant and child patient. (pp. 450–451)

6-2.6 Describe management of seizures in the infant and child patient. (pp. 450–451)

6-2.7 Discuss emergency medical care of the infant and child trauma patient. (pp. 446–447)

6-2.8 Summarize the signs and symptoms of possible child abuse and neglect. (pp. 452, 454)

6-2.9 Describe the medical-legal responsibilities in suspected child abuse. (pp. 452, 454)

6-2.10 Recognize need for First Responder debriefing following a difficult infant or child transport. (p. 454)

Affective

6-2.11 Attend to the feelings of the family when dealing with an ill or injured infant or child. (pp. 437–439, 451–452)

6-2.12 Understand the provider's own emotional response to caring for infants or children. (pp. 452, 454)

6-2.13 Demonstrate a caring attitude towards infants and children with illness or injury who require emergency medical services. (pp. 436–446)

6-2.14 Place the interests of the infant or child with an illness or injury as the foremost consideration when making any and all patient care decisions. (pp. 439, 442, 452, 455)

6-2.15 Communicate with empathy to infants and children with an illness or injury, as well as with family members and friends of the patient. (pp. 436–446)

Psychomotor

6-2.16 Demonstrate assessment of the infant and child. (pp. 440–446)

Enrichment

* Describe characteristics associated with the stages of infant and child development. (pp. 436–438)

* Discuss common respiratory emergencies in infants and children, including croup, epiglottitis, and asthma. (pp. 448–450)

* Identify the signs and symptoms of shock (hypoperfusion) in cases of trauma or dehydration in infants and children. (p. 447)

* Discuss the management of a patient with suspected sudden infant death syndrome (SIDS). (pp. 451–453)

SECTION 1:
THE PEDIATRIC PATIENT

There are times when determining the age of a young patient may be difficult. Even though age is a common benchmark for certain types of treatments, not all young patients physically mature at the same pace. For example, some 12-year-olds may be smaller than average. Some eight-year-olds may look older. Use your best judgment when the exact age of a patient is unknown.

DEVELOPMENTAL CHARACTERISTICS

Knowing the characteristics of children at each age can help you in an emergency. You will have a good idea of what to expect from them and how best to communicate. (See Table 26–1 for a summary.)

CASE STUDY

DISPATCH

My partner and I had just finished lunch as tones came over the speaker in the squad room. The dispatcher's voice followed. "Squad 2, respond to a third party call of a child struck by a car in the 200 block of Martin Luther King Boulevard. Be advised that an ambulance is being dispatched. Time of call is 1423 hours."

En route to the call, we were informed that the child's condition was unknown and the ambulance would be delayed.

SCENE SIZE-UP

Police led us through the crowd to the scene of the incident. We saw that the child was out of the roadway on the grass. A very upset father was beside the child. While my partner tried to introduce herself to the father and calm him down, I questioned a witness. She told me that the car had been traveling at about 15 mph when it hit the child. She said the child appeared to glance off the left front of the vehicle, fall to the ground, and roll onto the grass.

By that time my partner had calmed the father down, and gotten consent to provide emergency medical care.

INITIAL ASSESSMENT

The patient was on her side and not moving. She responded only to pain and had snoring respirations. She was little. Her father said she was six years old.

> Consider this patient as you read Chapter 26. Will assessment of the six-year-old be any different than assessment of an adult? How about treatment? Will that be different or about the same?

As a First Responder, your encounters with **pediatric patients** (infants and children) will be when they are ill or injured. They are apt to be frightened before you arrive. When you do get on scene, the presence of an unfamiliar person will add to what the patient already perceives as a frightening situation. Children pick up on anxiety easily. So it is very important to stay calm. Children, at any age, often take the lead from what they observe. So, if the adults on scene stay calm, a pediatric patient is likely to stay calm, too.

When dealing with younger children, it will help to get down to their eye level. Do not stare. Include them in your conversation. Do not make sudden movements when performing an assessment or providing emergency care. If a child is old enough to understand, ask permission to remove a piece of clothing or to touch his or her body. If a child holds out a hand or allows you to examine some part, seize the moment. The rule in pediatric care is to examine and palpate what you can when the opportunity presents itself.

TABLE 26-1
CHILDHOOD DEVELOPMENT BY AGE
▼

Common Term	Age	Characteristics and Behaviors
Infant	Birth to 1 year	Knows the voice and face of parents. Crying may indicate hunger, discomfort, or pain. Will want to be held by a parent or caregiver. Difficult to identify the precise location of an injury or source of pain.
Toddler	1–3 years old	Very curious at this age, so be alert to the possibility of poison ingestion. May be distrustful and uncooperative. Usually does not understand what is happening, which raises level of fear. May be very concerned about being separated from parents or caregivers. A stuffed toy may be helpful in gaining trust.
Preschooler	3–5 years old	Able to talk, but still may not understand what is being said to them. Use simple words. May be scared and believe what is happening in their fault. Sight of blood may intensify response. Sometimes a Band-Aid® helps.
School Age	6–12 years old	Should cooperate and be willing to follow the lead of parents and EMS provider. Have active imaginations and thoughts about death. Continual reassurance is important.
Adolescent	13–18 years old	Acts like adult. Able to provide accurate information. Modesty is important. Fears permanent scarring or deformity. May become involved in "mass hysteria." Be tolerant and do not get caught up in it.

With adolescents it is important to be sensitive to their feelings of modesty. In many ways they are young adults. Permanent disfigurement may be a major concern. Also, they are very sensitive to peer pressure and may need to be reassured that what they tell you will be held in confidence. Of course, you would still be free to include relevant information in your prehospital care report or in any report to emergency medical providers who have a need to know.

DEALING WITH CAREGIVERS

With pediatric patients it is important to understand that caregivers, especially parents, may be very upset and concerned. In fact, when a child is ill or injured, the First Responder should view the situation as one that involves a family, not just the child. Anticipate a variety of responses from caregivers. A few of the more common are crying, emotional outbursts, anger, guilt, and confusion.

Some of this emotion may be directed at EMS personnel. Do not take it personally. Caregivers need support and understanding.

As the assessment of the patient progresses, explain to the caregivers what is being done, and if time permits, tell them why. If appropriate, ask them to assist with emergency care. For example, a parent can hold an oxygen mask near the infant's face (Figure 26–1).

On occasion you may encounter a parent who will not let you help an ill or injured child. That parent may insist on remaining in control. Avoid becoming defensive. The parent's behavior has nothing at all to do with you. Remember, even though they may be coping in the only way they know how, ultimately the child is the patient. If you were called, you must make sure the patient is not in need of emergency medical care.

The following techniques may help in situations where parents are especially anxious:

- Your first priority is to protect the health and safety of the patient. If parents are making unsafe demands, try an approach of reserved confrontation. Explain that your opinion and procedures are based on sound medical knowledge and their demands are obstructing what is considered appropriate and in the child's best interest.

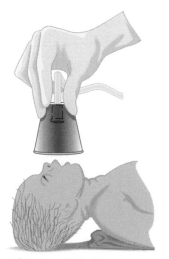

Figure 26–1
"Blow-by" oxygen using tubing and a paper cup. Never use Styrofoam.

- Realize that the parents may be correct. They usually know their children extremely well. A parent of a chronically ill child probably has a good grasp of what is going on.
- Regardless of how parents behave, treat them with courtesy, respect, and understanding. Avoid raising your voice. Tell them that you know they want help.
- Let parents stay as close to the patient as possible, as long as they are not interfering with care. If medically appropriate, a child can be held by a parent. Also, consider letting the parents do something for the child in order to help focus their attention away from you.
- Whatever you do, do not react with anger.

USING APPROPRIATE EQUIPMENT

Having the correct equipment in the correct size for the pediatric patient is extremely important to quality care. The following list of EMS equipment is appropriate for the different needs of infants and children:

- Adjunct airways in pediatric sizes.
- Face masks, oxygen masks, and nasal cannula in pediatric sizes.
- Bag-valve-mask (BVM) resuscitator with oxygen enrichment attachment. If the BVM has a pop-off valve, it must be able to be closed.
- Bulb syringe for suctioning.
- Blood pressure cuffs in pediatric sizes.
- Pediatric stethoscope.
- Cervical immobilization devices in various pediatric sizes.
- Backboards made especially for infants and children.
- New, clean stuffed animal to be used to comfort or distract the patient.

PATIENT ASSESSMENT

Scene Size-up

When entering a scene where there is an emergency involving a child, many EMS rescuers say, "90% of the assessment is done from the doorway." That is not really true. However, you can take a second or two to try to get the big picture. Observations you can make from "the doorway" in addition to your usual scene size-up include the interaction between the patient and parents, general appearance of the environment, and signs of possible **non-accidental trauma** (child abuse).

During scene size-up, see how caregivers are reacting and, if appropriate, consider how best to involve them in assessment and treatment of the patient. Note that you may be called to treat infant or child patients at a location other than where they were injured or became ill. It is not uncommon for adults to pick up a child in order to provide comfort or assistance. Understand they meant no harm. Ask caregivers specifically:

- Why was EMS called?
- What is the chief complaint?
- Has the child been moved? If so, where did the incident occur?

Be alert to the possibility of poison ingestion or a possible fall.

Initial Assessment

To assess an infant's or child's level of responsiveness, determine from the caregiver what is "normal." If a patient appears to be responsive but is unable to recognize his or her own parents, consider this a serious medical emergency.

Remember that an infant's or child's anatomy is not the same as an adult's (Figure 26–2). How-

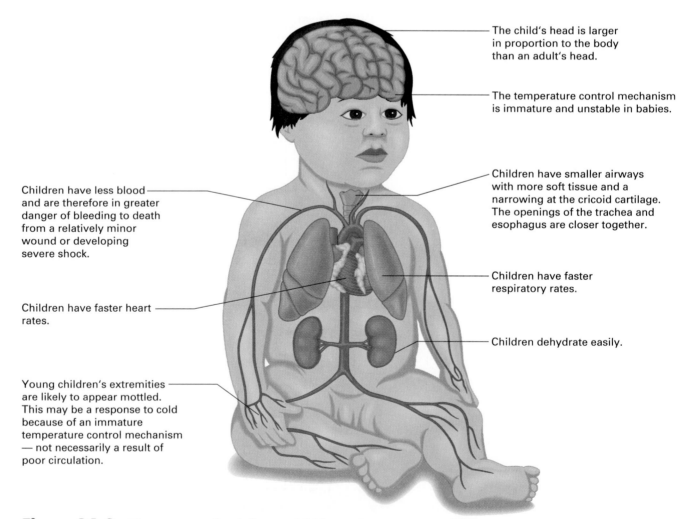

Children have less blood and are therefore in greater danger of bleeding to death from a relatively minor wound or developing severe shock.

Children have faster heart rates.

Young children's extremities are likely to appear mottled. This may be a response to cold because of an immature temperature control mechanism — not necessarily a result of poor circulation.

The child's head is larger in proportion to the body than an adult's head.

The temperature control mechanism is immature and unstable in babies.

Children have smaller airways with more soft tissue and a narrowing at the cricoid cartilage. The openings of the trachea and esophagus are closer together.

Children have faster respiratory rates.

Children dehydrate easily.

Figure 26-2   The anatomy of an infant or child is not the same as an adult's.

ever, assessment and treatment of the ABCs are as critical to the pediatric patient as to any other. The single most important maneuver is to ensure an open airway. When trauma is suspected, always use a jaw-thrust to open the airway. Never hyperextend the head and neck. The head of an infant or young child is large in proportion to the rest of the body. One way to properly position the head in a neutral position is to place a towel with a fold or two under the patient's shoulders.

Common signs in infants and children that indicate early respiratory distress are as follows (Figure 26–3):

- Noisy breathing, such as stridor, crowing, grunting.
- Cyanosis.
- Flaring nostrils.
- Retractions (drawing back) between the ribs or around the shoulders.
- Use of accessory muscles to breathe.
- Breathing with obvious effort.
- Altered mental status.

Immediately provide oxygen if any of these signs are evident. Continually monitor for signs of respiratory distress. If an infant's respirations are less than 20 per minute or a child's are less than 10, assist ventilations.

Assess circulation by palpating the infant's brachial pulse. Palpate the unresponsive child's carotid or femoral pulse. Palpate the responsive child's radial or brachial pulse.

When you assess the pediatric patient's circulation, remember that inadequate oxygen can slow the heart. Provide oxygen as soon as you detect a slow pulse. Use a mask that is the correct size for the patient. When the patient is not breathing and has no gag reflex, an oropharyngeal airway should be inserted to assist in maintaining an open airway. (See Chapter 6 for review of how to insert adjunct airways.)

Control external bleeding immediately. Remember that children have the ability to compensate for blood loss longer than an adult can. Decompensation (failure of the heart to maintain sufficient circulation of blood) is a very rapid process. It is imperative to monitor pediatric patients constantly.

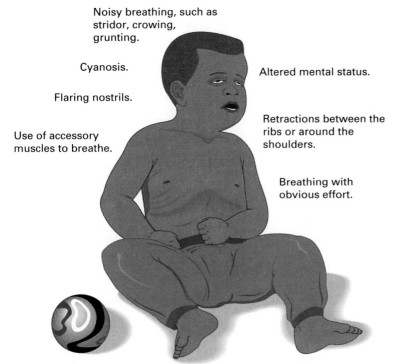

Figure 26-3 Signs of early respiratory problems.

After initial assessment and treatment, update EMS. For those patients with significant airway problems, respiratory or cardiac arrest, or the possibility of shock, rapid transport is indicated.

NOTE: The most important care you can give a pediatric patient is done in the initial assessment. Never stop required airway care to perform a physical exam or gather a patient history.

Patient History

If time permits, gather a medical history. Keep in mind that anxious, upset parents and a screaming child can be unnerving. If possible, talk to the child and involve the caregivers. Interview witnesses. Avoiding asking questions that require only yes-or-no answers. If responses to questions seem inconsistent or if they do not correspond to your initial assessment, try rephrasing the questions.

When you take a SAMPLE history for a medical patient, include questions such as: When did the signs and symptoms develop? How have they progressed? Is the problem a recurring one? If so, has the child been seen by a physician? If so, is the specific diagnosis known? What treatment was received?

When you take a SAMPLE history for a trauma patient, include the details of the accident, such as the time it occurred, mechanism of injury, and emergency care already given.

Physical Exam

It is difficult to assess pain in children. They may lack the body awareness and vocabulary necessary to describe it. Children also may not be able to separate the fear they feel from their physical condition. Ask the parent, if possible, how the child usually responds to pain. This may give you some idea of how the present condition compares.

The bodies of infants and children can hide injury for some time. Only after their compensatory abilities fail will you see changes in vital signs. The changes may occur very quickly, and the patient's condition may deteriorate very fast. So take the vital signs of infants and children more frequently than you would for an adult. (See Table 26–2.) Also, pay attention to your overall impression of how the patient looks and acts. Your observations may tell you more about the status of the child than any one vital sign.

TABLE 26-2
NORMAL VITAL SIGNS FOR INFANTS AND CHILDREN

Age	Weight Lb.	Weight Kg.	Pulse ( ) = Average	Respiration	Average Blood Pressure	
1–28 days	7.4	3.4	94–145 (125)	30–60	80	46
3 months	12.5	5.7	110–140 (120)	24–35	89	60
6 months	16.5	7.4	100–140 (120)	24–35	89	60
1 year	22.0	10.0	98–160 (120)	20–30	89	60
2 years	27.0	12.4	90–140 (110)	20–30	96	64
3 years	31.0	14.5	80–120 (100)	20–30	96	70
4 years	33.6	16.5	65–132 (100)	12–26	96	70
5 years	41.0	19.0	80–110 (100)	12–26	96–98	70
6 years	47.0	21.5	75–100 (100)	12–25	96–98	56
10 years	71.0	32.3	70–110 (90)	12–21	110	60

When you do assess a pediatric patient's vital signs, keep the following in mind:

- *Pulse*—Use the brachial pulse in an infant and the radial pulse in a child. If the radial pulse is not clear, check the brachial pulse. If the pulse is too rapid or too slow, immediately examine the patient for problems such as signs of respiratory distress, shock, or head injury.

  Rapid pulse may indicate oxygen deficiency, shock, or fever. It also may be normal in scared or overly excited children. A slow pulse in a child must first be presumed to be a sign of hypoxia (inadequate oxygen in the blood). Other causes of slow pulse may include pressure in the skull, depressant drugs, or a rare medical condition.

- *Respiration*—Children sometimes breathe irregularly. So monitor respirations for a full minute to determine rate. Do it frequently. (You also may need to place your hand on a "belly breather's" abdomen to get an accurate breathing rate.) Rates in children alter easily due to emotional and physical conditions. An increase over a previous rate can be significant.

  The quality of breathing also is important. Determine if it is adequate. Observe to see if the child is working to breathe and using accessory muscles. Look for retractions. Notice if breathing is noisy. Shortness of breath may indicate the need for you to assist ventilations.

- *Blood pressure*—A falling or low blood pressure in a pediatric patient can be a late indicator of shock. Be sure to use a blood pressure cuff that is the correct size for your patient. Use a pediatric stethoscope, if available. Do not take a blood pressure in children under three years of age.

- *Temperature*—Feel the arms and legs of infants and children to see if they are cold. The torso may be warm in comparison. Cold hands and feet may indicate shock, if your patient is not in a cold environment. Note that taking a rectal temperature and using a glass thermometer are not recommended for field use by First Responders.

- *Skin condition and capillary refill*—Always look at the pediatric patient's skin for signs of injury. Notice skin color. Though a newborn may have a mottled color on hands and feet, a child should not have a bluish discoloration. Be alert. Be sure to assess capillary refill (Figure 26–4). If it takes more than two seconds, the patient may be in shock. A delayed capillary refill should be considered an emergency in the pediatric patient.

Many children with head or spine injuries suffer nervous system damage as well. It is the cause of traumatic death at least two-thirds of the time. If the patient's history suggests trauma or if there is a significant mechanism of injury, then manually

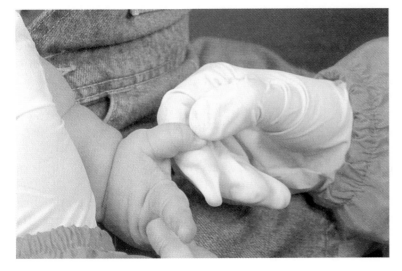

Figure 26-4 Assess capillary refill in infants and children less than 6 years of age.

stabilize the infant's or child's head and neck immediately. Assess for damage to the nervous system as follows. Remember that children do not have the same verbal skills as adults and their response to stimuli may be different. Parents may be able to describe a normal response.

- Determine the level of responsiveness. If the patient appears to have an altered mental status, ask parents to describe the normal level.
- Check the pupils. Find out if they are of equal size and, if practical, how they respond to light.
- Examine the head, neck, and spine for signs of injury.
- Check to see if the patient responds to verbal and painful stimuli. Pinch the skin between the thumb and forefinger.
- Check the ability to recognize familiar objects and people.
- Check the ability to move arms and legs purposefully.
- Check to see if there is clear or bloody fluid draining from ears.

If you suspect damage to the nervous system, keep your patient as still and calm as possible. Provide in-line stabilization of the patient's head and neck. Apply a cervical immobilization device if you are allowed to do so. Do not allow untrained people to move the patient. Activate the EMS system, if it has not already been done, and continue to assess vital signs.

When you care for an infant or child, be aware of the following special conditions and situations (Table 26–3):

- Monitor an infant's breathing continually. Infants have proportionately larger tongues, which if relaxed can easily block the airway.
- Head injuries are more likely in infants and children. When you suspect an injury above the clavicles or when the mechanism of injury is unknown, provide in-line stabilization. Apply a cervical immobilization device, if possible.
- Always support the head when you lift an infant. Before the age of nine months, an infant cannot fully support his or her own head.

- During the physical exam, check the anterior **fontanel** (soft spot) on top of an infant's skull. If you see a bulge, there may be pressure inside the skull. If you see a depression, the infant may be dehydrated and in shock. (The fontanel stays open for up to two years after birth.)
- Injuries to the extremities can damage the growth plates with long-term effects. Carefully assess extremities, including pulses, capillary refill, and skin condition. Be careful not to cause additional pain. Follow local protocols for splinting.
- Stop bleeding as quickly as possible. A comparatively small blood loss in an adult would be major for a child. Be alert to open fractures, which tend to bleed profusely.
- A child's skin surface is large compared to body mass. This makes children more susceptible to dehydration and hypothermia. Response to burns also can be more severe. Watch for signs of shock.
- Make sure cervical immobilization devices fit correctly. Note that some children have very short necks. Such a device may not work on them. Use a rolled towel instead.
- Children often get arms, legs, hands, feet, or heads trapped under or in rigid structures. The child is sometimes in pain and is almost always panicky. Calm the child first. Then see if he or she can move independently. Lubricate skin surface with baby oil or a water-soluble lubricant. Make sure it is not applied near the patient's mouth, nose, or eyes. If sawing or cutting is needed, make sure the child is protected with a heavy, fire resistant cover. Someone can talk to the child to provide encouragement. After the child is freed, perform a complete patient assessment.

Following are helpful hints for conducting a physical exam:

- If possible, assess the child while he or she is on the parent's lap (Figure 26–5).
- Prepare yourself so you can radiate confidence, competence, and friendliness. Remember that children between one and six seldom like strangers.

TABLE 26-3
ANATOMICAL DIFFERENCES IN INFANTS AND CHILDREN

Anatomical Differences	Impact on Assessment and Treatment
Larger tongue.	Can block airway.
Reduced size of airway.	Can become easily blocked.
Abundant secretions.	Can block airway.
"Baby" teeth.	Can easily dislodge and block airway
Flat nose and face.	Difficult to obtain good airway seal with face mask.
Proportionally large head.	Must maintain neutral position to keep airway open and in-line stabilization of head and neck. Higher potential for head injuries in cases of trauma.
"Soft spots" on head.	Bulging "soft spots" may indicate intracranial pressure; sunken ones may indicate dehydration.
Thinner and softer brain tissue.	Consider head injury more serious than in adults.
Short neck.	Difficult to stabilize and immobilize.
Shorter and narrower trachea, with more flexible cartilage.	Can close off trachea with overextension of the neck.
Faster respiratory rate.	Muscles fatigue easily, which can lead to respiratory distress.
Primarily nose breathers (newborns).	Airway more easily blocked.
Abdominal muscles used to breathe.	Difficult to evaluate breathing.
More flexible ribs.	Lungs are more easily damaged. May be significant injuries without external signs.
Heart can sustain faster rate for longer period of time.	Can compensate longer before showing signs of shock and usually decompensates more quickly than an adult.
More exposed spleen and liver.	Significant abdominal injury more likely. Abdomen more often a source of hidden injury.
Larger body surface.	Prone to hypothermia.
Softer bones.	Can easily bend and fracture.
Thinner skin.	Consider burns to be more serious than in an adult.

- Get as close as you can to a child's eye level. Sit next to the child if possible. When it comes time for a hands-on assessment, do it in the least threatening way. Consider starting at the toes and working your way up to the head.

- Explain what you are doing in terms a child can understand. Follow up on the child's questions. Maintain eye contact, but do not stare. Speak in a calm, quiet voice. Even infants will respond to a calm voice, and an apparently unresponsive child may absorb much of what you say.

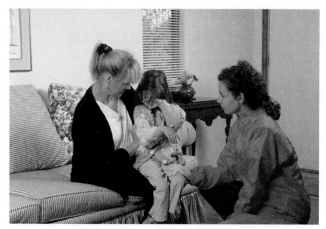

Figure 26-5 Having the child sit on a parent's lap can have a calming influence.

- Younger children tend to take statements literally. For example, if you say you want to take a pulse, they may think you mean to take something away from them. Watch your phrasing. Also older children do not like being talked about. Talk with them directly.
- Be gentle. Do everything you can to reduce the amount of pain that a child must endure. However, when there will be pain, be honest. "It will hurt when I touch you here, but it will last only a second. If you feel like crying, it's okay." Children can tolerate pain, if they are prepared for it and are given adequate support. With children under school age, keep the most painful parts of the assessment for the end. It will help if the child is kept on a parent's lap.
- Do not lie to a child. Always be honest. This does not mean you need to explain everything that is going on, but when you do answer questions or perform a procedure that could be uncomfortable, be candid.
- If a child is not calm enough to be treated, you must restrain the patient. But be sure it is absolutely necessary. Only when care is compromised should the child be separated from a parent.
- A stuffed animal may help to win the confidence of a young child. It also may help to distract the child during assessment and treatment. Also, very shy children sometimes "talk through" a stuffed animal. For example, they may not tell you where they hurt but might tell where the animal hurts, thereby giving you information about themselves.

Ongoing Assessment

The ongoing assessment is the same for infants and children as it is for adults. It never ends as long as you are caring for the patient.

Patient Hand-off

Just as you would for adult patients, include in your infant or child hand-off report:

- Age and sex of the patient.
- Chief complaint.
- Level of responsiveness (AVPU).
- Airway and breathing status.
- Circulation status.
- Physical exam findings.
- SAMPLE history.
- Treatment, interventions, and the patient's response to them.

SECTION 2: COMMON PEDIATRIC EMERGENCIES

TRAUMA

Injuries are the leading cause of death in infants and children. Blunt injury is the most common. Basic life support and trauma management in infants and children is similar to care provided to adults. Remember to treat as you go. That is, as you assess the patient's ABCs, take care of any problem you find. Remember that children may take longer to go into shock, but when they do, it usually develops more rapidly than in adults.

Always suspect trauma when infants and children are passengers in motor vehicle collisions. Suspect unrestrained passengers of head and neck injuries. Suspect blunt trauma to the abdomen if the child was wearing a lap belt without a shoulder belt. Fully restrained passengers often have abdominal and lower spine injuries. The car seats in which infants ride are often fastened improperly. So suspect head and neck injuries in these patients.

In some EMS systems, you may be allowed to immobilize a child right in his or her car seat.

This is done by applying a cervical immobilization device to the patient and placing padding between the child and seat to prevent movement. This procedure should not be used if the child has serious injuries or the potential for serious injuries, since the car seat may prohibit airway and other important emergency medical care.

If a child is immobilized in a car seat, never tip the seat back. The position may impair breathing by putting pressure on the child's diaphragm. Always make sure that the seat remains upright.

If a child riding a bicycle is struck by a car, suspect head, spine, and abdominal injuries. If the child was walking when struck, suspect head injury, abdominal injury, and pelvis or femur injury.

SHOCK

A major cause of shock in children is dehydration due to vomiting and diarrhea related to infection. Another cause is blood loss due to trauma.

Children tend to compensate more efficiently for shock. When they decompensate, it is a rapid process that can be devastating. Blood pressure may drop so far and so fast that the patient may go into cardiac arrest. So you must constantly monitor the injured patient for signs and symptoms of shock. Take his or her vital signs constantly, including capillary refill.

Signs and symptoms of shock in the pediatric patient include (Figure 26–6):

- Altered mental status, from anxiety to unresponsiveness.
- Apathy or lack of vitality. This may present as the inability of the child to identify a parent—an ominous sign.
- Delayed capillary refill.
- Rapid or weak and thready pulse.
- Pale, cool, clammy skin.
- Rapid breathing.
- Falling or low blood pressure (a late sign).
- Absence of tears when crying.

Hypothermia can intensify shock in infants. They usually cannot shiver to warm themselves. So be sure to keep them warm. Remember especially to cover an infant's head. While you are waiting for the EMTs to arrive on scene, follow these steps for emergency medical care of an infant in shock:

1. Have the patient lie flat. Make sure that the position does not interfere with breathing.
2. Be prepared to assist ventilations. Provide oxygen, if you are allowed.
3. Keep the patient warm and as calm as possible.
4. Monitor vital signs often.

Remember that a relatively small blood loss in a pediatric patient can be very dangerous. For example, a newborn usually has less blood than the contents of a soda can. When there is significant visible blood loss or suspected internal bleeding, rapid transport and constant monitoring are essential.

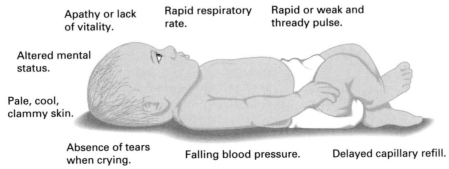

Figure 26-6 Signs of shock in an infant or child.

RESPIRATORY EMERGENCIES

There is nothing more important than controlling the airway and ensuring adequate breathing in a pediatric patient. The National Pediatric Trauma Registry has reported that 30% of all pediatric trauma deaths are related to inappropriate management of the airway. The American Heart Association reports that more than 90% of pediatric deaths from foreign body airway obstruction occur in children under five years of age. Of those, 65% are infants. It is estimated that most could be saved by early detection.

Note that there are some differences in the way you manage a child's airway. They are as follows (Figure 26–7):

- Children are more susceptible than adults to respiratory problems. They have smaller air passages and less reserve air capacity. A child's airway can be compromised by less trauma or infection. Be especially attentive to ensure a clear and open airway.
- A child's airway structures are not as long or as large as an adult's. A child's can close off if the neck is flexed or extended too far. The best position is a neutral or slightly extended position. If the child is flat on the back, place a thin pad or towel under the shoulders to keep the head and neck properly aligned. Monitor signs of breathing.
- Because of immature accessory muscles, children use their diaphragms to breathe. If there are no reasons to prevent you from doing so, place a child in a position of comfort. That usually is a sitting position.
- Children have a large tongue that can block the airway. Make sure the tongue is forward. If a jaw-thrust maneuver is used, make sure your hand stays on the bony part of the chin (Figure 26–8). If it falls below, the tongue could be pushed back to block the airway.
- Infants and children tend to breathe through their noses. They also have abundant secretions. So be prepared to suction often to make sure the nose stays clear (Figure 26–9).
- Apply oxygen, if you are allowed, by way of a mask. Humidified oxygen is preferred. But never withhold or delay oxygen in order to have it humidified. If a child will not tolerate a mask, then hold it slightly away from the patient's face.

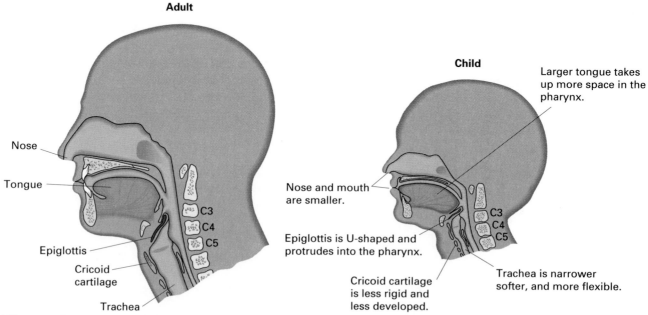

Figure 26-7 Comparison of airways of an adult and an infant or child.

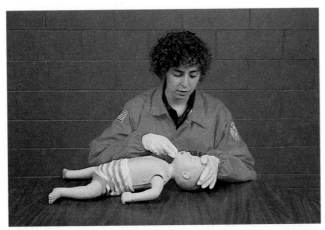

Figure 26-8 Airway obstruction may be relieved in an infant or child by keeping the head in a neutral or slightly extended position.

- If an infant or child is having a respiratory emergency, notify the incoming EMS unit and be sure an advanced life support (ALS) team is en route, if available.
- Even if the signs and symptoms of a respiratory emergency subside, it is still important for the child to be transported to a hospital.

For emergency care of infants and children with respiratory emergencies, see Chapter 6. For

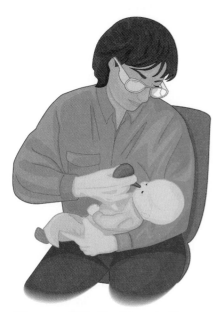

Figure 26-9 Use a bulb syringe for suctioning.

more information about respiratory problems in all patients, see Chapter 12.

Croup

Croup is a common viral infection of the upper airway. It is most common in children between the ages of one and five. With croup, swelling progressively narrows the airway. As the child breathes, he or she may produce strange whooping sounds or high-pitched squeaking. There may be hoarseness, with the child's cough typically described as a "seal bark." Episodes of croup occur more commonly at night.

As the child gets worse, he or she may experience the following signs of respiratory distress:

- Breathing with effort, including nasal flaring and retractions.
- Rapid breathing.
- Rising pulse.
- Paleness or cyanosis.
- Restlessness or altered mental status.

Severe attacks of croup can be dangerous. About 10% of all children with croup need to be hospitalized. Treat a child with croup the same way you would treat any respiratory emergency. Arrange for transport to the nearest hospital as quickly as possible.

Epiglottitis

Epiglottitis is caused by a bacterial infection that inflames the epiglottis. It often resembles croup but is more serious. Left untreated, epiglottitis can be life-threatening. Signs and symptoms may include:

- Occasional noise while inhaling.
- Anxious concentration on breathing. The child may try to stay very still.
- Sitting up and leaning forward, usually with chin thrust outward.
- Pain on swallowing and speaking.
- Drooling.
- Changes in voice quality.
- High fever (usually above 102°F).

If you suspect epiglottitis, do not ask the child to open his or her mouth. Do not try to examine the child's throat or place anything in the mouth. Touching the larynx can cause the airway to close completely. In all other ways, treat the child as you would for any respiratory emergency. Arrange for transport to the nearest hospital as quickly as possible.

Asthma

Asthma is common among children, especially those with allergies. However, it should always be considered a serious medical emergency. Parents usually know the child's history and recognize an asthma attack. Determine if the child is taking medication.

An acute asthma attack occurs when the bronchioles spasm and constrict. This causes the bronchial membranes to swell and get congested with mucus, which interferes with the ability to exhale. As a result, air gets trapped in the lungs, the chest gets inflated, breathing becomes impaired, and oxygen deficiency occurs.

Especially critical signs and symptoms include:

- Rapid irregular breathing, especially in younger children.
- Exhaustion.
- Sleepiness and changes in level of responsiveness.
- Cyanosis.
- Rapid pulse and dropping blood pressure.
- Signs of dehydration.
- Wheezing (high-pitched breathing sounds).
- Quiet or silent chest. (In the late stages of respiratory distress, respirations may become so shallow that they no longer cause noise. Do not be fooled into believing that the child has gotten better. The condition has worsened.)

Emergency care is the same as for any respiratory emergency. Be sure to monitor the airway and breathing constantly. Arrange for transport to the nearest hospital as quickly as possible.

CARDIAC ARREST

Most cardiac arrests in infants and children result from airway obstruction and respiratory arrest. It is therefore extremely important to assure an open airway and adequate breathing in your patients.

Signs and symptoms of circulatory failure in the pediatric patient are:

- Increased or decreased heart rate.
- Unequal central (femoral) and distal pulse rates.
- Poor skin color and delayed capillary refill.
- Altered mental status.

In cases of cardiac arrest in infants and children, provide CPR for one minute and then call for help if you are alone. Your goal is to keep your patient's brain alive. Remember that children have remarkable recuperative abilities. In cases of drowning, particularly cold-water drowning, and hypothermia, an extensive resuscitation effort may be needed. Do not stop or interrupt CPR. Arrange for transport to the nearest hospital as quickly as possible.

CPR techniques vary for adults, children, and infants. See Chapter 7 for the details of emergency care.

SEIZURES

Febrile seizures are seizures caused by high fever. They are the most common type of seizure in children. Seizures in children may be caused by infection, poisoning, trauma, decreased levels of oxygen, epilepsy, hypoglycemia, inflammation to the brain, or meningitis. They also may have unknown causes. However, all seizures, including febrile seizures, should be considered potentially life-threatening.

During most seizures, a child's:

- Arms and legs become rigid.
- Back arches.
- Muscles may twitch or jerk in spasm.
- Eyes roll up and become fixed, with dilated pupils.
- Breathing is often irregular or ineffective.
- Bladder and bowels lose control.

The child may be completely unresponsive. If the seizures lasts long enough, the child will show signs of cyanosis. The spasms will prevent the child from swallowing. He or she will push the saliva out of the mouth, which will appear to be frothing. If saliva is trapped in the throat, the child will make bubbling or gurgling sounds. This may mean the airway needs suctioning when the seizure has ended. After the seizures, the child often appears to be extremely sleepy.

To obtain a patient history, ask the parents the following questions:

- Has the child had seizures before? How often? Is this the child's normal seizure pattern? Have the seizures always been associated with fever or do they occur when the child is well? Did others in the family have seizures when they were children?
- How many seizures has the child had in the last 24 hours? What was done for them?
- Has the child had a head injury, a stiff neck, or a recent headache? Does he or she have diabetes?
- Is the child taking a seizure medication? Could the child have ingested any other medications?
- What did the seizure look like? Did it start in one part of the body and progress? Did the eyes go in different directions?

Emergency care of childhood seizures includes the following:

1. During the seizure, the tongue may relax and shift backward, decreasing the size of the air passage. To prevent this, as well as to encourage draining of mucus and frothing, place the patient in the recovery position. But do so only if there is no possibility of spine injury. Do not put anything in the patient's mouth.
2. Do not restrain the child during the seizure. Place the child where he or she cannot fall or strike something. An open space on the floor with furniture and other objects moved away is fine. If the child is on a bed that does not have sides, move the child to prevent a fall, if necessary.
3. Loosen any clothing that is tight and restricting, especially around the neck or face.
4. After the seizure, make sure that the airway is open. Be prepared to suction.
5. Administer high-concentration oxygen, if local protocol allows. Hold the mask slightly

away from the patient's face until the seizure is completely over. If breathing is diminished or absent and the airway is clear, assist ventilations with a bag-valve-mask (BVM) or pocket face mask with oxygen enrichment attachment. Follow local protocol.
6. Assess for injuries that may have occurred during the seizure.

If the seizure lasts longer than a few minutes and recurs without a recovery period, then the seizure may be status epilepticus. This condition is a true medical emergency. Notify the incoming EMS unit immediately. (See Chapter 13 for more information about seizures.)

SUDDEN INFANT DEATH SYNDROME (SIDS)

Sudden infant death syndrome (SIDS) is defined as the sudden death of infants in the first year of life. It used to be more commonly known as "crib death" or "cot death."

SIDS cannot be predicted or prevented. In fact, it is still not completely understood. It almost always occurs while the infant is sleeping. The infant is typically healthy, born prematurely, and between the ages of four weeks and seven months when he or she suddenly dies. No illness has been present, though there may have been recent cold symptoms. There is usually no indication of struggle.

Managing the SIDS Call

Unless the infant has rigor mortis (stiffness), immediately initiate basic life support, even if other signs make the effort appear futile. Begin CPR, and have someone activate the EMS system if it has not already been done.

The extreme emotional condition of the parents makes them victims as much as the baby. They will be in agony from emotional distress, remorse, and feelings of guilt. Avoid any comments that might suggest blame. Help them feel that everything possible is being done, but do not offer false hope. Follow local protocol.

When you can, obtain a brief medical history of the infant. This should not delay life-support efforts. If necessary, have other medical personnel find out the following: When was the child put in the crib? What was the last time the parents looked in on the baby? What were the circumstances concerning discovery of the infant? What was the position of the baby in the crib? What was the physical appearance of the infant and the crib? What else was in the crib? What was the appearance of the room and home? Is there medication present (even if it is for the adults)? What is the behavior of the people present? What is the general health of the infant, recent illnesses, medications, or allergies?

After ambulance personnel take over, encourage the parents to accompany their baby. Offer to stay with their other children until relatives arrive. Support the parents in any way possible.

Note that it is very common for First Responders to experience emotions such as anxiety, guilt, or anger after a SIDS call. Ignoring these feelings will not cause them to go away. They may even have serious, negative impact on your mental health. After a SIDS case, a critical incident debriefing session is very helpful. Talk out your feelings with colleagues and spouses. Do not hold them inside.

CHILD ABUSE AND NEGLECT

The definition of **abuse** is improper or excessive action so as to injure or cause harm. The term **neglect** refers to giving insufficient attention or respect to someone who has a claim to that attention and respect.

Child abuse, or non-accidental trauma, occurs in all parts of our society. The estimated number of children who are abused or neglected in the U.S. is staggering. Estimates range from 500,000 to 4 million cases annually with thousands of abused children dying. In fact, child abuse has been the only major cause of infant and child death to increase in the last 30 years. These are numbers that are cause for alarm.

During an emergency call, the adult (usually a parent) who abuses a child often behaves in an evasive manner. He or she may volunteer little information or give contradictory information about what happened. However, a call for child abuse may be a call for help. So do not be judgmental. Focus on the child.

Some forms of abuse are difficult to recognize on scene. For example, broken bones at various stages of healing can be identified only at the hospital. However, you may be able to recognize some forms of physical abuse and neglect (Figure 26–10). Signs and symptoms may include:

- Multiple bruises in various stages of healing.
- Injury that is not consistent with the mechanism of injury described by the caregivers.
- Patterns of injury that suggest abuse, such as cigarette burns, whip marks, or hand prints.
- Fresh burns such as scalding in a glove or dip pattern.
- Burns not consistent with the history presented by the caregivers.
- Untreated burns.

Also suspect possible abuse when there are repeated calls to the same address, when the caregivers seem inappropriately unconcerned or give conflicting stories, and when the child seems afraid to discuss how the injury occurred. If an infant or child presents with unresponsiveness or seizure or signs of severe internal injuries but no external signs, suspect central nervous system injuries, or shaken baby syndrome.

Signs and symptoms of neglect include the following:

- Lack of adult supervision.
- An appearance of malnourishment.
- Unsafe living conditions.
- Untreated chronic illness, such as no medication for asthma.
- Delay in reporting injuries.

If you suspect abuse or neglect, first and foremost make sure that the environment is safe for the patient. Provide all necessary emergency care. As time permits, observe the child and the caregivers. Look for objects that might have been used to hurt the child. Look for signs of neglect

CHILD ABUSE AND NEGLECT

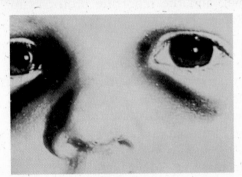

Figure 26-10a Child physical abuse.

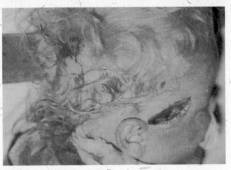

Figure 26-10b Child physical abuse.

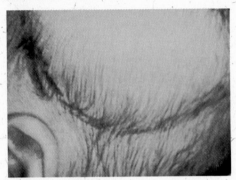

Figure 26-10c Child neglect from lack of appropriate medical care.

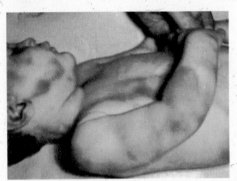

Figure 26-10d Child abuse death from multiple injuries.

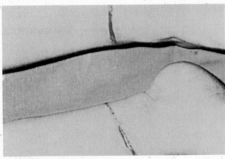

Figure 26-10e Physical abuse—restraining by tying.

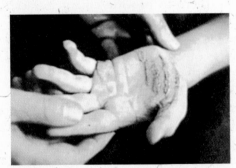

Figure 26-10f Physical abuse—burns from hand held on an electric stove.

in the general appearance of the child. Sometimes abuse and neglect are well hidden.

If you find yourself in a position of giving emergency care to a possible victim of child abuse or neglect, follow these guidelines:

- Gain entry to the home and access to the child, if it can be done safely. If the parents placed the emergency call, you will probably get in without any difficulty. If someone else called, the parents may resist. You may need to call the police.
- If you are asked to help the child, calm the parents. Tell them that if the child needs care, you will provide it. Tell them that is the only reason you are there. Speak in a low, firm voice.
- Focus attention on the child while you administer emergency care. Speak softly. Use the child's first name. Do not ask the child to recreate the situation while parents are present.
- Do a full patient assessment. Treat as you go. Note any suspicious abrasions, bruises, lacerations, and evidence of internal injury. Look also for signs of head injury. Remember that you are there to provide emergency care, not to determine child abuse.
- Update EMS in the same way you would for any other child in need of care and transport.
- You are not expected to deal with child abuse issues on the spot unless the child is in danger. In all suspected cases, the child should be transported.
- Never confront parents with a charge of child abuse. Being supportive and nonjudgmental with parents will help them be more receptive to others providing emergency care.
- Accusations can delay transport. Instead, report objective information to the transporting unit's crew. Report only what you see and what you hear. Do not comment on what you think.
- Maintain total confidentiality regarding the incident. Do not discuss it with your family or friends.

You must always report your suspicions of child abuse to the proper authorities. So, it is critical for you to learn the reporting laws in your own state and the reporting protocols for your EMS system. Find out:

- Who must report the abuse.
- What types of abuse and neglect must be reported.
- To whom the reports must be made.
- What information a First Responder must give.
- What immunity a First Responder is granted.
- Criminal penalties for failing to report.

TAKING CARE OF YOURSELF

Almost half of the children in the U.S. who die from accidents are pronounced dead either at the scene or at the hospital. The sudden and violent death of a child is emotionally wrenching, whether it occurs before you arrive or while you are giving care.

Recognize your reactions. Feelings of fear, rage, helplessness, anxiety, sorrow, and grief are common. It also is common for rescuers to feel shame and guilt, even if they did everything possible to help the child. These feelings are particularly intense if the child dies. Remember, some children will die despite your best efforts.

As a First Responder, you need to control your emotions while you are treating the child. In this way you can render the best assistance possible. After the case is over, however, you need to deal with your feelings. Talk them out. Use any critical incident stress debriefing (CISD) team that you have access to. CISD has been proven to be an excellent way to prevent or minimize long-term problems.

Not finding a way to talk through your feelings and resolve them can have a serious negative impact on your mental health. In addition to formal debriefing, it may be helpful to find a trusted friend who will listen. It is important to deal with the feelings and issues that can result from pediatric calls. Do not delay!

FIRST RESPONDER FOCUS

Some points to remember about the assessment and emergency care of pediatric patients follow. One EMS rescuer calls them "words for the wise":

- Maintaining a good airway and ensuring quality breathing are the two most important concerns for a First Responder when dealing with a pediatric emergency.
- When assisting ventilations, be sure to watch for chest rise. This is a good indicator of whether or not your breaths are effective.
- If you do not have an airway, you will not have a patient.
- With pediatric patients, all "roads" lead to the ABCs.
- Children tend to compensate longer before going into shock. Be alert! They decompensate rapidly.
- Children are prone to hypothermia. Keep them warm.
- When performing a patient assessment, take what you can when you can get it. For example, if a child holds out a hand, it is a good time to check the pulse or capillary refill.
- When the age of a child is unknown, use your best judgment based on the size of the child.
- In cases of abuse or neglect, EMS personnel may be the only advocates a child has.
- When you treat a traumatized child, you are treating a family.
- The interests of the infant or child must always be placed as the foremost consideration when making any and all patient care decisions. ■

CASE STUDY FOLLOW-UP

At the beginning of this chapter, you read that First Responders were on scene with an unresponsive six-year-old patient who had been hit by a car. To see how chapter skills apply to this emergency, read the following. It describes how the call was completed.

INITIAL ASSESSMENT (Continued)

We found the patient unresponsive with snoring respirations. My partner and I knew what we had to do in one word: airway. We got in position, applied manual stabilization, and turned her for better airway assessment and control. While my partner held her head and neck in-line, I applied a cervical immobilization device. A jaw-thrust stopped the snoring. Further examination of the mouth showed that two baby teeth had been knocked out and there was blood in the mouth. Suction took care of it. Breathing appeared to be adequate. I applied oxygen by way of a pediatric nonrebreather at 10 liters per minute.

Just then dispatch informed us that the ambulance would be on scene in about four to five minutes. We reported our general impression of the patient. "Six-year-old female was struck by vehicle. The airway is open, and she is breathing on her own. The patient is responsive to pain only." We advised the ambulance should continue to respond with red lights and sirens—priority one.

PHYSICAL EXAMINATION

We covered the patient with a blanket to maintain body heat and decided to proceed with a head-to-toe exam. Our findings included swelling with discoloration on the left forehead above the eye. Pupils were reactive but sluggish. The lower left arm was observed to be deformed and swollen. We found her respirations were 12 and shallow, which was slower than our last assessment, so we assisted ventilations.

PATIENT HISTORY

The father reported that the child was in good health and had no allergies.

ONGOING ASSESSMENT

We continued to assist ventilations until the ambulance crew arrived.

CASE STUDY FOLLOW-UP *(Continued)*

PATIENT HAND-OFF

When the paramedics got on scene, we gave them the hand-off report:

> "This is Tisa Kotto, six years old. She was hit by a car traveling approximately 15 mph about 20 minutes ago. We log-rolled her onto her back, applied a c-collar, and administered oxygen. She has an injury to the left forehead, two teeth knocked out, and a swollen deformed left arm. Her vitals are pulse 60, strong, regular; respirations 12 and shallow. We assisted ventilations. There is no medical history of allergies."

A few days later we went to the trauma center and asked about this patient. We were told that her head injury required surgery, but she was doing well and was expected to make a full recovery. One of the doctors asked what had happened and we gave him all the details. He listened intently. When we were done, he said that opening the airway and alerting the paramedics to the slowing respirations may have made the difference in the patient's outcome.

> Learn the unique aspects of providing emergency medical care to pediatric patients. One of the most important is that you are not treating the patient only. A calm, professional, reassuring approach can help to minimize the impact of the emergency on both the patient and the family.

REVIEW QUESTIONS

Page references where answers may be found or supported are provided at the end of each question.

Section 1

1. How is scene size-up for an emergency involving an infant or child different from that involving an adult? (pp. 439–440)
2. How is the initial assessment different? (pp. 440–442)
3. How is taking vital signs in an infant or child different from taking signs in an adult? (pp. 442–445)
4. What can an infant's fontanel tell you about his or her physical condition? (p. 444)
5. Why must you be more concerned about a small amount of blood loss in an infant or child than you would be about a small blood loss in an adult? (pp. 441, 444, 447)

6. What are some techniques you can use to help make the physical exam less threatening to the pediatric patient? (pp. 442–446)

Section 2

7. What are the signs and symptoms of shock in the pediatric patient? What is the emergency medical care? (p. 447)
8. What are some of the differences in the way you manage the airway of a pediatric patient? (pp. 448–449)
9. What are some of the common causes of seizures in the infant and child patient? Which ones are considered to be life-threatening? (pp. 450–451)
10. How would you manage a sudden infant death syndrome (SIDS) call? (pp. 451–452)
11. What are the signs and symptoms of possible child abuse and neglect? (pp. 452, 454)

CHAPTER 27

EMS OPERATIONS

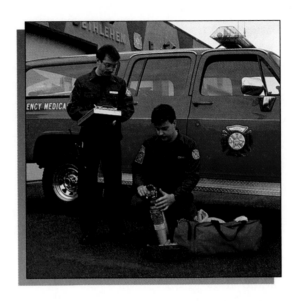

INTRODUCTION

The following chapter is meant to provide you with a brief overview of some of the operational aspects of out-of-hospital emergency care. Learn the six basic phases of an emergency response. Become familiar with the medical and non-medical equipment used on scene.

Even if you are not required to drive an emergency vehicle, become familiar with emergency vehicle safety. Since there may be a situation in which you are asked to travel in an ambulance, this chapter also provides related basic safety precautions.

Cognitive, affective, and psychomotor objectives are from the U.S. DOT's 1995 "First Responder: National Standard Curriculum." Enrichment objectives, if any, identify material that is supplemental to the DOT curriculum.

Cognitive

7-1.1 Discuss the medical and non-medical equipment needed to respond to a call. (pp. 458–459)

7-1.2 List the phases of an out-of-hospital call. (pp. 459–461)

Affective

7-1.11 Explain the rationale for having the unit prepared to respond. (p. 460)

Psychomotor

No objectives are identified.

Enrichment

* Discuss ways of driving an emergency vehicle safely, including how to use seat belts, lights, and sirens properly. (pp. 461–463)
* Describe how to stay safe in traffic on foot, including protective equipment and how to park, exit a vehicle, and channel traffic away from a scene. (pp. 463–465)
* Discuss safety tips for traveling in the passenger compartment of an ambulance, including how to brace oneself, secure a patient, secure equipment, and perform CPR. (pp. 465–467)

SECTION 1: RECOMMENDED EMS EQUIPMENT

When you are on duty, you should have EMS equipment at your disposal. This equipment will include the following items (Figure 27–1):

* Equipment for airway and breathing:
  - Adjunct airways.
  - Suction devices.
  - Pocket masks or other artificial ventilation devices.
* Equipment for bleeding control and bandaging:
  - Dressings of various types and sizes.
  - Bandages of various types and sizes.
  - Materials to stabilize impaled objects.
  - Sterile saline.
  - Scissors.
  - Adhesive tape.
* Equipment for patient assessment:
  - Stethoscope.
  - Wristwatch.
  - Pen light.
  - Sphygmomanometer (optional).
  - Prehospital care report forms.
  - Pen and notebook.

* Miscellaneous equipment:
  - OB (obstetric) kit.
  - Blankets.
  - Triage tags.
  - Chemical cold and heat packs.
  - Personal protective equipment for BSI precautions, such as disposable gloves, masks (including HEPA or N-95 respirator), eye wear, and gowns.
  - Antiseptic liquid or wipes, waterless hand-washing solution, and bags or containers for contaminated materials.

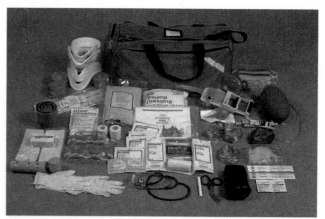

Figure 27-1 A basic First Responder jump kit.

CASE STUDY

DISPATCH
Our EMS unit was dispatched to the interstate highway for a motor vehicle collision.
That stretch of highway had the reputation for some really bad collisions.

SCENE SIZE-UP
We knew from experience that most crashes at this location were caused by lack of visi-
bility. There was a light grade that prevented drivers from seeing the road ahead. Cars
would go too fast and then couldn't stop for something in the road. This meant that one
crash usually turned into five or six.

Consider the scene as you read Chapter 27.
What can the First Responders do to keep it
safe for him- or herself, for other rescuers, and
for the patient?

- Turnout gear, heavy-duty and puncture-proof gloves, shatter-resistant eye protection, and other clothing—such as water-proof and reflective clothing—that will protect you from environmental hazards.
- Flares, cones, or reflective triangles for protection against traffic.
- Fire extinguisher.
- Flashlight and spare batteries.
- Local street maps.
- Latest edition of DOT's *North American Emergency Response Guidebook* for hazardous materials situations.
- Personal flotation device.
- Optional equipment—depending on the skills taught in your area, you may be trained to use some or all of the following:
  - Oxygen administration equipment.
  - Splints.
  - Backboards.
  - Automated external defibrillator (AED).
  - Body armor.

Even when a First Responder is off duty, he or she may come upon the scene of an injury or illness. That is why so many First Responders carry their own personal protective equipment in their vehicles and in their homes. Be sure you carry only equipment you are authorized to use.

Always use extra caution when off duty. You may not have radio contact or all the protective clothing you are used to having. You also may not be wearing clothing that identifies you as an EMS responder. Take extra time to explain to the patient who you are and that you are trained to help.

SECTION 2: PHASES OF A RESPONSE

There are six general phases of an EMS response. They are preparation, dispatch, en route to the scene, arrival on scene, transfer of care, and post-run activities.

PREPARATION

It is in the preparation phase of an EMS response that you report for duty and remain available for calls. Obviously, this phase is not the most exciting part of your job, but it may be the most important. That is because it also is the time when you must check and ready your equipment for service (Figure 27–2). Supplies should be checked each day. They also should be restocked, cleaned, or maintained after each run.

If you drive an EMS vehicle while on duty, inspect it daily. Your employer or volunteer organization should have a clear protocol for performing regular service and maintenance, reporting vehicle problems, and taking vehicles out of service when they are unsafe. Legally, you may be liable for damage caused by a malfunctioning vehicle if you were aware of the problem. So you also may be within your rights to refuse to use a vehicle you have reason to believe is unsafe.

DISPATCH

Dispatch is the formal beginning of an EMS response. Dispatchers get important information from callers who report an emergency. That information includes:

- Nature of the call.
- Name, exact location, and call-back number of the caller.
- Location of the patient.

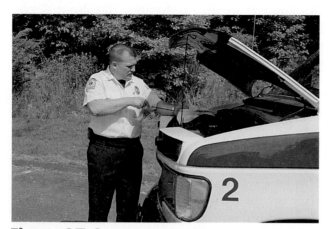

Figure 27-2 Check and ready your equipment.

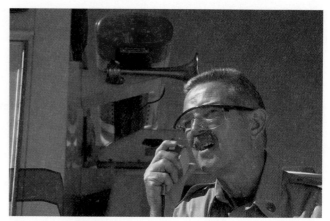

Figure 27-3 Dispatch is the formal beginning of an EMS response.

- Number of patients and the severity of the patient's problem.
- Any other special problems or considerations that may be pertinent.

As a First Responder, you may sometimes be the one who activates EMS by calling dispatch (Figure 27–3). Other times, a witness to the emergency will dial 9-1-1. He or she will provide the information to the dispatcher, who will in turn give it to you. Write the information down so you can refer to it en route. Use it to prepare yourself physically and mentally for the call. Do not hesitate to ask the dispatcher to repeat or restate information if anything is unclear.

Note that while you are en route to the scene, an emergency medical dispatcher may give specific, life-saving instructions to the caller to perform until you arrive.

EN ROUTE TO THE SCENE

Traveling to the scene involves much more than speed. Responses also must be safe. Excess speed or carelessness will result in a crash, which at least will prevent you from helping the people who need it.

When responding, be sure to know the exact location of the emergency. Have a route planned for your response. Wear your seat belts at all times in moving vehicles. Notify the dispatcher when you have begun your response, so that other emergency teams will be aware you are responding and so that the time may be logged.

ARRIVAL ON SCENE

Notify dispatch when you arrive on scene. Then approach cautiously. If you have driven to the scene, park your vehicle in a safe place. Then complete your scene size-up in a rapid, organized, and efficient manner. Once you have determined the scene safe to enter, proceed with your patient assessment plan.

TRANSFER OF CARE

By the time the responding EMTs arrive on scene you may already be performing an ongoing assessment and beginning to package your patient. (The term **package** refers to getting the patient ready to be moved and includes procedures such as stabilizing impaled objects and immobilizing injured limbs.)

Be prepared to give a concise and accurate patient hand-off report (Figure 27–4). Also be ready to assist the EMTs with packaging or lifting and moving, if they request your help.

POST-RUN ACTIVITIES

Report to dispatch when you return to your station. Then, after you turn in your prehospital care report, prepare for your next call. This means cleaning and disinfecting any equipment that may have become soiled as per your local protocols.

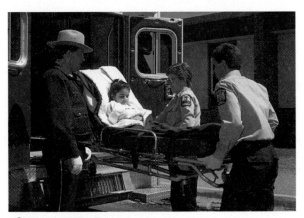

Figure 27-4 After hand-off, be prepared to assist the EMTs if you are asked to do so.

Replace any disposable supplies. Change any soiled clothing. Fuel your vehicle, if necessary. Then notify dispatch that you are in service and ready for another call.

SECTION 3: EMERGENCY VEHICLE SAFETY

Many rescuers spend a lot of time in traffic, both by driving and by moving around on foot at emergency scenes. If you have not had a basic safety course, check into the possibility of enrolling in one. It is a good idea to take advantage of refresher courses, too.

DRIVING SAFELY

Basic Safety Tips

Statistics show that haste is unnecessary in about 95% of all emergency runs. The experts maintain that only about 3% to 5% of all runs are true life-or-death situations. Yet, according to national data, approximately one in every ten ambulances is involved in an collision every year. Unless the situation is critical, travel at the posted speed limit. Excess speed makes an emergency vehicle less stable and poses a greater risk to you and others.

Much of driver safety depends on common sense and good judgment. The following basic tips can improve driver safety:

- Learn all local and state guidelines related to driving emergency vehicles before you drive one. By law you must always exercise due regard for the safety of others, and that includes yourself.
- When you can, travel in pairs. For example, the rescuer who is not driving can help the driver find the route, clear right-hand intersections, watch the road, and in case of litigation, act as a witness who can substantiate the record.
- If you need to back up your vehicle, do so slowly and carefully. Use all available mirrors. Have your partner take a position near the rear of the vehicle and act as a spotter (Figure 27–5).

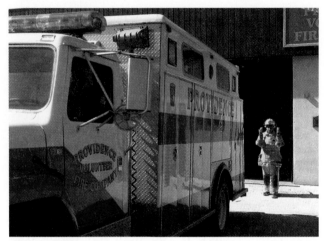

Figure 27-5 Travel in pairs. The rescuer who is not driving can help make sure patient and vehicle arrive safely.

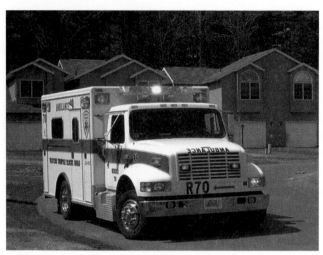

Figure 27-6 Use extra caution when on curves and hills.

- Know your territory. Take alternate routes whenever possible to avoid potential problems such as tunnels, bridges, and railroad crossings. Besides the obvious advantage of arriving on scene more quickly, when you know your territory you also can avoid collisions caused by trying to read a map while you drive.
- Exercise extra caution when traveling in congested traffic, such as rush-hour traffic in urban areas or areas just around industrial centers at shift change.
- Sudden braking is especially dangerous at high speeds. Remember that stopping time increases dramatically as speed increases. Plan for it.
- If the nature of the emergency requires you to drive at increased speeds, practice special caution on curves and hills. Brake to a safe and comfortable speed before you enter a curve. Then stay on the outside of the curve (Figure 27–6). Speed up carefully, gradually, and steadily as you leave the curve. When traveling down hills, use a lower gear instead of the brakes to maintain control of the vehicle.

Seat Belts

When in an emergency vehicle, always wear proper safety restraints, including lap and shoulder belts. Fasten them before you start the ignition. Keep them on until you have turned off the ignition. Even though seat belts are the law in

many states, a three-year study of ambulance collisions in one state showed a shocking rate of noncompliance. As many as 50% of those driving an ambulance failed to wear their seat belts.

Never take off safety restraints as you approach the emergency scene. Research shows that the last two intersections before arriving on scene are especially dangerous to rescue drivers, who try to save time by disengaging restraints.

Lights and Sirens

Whenever you respond to an emergency in a vehicle, use headlights and emergency lights even during the daytime. They can help to alert other drivers in case emergency lights blend in with traffic lights, the tail lights of cars traveling in opposite directions, the color of buildings, or holiday decorations. Use minimal lighting in heavy fog. Turn off headlights when you park. If you need to alert oncoming traffic while parked, leave the emergency lights on.

Always use emergency lights and sirens as required by your local protocols. Note, however, that a siren has a bizarre effect on the driver of an emergency vehicle. Some drivers are easily hypnotized by a siren and lose the ability to negotiate curves and turns. A siren also can disorient or panic drivers. (Never pull up behind another driver and blast the siren). Finally, a siren may not be effective, because often it is not heard. Insulation in newer vehicles can mask the sound of an approaching siren, as can a loud radio, conversation, pelting rain, thunder, dense shrubbery, trees, and buildings. To clear traffic quickly, use your vehicle's horn in conjunction with emergency lights and siren.

A significant safety advantage is to turn off your lights and siren as you approach the scene of an injury or illness. Lights and sirens attract crowds and can add to the chaos that already may exist. If there are hostile people on scene, you can take the first step toward calming and controlling the scene by arriving discreetly.

Remember that once you turn off your lights and siren, you are no longer driving an "authorized" emergency vehicle. You are subject to all the laws meant to govern regular traffic.

Hearing Protection

Chronic exposure to loud noises poses a danger to hearing. The trauma associated with repeated loud noise can cause permanent hearing loss. If your EMS system allows First Responders to drive or ride in emergency vehicles, take the following precautions to protect your hearing:

- Keep the windows closed while the siren is in use.
- Wear ear plugs or ear muffs to protect your ears. Be aware that these devices may prevent you from hearing other emergency vehicles as they approach. Use caution and always follow local protocol.
- If you can, move the siren speakers from the top of the cab to the front grille. This move can reduce the decibel level by about 5%.

Avoid prolonged or repeated loud noise off the job, too. Protect yourself against loud music, high-volume radios and televisions, loud chain saws, lawn mowers, hydraulic tools, generators, and other noise.

Driving an Ambulance

As soon as a patient is loaded into an ambulance, the driver is responsible for at least three lives—his or her own, a partner's, and the patient's. In many cases there may be multiple patients, family members, other helpers, or student riders. Most ambulances accommodate as many as six.

If your EMS system allows First Responders to drive ambulances, follow these guidelines to help assure a safe trip:

- Except in the most critical situations, do not exceed the posted speed limit. Excess speed is unsafe for everyone in the ambulance, especially for the patient. Speed poses special hazards at intersections and on curves.
- Start and stop smoothly. Make the transition from one speed to another gradually to avoid aggravating the patient's illness or injury.
- Drive at a steady but safe speed. If you keep your speed even, you often can time your approach to intersections and travel through with the green light. Also avoid weaving through traffic. It can compromise the patient.
- Whenever you can, avoid rough dirt roads, potholes, and other hazards that can jostle the patient. The inner two lanes of a four-lane highway are the smoothest. The lane closest to the gutter on city streets is the roughest. If you see that you are going to drive over a bump, railroad tracks or a stretch of rough road, warn those in the back so they can protect themselves.

As part of a driver training program, many drivers are required to lie on the stretcher while the instructor drives the ambulance. Even at low to moderate speeds, the experience from the point of view of the patient is often enlightening. (Do not use the lights or sirens or drive at increased speeds for training purposes unless you are at an approved training facility.)

STAYING SAFE IN TRAFFIC ON FOOT

As soon as you get out of your vehicle on scene, you are at risk from oncoming traffic. Even while your focus is on the patient, or the scene itself, you must never compromise your own safety.

Park for Maximum Safety

Turn off your headlights as soon as you park to prevent blinding oncoming drivers. If necessary, leave parking lights on or leave ambulance warning lights flashing to warn oncoming traffic.

Whenever you can, park on the shoulder of the road or in a driveway, in front of or behind the crash scene. Never park alongside a crash. If you are on a one- or two-lane road with no accessible parking areas, position your vehicle so that it blocks the entire roadway. This should prevent other vehicles from squeezing by. When the police are at the scene, follow their directions for vehicle placement.

An important part of ensuring your safety is to visually scan the scene as you approach. Notice areas of vulnerability or potential danger. Pinpoint places where you could seek concealment or protection. If you are with a partner, plan how you will approach before doing do. You may decide that your partner will go to the passenger who is still in the green car, for example, and you will go to the driver who is lying on the gravel.

Protect yourself from environmental hazards on scene by parking at a safe distance. Park at least 100 feet away from a burning vehicle and at least 2000 feet from an accident involving hazardous materials. Whenever possible, park uphill and upwind of any hazardous material or fire. Avoid parking on or driving over spilled liquids and broken glass.

Exiting a Vehicle Safely

A specific transition takes place as soon as you leave your vehicle. You move from your "sanctuary" to some else's turf, and that makes you vulnerable. Follow these tips for the greatest protection:

- Before you open the door, check the rear-view mirror to determine how much traffic is approaching from behind. If you can, wait a minute or two until traffic passes (Figure 27–7).
- Open your door slowly to alert passing motorists that you are getting out. Move carefully but quickly away from passing or oncoming traffic.
- If you have passengers in the rear compartment, have them get out through the rear doors instead of a side door, which might open into passing traffic.
- Be especially cautious about hazards at the scene, such as broken glass, twisted metal, or spilled gasoline. Immediately assess any crash involving trucks for hazardous materials.

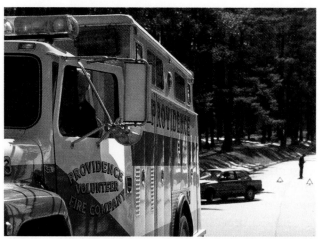

Figure 27–7 Slowly and cautiously open the door when exiting your vehicle.

- If the scene is safe to enter, walk purposefully to the patient. Running is a signal to others that you are out of control, and it causes your heart to race. The boost to your pulse and adrenaline levels can hinder your ability to effectively treat the patient.

Wear Protective Equipment

Plenty of rescues take place outdoors in the dark and in bad weather. An essential for every rescuer is reflective clothing. That includes reflective tape at least, a reflective vest, or other gear if you have access to it. If you are channeling traffic away from the crash scene while waiting for police, it is essential that you wear as much reflective gear as possible. It will help you to be visible to drivers who may have pitted windshields, frayed windshield wipers, or drug or alcohol impairment.

Depending on the situation, consider the following protective gear:

- In crashes involving hazardous materials, protect yourself with masks, gowns, and gloves as dictated by local protocol. In accidents involving grain, cement, or similar materials, wear a dust respirator.
- If there is any risk of falling debris, wear an impact-resistant protective helmet with reflective tape and a strap under the chin.

- In situations where splashing may occur (including splashing of blood and body fluids), wear safety goggles specified for work with power equipment. If you usually wear eyeglasses, get clip-on side shields.
- To protect yourself against the cold, wear gloves, a warm hat, long underwear, and several layers of medium weight clothing.
- Depending on the rescue situation, you may need rubber or waterproof boots and slip-resistant waterproof gloves.

Channeling Traffic Away from the Scene

While waiting for the arrival of law enforcement, you need to channel traffic away from the scene. This is not only for the safety of patients and bystanders, but it is also for your own safety and that of other rescuers. Your goals should be:

- To channel the regular flow of traffic around the scene, preventing additional collisions and injuries.
- To monitor traffic so that there is a minimum of disruption.
- To clear the scene so that other emergency vehicles can reach the patients quickly.

Unless there is a distinct hazard that dictates otherwise, keep traffic moving. Even if the roadway is blocked, try to reroute traffic to an alternate road rather than bring traffic to a standstill. To effectively channel traffic you need additional rescue personnel and attention-getting devices such as flares, chemical lights, or reflective cones. Follow these general guidelines:

- Make sure all those who are channeling traffic are wearing adequate reflective clothing or tape so that they can be clearly seen by approaching drivers.
- Visual signals given by rescuers must be clear. Approaching drivers need to understand quickly and exactly what you want them to do.
- Place flares, chemical lights, or reflective cones 10 to 15 feet apart and approximately 100 feet toward the oncoming traffic.

If the collision is on a two-lane highway, the flares or cones should be placed in both direc-

tions. On a curve or hill, place them at the beginning of the curve or at the crest of the hill. They should direct motorists around the crash scene, at least 50 feet from wrecked cars. Use this general rule: the flares or cones should begin far enough from the scene so that a car can safely stop before it hits the scene, even if the driver did not notice the flares or cones from a distance.

Many EMS systems recommend the use of reflective cones instead of flares because of possible burns while lighting or using flares, the need to keep lighting new flares as old ones extinguish, the difficulty of keeping flares working in bad weather, and the possibility of toxins from the smoke. Follow local protocol.

THE PATIENT COMPARTMENT

If you are part of an ambulance team, or if you assist other EMS providers, you face tremendous hazards every time you climb into the patient compartment. It is normal and necessary to move around in the compartment as you treat the patient. However, too few rescuers remember to protect their own safety. Using appropriate restraints and learning to position yourself can help to prevent injury en route to the hospital.

Whenever you do not need to move around in the patient compartment, wear proper restraints such as a safety harness.

Hanging on and Bracing

The principle of hanging on is one borrowed from rock climbers. You have four possible points of contact with the ambulance: two hands and two feet. At any one time, you must maintain at least three-point contact for optimum safety and stability. In other words, you should never have more than one hand or one foot at a time off a stable surface in the patient compartment. Do not forget your fifth point of contact—the seat of your pants. Follow these tips:

- To maintain the greatest stability, keep a wide base of support. Keep your feet at about shoulder width. Do not place your hands too close together.

- If you need to reach for something, keep both feet planted firmly on the floor. Grasp a stable object, such as the overhead bar, with your free hand.
- If you need to walk, even a single step, hold on to a stable object with both hands. Slide your hands along as you walk instead of moving arm-over-arm. If you need equipment, try putting it down and sliding it.
- Even when you are sitting, hook your feet under the stretcher bar to give yourself increased stability.

Bracing means to exert an opposing force against two parts of the ambulance with your body (Figure 27–8). It provides additional stability and protection. You can use your hands, feet, knees, or any combination of hip, shoulder, knees, and hands. You can exert yourself against any solid surface in the patient compartment, such as the squad bench or an interior wall. For greatest stability and safety, keep your center of gravity low. For women, the center of gravity is the hips, For men, it is the shoulders.

Securing the Patient

There are two reasons to firmly secure the patient in the compartment. First, you want to protect any patient from the risk of additional injury. Second, if the patient is hostile, you need to protect yourself and the patient from potential injury.

In the case of nonhostile patients, follow these guidelines:

- Secure anyone sitting on the squad bench in a seat belt.
- Place a pregnant woman in the captain's chair, since the lateral force from sudden stops is much less pronounced there than on the squad bench. Make sure she is wearing a seat belt.
- If the patient is on a stretcher, use snug but comfortable straps across the lower chest (but not over the arms) and just above the knees. Then secure the stretcher to the bar. If local protocol allows it, use additional straps. If the patient's medical condition allows, elevate the head of the stretcher slightly to ease the patient's anxiety over sudden stops.

In the case of hostile patients, follow these guidelines:

- Never apply restraints maliciously. Laws vary from one state to another about how and when restraints can be used. The use of restraints should always be a last-resort measure to protect your safety. If you do use restraints, document why you felt they were necessary in your written report.
- Once you restrain a patient, never remove the restraints, even if the patient calms down. The patient should stay restrained until you arrive at the hospital.
- Whenever possible, use soft restraints. A quick and easy one is made by folding a gauze bandage in half, slipping it over your hand, and

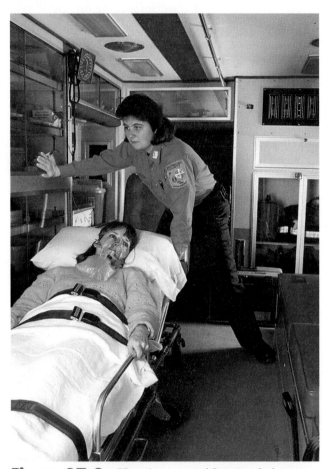

Figure 27-8 Hanging on and bracing help you to achieve optimum safety and stability inside the patient compartment.

turning it over on itself. You can then loop these over the patient's wrists and ankles. Secure the ends in a bow-tie knot far enough from the patient's hands so they cannot be untied. Combine regular strapping over the chest and knees with soft restraints at the ankles and wrists.

- If an extremely violent patient can break gauze bandages or leather straps, place him or her face-down on a stretcher. Put a scoop stretcher over the patient. Then buckle the stretcher belts securely over the scoop. Make sure to tie the patient's arms down. This method allows for natural drainage and gives EMS personnel access for intravenous lines or blood pressure cuffs. Monitor the patient's ABCs with extreme care.

Securing Equipment

If an ambulance is involved in a crash, especially a rollover, any unsecured piece of equipment could become a projectile that can injure you and the patient. As part of the cleanup at the end of each ambulance run, secure all equipment (Figure 27–9). Stow equipment in appropriate storage areas, and secure doors shut with latches. Clamp masks, oxygen equipment, and other heavy items to appropriate brackets. Use straps to secure portable gear. Devise hooks to keep bench tops closed.

Performing CPR in a Moving Ambulance

While you are performing CPR in an ambulance, you are in a risky position. You cannot maintain three-point contact. You cannot brace yourself adequately, and you cannot secure yourself in a seat belt. To improve your safety while performing CPR in a moving ambulance, follow these guidelines:

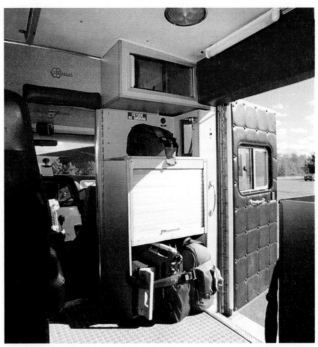

Figure 27-9 Make sure all equipment is secure before the emergency vehicle is in motion.

- Position your feet at least at shoulder width for the best possible base.
- If you can, have someone sit on the squad bench, secured by a seat belt, and grasp the back of your belt. If the ambulance suddenly changes direction or accelerates, the person hanging onto you can keep you from catapulting.
- Try for as much bracing as you can. Bend your knees into the side of the stretcher, wedge your feet against the squad bench, or brace one knee against the stretcher and the other against the squad bench.
- Do not brace yourself with your head. Your neck will not withstand the pressure.

FIRST RESPONDER FOCUS

The EMS adage "you can't help anyone if you don't get there" best describes the theme of this chapter. The time spent with a patient is perhaps the most notable and interesting part of being a First Responder. However, without a safe response, adequate protection from danger, and fully stocked and prepared equipment, there would be no patient care at all. Never ignore the basic tasks that make it possible for you to perform your job as a First Responder. ■

CASE STUDY FOLLOW-UP

At the beginning of this chapter, you read that First Responders had responded to the scene of a motor vehicle collision. To see how chapter skills apply to this emergency, read the following. It describes how the call was completed.

SCENE SIZE-UP *(Continued)*
Since we arrived before the state patrol, we set up a pattern of flares and reflectors over 1000 feet in front of the crash scene to protect ourselves. We placed the first response vehicle at the top of the grade so that it served as protection and extra warning. When we felt it to be safe, we exited our vehicle, watching our backs for traffic. Then we continued to size up the scene for other hazards, put on our gloves, and approached the crash vehicles. We saw a driver for each of the two vehicles present. There were no passengers.

INITIAL ASSESSMENT
Neither of the drivers wanted EMS, but we stuck around anyway until the EMTs arrived. Sometimes people realize they were injured once they calm down. There wasn't much damage to the cars. It was a minor sideswipe. The mechanism of injury certainly didn't seem severe.

PHYSICAL EXAMINATION
We led the drivers over to the guard rail and out of traffic. They allowed us to check their vital signs and for possible injuries. Neither had any complaints. The exams turned up nothing.

PATIENT HISTORY
The drivers refused to answer many questions.

ONGOING ASSESSMENT
We observed the drivers until the EMTs arrived on scene.

PATIENT HAND-OFF
When the ambulance arrived, we told the crew what we had—vital signs and a rough description of the incident. Neither of the patients wanted to be transported. Both patients refused all emergency care.

Bill Cerby, the first state trooper on scene, complemented us on the use of our reflectors, flares, and the positioning of our vehicle. No one had to tell us about the danger involved. We all had had too many calls to that location.

Most basic training programs for rescuers teach how to react safely to a variety of dangers. However, the most common threat to safety is likely to be something as simple as oncoming traffic or the way an emergency vehicle is driven. Be prepared. Have the knowledge, equipment, and skills that allow you to meet the standards set by your EMS system for each phase of an emergency response.

REVIEW QUESTIONS

Page references where answers may be found or supported are provided at the end of each question.

Section 1
1. What non-medical equipment should all First Responders have on hand? (pp. 458–459)
2. What medical equipment should all First Responders have on hand? (pp. 458–459)

Section 2
3. What are the six basic phases of an EMS response? (pp. 459–461)
4. When should you check, restock, clean, and maintain your supplies? (p. 460)
5. What information can you expect dispatch to give you when you are called to an emergency? (p. 460)

REVIEW QUESTIONS *(Continued)*

Section 3

6. Why is it recommended that First Responders travel in pairs? (p. 461)
7. Why should emergency lights be used during a daytime response? (pp. 462–463)
8. What are some reasons why it is a good idea to turn off your lights and siren when you approach an emergency scene? (pp. 462–463)

9. What way to exit an emergency vehicle would give you the greatest protection? (pp. 463–464)
10. What are the basic guidelines for setting up flares at the scene of a motor vehicle collision? (p. 465)
11. What are three goals of channeling traffic away from a scene? (p. 465)

CHAPTER 28

HAZARDOUS MATERIALS INCIDENTS AND EMERGENCIES

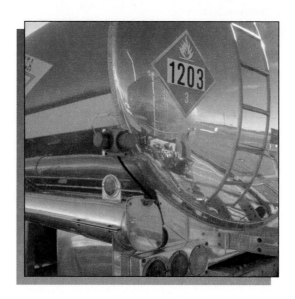

INTRODUCTION

Over 50 billion tons of hazardous materials are made in the U.S. every year. To manage the risk to the public, our government has developed specific regulations. They address nearly every aspect of the manufacturing, distribution, transportation, and use of such materials. Unfortunately, hazardous materials still may be spilled or released as a result of equipment failure, vehicle collisions, environmental conditions, and human error. The result can be the loss of life and property.

This chapter provides a brief overview of hazardous materials emergencies. As a First Responder, you are not required to deal with these materials. That takes specialized training and equipment. Instead, it is your job to recognize and report that a hazardous materials emergency exists.

Cognitive

7-1.6 Describe what the First Responder should do if there is reason to believe that there is a hazard at the scene. (p. 475)

7-1.7 State the role the First Responder should perform until appropriately trained personnel arrive at the scene of a hazardous materials situation. (p. 470)

Affective

No objectives are identified.

Psychomotor

No objectives are identified.

Enrichment

* Explain what hazardous materials are. (p. 471)
* Identify the training required to respond to a hazardous materials emergency. (pp. 474–475)
* Discuss how to recognize the presence of a hazardous material at the scene of an emergency. (pp. 471–472, 475–476)
* Describe the actions that need to be taken at the scene of a hazardous materials emergency. (pp. 474–478)
* Identify the resources that may be called upon once a hazardous materials incident is recognized. (pp. 472, 474)

SECTION 1: IDENTIFYING HAZARDOUS MATERIALS

WHAT IS A HAZARDOUS MATERIAL?

Hazardous materials are those that in any quantity pose a threat or unreasonable risk to life, health, or property if not properly controlled. Hazmats include chemicals, wastes, and other dangerous products. The principal dangers they present are toxicity, flammability, and reactivity. Those commonly shipped in the U.S. are:

* Explosives.
* Compressed and poisonous gases.
* Flammable solids and liquids.
* Oxidizers.
* Corrosives.
* Radioactive materials.

Hazardous materials are often transported to the user. While some travel by fixed pipeline (natural gas, for example), most go by rail or highway. That means hazardous materials, or **hazmats,** can be the cause of an emergency anywhere.

For example, is there a farm, business, or industry in your community that might have something hazardous on the premises? Do you have a hospital in your area? Do they practice nuclear medicine? Do you have a photo shop in town? What chemicals do they use to develop a photo? What about a lawn and garden company? Do they stock fertilizers, insecticides, or pesticides? Do your grocery stores refrigerate their produce with freezers cooled by ammonia?

PLACARDS AND SHIPPING PAPERS

U.S. Department of Transportation (DOT) requires packages and containers to be marked with specific hazard labels. Placards are required on the outside of vehicles carrying hazardous materials. The driver of the vehicle also must have shipping papers, which identify the exact substance, quantity, origin, and destination. (See Figures 28–1 and 28–2.)

A placard is usually a four-sided, diamond-shaped sign. Many are red or orange. A few are white or green. Whatever the color, the placard contains a four-digit number and a legend. They

CASE STUDY

DISPATCH

I was working security, patrolling the lower level of the mall when I received a radio call: "Team A, respond to the lower entrance near the restaurant. Investigate a report of fumes and people with trouble breathing. Time out 22:03."

SCENE SIZE-UP

As I approached the scene, I slowed my pace. Ahead I could see dozens of people streaming out of the restaurant. Many were bent over, trying to catch their breaths. Mike, the manager of the restaurant, ran over to me. He told me that the cleaning people were working in the kitchen. One of them mixed bleach, ammonia, and the "green stuff" together, which caused the problem.

> Consider this situation as you read Chapter 28. What may be done to ensure scene safety? Are all those people injured? How can they be treated appropriately?

identify the material as flammable, radioactive, explosive, or poisonous.

Shipping papers are sometimes called "manifests" or "waybills." They are another important means of identifying hazmats. If you can locate them, shipping papers have the name of the substance, the danger it presents, and a four-digit identification number. NOTE: Never endanger yourself or have others endanger themselves to retrieve shipping papers. The risk does *not* outweigh the benefit.

The National Fire Protection Association (NFPA) uses the NFPA 704 system (Figure 28–3). This system is generally used on fixed structures such as buildings. Its diamond-shaped symbol identifies danger with the use of color and numbers. The color blue indicates a health hazard. Red indicates a fire hazard. Yellow shows a reactivity hazard. Numbers used are 0 to 4. White is used for information such as the need for protective equipment. For example, 1 in a blue diamond and 4 in a red diamond mean the material presents a low health hazard but is very flammable.

AVAILABLE RESOURCES

A special resource is the *North American Emergency Response Guidebook*. (See Figure 28–4, p. 475.) It is available from the Government Printing Office. Carry it in your vehicle at all times. It includes a table of commonly used DOT labels and placards. That table is correlated with lists of chemicals. Each item in the lists is keyed to specific emergency action instructions.

Material safety data sheets (MSDS) offer another resource. Under federal regulations, all employees working with hazardous materials have a right to know about the dangers of those materials. So, all manufacturers are required to provide MSDS on hazardous materials. These sheets generally name the substance, physical properties, and fire, explosion, and health hazards. Emergency first aid also is usually listed.

The Chemical Transportation Emergency Center (CHEMTREC) is a toll-free 24-hour emergency phone service provided by chemical manufacturers. They advise rescuers on the nature of a product and

Hazardous Materials Warning Labels

DOMESTIC LABELING

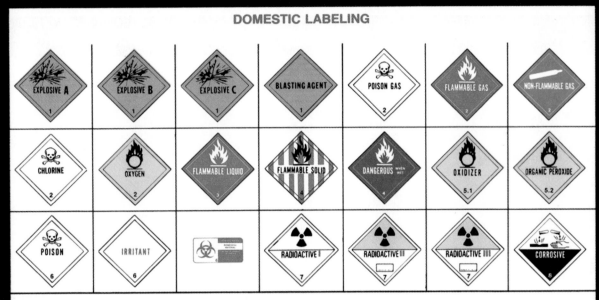

General Guidelines on Use of Labels
(CFR, Title 49, Transportation, Parts 100-177)

- Labels illustrated above are normally for *domestic shipments*. However, some air carriers *may* require the use of International Civil Aviation Organization (ICAO) labels.
- Domestic Warning Labels *may* display UN Class Number, Division Number (and Compatibility Group for Explosives only) [Sec. 172.407(g)].
- Any person who offers a hazardous material for transportation MUST label the package, if required [Sec. 172.400(a)].
- The Hazardous Materials Tables, Sec. 172.101 and 172.102, identify the proper label(s) for the hazardous materials listed.

- Label(s), when required, must be printed on or affixed to the surface of the package near the proper shipping name [Sec. 172.406(a)].
- When two or more different labels are required, display them next to each other [Sec. 172.406(c)].
- Labels may be affixed to packages (even when not required by regulations) provided each label represents a hazard of the material in the package [Sec. 172.401].

**Check the Appropriate Regulations
Domestic or International Shipment**

Additional Markings and Labels

HANDLING LABELS

Cargo Aircraft Only
172.402(b)

ORM-E
172.316

Package Orientation Markings
172.312(a)(c)

Bung Label
172.402(e)

INNER PACKAGES COMPLY WITH PRESCRIBED SPECIFICATIONS
173.25(a)(4)

Fumigation
173.9

EMPTY
173.427

Here are a few additional markings and labels pertaining to the transport of hazardous materials. The section number shown with each item refers to the appropriate section in the HMR. The Hazardous Materials Tables, Section 172.101 and 172.102, identify the proper shipping name, hazard class, identification number, required label(s) and packaging sections.

Poisonous Materials

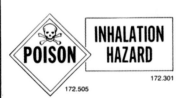
172.505

INHALATION HAZARD
172.301

Materials which meet the inhalation toxicity criteria specified in Section 173.3a(b)(2), have additional "communication standards" prescribed by the HMR. First, the words "Poison-Inhalation Hazard" must be entered on the shipping paper, as required by Section 172.203(k)(4), for any primary capacity units with a capacity greater than one liter. Second, packages of 110 gallons or less capacity must be marked "Inhalation Hazard" in accordance with Section 172.301(a). Lastly, transport vehicles, freight containers and portable tanks subject to the shipping paper requirements contained in Section 172.203(k)(4) must be placarded with POISON placards in addition to the placards required by Section 172.504. For additional information and exceptions to these communication requirements, see the referenced sections in the HMR.

Keep a copy of the DOT Emergency Response Guidebook handy!

Figure 28-1 DOT requires packages and storage containers to be marked with specific hazard labels.

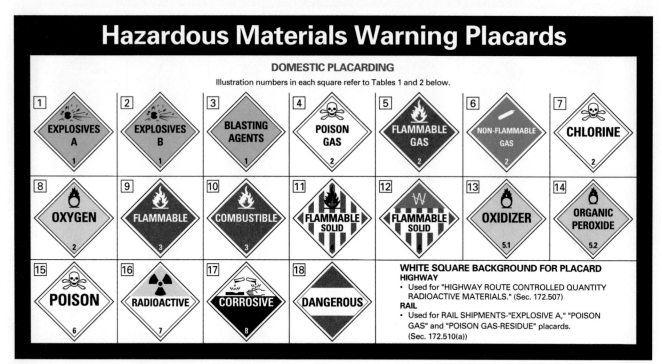

Figure 28-2 DOT also requires display placards to be put on the outside of vehicles carrying hazardous materials.

the steps that need to be taken to manage an incident. They also may contact the shipper who will provide detailed information and field assistance. The CHEMTREC number is 1-800-424-9300.

Another important resource is the regional poison control center and your own system's medical control. They can guide you in decontamination and treatment.

TRAINING REQUIRED BY LAW

People can get hurt or lose their lives at hazmat emergencies. So, the Occupational Safety and Health Administration (OSHA) and the Environmental Protection Agency (EPA) have developed safety regulations. See the OSHA publication "29 CFR 1910-120—Hazardous Waste

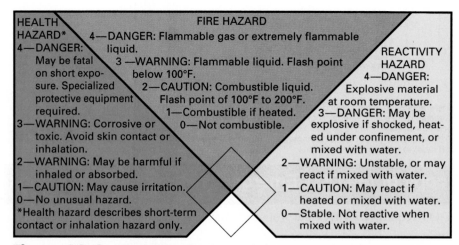

Figure 28-3 The NFPA 704 System helps you to identify healthy, reactivity, and fire hazards.

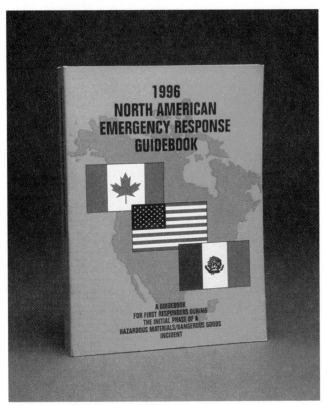

Figure 28-4 North American Emergency Response Guidebook.

Operations and Emergency Response Standards (1989)."

Four levels of training are identified:

- *First Responder Awareness.* This level of training is for those who are likely to witness or discover a hazardous materials emergency. They learn how to recognize a problem and how to call for the proper resources. No minimum training hours are required.
- *First Responder Operations.* This level of training is for those who initially respond to a hazmat emergency in order to protect people, property, and the environment. They learn how to keep at a safe distance and how to stop the emergency from spreading. A minimum of 8 hours of training is required.
- *Hazardous Materials Technician.* This level is for rescuers who actually plug, patch, or stop the release of a hazardous material. A minimum of 24 hours of training is required.
- *Hazardous Materials Specialist.* This level is for rescuers who want advanced knowledge and

skills. They learn to provide command and support activities at the site of a hazardous materials emergency. A minimum of 24 hours of additional training is required.

Note that the National Fire Protection Association (NFPA) has published Standard #473, which deals with competencies for EMS personnel at hazmat emergencies.

SECTION 2: GUIDELINES FOR A HAZARDOUS MATERIALS RESPONSE

Many hazmat incidents are dispatched as traffic accidents, poisonings, or unknown problem calls. Your initial actions build the crucial groundwork for the remainder of the incident. Your specific responsibilities include:

- Identifying the emergency as a hazmat incident.
- Identifying the hazardous materials.
- Establishing command and control zones.
- Establishing a medical treatment sector.

As always, your first priority is your own safety. *Never attempt a hazardous materials rescue unless you are properly trained and equipped.* If you have no training, radio immediately for help. While you are waiting, protect yourself and bystanders by keeping away from the danger. Avoid contact with any unidentified material, regardless of the level of protection offered by your clothing and equipment.

IDENTIFYING THE HAZMAT INCIDENT

Always consider the possibility of a hazmat incident. For example, if you are called to an unknown emergency, ask yourself: Is the call to the location of a previous hazmat incident? Is there an emergency plan for the location, which generally indicates that a risk exists? Use all the pre-arrival information available to you to decide on the best course of action.

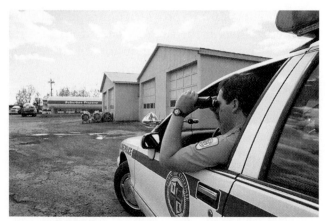

Figure 28-5 Use binoculars to identify hazmats from a distance.

As you approach the scene, use binoculars to begin to size up the scene (Figure 28–5). Identify any placards on vehicles, buildings, or containers (Figure 28–6). Proceed as always with caution. Too many First Responders discover a hazmat incident only after they are in the middle of it. Use all of your senses, coupled with a high index of suspicion. A number of visual clues can indicate a possible hazardous material:

- Smoking or self-igniting materials.
- Extraordinary fire conditions.
- Boiling or spattering of materials that have not been heated.
- Wavy or unusual vapors over a container of liquid material.
- Colored vapor clouds.
- Frost near a container leak (may indicate a liquid coolant).

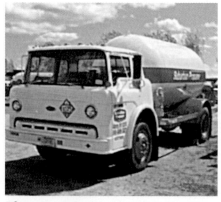

Figure 28-6 Hazmat placards displayed on a truck.

- Unusual condition of containers (peeling or discoloration of finishes, unexpected deterioration, deformity, or unexpected operation of pressure-relief valves).

Remember you may not be able to see or smell a hazardous material. Some are odorless and colorless. Others have properties that can deaden your senses. Always assume that the area surrounding a spill or leak is dangerous.

IDENTIFYING THE HAZARDOUS MATERIAL

After you identify an emergency as a hazmat incident, station yourself uphill and upwind of the scene. This vantage point should prevent the vapors from overwhelming you. Once stationed, report your position and the situation to dispatch. Your report should include:

- The nature and exact location of the incident.
- A description of the incident, including any potential for fire or explosion.
- Number of patients involved.
- Request for additional help, such as fire, police, EMS, and hazmat support.

Also suggest the best way other EMS responders can approach the scene. Include instructions for a staging area (the safe area where all responders should check in and get orders). If possible, identify the hazardous materials and the severity of the situation.

- What is the material, its properties, and dangers? Look for placards, NFPA numbers, or shipping papers. Then refer to your *Emergency Response Guidebook* for the name, properties, and dangers of the material.
- What are the sizes, shapes, kinds, and conditions of the containers?
- Is there imminent danger of the contamination spreading?

Although the hazmat team will be able to identify an unknown substance, you will be expected to make an initial identification.

ESTABLISHING COMMAND

Your agency should have a plan ready in case of a hazmat incident. Before a hazardous materials emergency ever develops, all appropriate agencies need to know how forces will be mobilized to handle it. Generally, the plan addresses the worst possible scenario. That way, the community will be able to handle any emergency that arises. The following should be included:

- One command officer responsible for all rescue decisions at every stage of the incident. All rescuers should be aware of who the command officer is. If the command officer hands over the decision-making power to someone else, all rescuers must be notified of the change.
- A clear chain of command from each rescuer to the command officer.
- An established system of communications used throughout the emergency. It should be one all rescuers are informed about, know how to use, and have access to.
- Receiving facilities. Choose facilities that are capable of handling large numbers of patients, have surgical capacity, and if possible have established decontamination procedures.

As the First Responder on scene, activate that plan and establish command. Stay in command until you are relieved by someone higher in the chain of command. The incoming incident command officer will want to know the following:

- Nature of the problem.
- Identification of the hazardous materials.
- The kind and condition of the containers.
- Existing weather conditions.
- Whether or not there is the presence of fire.
- Time elapsed since the emergency occurred.
- What has been done by people on scene.
- The number of victims.
- The danger of victimizing more people.

Once transfer of command has occurred, be prepared to care for decontaminated patients or to support rescue personnel as directed.

CREATING CONTROL ZONES

To prevent a hazmat incident from becoming worse, the danger area must be identified and iso-lated. That is usually done by designating three zones (Figure 28–7):

- *Hot zone*—This is the most dangerous area. It can be entered only with the correct personal protective equipment. Initial or gross decontamination will be performed here.
- *Warm zone*—This is the area immediately outside the hot zone. The proper protective equipment must be worn here (Figure 28–8). Once the immediate life-threats of the patient are managed, complete decontamination of the patient is performed.
- *Cold zone*—This is the outer perimeter. All contaminated clothing and equipment have been removed before entering it.

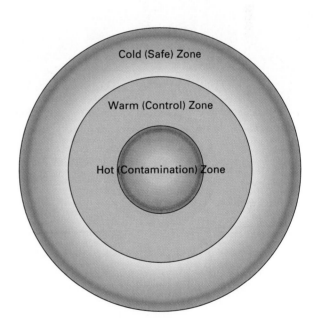

Hot (Contamination) Zone
Contamination is actually present.
Personnel must wear appropriate protective gear.
Number of rescuers limited to those absolutely necessary.
Bystanders never allowed.

Warm (Control) Zone
Area surrounding the contamination zone.
Vital to preventing spread of contamination.
Personnel must wear appropriate protective gear.
Life-saving emergency care is performed.

Cold (Safe) Zone
Normal triage, stabilization, and treatment are performed.
Rescuers must shed contaminated gear before entering the cold zone.

Figure 28-7 Establish control zones.

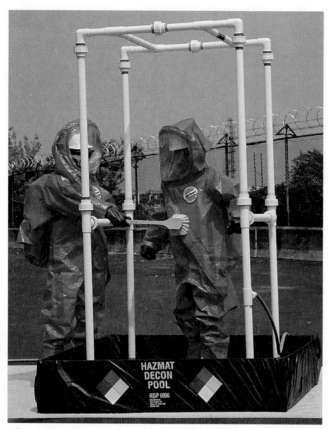

Figure 28-8 Rescuers in decontamination process.

Do not enter the warm zone unless you are trained and equipped to do so. Instead, patients should be brought to you for emergency medical treatment in the cold zone. Note that all people not necessary to the rescue should be kept away from the zoned areas.

ESTABLISHING A MEDICAL TREATMENT SECTOR

All EMS personnel and equipment must be staged in the cold zone. The establishment of a definable perimeter cannot be overstressed. In even relatively small incidents, victims may scatter and spread the contamination with them. The result can be an ever-increasing scene that quickly becomes unmanageable. Note that anyone exiting the hot zone should be considered contaminated until proven otherwise.

If the hazardous materials can be identified, follow the treatment instructions given in your *Emergency Response Guidebook* or by the regional poison control center.

FIRST RESPONDER FOCUS

Understand that hazardous materials are everywhere. They can be found in more places than in tractor trailers with signs that warn of highly corrosive materials. Remember that even household cleaners can cause as deadly a reaction as most you can find on the highway.

The first way to stay safe from hazardous materials is to realize that you will encounter them. Sooner or later, it will happen. Be prepared. ■

CASE STUDY FOLLOW-UP

At the beginning of this chapter, you read that a First Responder was on the scene of a possible hazmat emergency. To see how chapter skills apply, read the following. It describes how the call was completed.

SCENE SIZE-UP *(Continued)*
I radioed communications immediately. "Team A, we have a possible hazardous materials spill at the restaurant. Please begin the Chemical Inci-

dent Plan." Then I went on to report, "I will be incident command. Please have emergency services respond to my location at the lower entrance of the mall. Advise them that we have chemical fumes from a mixture of bleach, ammonia, and a green-soap solution." Scanning the area quickly, I added, "We have about 26 people with trouble breathing. Medical assistance is needed immediately."

CASE STUDY FOLLOW-UP *(Continued)*

At this point I realized I had a large number of people who could scatter, so I asked several other security guards to do several things.

First, we had to get all of the injured people to go down the hall until help could arrive. Someone suggested that we ask them to wait outside, but I disagreed. I thought that if we let them outside, they would go to their cars and leave. Plus, that was where emergency services were staging. What with people leaving and EMS responding, well, I was afraid things would get out of hand.

Second, I asked the other guards to set up a perimeter at least 100 yards down the hall. I was amazed at the number of people who insisted that they had to get through to go shopping or get to work. Some even thought we were conducting a drill.

We were just getting things set up when the police arrived. I quickly explained what happened and what had been done. The fire chief joined us and declared a hazardous materials incident. He requested the hazmat team. After consulting with poison control, firefighters proceeded to treat the patients with high-flow oxygen and move them to a triage point.

Several weeks after the incident I was commended by my employer for quick thinking and decisive action at the scene of an emergency.

> A hazardous materials incident challenges the best in First Responders. Besides the usual patient-care issues, there is the additional safety problem. Be sure to learn and follow all of your local protocols for such emergencies.

REVIEW QUESTIONS

Page references where answers may be found or supported are provided at the end of each question.

Section 1

1. What is a hazardous material? (p. 471)
2. To what do the terms "placards" and "shipping papers" refer? (pp. 471–472)
3. What is the NFPA 704 System? (p. 472)
4. What are some of the resources available to responders on the scene of a hazmat incident? (pp. 472, 474)
5. What are the four levels of hazmat training described by OSHA? (pp. 474–475)

Section 2

6. What is a First Resonder's first priority upon arrival at the scene of a hazmat incident? (p. 475)
7. What are some examples of visual clues that indicate a possible hazardous material? (p. 476)
8. After identifying an emergency as a hazardous materials incident, what information should your report to EMS dispatch include? (p. 476)
9. What are "control zones"? Briefly describe them. (pp. 477–478)

CHAPTER 29

MULTIPLE-CASUALTY INCIDENTS AND INCIDENT COMMAND

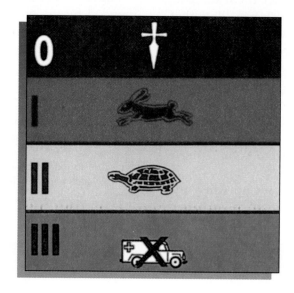

INTRODUCTION

Multiple-casualty incidents range from a car crash to hurricanes, floods, earthquakes, and bombings. This chapter will introduce you to ways in which EMS systems respond to such emergencies. It also will give you an overview of your role as a First Responder, including how you can provide the best emergency care to the greatest number of patients.

Cognitive, affective, and psychomotor objectives are from the U.S. DOT's 1995 "First Responder: National Standard Curriculum." Enrichment objectives, if any, identify material that is supplemental to the DOT curriculum.

Cognitive

7-1.8   Describe the criteria for a multiple-casualty situation. (p. 481)

7-1.9   Discuss the role of the First Responder in the multiple-casualty situation. (pp. 483–485)

7-1.10   Summarize the components of triage. (pp. 485–487)

Affective

No objectives are identified.

Psychomotor

7-1.2   Given a scenario of a mass casualty incident, perform triage. (pp. 485–487)

Enrichment

*   Describe the role of command in a multiple-casualty incident. (pp. 481–483)
*   Identify the procedure for transferring command. (pp. 484–485)
*   Identify communications as a key component of any MCI. (pp. 484–485)
*   Describe the incident command system (ICS). (p. 481)
*   Describe commonly used EMS sector functions. (pp. 481–483)
*   Discuss three-level and two-level triage systems. (pp. 485–487)
*   Identify a triage tag. (pp. 486–487)
*   Discuss ways to reduce the psychological impact of disasters on patients and rescuers. (pp. 487–489)

SECTION 1: INCIDENT COMMAND SYSTEM

One of the most challenging situations for a First Responder is a **multiple-casualty incident** or **MCI**. An MCI is any event where three or more patients are involved. Most communities have a plan in place for handling an MCI. However, for any plan to be effective, it must be flexible enough to work with a three-person car crash (the most common MCI) as well as a large-scale disaster involving 15 or more patients.

One widely used plan is the Federal Incident Command or Management System. Originating in California, it was designed to handle large-scale fires that involve multiple agencies. It now gives us a framework for all types of MCIs.

How resources are used is basic to the incident command system (ICS). Not every MCI will need every community resource. In fact, most MCIs use only limited resources. Sometimes this fact is referred to as the "toolbox approach." Think of a community's resources as a toolbox.

Instead of emptying it at every MCI, only the tools that are needed are used. That is, instead of calling for police, fire service, EMS, hazmat teams, and all other rescuers just in case they may be needed, call for only the resources that are necessary.

As a First Responder, find out what your EMS system requires you to do in those first crucial minutes of an MCI. As the first medically trained rescuer on scene, you will "set the stage" for how the incident will be handled.

EMS SECTOR FUNCTIONS

Command is established at all incidents (Figure 29–1). That person stays in command until it is transferred to someone else or until the incident comes to an end.

If an incident is large or complex, command can designate sector officers to help (Figure 29–2). When needed, the EMS sector may include the following:

CASE STUDY

DISPATCH

Last week while on duty for the fire department, I was assigned to the medical first response unit. Shortly after checking out our equipment and supplies, my partner and I were dispatched to an explosion with fire at a small factory.

SCENE SIZE-UP

Our response time was five minutes. When we reached the scene, we were told where to park our vehicle. I also was told to establish EMS command and determine the number and extent of injuries. My partner and I immediately donned our identification vests. I wore the EMS command vest. She put on the triage sector vest.

A plant security guard told me that nine people were working in the area when the explosion occurred. Eight people escaped with their lives. One was still unaccounted for. I radioed this information to the incident commander.

Emotions were running high among the patients. I knew that many patients take the lead of the rescuers. So calm was the rule.

Consider this situation as you read Chapter 29. What can be done to assure that all patients get timely and appropriate emergency medical care?

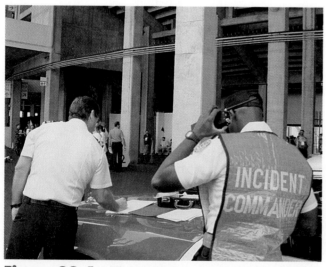

Figure 29-1 The incident commander directs the response and coordinates resources at an MCI.

- *Triage officer.* This officer supervises patient assessment, tagging, and removal of patients to a designated treatment area.
- *Treatment officer.* This officer sets up a treatment area and supervises treatment. Generally, one EMS rescuer is assigned to each patient. The treatment and transportation officers make sure the most seriously injured are transported first.
- *Transportation officer.* This officer arranges for ambulances. He or she also tracks the priority, identity, and destination of all patients leaving the scene (Figure 29–3). The transportation and staging officers make sure resources are available as needed.
- *Staging officer.* This officer releases and distributes resources when they are needed. He or she also sees that "gridlock" does not occur in the transportation area.

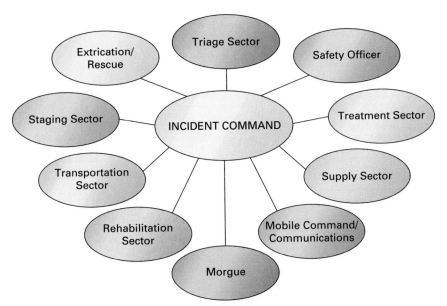

Figure 29-2   After an incident manager is identified, EMS sectors are established as needed.

- *Safety officer.* This officer maintains scene safety. He or she identifies potential dangers and takes action to prevent them from causing injury to patients and rescuers.

When there are many patients who need special rescue or extrication from wreckage, an extrication sector should be established.

In large-scale operations where a great many resources are used for long periods of time, a *logistics officer* may be needed. This officer makes certain that medical supplies, communications equipment, transportation units, food, and any other supplies are available when needed. This officer also may set up a rehabilitation sector where emergency personnel can go for evaluation and treatment as well as food and water.

When there are deceased victims, a morgue may be set up. This sector should be overseen by the police along with a medical examiner or coroner.

FIRST RESPONDER'S ROLE

The most senior First Responder arriving at an MCI is responsible for carrying out the MCI plan. Your major goals are then to:

- Establish command.
- Size up the scene.
- Request additional resources.
- Begin triage.

(See Table 29–1 for a summary of command responsibilities.) Note that once you identify an incident as an MCI, resist the urge to jump in and provide treatment. Remember that patients with loud voices have open airways. Quiet patients may not be breathing.

During your scene size-up, identify the following:

- Scene safety.
- Number of patients, including the "walking wounded."
- Needs for extrication.
- Estimated number of ambulances needed.
- Other factors affecting the scene and resources, such as weather or terrain.
- Number of sectors needed.
- Area to stage resources.

Make an initial scene report to EMS dispatch. Keep it short and to the point. Be sure to give the information necessary for other rescuers to react to the MCI appropriately. For example:

THE COMMAND TOOLBOX

MULTICASUALTY RECORDER WORKSHEET

Ambulance Company	Ambulance ID Number	Patient Triage Tag Number	Patient Status	Hospital Destination	Off-Scene Time

Figure 29-3 Sample of a tracking sheet for the transportation officer at an MCI.

TABLE 29-1

COMMAND OFFICER RESPONSIBILITIES

- Assume an effective command mode and position. Provide continuing command until relieved by a higher-ranking official.
- Transmit a brief preliminary report to EMS dispatch.
- Rapidly evaluate the situation.
- Request additional resources.
- Quickly develop a safe management strategy.
- Delegate authority.
- Review and evaluate effectiveness of sector operations through frequent progress reports from sector officers.
- Modify sector operations as required.
- As incident winds down, return units to service and secure incident when appropriate.

"Firecom, this is Engine 405. We are on the scene of a two-car collision with entrapment of three priority-one patients. Dispatch a rescue company and three paramedic ambulances. Alert the trauma center. I will now be called Central Avenue Command. Police are needed to assist with traffic and crowd control ASAP. Approach from the north. Staging is on Central between Kennedy and 67th Street."

Some MCI plans call for the command vehicle to have two traffic cones on top of it. Whatever method you use, make sure command can be identified easily. Bibs or vests should be worn by command personnel and sector officers for easy recognition.

Communication is a key component of any MCI plan. Keep calm when making radio transmissions. Use plain English and common terms. Try to keep radio traffic to a minimum. Encourage face-to-face communication.

When you are relieved by someone higher in the chain of command, report the following to him or her:

- Nature of the problem.
- Potential hazards.
- Number of patients.
- Time elapsed since the emergency occurred.
- What already has been done.

If you respond to an MCI where command is already established, report immediately to the command sector. Identify the incident commander. Introduce yourself and your level of training and ask for instructions. Be prepared to care for patients or to support rescue personnel as directed.

SECTION 2: TRIAGE AND EMERGENCY CARE

Triage is a French word meaning "pick" or "sort." It is a process of classifying sick and injured patients that was first used by the military. During the Korean and Vietnam Wars, it resulted in a big improvement in the survival rates of the injured. Today, triage is used to determine the order in which patients receive medical care and transport.

TRIAGE SYSTEMS

In triage, the most critical but salvageable patients are treated and transported first. Different areas may have their own ways of performing triage. So know what your EMS system expects of you. Follow all local protocols.

Three-Level Triage Systems

Three-level triage systems are the most common (Figure 29–4). One that has proven very successful is "START," which stands for "Simple Triage and Rapid Treatment." START categories include:

- *Priority-1 Red.* This is the highest priority given to patients.
- *Priority-2 Yellow.* This is the second priority or urgent-care category.
- *Priority-3 Green.* This is the lowest priority or delayed-care category.

For the Priority-1 Red category, patients are given a red tag if they meet three criteria. First, their injuries must be life-threatening and risk of asphyxiation or shock is imminent or present. Second, they can be stabilized without constant care. Third, they have a very good chance of survival if treated and transported immediately. (Patients with catastrophic injuries of the head or chest are not included in this category. They have little chance of recovery.) This priority goes to patients with:

- Airway problems.
- Respiratory arrest.
- Severe uncontrolled bleeding.
- Pneumothorax.
- Respiratory-tract burns.
- Major or complicated burns.
- Cervical-spine injury.
- Open abdominal wounds.
- Severe or impending shock.
- Hyperthermia or hypothermia.
- Unresponsiveness without head injury.
- Medical conditions such as diabetes and poisoning.
- Open—but not catastrophic—chest wounds and severe head injuries or head injuries accompanied by decreasing levels of responsiveness.

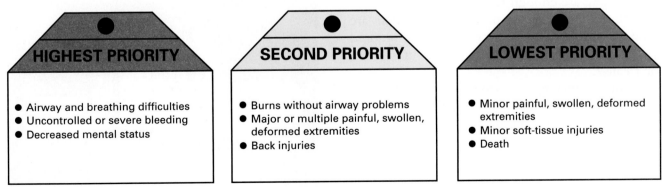

Figure 29-4 An example of a three-level triage system identified in the U.S. DOT "First Responder: National Standard Curriculum."

Priority-2 Yellow patients are treated and transported next. They include patients with:

- Seizures.
- Stable abdominal injuries.
- Emergency childbirth.
- Eye injuries.
- Uncomplicated burns.
- Major open and multiple painful, swollen, deformed extremities.

Priority-3 Green is given to the patients who are not seriously injured, need minimal care, and can wait for treatment without getting worse. Their injuries include:

- Minor painful and swollen extremities.
- Minor burns.
- Minor soft-tissue injuries such as small scrapes, cuts, and bruises that do not involve significant bleeding.

A fourth category may be included in a START system. It is Priority-0 Black. This is the no-care category. Black tags are given to individuals who are dead or who have injuries that would be fatal even if they receive treatment. Their injuries include:

- Catastrophic head or chest injuries.
- Injuries certain to cause death such as decapitation, severed trunk, and total incineration.
- Unresponsiveness and pulselessness.

Cardiac-arrest patients are treated as dead unless there are enough rescuers to care for them as well as other injured patients. If rescuers are limited in number, these patients must be ignored so that patients with better chances of survival can be treated.

Note managing a cardiac-arrest patient in triage is controversial. The decision to try to resuscitate depends on the number of patients involved and the resources available. However, when there are multiple patients of lightning strike, resuscitation efforts should be made. These patients tend to have a very good chance of survival.

Two-Level Triage Systems

A different system that can cut down on confusion uses only two categories. They are "immediate" and "delayed." Patients in the "immediate" category have life-threatening injuries but are salvageable if cared for immediately. They receive priority for treatment and transport.

Patients in the "delayed" category include all the rest of the patients on scene. That includes patients with minor injuries, patients with injuries so critical that they will die even with aggressive treatment, and patients who are dead.

Triage Tags

After patients are assessed and sorted, they must be tagged for rapid identification. Triage tags comes in a variety of sizes, shapes, and colors (Figure 29–5). Generally, use them only if more than 10 patients are involved in a single incident. Avoid tags that need a ball-point pen or carbons. Avoid tags that are too detailed. Be sure there is a method of securing the tags so that they do not come loose or drop off.

Once a patient is given a tag, do not remove it. If the patient changes status before being treated, draw a bold line through the original tag, note the time, and put a new tag on the patient. This procedure helps rescuers know that the patient has had a change in status.

One of the most popular tags is the Mettag. It uses symbols instead of words for rapid identifi-

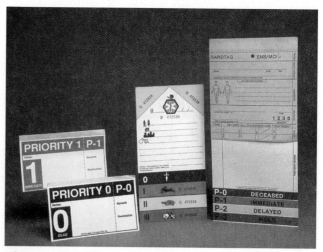

Figure 29-5 Commonly used triage tags.

cation. It also is highly visible. With perforated divisions, it contains a strip for each of the categories: red (rabbit) for the highest priority, yellow (turtle) for second priority, green (ambulance with X through it) for those not in need of transport, and black (shovel and cross) for the dead. Rescuers simply tear off the strips not needed so that the applicable strip is on the outside edge.

Conducting Triage

To perform triage at an MCI, you must assess each patient's condition, determine the urgency of the condition, and assign a priority for treatment. In general, begin triage with an initial assessment as follows:

- If the patient is alert and talking and has no major bleeding, reassure him or her and move on.
- If the patient is unresponsive and there is an airway obstruction, perform the Heimlich maneuver. If breathing is absent, perform artificial ventilation (if local protocols allow it). If there is no pulse, move on to the next patient.
- If the patient has severe bleeding, quickly apply a pressure dressing and elevation. Then move on to the next patient.

In the START system, first tell all patients who can walk to get up and walk unassisted to a specified area. Give these patients—the "walking wounded"—a Priority-3 Green (delayed care). Then turn your attention to the patients who could not walk away. Begin triage with an initial assessment as follows:

- Breathing:
  - If breathing is faster then 30 breaths per minute, give the patient a Priority-1 Red.
  - If the patient is not breathing, quickly clear foreign matter from the mouth and open the airway. If breathing resumes, give the patient a Priority-1 Red. If breathing does not resume, tag with a Priority-0 Black.
  - If breathing is less than 30 breaths per minute, perform the next assessment.
- Circulation:
  - If there is no carotid pulse, tag the patient as a Priority-0 Black.

  - If the carotid pulse is weak or irregular, give the patient a Priority-1 Red.
  - If the carotid pulse is strong, perform the next assessment.
- Mental Status:
  - If there is no response to a simple command such as "close your eyes," give the patient a Priority-1 Red.
  - If the patient can respond to a simple command, give him or her a Priority-2 Yellow.

PSYCHOLOGICAL IMPACT OF AN MCI

Psychological injuries can be severe, too. Almost all the people involved in an MCI experience fear. Many also feel shaky, perspire profusely, and become confused, irritable, anxious, suspicious, moody, restless, and fatigued. Many will have sleep problems, concentration problems, depression, nausea, vomiting, and diarrhea. Survivors often experience anger, guilt, shock, denial, and feelings of isolation and vulnerability. All of these reactions are normal.

The reactions of children depend on age, disposition, and family and community support. Generally, preschoolers cry, lose control of bowels and bladder, become confused, and suck their thumbs. Older children suffer from extreme fears about their safety. They may show confusion, depression, headache, inability to concentrate, withdrawal, poor performance, and a tendency to fight with peers. Older children and adolescents may show extreme aggression. Their stress may be severe enough to disrupt their lives.

Others at risk for severe reactions are the elderly, those in poor physical or emotional health, the handicapped, and those who have unresolved past losses or crises.

Rescuers react, too. Often they react in the same way their patients do. Common reactions are fear about personal safety, crying, anger, guilt, numbness, preoccupation with death, frustration, and fatigue. Most reactions peak within about one week and then diminish. About half have dreams of the disaster for weeks or months afterward. In some cases, rescuers suffer long-term reactions. A critical incident stress debriefing (CISD) is one of the best ways for rescuers to deal with reactions to an MCI. (See Chapter 2 for details.)

General Guidelines for Rescuers

General guidelines for any type of MCI are as follows:

- Do not let yourself become overwhelmed by the size of the emergency. Learn your local MCI plans well. Follow them. They will help you keep calm and effective.
- Families of patients deserve accurate information. As soon as possible, assign several workers to provide it to the properly authorized person only. That usually is the chief town executive, the public relations officer, or the incident commander.
- Reunite patients with their families as soon as possible. They will feel less stressed once they are together. Families also can provide medical histories that will increase your ability to care for patients. A separate area away from the scene, onlookers, and the press should be identified for this purpose.
- If the MCI involves a large number of patients, group them with their families and neighbors. This will help reduce feelings of fear and isolation.
- Identify high-risk patients. Target them for immediate crisis intervention services.
- Provide a structure. Tell patients exactly what is happening.
- Work can be therapeutic. Encourage the "walking wounded" to do necessary chores. Explain the tasks simply and clearly. Consider having the patients support each other until medical personnel are available.
- Help patients confront the reality of the disaster. Encourage them to talk about it and what they feel. If you sense that they are not facing reality or that their expectations are much worse than reality, help them adjust their views. If you engage a patient in this type of talk, make sure you have time to listen and respond.
- Do not give false assurances. If you do, patients may resist any further outside help. Honestly appraise the situation. Offer help where it is needed.

- Patients may refuse help. There are many reasons why, including how they were brought up. Explain that accepting help is not admitting weakness. Make sure they understand help is only temporary and that as soon as things are under control they can help someone else.
- Arrange for a group discussion where patients can share ideas as soon as physical needs are taken care of.
- Encourage all those involved—including rescuers—to get good follow-up care and support.

Also consider using the help of the American Red Cross or a similar organization. They may be able to assist with psychological counseling and other support services to patients and families. Such organizations should be identified in the disaster plan and alerted as soon as possible in a large-scale MCI.

Reducing Stress in Rescuers

Once the rescue operation is underway, a new danger arises. Rescuers may begin to suffer from stress. If measures are not taken immediately, rescue workers can become inefficient and, at worst, become victims themselves. To help reduce stress, the following guidelines may be useful:

- Make sure rescuer workers are fully aware of their exact assignments. Well defined limits help to reduce stress.
- Assign rescue workers to tasks according to their skills and experience. If there are any questions, do not gamble. Give workers the tasks you are certain they can do.
- Tell rescuers to rest at regular intervals away from the hub of the disaster. They should sit or lie down, have something to eat or drink, and relax as much as possible. Have counseling available for those who need "defusing." If rest periods are effectively rotated, there will be enough workers to carry on disaster assistance.
- Have several workers circulate among rescuers to watch for signs of physical exhaustion and stress. If one worker appears to be having problems, he or she should rest for a longer period than usual. After rest, give him or her a less stressful task. If appropriate, trained psy-

chological support personnel can evaluate workers if a high level of stress is suspected.

- Provide plenty of nourishing drinks and food. Encourage rescue workers to eat and drink to keep up their strength. Avoid foods high in fat, sugar, and caffeine.
- Encourage rescue workers to talk among themselves. Talking helps to relieve stress. Discour-age lighthearted conversation and joking. Some patients and workers may be offended, which can increase stress on scene.
- Make sure that rescuers have a chance to talk with trained counselors after the incident. If your team has access to critical incident stress debriefing (CISD), make sure all rescuers who worked the scene take advantage of it.

FIRST RESPONDER FOCUS

▼

Most people consider multiple casualty incidents to be the plane crashes and commuter train wrecks. While these certainly qualify, the most common MCIs are the two cars that collide, each with three injured passengers. Most EMS systems would have to stretch resources to take care of these six patients. Learn what your EMS system expects of you.

In the first few minutes of an MCI, the most important task that the first trained person on the scene can perform is to *plan,* not rush in. ■

CASE STUDY FOLLOW-UP

At the beginning of this chapter, you read that First Responders were on the scene of an MCI. To see how chapter skills apply to this emergency, read the following. It describes how the call was completed.

INITIAL ASSESSMENT AND TRIAGE

Jan, my partner, started triage. When another First Responder arrived, I assigned him to establish a transport sector and gave him a staging vest. I reminded him to make sure that he identified a safe area where ambulances could enter and exit quickly and safely.

Jan soon reported that two patients were Priority 1, three were Priority 2, and three were Priority 3. I updated the incident commander and requested seven ambulances, three of which were to be equipped for advanced life support (ALS). I also requested that he alert the trauma center.

A minute or so later it was confirmed that one patient was still inside the plant. We believed that patient to be a Priority 0. At that moment, the para-medic EMS supervisor arrived. I provided a full report and turned over EMS command to him. I was then assigned to assist in the treatment area.

Over the next half hour all eight patients were transported to a hospital. A police officer was assigned to guard the one dead body until the coroner arrived. Triage and transport for the injured patients had taken 45 minutes.

When EMS command was terminated, the incident commander told us that a critical incident stress debriefing would be organized for all rescue personnel involved.

For you to be an effective member of EMS response to an MCI, you must learn your local plans and protocols. Review them often. Practice them whenever you are given the opportunity.

REVIEW QUESTIONS

Page references where answers may be found or supported are provided at the end of each question.

Section 1

1. What is a multiple-casualty incident? (p. 481)
2. What is the Incident Command System (ICS)? (p. 481)
3. What are some common EMS sector functions? (pp. 481–483)

4. What are the first critical steps that must be completed at an MCI? (p. 483)

Section 2

5. What information must you report to EMS dispatch after your scene size-up? (pp. 483–484)
6. What are the possible categories in two-level and three-level triage systems? (pp. 485–487)

CHAPTER 30

WATER EMERGENCIES

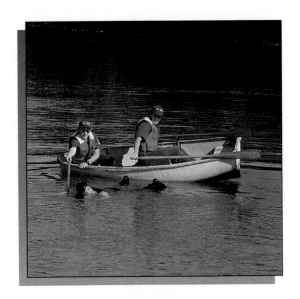

INTRODUCTION

Water is everywhere. Oceans, lakes, and streams are only the most obvious sites of possible water emergencies. Drownings also occur in home pools, which are numerous. Many industries have vats or pools large enough to drown several men. Even bathtubs and toilets present a danger to small children.

This chapter offers an overview to water rescue. It introduces you to the challenge of providing emergency care in water and to some of the common hazards of water rescue.

OBJECTIVES

Cognitive, affective, and psychomotor objectives are from the U.S. DOT's 1995 "First Responder: National Standard Curriculum." Enrichment objectives, if any, identify material that is supplemental to the DOT curriculum.

Cognitive

No objectives are identified.

Affective

No objectives are identified.

Psychomotor

No objectives are identified.

Enrichment

* Understand how drowning and near-drownings occur. (pp. 493–494)
* Describe key components of scene size-up in a water emergency. (pp. 494–495)
* Discuss some of the difficulties of assessing a patient who is in the water. (pp. 495–496)
* Describe emergency care of a near-drowning patient with no injuries to the spine. (p. 496)
* Describe emergency care of a near-drowning patient with suspected spinal injuries. (pp. 496–497)
* List the hazards commonly associated with fast-moving water. (pp. 500–502)
* Discuss the differences between warm-water and cold-water rescues. (p. 502)
* Describe the assessment and emergency medical care of a patient with a diving emergency, including air embolism and decompression sickness. (pp. 503–504)

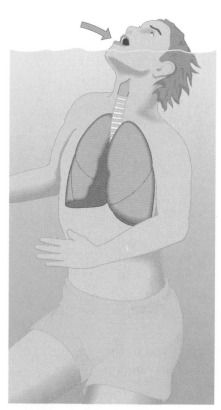

Drowning can be the result of cold, fatigue, injury, disorientation, intoxication, or limited swimming abilities.

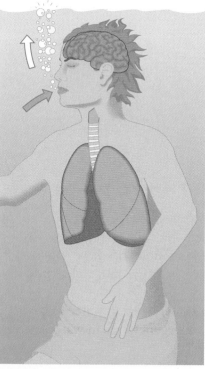

The drowning victim struggles to inhale air as long as possible. Eventually the victim inhales water or a muscle spasm of the larynx closes the airway.

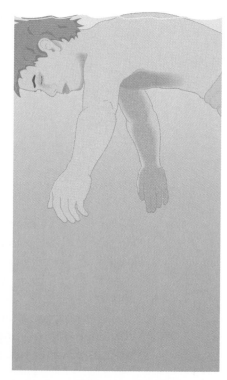

Loss of consciousness, convulsions, cardiac arrest, and death may follow.

Figure 30-1   Drowning.

CASE STUDY

DISPATCH

I spend my summers working as a life guard at the town pool. I was on scene when a water emergency occurred.

SCENE SIZE-UP

The pool was crowded that day. It was blindingly bright and very hot. I was on the stand watching some youngsters use the low diving board, when I heard people start to yell. I looked towards the middle of the pool and saw a young male floating face down on the far side. I knew him. It was Jimmy. I jumped in and swam over to him. Everyone was yelling. One bystander shouted that he had a seizure.

I thought quickly. I didn't see him dive. I didn't know if he'd been in a fight. All I knew was that he appeared to be unresponsive. I decided I better not move him from the water.

> Consider this patient as you read Chapter 30. What should be done to assess and treat his condition?

SECTION 1: DROWNING AND NEAR-DROWNING

Drowning is defined as death from suffocation due to submersion. It is the third leading cause of accidental death in the United States. After auto collisions, drowning is the most common cause of preventable death among children.

WHAT HAPPENS IN DROWNING?

Drowning can be the result of cold, fatigue, injury, disorientation, intoxication, or limited swimming ability. (See Figure 30–1.) However, survival from a near-drowning can depend on many factors, including whether or not the water is fresh or salty, warm or cold, clear or murky, still or moving.

Fresh Water vs. Saltwater

In fresh-water drowning, water passes through the patient's lungs into the bloodstream. There it can cause hemodilution (thinning of the blood by excess water) and destruction of red blood cells. More commonly, simple asphyxia (suffocation) is the cause of death.

In saltwater drownings, aspirated water is saltier than body fluids. So water leaves the blood and enters the lungs to help dilute the salt. The air in the lungs mixes with the fluids and forms a frothy foam, which acts as a barrier to oxygen exchange. The result can be death.

"Wet" and "Dry" Drownings

"Wet" drowning occurs when fluid is aspirated into the lungs. "Dry" drowning occurs when a severe muscle spasm of the larynx closes it, preventing aspiration and respiration. About 10% to 40% of all drownings are estimated to be "dry." Autopsies reveal that only about 15% aspirate a significant amount of water.

Warm- vs. Cold-Water Drownings

There is a significant difference between warm- and cold-water drownings. Unlike warm-water ones, drownings that occur in cold water (below 68°F) have resulted in successful resuscitations, even up to an hour after submersion. Hypothermia and the "diving reflex" have something to do with this. Both slow down the body's metabolism and reduce the need for oxygen.

Muscles do not function properly when cold, so it becomes difficult for the patient to keep himself afloat. The hypothermic patient also may be unable to follow directions or assist with the rescue. Note that cold water temperatures affect rescuers, too.

SECTION 2: WATER RESCUE

GENERAL GUIDELINES FOR EMERGENCY CARE

Scene Size-up

In a water-related emergency, you obviously need to reach the patient. However, you must do so with the utmost concern for your own safety. Remember that water can conceal many hazards. Holes, sharp drop-offs, and underwater entanglements such as fallen trees or wire fences may not be visible from shore. The force of moving water also can be very deceptive. Do not walk in fast-moving water over knee depth. It is not safe. Moving water in streams, rivers, even storm drains can push you over and hold you down.

Hazardous materials are also a concern in water emergencies. For example, a car in the water could leak oil or gas, which float on the sur-face. Such hazards pose a respiratory risk for both patients and rescuers. Floods can cause sewage to be released in normally safe waters. Risk of electrocution exists in flooded buildings or grounds. Severe bleeding of the patient also can pose the risk of infection to other patients and rescuers.

When determining how to respond to a water emergency, take into account the patient's condition, water conditions, and the resources on hand.

- *Patient condition.*
  - Is the patient responsive and able to assist in the rescue? If so, reaching out with a pole or throwing a rope may be the safest method of rescue.
  - Does the patient have any obvious injuries? If the patient is unstable, you may have to extricate him or her from the water before beginning care.
  - Is the patient on the surface or is he or she submerged? The submerged patient may need basic life support immediately. He or she also may be difficult to locate.
- *Water condition.*
  - *Visibility*—Can you see any potential hazards under the water? Can you see the patient and his or her injuries?
  - *Temperature*—For a cold-water drowning, you must continue resuscitation until the patient is rewarmed at the hospital. Note that even when the air is warm, the water may still be cold.
  - *Moving water*—Will the location of the victim change? Is it safe for you to enter it?
  - *Depth of the water*—Can your feet touch the bottom so you can stand, or will additional equipment be needed?
  - *Other hazards*—Are there hazardous materials present, such as oil, gas, or sewage? Is there any risk of electrocution?
- *Resources on hand.* How may rescuers are on scene? Are they trained in water rescue? Can they all swim? Does each have a personal flotation device? Do you need any special rescue teams such as a dive team?

If a water emergency occurs in open, shallow water that has a stable, uniform bottom, attempt a rescue. However, never try a water rescue unless you meet all of the following criteria:

- You are a good swimmer *and* . . .
- You are specially trained in water rescue *and* . . .
- You are wearing a personal flotation device *and* . . .
- You are accompanied by other rescuers.

If you meet all four criteria and your patient is responsive and close to shore, attempt a rescue. Use the "reach, throw, row, and go" strategy in the following order:

- *Reach*—Hold out an object for the patient to grab. Anything that will extend your reach will work. You can use a towel, shirt, backboard, or other strong object that will not break. Before holding out the object, make sure you have solid footing and will not slip in the water. Once the object is grabbed, pull the patient to shore.
- *Throw*—If the patient is too far to reach, then throw an object that floats (Figure 30–2). Use anything that will float and is heavy enough to throw. A thermos jug, a picnic cooler, or capped empty milk jug will do. This will give the patient support and give you more time to make the rescue. If possible, tie a rope to the object you throw. Toss the object to the patient, and pull on the rope to tow the patient in. Again, be sure of your own footing and stability.

- *Row*—If the patient is too far to reach or throw an object to from shore, then use a boat to get closer to the patient.
- *Go*—If reaching, throwing, and rowing are not possible, then swim to the patient. However, do this only if you are a good swimmer, specially trained in water rescue, wearing a personal flotation device, and accompanied by other rescuers.

Patient Assessment

Any injury that can occur on land also can occur in water. However, it can be more difficult to detect and treat injuries in water.

Bleeding, for example, is easy to spot on land. In the water any bleeding that occurs may be immediately diluted and dispersed. So not only may it be difficult to judge how severe the bleeding is, it also may not be possible to recognize that the patient is bleeding. Also, if the patient is wearing a wet suit, a large amount of blood can pool inside it before bleeding is recognized.

Broken bones, too, are difficult to identify. The water may be murky or dark. The surface of water also can distort visual images. Limbs, for example, can appear angulated or straight when they are not, just by the refraction. One way to

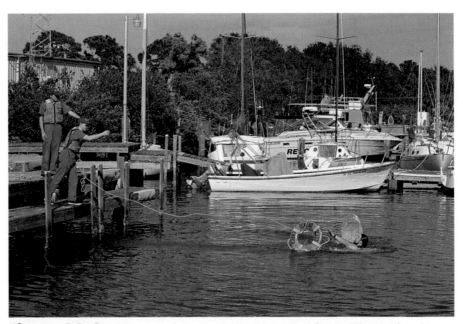

Figure 30-2 Tie a sturdy rope to an object that floats. Throw the object and pull the patient in.

deal with this problem is to assume fractures until proven otherwise in any unresponsive patient.

If the emergency is the result of a diving accident or if the patient has been struck by a boat, water skier, surfboard, or other object, suspect spine injury. Also suspect spine injury in any swimmer who is unresponsive, especially one in shallow, warm water.

Emergency Medical Care

If the patient is responsive and you are sure there is no spine injury, follow these guidelines:

1. Remove the patient from the water as quickly as you can by any safe method possible.
2. Complete the initial assessment. Administer high-flow oxygen, if you are allowed to do so. Be prepared to suction.
3. Conserve the patient's body heat. Remove wet clothing. Place the patient on a blanket. Then cover him or her with another blanket. If possible, move the patient to a warm environment. Do not allow the patient to walk.
4. While you are waiting for the ambulance, perform a physical exam and gather a patient history.

If your patient is unresponsive and in shallow, warm water, maintain the airway but do not move the patient. If the patient is breathing, keep him or her in a face-up position. Support the patient's back (Figure 30–3). If there is a second rescuer present, also stabilize the patient's head and neck (Figure 30–4).

If you find the unresponsive patient face-down in shallow water, you have to turn him. Perform the head-splint technique by following these steps (Figure 30–5):

1. Get alongside the patient.
2. Extend the patient's arms straight up alongside his or her head. Press the arms against the patient's head to create a splint.
3. If necessary, move the patient forward to a horizontal position.
4. Rotate the patient by bringing the hand farthest away towards you and pushing away the hand that was closest. As you rotate the patient, lower yourself in the water until the water is at shoulder level.
5. Maintain stabilization of the patient's head. Do this with one hand by holding the patient's head between his arms. With your

HIP AND SHOULDER SUPPORT

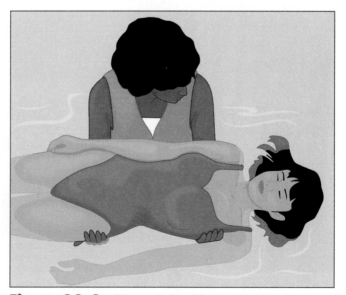

Figure 30-3 Hip and shoulder support.

HEAD-CHIN SUPPORT WITH TWO RESCUERS

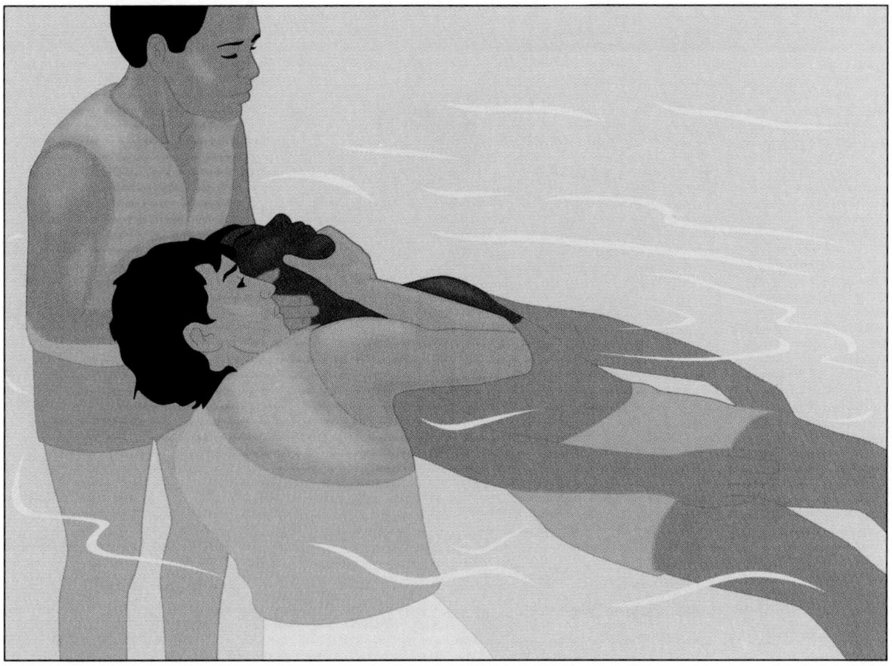

Figure 30-4 In-line stabilization with two rescuers.

other hand, support the patient's lower back until help arrives.

If the unresponsive patient is in water that is unsafe (deep, cold, or moving) or if the patient needs CPR, qualified rescuers should position the patient on a backboard. Once immobilized, the patient should be removed from the water. Note that ventilations can start in the water. Chest compressions cannot. Patients who need CPR must be removed from the water first.

To turn a patient to a face-up position in deep water, perform the head-chin support technique. Follow these steps (Figure 30–6, p. 500):

1. Position yourself alongside the patient.
2. Position one arm along the patient's spine, supporting the patient's head with your hand. Place your other arm along the patient's chest in line with the sternum, supporting the mandible with your hand.
3. If necessary, move the patient forward to a horizontal position.
4. Then rotate the patient by ducking under his body.

5. Continue to maintain in-line stabilization until a backboard is used to immobilize the spine.

To immobilize a patient, use a long backboard or other rigid support such as a water ski or surf board. Slide it under the patient. Let it float up until it is snugly against the patient's back. Apply a rigid cervical immobilization device. Then secure the patient to the backboard. Never try to support the patient's spine with anything that might bend or break, such as an air mattress or a Styrofoam float. As you are backboarding the patient, be sure to have enough rescuers helping. They need to make sure the patient's face does not become submerged. After immobilization, lift the patient from the water head first. If the patient is wearing a lifejacket, leave it in place. Remember to pad under the patient's head to keep the spine in alignment.

NOTE: Always have a near-drowning patient taken to a hospital, even if you believe the danger has passed. Complications can develop and may be fatal as long as 72 hours after the incident.

HEAD-SPLINT TECHNIQUE

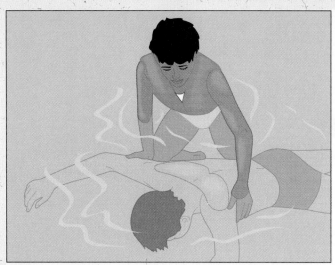

Figure 30-5a   Position yourself alongside the patient.

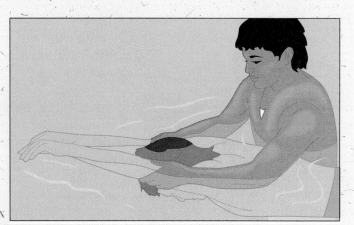

Figure 30-5b   Extend the patient's arms straight up alongside his or her head to create a splint.

HEAD-SPLINT TECHNIQUE *(Continued)*

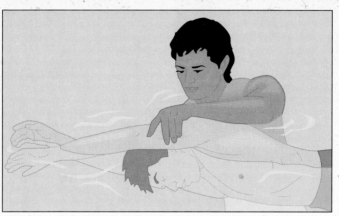

Figure 30-5c   Begin to rotate the torso toward you.

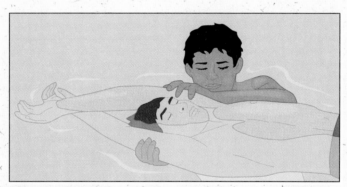

Figure 30-5d   As you rotate the patient, lower yourself in the water.

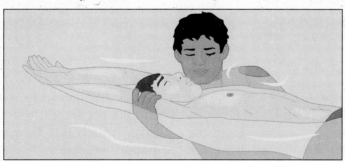

Figure 30-5e   Maintain stabilization by holding the patient's head between his or her arms.

HEAD-CHIN SUPPORT TECHNIQUE

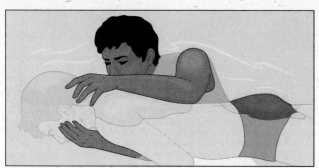

Figure 30-6a Position yourself. Support the patient's head with one hand and the mandible with the other.

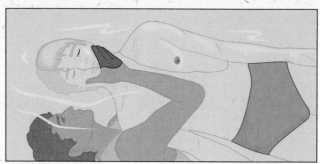

Figure 30-6b Then rotate the patient by ducking under him or her.

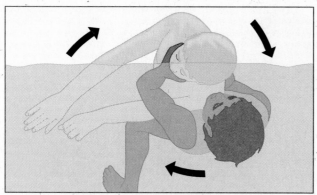

Figure 30-6c Continue to rotate until the patient is face up.

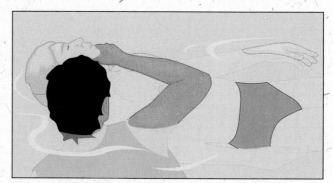

Figure 30-6d Maintain in-line stabilization until a backboard is used to immobilize the spine.

MOVING-WATER RESCUE

Many people are drawn to moving water, or "white water," for recreation. Those who are trained and experienced, know how to read moving water. They understand the hazards and manage them. It is all part of their sport. Moving-water incidents usually occur when someone who is unaware of the dangers gets into the water. This is true of both victims and rescuers.

The force of moving water is measured by its depth, width, and velocity. For example, a river that is 200-feet wide, 4-feet deep, and moving at 20-feet per second will move about 16,000 cubic feet per second. That is roughly equal to 550 pounds of force.

Fast-moving water is dangerous. Certain river features make it even more so. They include the following:

• *Strainers.* These are obstructions that allow water to pass through but catch people and other objects. Some of the most common are trees and branches. If a strainer catches a swimmer, the force of the water can hold the swimmer there until hypothermia sets in and he or she tires and drowns.

• *Obstructions.* Another problem is any type of obstruction in the river that a person can get pinned against, such as a bridge abutment. A person can easily become trapped against the object and be held there by the force of moving water. Again, hypothermia can set in and he or she can tire and drown.

• *Holes.* Not all the water in a fast-moving river flows downstream. When water flows over a large object, a recirculating current or "hole" may form. When this happens, the current can keep recirculating a swimmer in its backwash until he or she tires and drowns. Holes are difficult to see from upstream. Large ones are very difficult to escape from.

• *Low-head dams* (Figure 30–7). These dams are only a few feet high. They are built from concrete and have vertical abutments on each side. They are very difficult to see from upstream and often tend to be very wide. Water that flows over these dams can form a very large and uniform "hole" that extends across the river. If a boater gets too close to the "boil line," he or she can get caught in the recirculating current and capsize. The person and the boat then can get pushed to the bottom and back to the surface again and again.

• *Extremity entrapment* (Figure 30–8). Legs can get trapped between rocks or in other obstructions, especially in fast-moving water above a person's knees. Typically, this occurs to inexperienced folks who fall out of a boat and try to stand up. When this happens, the best thing to do is a back stroke with feet pointed downstream. Note that when an extremity gets caught, it must be extracted exactly in the same direction that it went in.

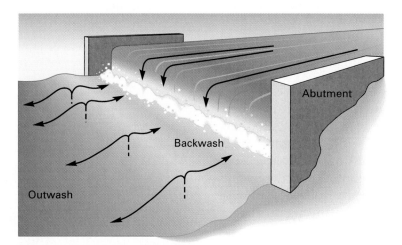

Figure 30-7a   A low-head dam.

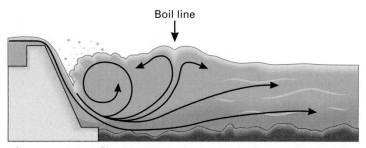

Figure 30-7b   A "hole" formed by the waters flowing over a low-head dam.

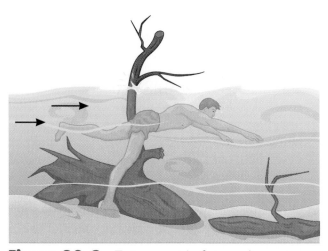

Figure 30-8 Entrapment in fast-moving water.

The basic, time-honored model for all water rescues is to reach, throw, row, and go. Remember, if you cannot easily effect a rescue using a simple shore-based technique (reach or throw), call for a team specializing in water rescue. Do not enter the water! Even special teams only try swimming or "live-bait" rescues as a last resort.

ICE RESCUE

Judging the thickness of ice and overall safety is very tricky. The old rule-of-thumb—"one inch, keep off; two inches, one may; three inches, small groups; four inches, okay"—is *not* accurate. Many factors can alter the thickness of the ice over large and small areas. For example, underground springs cause water turbulence from beneath and thinner ice above. So do decaying plant matter, schools of fish, and so on.

The "reach, throw, row, and go" method is used for all water rescues, including ice rescue. However, there are some differences you should note:

- *Reach and throw.* As a drowning patient becomes more hypothermic, he or she will be less and less able to hold onto a rope. An alternative technique is to throw an inflated fire hose. By using modified end caps and air from a SCBA tank, a fire hose can be inflated quickly and pushed out to the patient.

- *Row.* A conventional boat may not be able to break the ice as it moves, unless the ice is very thin. An option may be to use a small inflatable craft with ropes to tether it and pull it from shore. Perhaps the best crafts for ice rescues are the air boat and hover craft. Either can be maneuvered over ice, water, or dry land.

- *Go.* When patients are too hypothermic to hang on, rescuers must go in to get them (Figure 30–9). This usually involves wearing a "dry" neoprene ice-rescue suit, which is tethered to shore. The rescuer then crawls, shuffles, or swims out to grab and pull the patient in.

When a person falls through ice, a First Responder must immediately call for a special ice-rescue team. Then, don a personal flotation device and make reasonable attempts to reach or throw something to the patient from shore. If you are successful, the team can be canceled. If not, the team already on the way will have a chance to get to the scene in time to help the patient. Remember to prevent well intentioned bystanders from going onto the ice. More people to save may lead to more lives being lost.

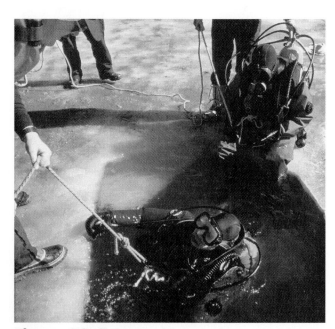

Figure 30-9 An ice rescue.

SECTION 3: BAROTRAUMA

The term *barotrauma* refers to several conditions. It occurs when scuba or deep-water divers experience increasing underwater pressures or when they ascend in deep water improperly. Such patients may need both basic life support and transport to a treatment center that specializes in diving injuries.

Note that patients with diving emergencies require specialized medical knowledge and care. If needed, Duke University's "Divers Alert Network" is a source of free medical consultation services for dive-related emergencies. Their 24-hour emergency hot line number is 919-684-8111.

AIR EMBOLISM

An air embolism is one or more air bubbles that block a blood vessel. It occurs when a diver holds his or her breath during the ascent from a dive. Air in the lungs then expands rapidly, rupturing the alveoli and damaging nearby blood vessels. As a result, air bubbles enter the bloodstream. The most dangerous places for air bubbles to lodge are in the heart, brain, or spinal cord.

Signs and symptoms have rapid onset. Within 15 minutes of surfacing, the diver may have any of the following:

- Difficulty breathing.
- Blotching or itching skin.
- Frothy blood in the nose and mouth.
- Pain in the muscles and joints.
- Chest pain or pain in the abdomen.
- Swelling and a grating sound in the neck.
- Numbness or tingling in the extremities.
- General weakness, paralysis.
- Possible convulsions.
- Dizziness.
- Vomiting.
- Blurred or distorted vision.
- Loss or distortion of memory.
- Slurred speech, lack of coordination.
- Unresponsiveness.
- Cardiac or respiratory arrest.
- Behavioral changes (this may be the only sign).

The patient needs recompression treatment at the hospital. Be sure to arrange for transport as soon as possible. To provide emergency care, treat all life-threats first. Assure an adequate airway, and administer 100% oxygen if you are allowed. If there is no sign of spine injury, position the patient on the left side with head and chest lower than the feet (Figure 30–10). Be prepared to provide ventilations or CPR.

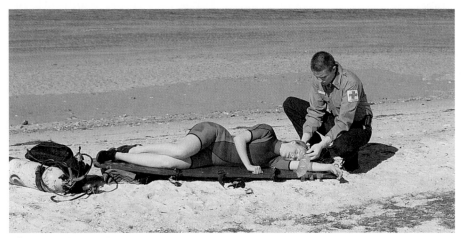

Figure 30-10 Proper positioning of a diving-accident patient.

DECOMPRESSION SICKNESS

Decompression sickness, or "the bends," usually occurs when a diver comes up too quickly from a deep prolonged dive. It can happen to anyone who is exposed to increasing pressure while breathing compressed air. It can range from mild to severe. It is more common than air embolism. The risk of decompression sickness increases if the diver flies within 12 hours of a dive.

Decompression sickness occurs when certain gases (usually nitrogen) are breathed by the diver over time. When the diver ascends, the nitrogen turns into tiny bubbles that lodge in the tissues throughout the body and eventually enter the bloodstream. The worst injuries occur when the nitrogen bubbles lodge in the brain, lungs, heart, or spinal cord. A burst lung is the most dire injury associated with this problem.

Signs and symptoms are gradual in onset. They usually occur 12 to 24 hours after the dive, but can occur up to 48 hours later. They include:

- Difficulty breathing, choking or coughing.
- Chest pain.
- Itchy, mottled skin with a minor skin rash that can change in appearance.
- Swelling of tissues, with pits in the swelling.
- Severe, deep aching pain in the joints and muscles.
- Nausea and vomiting with abdominal pain.
- Fatigue, dizziness, collapse sometimes leading to unresponsiveness.
- Headache.
- Blurred vision.
- Hallucinations.
- Ringing of the ears or partial deafness.
- Staggering gait.
- Numbness, paralysis.
- Inability to urinate.

The patient needs to be taken to a facility with a recompression chamber for rapid treat-ment. Arrange for transport immediately. To provide emergency care, treat life-threats first. Assure an adequate airway, and administer 100% oxygen if you are allowed. Be prepared to provide CPR. If there is no sign of spine injury, position the patient on the left side with head lower than the feet. Slant the patient's entire body about 15° to help prevent gas bubbles from injuring the brain or lungs.

THE SQUEEZE

The "squeeze" and the "reverse squeeze" can involve any part of the body that is filled with air. When divers descend or ascend, air pressure must be equalized to maintain proper pressure in the body's air cavities. If proper pressure is not maintained, injury to the tissues of the air cavities results. If there is an air pocket in a tooth due to decay or a defective filling, the tooth may rupture. Divers are at increased risk of the squeeze and reverse squeeze if they have an upper respiratory infection or an allergy that obstructs the sinuses.

Signs and symptoms include:

- Mild to severe pain in the affected area.
- Blood or fluid discharge from the nose or ears.
- Bleeding from the tiny blood vessels in the eyes.
- Extreme dizziness, disorientation.
- Nausea.
- Ear pain (most common), ringing in the ears, possible deafness.

The patient needs to be cared for immediately at a medical facility to prevent permanent blindness, deafness, dizziness, or the inability to dive in the future. Arrange for transport immediately. To provide emergency care, treat life-threats first. Suction to assure an adequate airway. Administer oxygen if you are allowed. Keep the patient calm while waiting for medical help to arrive.

FIRST RESPONDER FOCUS

Water emergencies can be surprisingly dangerous, even for good swimmers. Many people do not realize that the currents or water temperatures affecting the victim will affect them, too.

Television portrays water rescues as a simple matter of swimming out to the grateful victim and casually bringing them to shore. In real life, victims are frantic. In their effort to save themselves, they can drown the rescuer.

This chapter presented several ways of effecting a water rescue from the safety of shore. Do not attempt a rescue without the proper resources and a proper assessment of the dangers you will face. ■

CASE STUDY FOLLOW-UP

At the beginning of this chapter, you read that a First Responder was on scene of a possible drowning. To see how chapter skills apply to this emergency, read the following. It describes how the call was completed.

INITIAL ASSESSMENT

I moved to Jimmy's head and carefully turned him over without stressing his spine. Then I opened his airway and checked to see if he was breathing. He wasn't. But he had a pulse.

We were pretty close to the side of the pool. Two other lifeguards arrived just above us, and one was quick enough to open the first-aid kit and hand me a pocket mask. She jumped in to help, while the other lifeguard went to call 9-1-1.

Even though I had never done it before on a real person, I put the face mask in place and started ventilations—one breath every five seconds. It felt as if we were working on him for a while, but I guess it was only a few minutes when he started to cough. He brought up a little water, not much. All of a sudden there was an ambulance crew above us.

PHYSICAL EXAMINATION

The lifeguard who had jumped in the water to help visually inspected the patient from head to toe. She reported that she found no signs of injury.

PATIENT HISTORY

I knew Jimmy had seizures before. He told me so. But I never actually witnessed one.

ONGOING ASSESSMENT

The paramedics took over care before we had a chance to do anything but provide basic life support.

PATIENT HAND-OFF

Our hand-off report was brief. We told the crew chief that Jimmy was unresponsive when we found him, and that we had no evidence that he had hurt his neck or back. But since we didn't know for sure, we had held manual stabilization of his head and neck. We reported that Jimmy had a history of seizures, and that according to an unknown bystander he may have experienced one.

The paramedics positioned a backboard under Jimmy, secured him, and lifted him from the water. He still wasn't wide awake, but we told him he was in good hands and that we'd contact his family.

> Water-related emergencies pose a special challenge to First Responders. Patients in such emergencies often need immediate life-saving care. However, the same hazards that caused the emergency can endanger rescuers, too. Remember, your safety must come first. Do only what you are trained and equipped to do.

REVIEW QUESTIONS

Page references where answers may be found or supported are provided at the end of each question.

Section 1

1. What happens when a person drowns? Briefly describe fresh-water and saltwater drowning, wet and dry drowning, and cold-water drowning. (pp. 493–494)
2. What are some of the hazards a water emergency may pose for the rescuer? (pp. 494–495)
3. What criteria must you meet before you can attempt a water rescue? (pp. 494–495)
4. What is the "reach, throw, row, and go" strategy for water rescue? (p. 495)

5. What are the general guidelines for emergency care of a near-drowning patient? (pp. 496–497)

Section 2

6. What are the hazards commonly associated with fast-moving water? (pp. 500–501)

Section 3

7. What are the general guidelines for the emergency care of a patient with a diving-related emergency such as air embolism or decompression sickness? (pp. 503–504)

CHAPTER 31

VEHICLE STABILIZATION AND PATIENT EXTRICATION

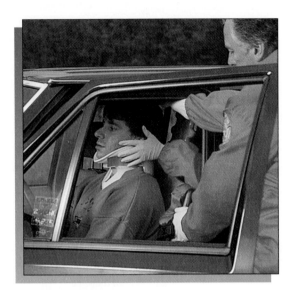

INTRODUCTION

Most of the time you will find your patients in safe, easily accessible locations where gaining access is no more than a knock on a door. However, there will be times when advanced rescue techniques must be used. By far the most common involve motor vehicle collisions.

When you arrive on scene of a collision, you may find anything from an unhurt occupant and a stable vehicle to multiple vehicles with pinned occupants. This chapter provides an overview of how you can proceed safely and effectively. In practice, be sure to follow all local protocols.

O B J E C T I V E S

Cognitive, affective, and psychomotor objectives are from the U.S. DOT's 1995 "First Responder: National Standard Curriculum." Enrichment objectives, if any, identify material that is supplemental to the DOT curriculum.

Cognitive

7-1.3 Discuss the role of the First Responder in extrication. (pp. 510–511)

7-1.4 List various methods of gaining access to the patient. (pp. 511–514)

7-1.5 Distinguish between simple and complex access. (pp. 511–512)

Affective

No objectives are identified.

Psychomotor

No objectives are identified.

Enrichment

* Describe the types of personal protective equipment recommended for rescue at the site of a vehicle collision. (p. 508)
* Discuss how to determine the number of patients at the scene of a vehicle collision. (pp. 508–509)
* Describe basic goals of traffic control at the scene of a collision. (pp. 509–510)
* State how a rescuer can recognize whether or not a vehicle is stable. (p. 510)
* Describe the basic steps of stabilizing an upright vehicle and an overturned vehicle. (p. 510)
* List simple, basic tools that can be used in extrication. (p. 514)

SECTION 1: SCENE SAFETY

PERSONAL PROTECTIVE EQUIPMENT

All EMS responders working in or around a wrecked vehicle and an extrication in progress must wear the following:

* *Eye protection.* Goggles or safety glasses with side shields are best to prevent flying metal shards from penetrating the eyes. Safety glasses with side shields also can be used to protect you from blood-borne pathogens. The flip-down shield on a firefighter helmet is not adequate protection for the eyes.
* *Hand protection.* While firefighter gloves provide the best puncture protection, they allow for poor manual dexterity. Although not offering as much protection, a pair of snugly fitting leather work gloves is a good alternative.
* *Body protection.* A flame-retardant outer shell such as firefighter turnout gear, brush-fire garment, or jumpsuit provide some protection from fire and limited protection from sharp objects. All garments should have reflective trim to improve night recognition.
* *Foot protection.* Wear turnout pants with either short rubber or leather boots with lug soles to prevent slippage. Boots should be above ankle height to prevent glass from dropping in.

DETERMINE THE NUMBER OF PATIENTS

In a vehicle collision—just as for every other type of emergency—assess personal safety. Then identify the mechanism of injury or nature of illness, and determine necessary resources. To determine the resources you need on scene, find out how many patients are involved. It may be difficult to locate all patients at first, but it is critical that you do. Use a systematic approach.

* If it is safe to enter the scene, ask a responsive patient to tell you how many others were involved in the crash.

CASE STUDY

DISPATCH

My partner and I are police officers with First Responder training. We were called to Smith Road just north of Peacham for a vehicle collision involving multiple casualties. Time out was 10 p.m.

SCENE SIZE-UP

As we approached, we saw a small red sports car sitting nose to nose with a large dump truck. The front of the little car was collapsed like an accordion under the front axle of the truck. The front bumper of the truck was even with the windshield of the car. We saw a driver and a passenger in the truck, both appeared to be responsive. We also saw two motionless young people in the front seat of the car. There was a considerable amount of blood coming from multiple face wounds.

> Consider this emergency as you read Chapter 31. How would you proceed?

• Question witnesses to see if a victim walked away from the scene.

• In case of a high-impact crash, search the surrounding area carefully. Look in ditches and tall weeds.

• Look for tracks in the earth or snow. A person who could get free from wreckage may be wandering aimlessly.

• Search the vehicle itself carefully. A patient may be wedged under the dashboard, for example.

• Look quickly for items that give clues to unaccounted for children, such as a lunch box, diaper bag, or extra jacket.

Combine this information with your evaluation of scene safety. Are there enough rescue personnel on scene? If not, send for help immediately. Continue to evaluate the situation for the most efficient, safest ways to help patients and protect rescue teams.

If a car is on fire, decide if you can remove the passengers quickly enough or if you should fight the fire. If the passengers are not trapped, move them first. If they cannot be extricated quickly, deal with the fire. That is, safely do what you can within your training and with the available equipment.

CONTROL THE SCENE

The crash scene can involve environmental hazards as well as a great deal of confusion. Send for law enforcement and fire services to help control the scene. While you wait for them to arrive, begin scene control. Quickly deal with bystanders by having them move out of the danger zone.

Spilled gasoline often is present at an auto crash. Allow no smoking on scene. Turn off all vehicle ignitions. If possible, get a fire crew with hoses to stand by during rescue.

CONTROL TRAFFIC

The basic goals of traffic control at the scene of a collision, are:

- To clear the scene so that emergency vehicles can get through quickly.
- To monitor regular traffic around the scene so no further crashes or injuries occur.
- To monitor traffic so that passing vehicles have a minimum of inconvenience.

Unless a distinct hazard justifies stopping all traffic, keep traffic moving. If the road is blocked, try to move traffic to an alternative route. Whatever you choose to do, make sure that motorists and pedestrians in the area know exactly what you want them to do. Keep rescue personnel well positioned along the roadway. If possible, rescuers should wear reflective clothing so they can be seen easily before and after dark. Use clear visual signals coupled with attention-getting devices such as flares or cones.

Fuses should be set 10-15 feet apart and extend 100 feet toward traffic. The pattern of fuses should lead traffic around the emergency. The danger zone includes at least a 50-foot radius around the wrecked cars. When the crash occurs on a curve, consider the start of the curve as the edge of the danger zone. On a hill, one edge of the danger zone should be the crest of the hill. If the highway has two lanes, position flares in both directions. If heavy trucks travel the road, extend the flare string, because trucks take much longer than cars to stop.

VEHICLE STABILIZATION

After all possible outside hazards are controlled, make the rescue setting as safe as possible. Always suspect that a vehicle is unstable until you have made it stable. Assume the vehicle is not stable if:

- It is on a tilted surface such as a hill.
- Part of it is stacked on top of another vehicle.
- It is on a slippery surface such as ice, snow, or spilled oil.

- It is overturned.
- It rests on its side.

Basic to stabilization is **cribbing** (Figure 31–1). Cribbing is a system of wood or other supports used to prop up a vehicle. Wood is stacked in box-like squares and wedges to keep pressure uniform. To create a stable environment, the cribbing is arranged diagonally to the vehicle frame. Do not crib under wheels or tires, because the vehicle will tend to roll. Never stack cribbing higher than its own length. There should never be more than one or two inches between the cribbing and the vehicle.

Any vehicle that can be moved easily during extrication or patient care needs to be stabilized by the placement of cribbing or step blocks under the frame and by clipping the valve stems of the tires. Excess movement of the vehicle could prove fatal for a patient with severe spinal injuries and may injure the rescue team. To stabilize vehicles:

- *Upright vehicles.* For a vehicle that rests on all four wheels, place the gear selector in park, or, if a standard shift, into reverse. Use blocks or wedges at wheels to prevent unexpected rolling. Chock wheels tightly against the curb when possible. To reduce the amount of movement even when you are using power tools, cut the tire valve stems so that the car rests on the rims.
- *Overturned vehicles.* To stabilize an overturned vehicle, place a solid object between the roof and the roadway. Use an object such as a wheel chock, spare tire, cribbing, or timber. If necessary, use a bumper jack to angle the vehicle against the solid object until it is stable. Hook a chain to the vehicle's axle. Then loop the chain around a tree or post.

SECTION 2: EXTRICATION OF THE PATIENT

Generally, emergency medical care is done before patient extrication, unless a delay would endanger the life of the patient or rescuer. The role of the First Responder is to administer emergency med-

STABILIZING WITH CRIBBING

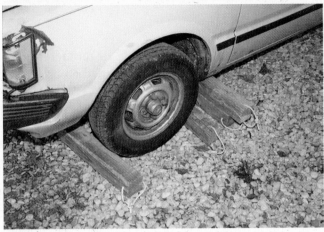

Figure 31-1a

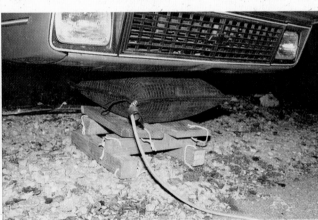

Figure 31-1b

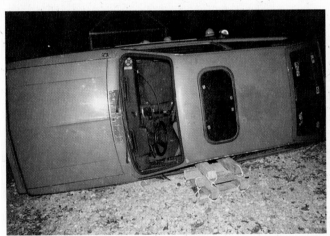

Figure 31-1c

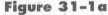

Figure 31-1d

ical care. The First Responder also is to assure that the patient is removed in a way that minimizes further injury.

In certain circumstances First Responders are required to take steps to gain access to the patient in a vehicle. Take only the steps you are trained to take. Call for additional assistance and rescue personnel if needed. In such cases, a chain of command should be established to ensure patient care priorities.

GAINING ACCESS

There are two basic ways a rescuer can gain access to a patient. **Simple access** is access by which no tools are needed. **Complex access** is access that requires tools and specialized equipment.

Most emergencies do not present access problems. However, when you are confronted with one, quickly evaluate the situation and decide if a simple or complex access is needed. If complex access is needed, call for rescuers who have the training and equipment. Remember that getting to the patient safely is critical. A lot of emotion can be involved at a crash scene. Do not allow that to hurry you into a setting that is not safe to enter. Enter the wreck to administer emergency care only when the vehicle is stabilized and safe.

Doors

A door is always the access of choice. This is because it is the largest uncomplicated opening in a vehicle. Always start by testing the door handles.

First try to open the door nearest the patient. If the doors are locked, try to open the lock by either having the patient in the car do so or by using a coat hanger or other device between the door frame and window. Routinely unlock all other doors to allow access by other rescuers. If the doors cannot be opened, determine the best point of entry and proceed accordingly. For instructions on how to expose a lock mechanism, see Figure 31–2.

Since 1983 cars are made with a collision beam inside the door, which makes it tougher for a door to cave in. Beware that the beam can buckle after impact, and a sharp end may stick into the passenger compartment. As you try to gain access through a door, be sure that the angle of force does not propel the beam further into the vehicle.

Windows

Car windows usually are made of tempered glass. Rear and side windows are designed to break into small granules. If you can, remove the window without breaking it. Fine particles of glass can stay unnoticed in a deep wound and cause damage after it closes. So cover the patient with a heavy safety blanket before breaking a window or as soon as possible.

If fixed windows are installed in U-shaped black plastic or rubber, remove the rim. Insert the point of a linoleum knife or similar tool into the molding at the midpoint of the glass. Keep the blade as flat against the glass as you can. Draw the knife across the top and down the side. Repeat on the other side. Soapy water will keep the blade moving easily. Work the end of a short pry bar behind the glass and pry it loose from the top. The window will pivot on its bottom edge.

EXPOSING A LOCK MECHANISM

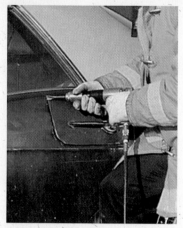

Figure 31–2a Cut around the handle and lock.

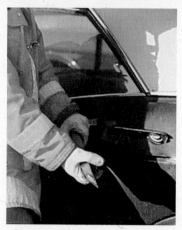

Figure 31–2b Pry open the cut area.

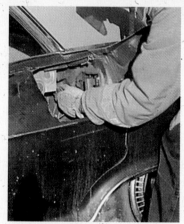

Figure 31–2c Operate rods and levers to pop open the lock.

If you must break a window, locate the window farthest from the patient. Give a quick hard thrust in the lower corner with a spring-loaded punch, screwdriver, or other sharp object. (See Figure 31–3.) If you can, put strips of broad tape or a sheet of contact paper over the glass to prevent broken pieces from spraying on the patient. Use your gloved hand to carefully pull the glass outside the vehicle. Clear all glass away from the window opening. Before you crawl in, drape a heavy tarp or blanket over the door edge and the interior of the car just below the window.

Windshield

Windshields usually are made of laminated safety glass, which cannot be broken safely. If the windshield is largely intact, pry up the chrome trim at the joints using a baling hook, pry bar, or screwdriver.

To remove the rubber seal that sets the windshield in the car, use a linoleum knife to slice the rubber bead. Drive the point into the channel and keep the blade flat against the glass. Then force a screwdriver behind the glass and simply pop out the windshield. For a Mastic-set windshield, remove the molding. Then use a Mastic cutter to free the windshield. The Mastic cutter may be obtained from an auto parts store or an auto windshield business.

Removal of a broken Mastic-set windshield may cause a great deal of splintering. Therefore, as with any extrication, you and the patient must be protected properly. Cover the patient with a safety blanket. Make sure each rescuer has full facial protection and wears a long-sleeved shirt and heavy gloves. Always consider using an alternative entry method before breaking or cutting glass.

Airbags

If the airbag has released, there may be some residue. This is not harmful and can be washed off. If the airbag was not triggered by the crash, disconnect the negative side of the battery and the yellow airbag connector. Do not cut the connector or its wires. They will keep the shorting bar activated, preventing accidental triggering.

BREAKING A CAR WINDOW

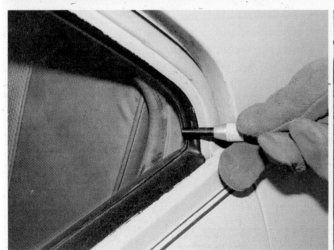 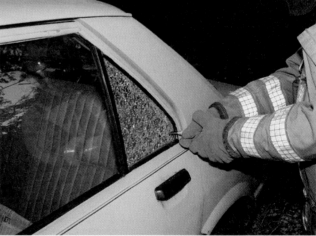

Figure 31-3a Position a punch in the corner of the side window farthest away from the patient.

Figure 31-3b Push in the shattered tempered glass, and reach in to open the door or roll down the window.

Pinned Patients

Always summon a rescue unit when a patient is pinned beneath a vehicle. To raise the vehicle use a sturdy jack, but not with a completely overturned vehicle. A pry bar and blocks may be used. A large group of bystanders can assist in lifting the vehicle off a patient. Be sure to shore up the vehicle so that it will not fall on the patient.

If a patient has a body part through a window, pad the extruded part well with bandaging material. Then carefully use pliers or a knife to break or fold away the glass. Once the body part is free, care for it.

If a patient is jammed or pinned inside the vehicle, consider the following simple procedures:

- Remove a shoe or other piece of clothing that may be pinning the patient.
- Move the front seat to give additional working space. It may be possible to lift the back seat entirely.
- Seat belts that will not open can be cut with shears or a knife. Support the dangling patient as you cut the belt.

EMERGENCY CARE OF THE PATIENT

As in any emergency, your first priority is always your own safety. (You are not good to the patient if you become another casualty.) Be sure the scene is safe, the vehicle is stable, and you are wearing the appropriate personal protective equipment before you try to reach the patient.

After gaining safe access, provide the same care you would give to any trauma patient. Stabilize the head and neck. Complete an initial assessment. Provide critical interventions. Be sure you have called for the necessary resources.

Remain with the patient during a complex extrication. Continually monitor his or her condition. If it begins to deteriorate, advise the rescue crew. They may be able to change the approach to the incident and get the patient out more quickly. During the process, be sure to protect yourself and the patient from the glass and flying debris. Use heavy blankets, a tarp, or even a solid object like a backboard.

Try to keep the patient calm during rescue. Even with an altered mental status, the patient may get very frightened. So keep him or her informed about what is being done to help. For example, let the patient know when a loud noise will occur and what is being done to cause it.

Immobilize the patient's spine during rescue. (Follow the precautions and procedures described in Chapter 23, "Injuries to the Spine.") The only exception to this rule occurs when there is an immediate threat to life, such as fire, and an emergency move is required.

EXTRICATION TOOLS AND EQUIPMENT

The majority of states in the U.S. have specially designed systems of patient extrication. The equipment is costly and requires special training. Where possible and appropriate, contact the local rescue squad immediately after a collision in which someone is trapped. They will be able to get to the patient quickly and safely.

It is important to be prepared in case a rescue squad is not available. Basic tools that can be used include hammer, screwdriver, chisel, crowbar, pliers, linoleum knife, work gloves and goggles, shovel, tire irons, wrenches, knives, car jacks, and ropes or chains. Ingenuity can put these tools to work in a safe and effective way.

FIRST RESPONDER FOCUS

▼

Whether on or off duty, you will come across a motor vehicle collision at some point in your career as a First Responder. Most of the decisions you make involving vehicle access and stabilization will be made during the scene size-up.

For your own safety consider:

- Whether or not the vehicle is stable. Remember, unstable vehicles can shift and injure you.
- Whether or not there are hazardous materials present. This includes transported substances and leaking gasoline.

Patient care considerations include:

- Can access to the patient be gained?
- Can access be gained by simple or complex procedures?

- What is the priority of the patient? What are his or her injuries?
- Can the patient be removed from the vehicle while immobilized on a backboard? Or will extrication require cutting or moving parts of the vehicle?

Careful consideration early in the call will help the rest of the call flow smoothly. It also will prevent unnecessary delays in patient access and transport. ■

CASE STUDY FOLLOW-UP

At the beginning of this chapter, you read that First Responders were on the scene of a collision with multiple patients. To see how chapter skills apply to this emergency, read the following. It describes how the call was completed.

SCENE SIZE-UP *(Continued)*
This was a complex-access rescue situation. We immediately updated dispatch and requested specialized rescue crews and an ambulance for each patient. Then we positioned our vehicle about 100 feet from the wreckage to give the rescue units space to pull in.

As soon as we determined it was safe to approach, we saw that both vehicles had all four wheels on solid ground and appeared to be stable. We made sure that both engines were turned off and brakes were on. We also looked for any smoke or leaks.

INITIAL ASSESSMENT
Then we attempted to gain access to the patients and perform triage. We did as much of an initial assessment as we could on the patients in the sports car from the open windows. The occupants of the truck did not appear to be seriously injured. They were alert with minor complaints. We instructed them to remain in their seats until more help arrives. Most of the damage and injuries were to the sports car and its occupants.

We were taking spinal precautions and attempting to maintain airways and control serious bleeding of the patients when the first ambulance arrived.

PATIENT HAND-OFF
We reported the number of patients and our initial observations to the EMTs, including which patients we believed were a first priority. While they proceeded to assess and care for the patients, we provided direction to the other responding units.

It took a while for the patients to be disentangled from the wreckage. We assisted in every way we could—from redirecting traffic to holding manual stabilization of a patient's head and neck during extrication.

After the patients were freed, we helped the EMTs quickly reassess them and move them into the ambulances.

> As in all emergency situations, remember that your first priority is your own safety. Do not enter the scene of an emergency until you have determined that it is safe. Do not attempt a complex rescue, unless you are trained and equipped to do so. Follow your local protocols.

REVIEW QUESTIONS

Page references where answers may be found or supported are provided at the end of each question.

Section 1

1. What are some types of personal protective equipment a rescuer should wear at the site of a vehicle collision? (p. 508)
2. What are the basic goals of traffic control at the scene of a collision? (p. 510)
3. How can a rescuer recognize whether or not a vehicle is stable? (p. 510)
4. What are some basic methods of stabilizing an upright vehicle? An overturned vehicle? (p. 510)

Section 2

5. In general, what is the role of the First Responder in extrication? (pp. 510–511)
6. What is the difference between simple and complex access? (pp. 511–512)
7. What is always the access of choice? Explain your answer. (p. 512)
8. What are some basic guidelines for the emergency medical care of patients who are trapped in wreckage? (p. 514)

CHAPTER 32

SPECIAL RESCUE SITUATIONS

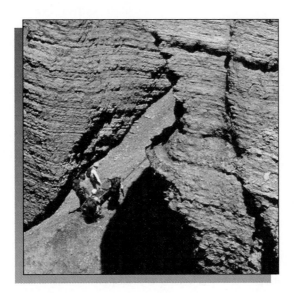

INTRODUCTION

People who are drawn to public safety and emergency work tend to be very action-oriented. They almost always rather *do* something than just stand and watch. The problem is that taking action in situations where you may be unaware of the hazards can result in serious injury or even death. This chapter will introduce you to some of the hazards of special rescue, hazards which could go unnoticed until it is too late.

Cognitive, affective, and psychomotor objectives are from the U.S. DOT's 1995 "First Responder: National Standard Curriculum." Enrichment objectives, if any, identify material that is supplemental to the DOT curriculum.

Cognitive

No objectives are identified.

Affective

No objectives are identified.

Psychomotor

No objectives are identified.

Enrichment

* Define the term "confined-space emergencies." (p. 518)
* Describe some of the hazards involved in rescues of patients having confined-space emergencies. (pp. 518–519)
* Identify the role of the First Responder in a confined-space emergency. (pp. 519–520)
* Discuss the general guidelines for performing safe litter carries over distances on rough terrain. (pp. 520–521)
* State the criteria for identifying a rescue as a low-angle or high-angle rescue. (p. 521)
* Describe the basic capabilities of a helicopter in rescue operations. (pp. 521–523)
* List the characteristics of a safe helicopter landing zone. (p. 524)
* Describe the procedure for safely approaching a helicopter that has just landed. (p. 524)

SECTION 1: CONFINED-SPACE EMERGENCIES

Most of the time we do not think about the air we breathe, unless it has a bad odor or it is irritating in some way. Unfortunately, not all hazards in the environment warn us away with odors. Confined spaces can be especially dangerous to rescuers as well as patients.

A confined space is defined as a place with limited access and egress that is not designed for human occupancy. Some examples of confined spaces are (Figure 32–1):

* *Silos.* Silos are used in agriculture to store solid materials. Some are designed specifically to limit the presence of oxygen. Hazards include poisonous gases emitted during the natural fermentation of crops, as well as engulfment and suffocation. Silos are perhaps the most common sites of confined-space emergencies.
* *Storage bins.* These include both grain bins and grain elevators. Like silos, they present the hazards of low oxygen levels and engulfment.
* *Underground vaults.* These include utility vaults for water, sewer, electrical power, telephone, and other communications cables. Hazards include poisonous gases and electrocution.
* *Wells, culverts, and cisterns.* These offer little oxygen and a high risk of drowning or entrapment.

A low oxygen level is a significant, common hazard in confined spaces. Also common are poisonous gases such as hydrogen sulfide, carbon dioxide, carbon monoxide, and methane. Note that sometimes atmospheres are explosive as well as poisonous.

SAFETY PRECAUTIONS

The U.S. Occupational Safety and Health Administration (OSHA) has taken an aggressive approach to safety for workers in confined spaces. Among its rules are the following:

* The atmosphere must be properly ventilated and monitored for oxygen, carbon monoxide, and hydrogen sulfide.

CASE STUDY

DISPATCH

My first response unit was dispatched for an automobile crash on County Route 402—the farthest part of our district. The report was that one car left the road and rolled over.

SCENE SIZE-UP

We approached the scene. There were no signs of wires down, leaking gas, or hazardous materials. The car looked like it was bounced around a lot but somehow ended up on its wheels. There was one passenger inside the vehicle. We put on our gear and gloves and approached. There was a star in the windshield where the driver hit his head. The steering wheel was bent. We were unable to open the doors because the roof was pushed down on them. Rescue was notified.

Consider this situation as you read Chapter 32. How would you proceed?

- Electrical systems must be locked and lagged out.
- Stored energy must be dissipated.
- Pipes must be disconnected or blanked out.
- A person who plans to enter a space must use the appropriate respiratory protection, such as a self-contained breathing apparatus (SCBA).

A call to a confined-space emergency is usually for a fall, medical problem, asphyxia, explosion, or machinery entrapment. As a First Responder, your responsibility is to recognize the emergency and call for the proper help as soon as possible. Do not enter a scene unless you know that it is safe. Only members of specialized teams that are trained and equipped for the emergency should enter.

When you are called to a confined-space emergency, proceed with scene size-up as follows:

1. Determine the nature of the emergency.
   - Obtain a copy of the permit for the site and assess the type of work being done.
   - Determine how many workers are inside the confined space.
   - Without entering the space, determine what the hazards are.
2. Call for a specialized rescue team, as well as for emergency medical personnel and transport.
3. Establish a perimeter, and do not allow anyone to enter.
4. When they arrive, assist medical or rescue personnel if you trained to do so and if you can do so safely.

CAVE-INS AND RESCUES FROM TRENCHES

OSHA requires a "trench box" or "shoring" in any trench that is deeper than five feet. Trench boxes are now commonly used all over the U.S. Unfortunately, a contractor or a do-it-yourselfer sometimes does not use one. Dirt may be too close to the top edge of a trench and ground vibration, water seepage, or an intersecting trench causes one of the walls to give way.

Most trench collapses occur at sites that are less than 6-feet wide and 12-feet deep. Usually, a

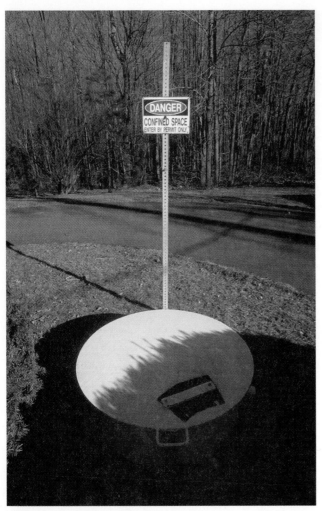

Figure 32-1 A confined-space.

worker was inside the trench when the walls collapsed, burying the worker either completely or partially. If someone jumps into the trench to try to rescue the worker, a secondary collapse occurs and he or she gets buried too.

Soil weighs about 100 pounds per cubic yard. That is, two feet of soil piled on top of a person's back or chest is equal to about a 1000 pounds. So even if a person is only partially buried, the weight of the soil on his or her chest can cause respiratory difficulties. To rescue such a victim safely requires methodical and strenuous effort. It can be a slow process.

No matter how the cave-in occurs, if the trench is more than waist-deep, a specialized trench rescue team is needed. As a First Responder, your job is to secure the scene by establishing a perimeter. Do not allow anyone to enter the trench or its immediate area. Call for the rescue team as soon as possible. Remember, if a collapse has occurred, another one is very likely.

SECTION 2: ROUGH-TERRAIN EVACUATIONS

More people are engaging in—and getting injured in—mountain biking, skiing, rock climbing, and other types of rough-terrain sports. As a First Responder, you may be required to assist in evacuation of these patients.

LITTER CARRIES

It takes 18–20 people to carry a litter, or portable stretcher, for one mile. Wheels may be attached to some types of portable stretchers, but they only work well on fairly flat terrain.

To perform a litter carry over rough terrain for some distance, follow these general guidelines:

• Select teams of four to six bearers each (Figure 32–2). Members of each team should be about equal in height.

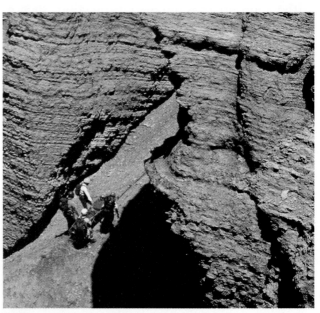

Figure 32-2 Litter carry over rough terrain.

- After a team carries the portable stretcher a short distance, team members should change positions and then sides.
- After another short distance, a fresh team should rotate into position and take over.

HIGH- AND LOW-ANGLE RESCUES

When the angle of the terrain increases, the risk of falling and dropping a patient on a litter increases. One way to manage this risk is to use a rope system to lift or lower the stretcher while rescuers hold and guide it (Figure 32–3).

In most cases, a high-angle rescue is obvious. It would involve moving up or down a cliff, gorge, or side of a building, for example. If you have any doubt, a high-angle rescue team would be needed under the following conditions:

- The slope forms more than a 40-degree angle.
- Slips or falls would likely result in serious injury or death due to the dangerous terrain below the slope.
- The terrain is so hazardous, it requires rappelling. (Rappelling is a special technique of getting down a cliff by means of a secured rope.)

A low-angle rescue generally does not need a rope system. You can identify a low-angle rescue by the following conditions:

- The slope forms less than a 40-degree angle.
- The rescuers' hands are not needed for balance or scrambling.
- Slips or falls would not likely result in serious injury or death.

As soon as you recognize a low- or high-angle emergency, call immediately for specialized personnel to perform the rescue. Follow your local protocols.

SECTION 3: HELICOPTERS IN RESCUE OPERATIONS

A helicopter's ability to hover, land in small places, and carry people and equipment make it a logical rescue platform. Over the years, search-and-rescue operations have come to depend on helicopters (Figure 32–4). However, ground-based rescue efforts should never wait for air support. Weather conditions or other aircraft limitations can result in significant delays. So when calling for air support, make sure you have a back-up plan in case air rescue is delayed or impossible. (See Table 32–1 for guidelines for when to request air support.)

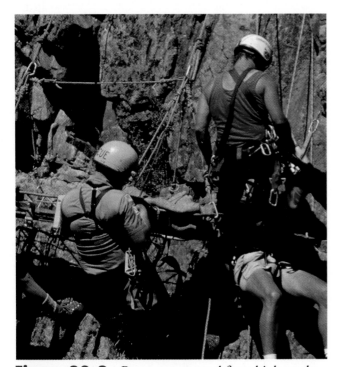

Figure 32-3 Rope system used for a high-angle rescue.

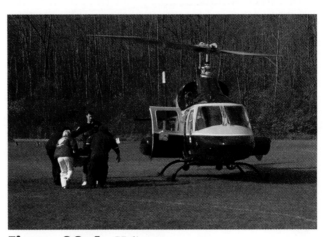

Figure 32-4 Helicopter rescue.

TABLE 32-1

WHEN TO CALL FOR A HELICOPTER

▼

Operational Reasons	Medical Reasons
- Normal ground travel to the appropriate medical facility would take more than 30 minutes. - Extrication will be prolonged. - Location of the emergency is at a remote site. - Patient needs paramedic-level care.	- The patient has a life- or limb-threatening condition. - The patient's condition is unstable (shock, head injury with altered mental status, chest trauma with respiratory distress, penetrating injuries to body cavity, amputations, burns over 15% of the body or to the face). - There is a serious mechanism of injury (fall of 15 feet or more, blow from a vehicle traveling over 20 mph, ejection from vehicle, a rollover without restraints, major deformity to passenger compartment or to vehicle's front end, a death of one of the car passengers).

HELICOPTER CAPABILITIES

Weather Limitations

An aircraft can take off and land either visually or by way of instruments. However, instrument flight rules, or IFR, are used only to fly from one airport to another. Sometimes they are used to guide a pilot to safety when weather suddenly turns bad.

Visibility is crucial to rescue operations. The pilot and crew must be able to see the ground team for flight instructions. Since visibility is needed, an aircraft would not be able to launch if the weather is below minimum standards. A good rule of thumb to follow to estimate visibility at the rescue site is:

- *Day*—500-foot cloud ceiling and one mile of visibility.
- *Night*—1000-foot cloud ceiling and three miles of visibility.

Altitude also plays an important role. The ability of a helicopter to hold a hover is key to a rescue operation. As the altitude of a craft increases, air density decreases. In addition, the warmer the air, the less dense it is. As air density decreases, more power is needed for the aircraft to hold a hover. At some point, altitude or air temperature may make it impossible to accomplish a mission.

Control Systems

Piloting a helicopter is complex. The pilot must be able to operate three main control systems:

- The "collective" controls the angle of the main rotor blades. It also controls the vertical motion of the craft. By using the collective and a great deal of power, the aircraft can lift off the ground.
- The "cyclic" tilts the spinning rotors and produces the forward, backward, and side movements of the craft.
- The "rudder pedals" control the pitch of the tail rotor and the rotation of the aircraft.

During takeoff, the helicopter pilot must increase the power and rotor speed. Then he or she uses the collective to increase the angle of the rotor blades and lift off. The cyclic is moved forward to make the transition from vertical lift to forward flight. As the aircraft moves forward, additional air speed is needed for more lift. Once the craft is at the proper altitude, the need for power is reduced. Because of the engine power needed, take-offs and landings are dangerous times.

The controls of the helicopter are very sensitive. A small movement of one of them can mean a major change in the attitude of the craft. To pilot a helicopter during a hover is especially strenuous and stressful. It has been compared to rubbing your belly, patting the top of your head, and reciting the Gettysburg address all at once.

In addition, when in a hover, the pilot cannot see the target below. The crew chief watches the spot and verbally guides the pilot. The pilot also needs to spot a reference point. Normally, this is tricky. At night or in low-light conditions, it can be very difficult.

Space and Load

Some crafts are large enough to carry a whole squad of people. Others are small and cannot hold many more than a pilot, patient, and one crew member. In general, helicopters are very weight sensitive.

When the capacity of a craft is listed, it usually does not take into account the fuel load, crew, equipment, altitude, and air temperature. All of these factors have a major influence on the performance of the craft. If a craft is heavily weighted, for example, it may be able to land in a tight spot, but it may not be able to take off without getting rid of unnecessary gear or crew.

SPECIAL TACTICS

One of the main reasons to choose a helicopter for rescue is its ability to pick up and extract people without landing. That involves hoisting, rappelling, and flying with external loads. All of these tactics are risky. Because of the danger and stress of hovering, special tactics are almost always aimed at reducing hover time.

Hoisting

Some aircraft are equipped with mechanical hoists. They are made to insert or to extract people from the ground. They are most commonly found on military craft and on some public safety aircraft.

Hoisting operations require hover time, which will vary depending on the speed of the hoist and the amount of cable out. Operations also are limited by the safe working load of the cable and by the number of duty cycles of the system.

If you work around helicopters that have hoists, become familiar with the ground safety procedures. One that applies to all hoist cables relates to static electricity. When a cable is lowered, it must touch the ground to allow its electrical charge to dissipate. If the cable is touched before that happens, the first person who touches it will get an electrical jolt.

SPIE Line

The use of a special insertion and extrication (SPIE) line is called the "short-haul technique." It was developed by mountain rescue teams in Europe and by Parks Canada. It involves flying beneath the helicopter as an external load. It is commonly used with light duty aircraft without hoists to both insert and extract rescuers and patients.

Generally, a weighted and backed up rope system is attached to the cargo hook or belly band of a helicopter. At the other end of the rope, rescuers in flight helmets with communications and harnesses are clipped in. When the helicopter ascends, they dangle beneath the craft as they are flown to the target area and gently lowered to the ground.

To extract, the craft flies into position and the ground team clips the litter or patients into the SPIE line. They are then flown back to a staging area and gently lowered into position.

Both insertion and extraction are risky operations. They should be undertaken only by specialized rescue teams. Note that if an external load becomes destabilized during flight or if an emergency occurs where the helicopter and crew are in jeopardy, an external load may be jettisoned.

LANDING ZONES

The helicopter landing zone should be at least 100 feet by 100 feet square. The landing zone, or LZ, should be flat or have no more than an eight-degree slope. The LZ also should be (Table 32–2):

- *Free of obstructions.* That includes wires, trees, buildings, and other obstructions. If it is surrounded by obstructions, the pilot will be forced into a vertical take off, which takes tremendous power and is very dangerous. If there are any obstructions near the LZ, inform the pilot by radio.
- *No loose objects.* Anything on the ground that is loose will blow around in the 100-mile-per-hour rotor wash of the helicopter. Stones, dirt, and other objects are easily picked up and blown into people and vehicles causing both injury and property damage.
- *Scene lighting.* Keep emergency lights on to help the pilot locate the scene. Also place markers on all four corners of the LZ. Chemical light sticks or small strobe lights work well. Avoid shining spotlights on the helicopter because they can blind the pilot.
- *Traffic control.* The LZ must be absolutely secure. There should be no traffic within 100 feet of the aircraft.

Both the main and tail rotors on a helicopter are extremely dangerous. Do not approach the

---

TABLE 32-2

LANDING ZONE GUIDELINES

▼

- Approximately 100 × 100 foot area.
- Free of all obstructions.
- Clear of wires, towers, vehicles, people, and loose objects.
- Firm ground with less than 8° slope.
- Markers on all four corners.
- All emergency red lights should be on.
- No white lights, spotlights, or blue lights directed toward the helicopter or landing zone.
- No smoking.

---

craft until the pilot or crew chief signals you to approach or escorts you to the ship. Never approach from the rear. The tail rotor is spinning so fast, it is nearly invisible and it can kill. In addition, the main rotor may be lower than it appears to be. Depending on the grade of the LZ, the spinning blade may be no more than a few feet above the ground.

If you are signaled to approach the helicopter, maintain eye contact with the pilot or crew chief. Approach only from the front. Stay low. Avoid carrying anything above your head. Avoid wearing anything loose that can be blown away by the rotor wash.

FIRST RESPONDER FOCUS
▼

One of the reasons you have decided to become a First Responder may be the varied situations you will encounter. This chapter may cover the most unusual. However, times change. And so have the situations in which people find themselves in need of rescue.

Rescue technology and procedures have kept up with those changes. They have advanced dra-matically in the past several years. It is now possible to rescue a person safely from a confined space or mountain slope and transport to a trauma center capable of handling the most complex and serious injuries.

Know the resources and special teams available in your area before you need to call. ■

CASE STUDY FOLLOW-UP

At the beginning of this chapter, you read that First Responders were at the scene of a car crash. To see how chapter skills apply to this emergency, read the following. It describes how the call was completed.

INITIAL ASSESSMENT

The patient was moaning. He seemed to know who we were but he wasn't alert. He was moving air and had no blood or other airway obstructions. We didn't see any obvious bleeding. The man's skin was pale and moist. My partner stabilized his head, and I checked his pulse. It was 110 and weak.

We were concerned about the mechanism of injury and the signs of shock. I radioed for the MedFlight helicopter. They were available and had an ETA of less than 20 minutes.

PHYSICAL EXAMINATION

We couldn't get the man out of the car so we continued stabilization. I began an assessment. He appeared to have a chest injury and a contusion to his forehead. His level of responsiveness had diminished somewhat from the time we arrived. We had oxygen with us, so we applied it via nonrebreather mask.

PATIENT HISTORY

We were unable to obtain a history.

ONGOING ASSESSMENT

We monitored the patient closely until the EMTs arrived.

PATIENT HAND-OFF

After reporting what little we knew, the EMTs began emergency care. I went across the street to a level area and checked out a landing zone for the helicopter. I radioed dispatch with the exact location. There were wires on our side of the road so I wanted them to be careful.

Rescue had begun to extricate the patient. It didn't take that long once they got there. The helicopter arrived just as the EMTs, with help from my partner, performed a rapid extrication since the patient was unstable. They turned him over to the crew from the helicopter. The travel time to the hospital was about 10 or 12 minutes. It would have been at least 30 minutes for us.

The patient survived. I called the other day. It was close, they said. He almost didn't make it to surgery. The helicopter saved time—and his life.

> Know the area you are assigned to. Find out how people live, work, and play there. Then learn about the hazards common in your community and the resources available to handle them.

REVIEW QUESTIONS

Page references where answers may be found or supported are provided at the end of each question.

Section 1

1. What are some of the hazards involved in rescues of patients with confined-space emergencies? (pp. 518–519)

2. What is the role of the First Responder in a confined-space emergency? (pp. 519–520)

Section 2

3. What are the general guidelines for performing safe litter carries over distances on rough terrain? (pp. 520–521)

REVIEW QUESTIONS *(Continued)*

4. What are the criteria for identifying a rescue as a low-angle or high-angle rescue? (p. 521)

6. How should you approach a helicopter safely? (p. 524)

Section 3

5. What are the characteristics of a safe helicopter landing zone? (p. 524)

GLOSSARY OF ABBREVIATIONS

A

ABCs: airway, breathing, circulation.
ACLS: advanced cardiac life support.
ADA: Americans with Disabilities Act.
AED: automated external defibrillator.
AHA: American Heart Association.
AIDS: acquired immune deficiency syndrome.
ALS: advanced life support.
ATV: all-terrain vehicle.
AVPU: alert, verbal, painful, unresponsive.

B

BLS: basic life support.
BSA: body surface area.
BSI: body substance isolation.
BVM: bag-valve-mask device.

C

CDC: Centers for Disease Control.
CHEMTREC: Chemical Transportation Emergency Center.
CISD: critical incident stress debriefing.
COPD: chronic obstruction pulmonary disease.
CPR: cardiopulmonary resuscitation.
CVA: cerebral vascular accident.

D

DNR orders: do not resuscitate orders.
DOT: U.S. Department of Transportation.
DOTS: deformities, open injuries, tenderness, swelling.

E

EKG: electrocardiogram.
EMD: emergency medical dispatcher.
EMS: emergency medical services.
EMT: emergency medical technician.
EMT-B: EMT-Basic.
EMT-I: EMT-Intermediate.
EMT-P: EMT-Paramedic.
EPA: Environmental Protection Agency.
ERT: emergency response team.
ETA: estimated time of arrival.

F

FBAO: foreign body airway obstruction.
FCC: Federal Communications Commission.

H

hazmat: hazardous material.
HBIG: hepatitis B immunoglobulin.
HBV: hepatitis B virus.
HEPA respirator: high efficiency particulate air respirator.
HIV: human immunodeficiency virus.

I

ICS: incident command system.

L

LZ: landing zone.

M

MCI: multiple-casualty incident.
ml: milliliters.
MOI: mechanism of injury.
MSDA: material safety data sheets.

N

NFPA: National Fire Protection Association.
NHTSA: National Highway Traffic Safety Administration.
NIOSH: National Institute of Occupational Safety and Health.
NOI: nature of illness.

O

O$_2$: oxygen.
OB kit: obstetrical kit.
OPQRRRST: onset, provocation, quality, region, radiation, relief, severity, time of pain.
OSHA: Occupational Safety and Health Administration.

P

PCR: prehospital care report.
PEA: pulseless electrical activity.
PPE: personal protective equipment.
psi: pounds per square inch.
PTO: power takeoff shaft of a tractor.

S

SAED: semi-automated external defibrillator.
SAMPLE: signs and symptoms, allergies, medications, pertinent past history, last oral intake, events.

SCBA: self-contained breathing apparatus.
SIDS: sudden infant death syndrome.
START system: simple triage and rapid treatment system.

T

TB: tuberculosis.
TIA: transient ischemic attack.

GLOSSARY OF TERMS

A

abandonment: a legal term referring to discontinuing emergency medical care without making sure that another health-care professional with equal or better training has taken over.

abdominal cavity: the space below the diaphragm and continuous with the pelvic cavity.

abrasion: an open wound caused by scraping, rubbing, or shearing away of the epidermis.

abuse: improper or excessive action so as to injure or cause harm.

accessory muscles: additional muscles; in regard to breathing, these are the muscles of the neck and the muscles between the ribs.

activated charcoal: a finely ground charcoal that is very absorbent and is sometimes used as an antidote to some ingested poisons.

acute abdomen: a sharp, severe abdominal pain with rapid onset.

advance directive: a patient's instructions, written in advance, regarding the kind of resuscitation efforts that should be made in a life-threatening emergency.

afterbirth: the placenta after it separates from the uterine wall and delivers.

agonal respirations: reflex gasping with no regular pattern or depth; a sign of impending cardiac or respiratory arrest.

airway adjunct: an artificial airway.

alimentary tract: the food passageway that extends from the mouth to the anus.

altered mental status: a change in a patient's normal mental status.

alveoli: the air sacs of the lungs. *Singular* alveolus.

amniotic sac: a sac of fluid in which the fetus floats.

amputation: an injury that occurs when a body part is severed from the body.

anaphylactic shock: *See* anaphylaxis.

anaphylaxis: an acute allergic reaction with severe bronchospasm and vascular collapse, which can be rapidly fatal.

anatomical position: a position in which the patient is standing erect with arms down at the sides, palms facing front.

aneurysm: an enlarged or burst artery.

antecubital space: the hollow, or front, of the elbow.

anterior: a term of direction or position meaning toward the front. *Opposite of* posterior.

aorta: major artery that starts at the left ventricle of the heart and carries oxygen-rich blood to the body.

apical pulse: an arterial pulse point located under the left breast.

arterial bleeding: recognized by bright red blood spurting from a wound.

arteries: blood vessels that take blood away from the heart.

arterioles: the smallest arteries.

artificial ventilation: a method of assisting breathing by forcing air into a patient's lungs.

asphyxia: suffocation.

aspirate: to inhale materials into the lungs.

atria: the two upper chambers of the heart. *Singular* atrium.

auscultation: a method of examination that involves listening for signs of injury or illness.

autonomic nervous system: the part of the nervous system that handles involuntary activities.

avulsion: an open wound that is characterized by a torn flap of skin or soft tissue that is either still attached to the body or pulled off completely.

B

bag of waters: amniotic sac.

barotrauma: an injury caused by a change in the atmospheric pressure between a closed space and the surrounding area.

behavior: the way a person acts or performs.

behavioral emergency: a situation in which a patient exhibits behavior that is unacceptable or intolerable to the patient, family, or community.

birth canal: a passage made of the cervix and vagina.

blanch: to lose color.

blood pressure: the amount of pressure the surging blood exerts against the arterial walls.

blood vessels: a closed system of tubes through which blood flows.

bloody show: the mucous plug that is discharged during labor.

blunt trauma: injuries caused by a sudden blow or force that has a crushing impact.

body armor: a garment made of a synthetic material that resists penetration by bullets.

body mechanics: the safest and most efficient methods of using the body to gain a mechanical advantage.

body substance isolation (BSI): a strict form of infection control based on the premise that all blood and body fluids are infectious.

brachial pulse point: an arterial pulse that can be felt on the inside of the arm between the elbow and the shoulder.

bracing: exerting an opposing force against two parts of a stable surface with your body; in EMS, usually refers to a safety precaution taken while riding in an ambulance patient compartment.

bronchi: the two main branches of the trachea, which lead to the lungs. *Singular* bronchus.

burn center: a medical facility devoted to treatment of burns, often including long-term care and rehabilitation.

burnout: a state of exhaustion and irritability caused by the chronic stress of work-related problems in an emotionally charged environment.

C

capillaries: the smallest blood vessels through which the exchange of fluid, oxygen, and carbon dioxide takes place between the blood and tissue cells.

capillary bleeding: recognized by dark red blood that oozes slowly from a wound.

capillary refill: the time it takes for capillaries that have been compressed to refill with blood.

cardiac arrest: the sudden cessation of circulation.

cardiac muscle: one of three types of muscles; makes up the walls of the heart.

carotid pulse point: an arterial pulse that can be felt on either side of the neck.

catheter: a hollow tube that is part of a suctioning system. *Also called* tonsil tip *or* tonsil sucker.

central nervous system: the brain and the spinal cord.

cerebrospinal fluid: a water cushion that helps to protect the brain and spinal cord from trauma.

cervical spine: the neck, formed by the first seven vertebrae.

cervix: the neck of the uterus.

chain of survival: term used by the American Heart Association for a series of interventions that provide the best chance of survival for a cardiac-arrest patient.

chief complaint: the reason that EMS was called stated in the patient's own words.

child: according to AHA standards, any patient who is age one to eight years old.

chronic: of long duration.

circulatory system: the system that transports blood to all parts of the body.

clamping injury: a soft-tissue injury usually caused by a body part being stuck in an area smaller than itself.

clavicle: the collarbone.

cleaning: the process of washing a soiled object with soap and water. *See* disinfecting *and* sterilizing.

closed wound: an injury to the soft tissues beneath unbroken skin.

coccyx: the tail bone, formed by four fused vertebrae. *Also called* coccygeal spine.

colicky pain: cramps that occur in waves.

competent: in EMS a competent adult is one who is lucid and able to make an informed decision about medical care.

complex access: the process of gaining access to a patient which requires the use of tools and specialized equipment.

consent: permission to provide emergency care. *See* expressed consent *and* implied consent.

constrict: get smaller.

contusion: a bruise; a type of closed soft-tissue injury.

cornea: the anterior part of a transparent coating that covers the iris and pupil.

cranium: the bones that form the top (including the forehead), back, and sides of the skull.

crepitus: the sound or feeling of bones grinding against each other.

cribbing: a system of wood or other materials used to support an object.

cricoid cartilage: shaped like a ring, this is the lowermost cartilage of the larynx.

critical incident: any situation that causes a rescuer to experience unusually strong emotions which interfere with the ability to function either during the incident or later.

critical incident stress debriefing (CISD): a session usually held within three days of a critical incident in which a team of peer counselors and mental health professionals help rescuers work through the emotions that normally follow a critical incident.

cross-finger technique: a method of opening a patient's clenched jaw.

crowing: a sound made during respiration similar to the cawing of a crow, which may mean the muscles around the larynx are in spasm.

crowning: the appearance of the baby's head or other body part at the opening of the birth canal.

crushing injury: an open or closed injury to soft tissues and underlying organs that is the result of a sudden blow or a blunt force that has a crushing impact.

cyanosis: bluish discoloration of the skin and mucous membranes; a sign that body tissues are not receiving enough oxygen.

D

debriefing: a technique used to help rescuers work through their emotions within 24 to 72 hours after a critical incident.

deep: a term of position, meaning remote or far from the surface. *Opposite of* superficial.

defibrillation: the process by which an electrical current is sent to the heart to correct fatal heart rhythms.

defusing: a short, informal type of debriefing held within hours of a critical incident.

dermis: second layer of skin. *See* epidermis *and* subcutaneous tissue.

diabetes: a disease in which the normal relationship between glucose (sugar) and insulin is altered.

diaphragm: a muscle, located between the thoracic and abdominal cavities, that moves up and down during respiration.

diastolic pressure: the result of the relaxation of the heart between contractions. *See* systolic pressure.

dilate: enlarge.

direct medical control: refers to an EMS medical director or another physician giving orders to an EMS rescuer at the scene of an emergency via telephone, radio, or in person. *See* indirect medical control.

disinfecting: the process of cleaning plus using a disinfectant, such as alcohol or bleach, to kill microorganisms on an object. *See* cleaning *and* sterilizing.

distal: a term of direction or position, meaning distant or far away from the point of reference, which is usually the torso. *Opposite of* proximal.

diving reflex: the body's natural response to submersion in cold water in which breathing is inhibited, heart rate decreases, and blood vessels constrict in order to maintain blood flow to the brain and heart. *Also called* mammalian diving reflex.

Do Not Resuscitate (DNR) orders: documents that relate the wish of the chronically or terminally ill patient not to be resuscitated. *See* advance directive.

dorsalis pedis pulse: an arterial pulse point that can be felt at the top of the foot on the great toe side.

dressing: a covering for a wound.

drowning: death from suffocation due to immersion in water.

drug abuse: self-administration of one or more drugs in a way that is not in accord with approved medical or social practice.

duty to act: the legal obligation to care for a patient who requires it.

dyspnea: shortness of breath.

E

ecchymosis: black and blue discoloration.

embolus: a mass of undissolved matter in the blood. *Plural* emboli.

emergency move: a move made when there is immediate danger to the patient, usually performed by a single rescuer.

EMT-Basic (EMT-B): an emergency medical technician trained to the level above the EMS First Responder.

EMT-Intermediate (EMT-I): an emergency medical technician trained to a higher level than the EMT-Basic and First Responder.

EMT-Paramedic (EMT-P): the most highly trained emergency medical technician in EMS.

epidermis: outermost layer of skin. *See* dermis *and* subcutaneous tissue.

epiglottis: a leaf-shaped structure that prevents foreign objects from entering the trachea during swallowing.

epiglottitis: a bacterial infection of the epiglottis.

esophagus: a passageway at the lower end of the pharynx that leads to the stomach.

evisceration: the protrusion of organs from an open wound.

expiration: breathing out; exhaling.

expressed consent: permission that must be obtained from every responsive, competent adult patient before emergency medical care may be rendered.

external: a term of position, meaning outside. *Opposite of* internal.

extremities: the limbs of the body.

extrude: to push or force out.

eye orbits: eye sockets; the bones in the skull that hold the eyeballs.

F

fallopian tube: the tube or duct that extends up from the uterus to a position near an ovary.

femoral pulse point: an arterial pulse that can be felt in the area of the groin in the crease between the abdomen and the thigh.

femur: the bone in the thigh, or upper leg.

fibula: one of the bones of the lower leg.

finger sweep: a technique used to remove a foreign object from the mouth.

First Responder: the first person on the scene with emergency medical care skills, typically trained to the most basic EMS level.

flail chest: a closed chest injury resulting in the chest wall becoming unstable.

flail segment: an area of chest wall between broken ribs that becomes free-floating.

fontanel: a soft spot lying between the cranial bones of the skull of an infant.

frostbite: freezing or near freezing of a specific body part. *Also called* local cold injury.

full thickness burn: a burn that extends through all layers of skin and may involve muscles, organs, and bone.

G

gastric distention: inflation of the stomach.

genitalia: reproductive organs.

globe: eyeball.

glucose: a type of sugar.

grieving process: the process by which people cope with death.

guarding position: a position in which the patient is on his or her side with knees drawn up toward the abdomen.

H

hand-off report: a report of the patient's condition and the care that was given, made to the EMS personnel who take over patient care.

hazardous material: a substance that in any quantity poses threat or unreasonable risk to life, health, or property if not properly controlled.

hazmat: hazardous material.

head-tilt/chin-lift maneuver: a manual technique used to open the airway of an uninjured patient. *See* jaw-thrust maneuver.

Heimlich maneuver: a technique used to dislodge and expel a foreign body airway obstruction. *Also called* subdiaphragmatic abdominal thrusts *and* abdominal thrusts.

hematoma: a collection of blood beneath the skin.

hemodilution: an increase in volume of blood plasma resulting in reduced concentration of red blood cells.

hemothorax: collapse of the lungs caused by bleeding in the chest.

humane restraints: padded soft leather or cloth straps used to tie a patient down in order to keep the patient from hurting him- or herself and others.

humerus: the bone that extends from the shoulder to the elbow.

hyperthermia: fever or raised body temperature.

hyperventilation: rapid breathing common to diseases such as asthma and pulmonary edema; the syndrome is common to anxiety-induced states.

hypoglycemia: low blood sugar.

hypoperfusion: *See* shock.

hypothermia: the overall reduction of body temperature. *Also called* generalized cold emergency.

hypoxemia: a condition caused by a deficiency of oxygen in the blood.

hypoxia: decreased levels of oxygen in the blood.

I

ilium: one of the bones that form the pelvis. *Plural* ilia.

immobilize: to make immovable.

impaled object: an object that is embedded in an open wound.

implied consent: the assumption that in an emergency a patient who cannot give permission for emergency medical care would give it if he or she could.

incontinent: unable to retain.

index of suspicion: an informal measure of anticipation that certain types of mechanisms produce specific types of injury.

indirect medical control: refers to EMS system design, protocols and standing orders, education for EMS personnel, and quality management. *See* direct medical control.

infant: according to AHA standards, a patient from birth to one year old.

infectious disease: a disease that can spread from one person to another.

inferior: a term of direction or position, meaning toward or closer to the feet. *Opposite of* superior.

inferior vena cava: the great vein that collects blood from the lower body and delivers it to the heart.

initial assessment: part of patient assessment, conducted directly after the scene size-up, in which the rescuer identifies and treats life-threatening conditions.

inspection: method of examination that involves looking for signs of injury or illness.

inspiration: breathing in; inhaling.

insulin: a hormone secreted by the pancreas, essential to the metabolism of blood sugar.

intercostal: between the ribs.

internal: a term of position, meaning inside. *Opposite of* external.

internal bleeding: bleeding that occurs inside the body.

involuntary muscle: *See* smooth muscle.

ischium: the lower portion of the pelvis or hip bone. *Plural* ischia.

J

jaw-thrust maneuver: a manual technique used to open the airway of an unresponsive patient who is injured or any patient who has suspected spine injury. *See* head-tilt/chin-lift maneuver.

K

kinematics of trauma: the science of analyzing mechanisms of injury.

kinetic energy: the total amount of energy contained in an object in motion.

L

labor: the term used to describe the process of childbirth.

laceration: an open wound of varying depth.

larynx: the voice box.

lateral: a term of direction or position, meaning to the left or right of the midline. *See* medial.

lateral recumbent position: the patient is lying on the left or right side.

level of responsiveness: mental status, usually characterized as alert, verbal, responsive to pain, or unresponsive.

ligaments: tissues that connect bone to bone.

litter: portable stretcher or cot.

local cold injury: freezing or near freezing of a specific body part. *Also called* frostbite.

log roll: a method of turning a patient without causing injury to his or her spine.

lumbar spine: the lower back, formed by five vertebrae.

M

manual traction: applying a pulling force to a body part in order to align it.

mechanism of injury (MOI): the force or forces that cause an injury.

meconium staining: a greenish or brownish color to the amniotic fluid, which means the unborn infant had a bowel movement.

medial: a term of direction or position, meaning toward the midline or center of the body. *See* lateral.

medical director: in EMS this person is the physician legally responsible for the clinical and patient-care aspects of an EMS system.

medical patient: a patient who is ill, not injured.

minor: any person under the legally defined age of an adult; usually under the age of 18 or 21.

mouth-to-barrier device ventilation: a technique of artificial ventilation that involves the use of a barrier device such as a face shield to blow air into the mouth of a patient.

mouth-to-mask ventilation: a technique of artificial ventilation that involves the use of a pocket mask with one-way valve to blow air into the mouth of a patient.

mouth-to-mouth ventilation: a technique of artificial ventilation that involves blowing air directly from the rescuer's mouth into the mouth of a patient.

multiple-casualty incident (MCI): any emergency where three or more patients are involved.

musculoskeletal system: a system made up of the skeleton and muscles, which help to give the body shape, protect the organs, and provide for movement.

myocardial infarction: heart attack.

N

nasal airway: *See* nasopharyngeal airway.

nasal cannula: an oxygen delivery device characterized by two soft plastic tips, which are inserted a short distance into the nostrils.

nasopharyngeal airway: an artificial airway positioned in the nose and extending down to the larynx. *Also called* nasal airway.

nasopharynx: the nasal part of the pharynx.

nature of illness (NOI): the type of medical condition or complaint a patient may be suffering.

neglect: refers to giving insufficient attention or respect to someone who has a claim to that attention and respect.

negligence: the act of deviating from the accepted standard of care through carelessness, inattention, disregard, inadvertence, or oversight that was accidental but avoidable.

nervous system: the body system that controls the voluntary and involuntary activity of the body; includes the brain, spinal cord, and nerves.

non-accidental trauma: injuries such as those caused by child abuse.

non-emergency move: a move made by several rescuers usually after a patient has been stabilized. *Also called* non-urgent move.

nonrebreather mask: an oxygen delivery device characterized by an oxygen reservoir bag and a one-way valve.

O

occlude: to block, close up, or obstruct.

occlusive dressing: a dressing that can form an airtight and sometimes water-tight seal.

open injury: an injury to the soft tissues that is caused by a blow and results in breaking the skin.

oral airway: *See* oropharyngeal airway.

orbit: eye socket; the bones in the skull that hold the eyeball.

oropharyngeal airway: an artificial airway positioned in the mouth and extending down to the larynx. *Also called* oral airway.

oropharynx: the central part of the pharynx.

overdose: an emergency that involves poisoning by drugs or alcohol.

P

packaging: refers to getting the patient ready to be moved and includes procedures such as stabilizing impaled objects and immobilizing injured limbs.

palmar surface method: a method used to estimate the percent of body surface area involved in a burn injury.

palpation: method of examination that involves feeling for signs of injury or illness.

palpitations: a sensation of abnormal rapid throbbing or fluttering of the heart

paradoxical breathing: a segment of the chest moves in the opposite direction to the rest of the chest during respiration; typically seen with a flail segment.

paramedic: *See* EMT-Paramedic.

parietal pleura: the membrane that covers the internal chest wall.

partial thickness burn: a burn that involves both the epidermis and dermis.

patella: the knee cap.

patent airway: an airway that is open and clear of obstructions.

pathogens: microorganisms such as bacteria and viruses, which cause disease.

patient history: facts about the patient's medical history that are relevant to the patient's condition.

pediatric center: medical facility devoted to the treatment of infants and children.

pediatric patients: patients who are infants or children.

pelvic cavity: a space bound by the lower part of the spine, the hip bones, and the pubis.

pelvis: the hips.

penetration/puncture wound: an open wound that is the result of a sharp, pointed object being pushed or driven into soft tissues.

perfusion: refers to the circulation of blood throughout a body organ or structure.

perinatal center: medical facility devoted to the treatment of high-risk pregnant patients.

peripheral nervous system: the portion of the nervous system that is located outside the brain and spinal cord; the nerves.

personal protective equipment (PPE): equipment used by a rescuer to protect against injury and the spread of infectious disease.

pharynx: the throat.

placenta: a disk-shaped inner lining of the uterus that provides nourishment and oxygen to a fetus.

pleura: the membranes that enfold both lungs.

pleural cavity: the space between the visceral pleura and the parietal pleura.

pneumothorax: collapse of the lungs caused by air in the chest.

poison center: medical facility devoted to providing information for treatment of poisoning victims.

posterior: a term of direction or position, meaning toward the back. *Opposite of* anterior.

posterior tibial pulse: an arterial pulse point that can be felt behind the medial ankle bone.

power grip: a technique used to get maximum force from hands while lifting and moving.

power lift: a technique used for lifting, especially helpful to rescuers with weak knees or thighs.

prehospital care: emergency medical treatment in the field before transport to a medical facility. *Also called* out-of-hospital care.

priapism: a constant erection of the penis.

prone: a position in which a patient is lying face down on his or her stomach. *Opposite of* supine.

protocols: written orders issued by the medical director that may be applied to patient care; a type of standing order.

proximal: a term of direction or position, meaning close or near the point of reference, which is usually the torso. *Opposite of* distal.

pubis: bone of the groin; the anterior portion of the pelvis.

pulmonary: concerning or involving the lungs.

pulmonary vein: vessel carrying oxygen-rich blood from the lungs to the left atrium of the heart.

pulse pressure: the difference between systolic blood pressure and diastolic blood pressure.

pulse: the wave of blood propelled through the arteries as a result of the pumping action of the heart.

pustules: raised areas of the skin that are filled with pus.

R

radial pulse point: an arterial pulse that can be felt on the palm side of the wrist.

radius: one of the bones of the forearm.

rape: sexual intercourse that is performed without consent and by compulsion through force, threat, or fraud.

rape trauma syndrome: a reaction to rape that involves four general stages: acute (impact) reaction, outward adjustment, depression, and acceptance and resolution.

rappelling: a special technique of getting down a cliff by means of a secured rope.

reasonable force: the minimum amount of force needed to keep a patient from injuring him- or herself and others.

recovery position: lateral recumbent position; used to allow fluids to drain from the patient's mouth instead of into the airway.

referred pain: pain felt in a part of the body that is different from its actual point of origin.

relative skin temperature: an assessment of skin temperature obtained by touching the patient's skin.

respiration: the passage of air into and out of the lungs.

respiratory arrest: the cessation of spontaneous breathing.

respiratory distress: shortness of breath or a feeling of air hunger with labored breathing.

respiratory system: organs involved in the interchange of gases between the body and the environment.

responsive: conscious; acting or moving in response to stimulus.

retraction: a pulling inward.

rule of nines: a method used to estimate the percent of body surface area involved in a burn injury.

S

sacrum: the lower part of the spine, formed by five fused vertebrae.

scapulae: the shoulder blades. *Singular* scapula.

scene size-up: an overall assessment of the emergency scene.

scope of care: actions and care legally allowed to be provided by a First Responder.

seizure: a sudden and temporary change in mental status caused by massive electrical discharge in the brain.

septum: a wall that divides two cavities.

sexual assault: any touch that the victim did not initiate or agree to and that is imposed by coercion, threat, deception, or threats of physical violence.

shock: a life-threatening, progressive condition that results from the inadequate delivery of oxygenated blood throughout the body.

shoulder girdle: consists of the clavicles and scapulae.

sign: any injury or medical condition that can be observed in a patient.

simple access: the process of gaining access to a patient without the use of tools.

skeletal muscle: one of three types of muscles; makes possible all deliberate acts such as walking and chewing. *Also called* voluntary muscle.

skull: a bony structure that houses and protects the brain.

smooth muscle: one of three types of muscles; found in the walls of tubelike organs, ducts, and blood vessels. *Also called* involuntary muscle.

sniffing position: position of a patient's head when the neck is flexed and the head is extended.

soft-tissue injuries: injuries to the skin, muscles, nerve, and blood vessels.

sphygmomanometer: instrument used to measure blood pressure. *Also called* blood pressure cuff.

spinal column: the column of bones, or vertebrae, that houses and protects the spinal cord.

spinal precautions: methods used to protect the spine from further injury; for First Responders, usually refers to the manual stabilization of the patient's head and neck until the patient is completely immobilized.

splint: a device used to immobilize a body part.

spontaneous abortion: miscarriage, or the loss of pregnancy before the twentieth week.

stabilize: to hold firmly and steadily.

standard of care: the care that would be expected to be provided to the same patient under the same circumstances by another First Responder who had received the same training.

standing orders: advance orders, rules, regulations, or step-by-step procedures to be taken under certain conditions; a type of indirect medical control.

status epilepticus: a seizure lasting longer than 10 minutes or seizures that occur consecutively without a period of responsiveness between them.

sterile: free of all microorganisms and spores.

sterilizing: process in which a chemical or other substance, such as superheated steam, is used to kill all microorganisms on an object. *See* cleaning *and* disinfecting.

sternum: breastbone.

stethoscope: instrument that aids in auscultating (listening) for sounds within the body.

stoma: a permanent surgically created opening that connects the trachea directly to the front of the neck.

stress: any change in the body's internal balance; occurs when external demands become greater than personal resources.

stridor: harsh, high-pitched sound made during inhalation, which may mean the larynx is swollen and blocking the upper airway.

stroke: loss of brain function caused by a blocked or ruptured blood vessel in the brain.

subcutaneous tissue: layer of fat beneath the skin.

sucking chest wound: open wound to the chest or back that bubbles or makes a sucking noise.

suctioning: using negative pressure created by a commercial device to keep the patient's airway clear.

superficial: term of position, meaning near the surface. *Opposite of* deep.

superficial burn: a burn that involves only the epidermis.

superior: a term of direction or position, meaning toward or closer to the head. *Opposite of* inferior.

supine: a position in which a patient is lying face up on his or her back. *Opposite of* prone.

symphysis pubis: the junction of the pubic bones on the midline in front; the bony eminence under the pubic hair.

symptom: any injury or medical condition that can only be described by the patient.

syrup of ipecac: a drug used to induce vomiting, usually in a patient who has ingested poison.

systolic pressure: the result of a contraction of the heart, which forces blood through the arteries. *See* diastolic pressure.

T

tendons: tissues that connect muscle to bone.

tension pneumothorax: a condition that is the result of an open chest wound, in which a severe build-up of air compresses the lungs and heart toward the uninjured side of the chest.

thoracic cavity: the space above the diaphragm and within the walls of the thorax. *Also called* chest cavity.

thoracic spine: the upper back, formed by 12 vertebrae.

thorax: the chest. *Also called* rib cage.

thrombus: a blood clot that obstructs a blood vessel.

tibia: one of the bones of the lower leg.

tongue-jaw lift: a technique used to draw the tongue away from the back of the throat and away from a foreign body that may be lodged there.

tourniquet: a constricting band used as a last resort on an extremity to apply pressure over an artery in order to control bleeding.

trachea: windpipe.

trauma center: a medical facility devoted to the treatment of injuries.

trauma patient: a patient who is injured.

triage: the process of sorting patients to determine the order in which they will receive care.

trimester: a three-month period.

tripod position: a position in which the patient is sitting upright, leaning forward, fighting to breathe.

U

ulna: one of the bones of the forearm.

umbilical cord: an extension of the placenta through which the fetus receives nourishment while in the uterus.

universal number: a phone number—usually 9-1-1—used in many areas to access emergency services including police, fire, rescue, and ambulance.

universal precautions: a form of infection control used against diseases spread by way of blood.

unresponsive: unconscious; not acting or moving in response to stimulus.

uterus: the organ that contains the developing fetus.

V

veins: blood vessels that carry blood back to the heart from the rest of the body.

velocity: the speed at which an object moves.

venous bleeding: recognized by dark red blood that flows steadily from a wound.

ventilation: a method of assisting breathing by forcing air into a patient's lungs.

ventricles: the two lower chambers of the heart.

venules: the smallest kind of veins.

vertebrae: the 33 bone segments of the spinal column. *Singular* vertebra.

vesicles: small blisters or cysts that contain moisture.

visceral pleura: the membrane that covers the outer surface of the lungs.

vital signs: signs of life; assessments related to breathing, pulse, skin, pupils, and blood pressure.

voluntary muscle: *See* skeletal muscle.

W

wheals: itchy, raised, round marks on the skin that are red around the edges and white at the center.

withdrawal: a syndrome that occurs after a period of abstinence from the drugs or alcohol to which a person's body has become accustomed.

wound: a soft-tissue injury.

X

xiphoid process: the lowest portion of the sternum.

*[Italic page references = Illustrations/tables]